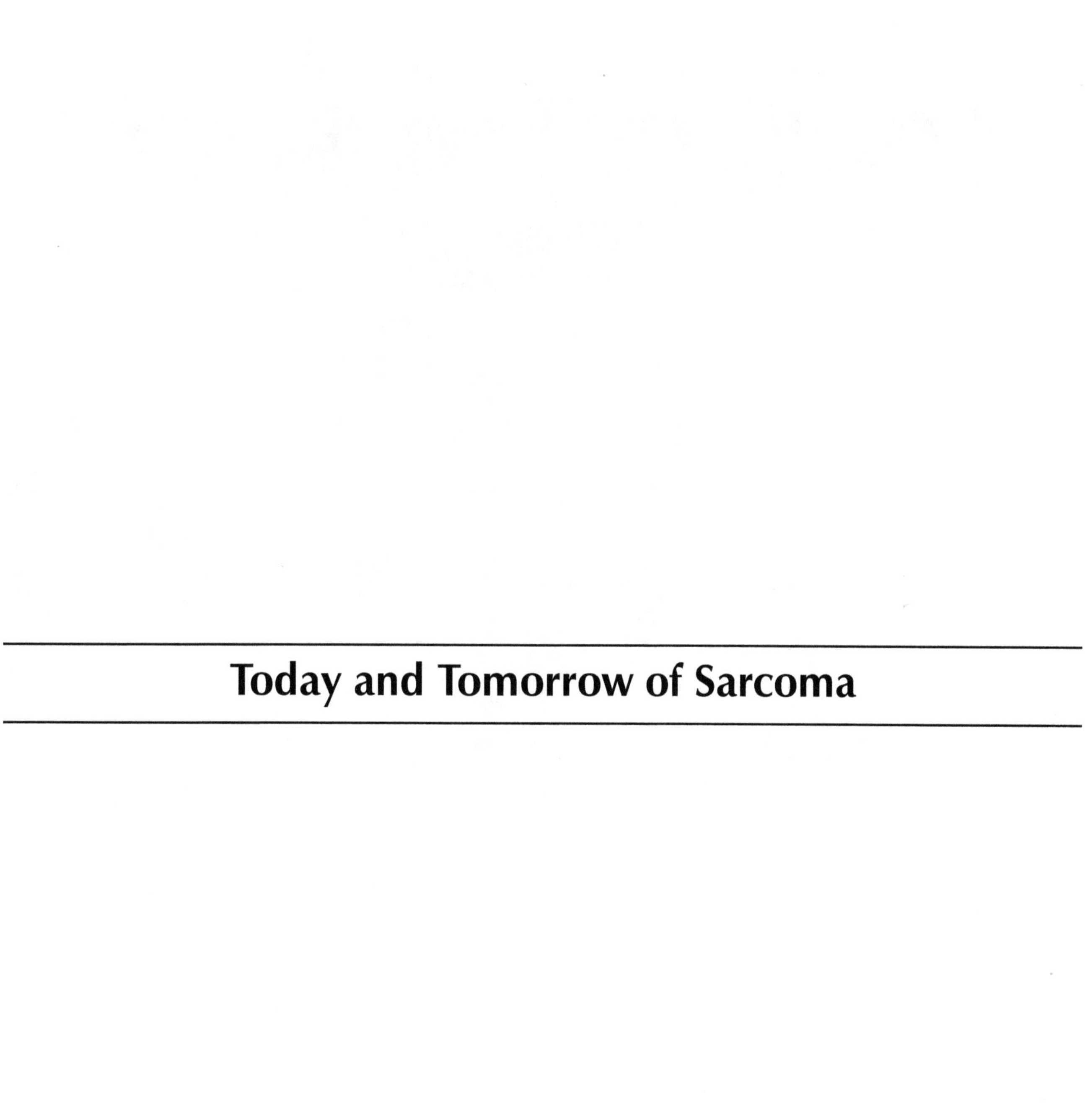

Today and Tomorrow of Sarcoma

Today and Tomorrow of Sarcoma

Editor: Serenity Hodges

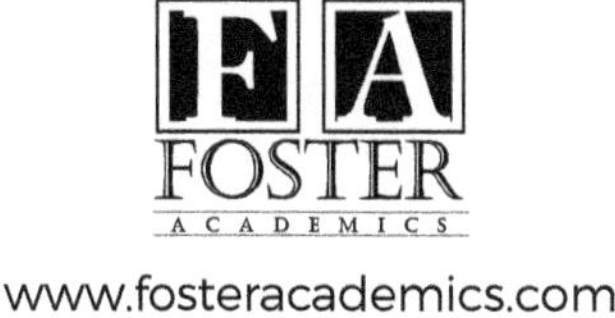

www.fosteracademics.com

www.fosteracademics.com

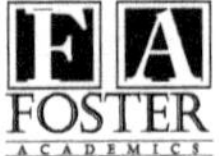

Cataloging-in-Publication Data

Today and tomorrow of sarcoma / edited by Serenity Hodges.
p. cm.
Includes bibliographical references and index.
ISBN 978-1-63242-913-1
1. Sarcoma. 2. Sarcoma--Diagnosis. 3. Sarcoma--Treatment. 4. Cancer. 5. Tumors. I. Hodges, Serenity.
RC270 .T63 2020
616.994--dc23

Foster Academics,
118-35 Queens Blvd., Suite 400,
Forest Hills, NY 11375, USA

ISBN 978-1-63242-913-1 (Hardback)

Contents

Preface

Sarcoma is a rare form of cancer. It grows in connective tissue. It can affect all age groups of people. Some sarcomas such as chondrosarcoma, leiomyosarcoma and gastrointestinal stromal tumor occur more commonly in adults than children, while high-grade bone sarcomas such as osteosarcoma and Ewing's sarcoma occur more in children and young adults. Scientists have made remarkable progress in the understanding of how gene changes cause sarcomas to develop. Such insights are crucial in developing tests for the diagnosis and classification of sarcomas. Active research is being conducted in the formulation and combinations of different therapies for the treatment of sarcomas. Vaccines, T-cell therapies, hyperthermia and cryosurgery are being explored for the destruction of tumors. This book explores all the important aspects of sarcoma in the present day scenario. The various studies that are constantly contributing towards the management of sarcoma are examined in detail. The readers would gain knowledge that would broaden their perspective about oncology and oncological medicine.

All of the data presented henceforth, was collaborated in the wake of recent advancements in the field. The aim of this book is to present the diversified developments from across the globe in a comprehensible manner. The opinions expressed in each chapter belong solely to the contributing authors. Their interpretations of the topics are the integral part of this book, which I have carefully compiled for a better understanding of the readers.

At the end, I would like to thank all those who dedicated their time and efforts for the successful completion of this book. I also wish to convey my gratitude towards my friends and family who supported me at every step.

Editor

1

Epidemiology, Treatment Patterns, and Outcomes of Metastatic Soft Tissue Sarcoma in a Community-Based Oncology Network

Clara Chen,[1] Rohit Borker,[2] James Ewing,[1,3,4,5] Wan-Yu Tseng,[1] Michelle D. Hackshaw,[2] Shanmugapriya Saravanan,[1] Rahul Dhanda,[1] and Eric Nadler[1,3,4,5,6]

[1] *Department of Information Technology, Health Economics and Outcomes Research, McKesson Specialty Health, The Woodlands, TX, USA*
[2] *GlaxoSmithKline, Philadelphia, PA 19112, USA*
[3] *Texas Oncology, Dallas, TX, USA*
[4] *Baylor Charles A. Sammons Cancer Center, Dallas, TX, USA*
[5] *Baylor University Medical Center at Dallas, Dallas, TX, USA*
[6] *Texas Oncology, Baylor Sammons Cancer Center, 3410 Worth Street, Dallas, TX 75246, USA*

Correspondence should be addressed to Eric Nadler; eric.nadler@usoncology.com

Academic Editor: Charles Catton

Purpose. To assess epidemiology, treatment patterns, and outcomes of metastatic soft tissue sarcoma (mSTS) patients in USA community oncology practices. *Methods.* This retrospective, descriptive study used US Oncology's iKnowMed electronic health records database. Adults (≥18 years) with mSTS and at least two visits between July 2007 and June 2010 were included. Key outcomes were practice patterns, overall survival (OS), and progression-free survival (PFS). *Results.* 363 mSTS patients (174 treated and 189 untreated) met the prespecified exclusion/inclusion criteria. The most common subtypes were leiomyosarcoma ($n = 104$; 29%), liposarcoma ($n = 40$; 11%), and synovial sarcoma ($n = 12$; 3%); the remainder ($n = 207$; 57%) comprised 27 histologic subtypes. Treated patients were younger and had lower ECOG scores; 75% and 25% received first-line combination or monotherapy, respectively. Median OS of treated and untreated patients was 22 and 17 months, respectively, and 29 months in patients with the three most common subtypes. Before controlling for effects of covariates, younger age and lower ECOG scores were associated with better OS and PFS. *Conclusion.* This study provides insights into mSTS epidemiology, treatment patterns, and outcomes in a large community-based oncology network. These results warrant further studies with larger cohorts.

1. Introduction

Soft tissue sarcomas (STS) are rare mesenchymal tumors that account for 1% of adult cancers [1–7] and comprise over 50 different histologic subtypes that differ in pathogenesis and outcomes [1–3, 6, 7]. Collectively, they are associated with a mortality rate of over 4,000 patients per year [2]. The treatment of STS is dependent upon several factors, including histologic subtype, disease stage, and patient performance status; the treatment options include surgery, radiotherapy, and/or chemotherapy [1, 3, 6–10]. Although localized resected disease can often be cured, the prognosis of patients with metastatic STS (mSTS) remains poor, with median survival of approximately one year [1, 3, 6, 11–15]. Good prognostic factors for mSTS include younger patients with good performance status and low tumor grade [3, 6, 16].

Most of our insights regarding factors that influence the outcomes following chemotherapy in mSTS have been obtained mainly from clinical trials [11–14, 16]. The purpose of this study was to gain an improved understanding of the "real-world" epidemiology as well as treatment patterns and outcomes of mSTS in the setting of community oncology clinics.

2. Methods

Data was obtained from the McKesson Specialty Health (MSH)/US Oncology (USON) iKnowMed (iKM) electronic health record (EHR) and electronic chart review. The study period was from July 1, 2007, to June 30, 2010, with follow-up through June 30, 2011. Adults (≥18 years) with mSTS were included if they received care at practice sites with the full capabilities of the iKM EHR system and had at least two visits during the study period. Patients were excluded if during the study period they were diagnosed with or treated for a primary cancer other than mSTS or were enrolled in a randomized clinical trial. Electronic chart review was conducted to validate and supplement EHR data for critical parameters, including cell morphology and histology. For the measurement of progression-free survival (PFS), an escalation in the line of therapy (LOT) from first-line to second-line was used as a proxy measurement for disease progression. Thus, PFS in this study was defined as the time in months from the initiation of first-line chemotherapy to the initiation of second-line chemotherapy, or death from any cause, whichever occurred first. Patients who were progression-free were censored at the end of the study follow-up period or at the date they were last known to be alive, whichever occurred first.

Descriptive analyses were conducted on patient demographics and clinical characteristics, as well as treatment patterns. Overall survival (OS) and PFS were estimated using Kaplan-Meier plots. Mean and median survival time and survival rates were derived with 95% confidence intervals (CI). SAS 9.2 and STATA 11.2 were used for data management and statistical analysis.

3. Results

3.1. Study Population. In the iKnowMed EHR, 4,245 individuals had histologically confirmed STS, of which 1,286 (30%) had metastatic disease. Supplementary Figure 1 depicts the patient consort diagram; based upon the inclusion/exclusion criteria employed, we selected 363 mSTS patients for further evaluation: 174 of the 329 treated and 189 of the 957 untreated patients (see Supplementary Material available online at http://dx.doi.org/10.1155/2014/145764).

Table 1 describes the demographic and clinical characteristics of our study sample. The mean age (standard deviation) at diagnosis of mSTS in the entire study population was 61 (16) years. Forty-eight percent were female and 52% were male. Based on the histology of their tumors, the study population (n = 363) was categorized into four major groups: those with leiomyosarcoma (n = 104; 29%), liposarcoma (n = 40; 11%), and synovial sarcoma (n = 12; 3%), and the remainder were designated as "other" (n = 207; 57%) as they comprised subjects with 27 histologic subtypes, each with small sample sizes. The frequency of the histology subtypes was similar in treated and untreated patients (Table 1). We adopted this categorization schema as these were the most prevalent groups based on histology, and recent studies used similar groupings [17]. The most common primary tumor sites in the treated population were the extremities (33%), retroperitoneal (19%), and the trunk and viscera (14%).

Among treated and untreated patients with available clinical data, presentation in both groups was most commonly with stage IV disease (54% and 67%, resp.), grade 3 tumor (69% each), resectable tumor (50% and 61%, resp.), and ECOG score of 1 (49% and 47%, resp.) (Table 1). Treated patients were younger (median = 58 yr) than untreated patients (median = 65 yr) and the overall ECOG performance at study entry between treated and untreated patients differed (Table 1). In addition, male patients were more likely to receive chemotherapy when compared with female patients (60% versus 40%, resp.).

3.2. Treatment Patterns. Of the 174 treated patients, 173 (99%) and 42 (24%) received first- and second-line therapies, respectively, and only 14 (8%) continued with third-line therapy. (Note: one of the 174 treated patients received second-line therapy as initial therapy.) The most frequently used chemotherapy regimens in first-, second-, and third-line therapies were as follows: for first-line chemotherapy, doxorubicin plus ifosfamide (29%), docetaxel plus gemcitabine (24%), or doxorubicin alone (12%) was used. For second-line chemotherapy, docetaxel plus gemcitabine (52%) was used the most, followed by doxorubicin alone (17%). For third-line chemotherapy, liposomal doxorubicin alone (29%) or docetaxel plus gemcitabine (21%) was given.

Of the treated patients, 64 (37%) received monotherapy, whereas 135 (78%) received combination therapy; approximately 14% received both monotherapy and combination therapies. Among those receiving first-line therapy (n = 173), 28% received monotherapy and 72% combination therapy, and similar proportions were observed for those receiving second-line therapy (29% and 71%, resp.). Of the 14 patients who continued chemotherapy into third-line, 57% and 43% received monotherapy and combination therapy, respectively. These data suggested that among those receiving first- or second-line chemotherapies, a greater proportion received combination compared with monotherapy. In contrast, the reverse pattern was observed in those receiving third-line therapy.

The following treatment patterns were observed. Among the 49 patients who received monotherapy as first-line therapy, doxorubicin (43%), gemcitabine (27%), and liposomal doxorubicin (14%) were the more frequently used agents, while among the 126 patients receiving first-line combination therapy the most common regimens were doxorubicin plus ifosfamide (41%), docetaxel plus gemcitabine (35%), and doxorubicin plus dacarbazine (6%). Among the 12 patients who received monotherapy as second-line therapy, doxorubicin (58%) was most often used, while in the 30 subjects receiving combination second-line therapy, docetaxel plus gemcitabine (73%) was used most frequently. Ninety-five patients received anthracycline-containing first-line therapy, and of these 37 continued with second-line chemotherapy; among these patients docetaxel plus gemcitabine (70%) was most commonly used.

We examined the usage of monotherapy versus combination therapy according to histology subtype (Supplementary Table 1). Among those receiving combination (n = 129) and monotherapy (n = 50), 56% and 40%, respectively, were patients with the top three subtypes. Reflecting that a lower proportion of patients with the other subtypes received combination therapy, 72 of the 92 subjects with the top three subtypes (78.3%) versus 57 of the 87 individuals with

TABLE 1: Demographic and clinical characteristics of treated and untreated metastatic STS patients.

Characteristic	Total (N = 363)	Treated patients (N = 174)	Untreated patients (N = 189)	P
Age at treatment, N (%)				
Mean (SD)	61 (16)	58 (14)	63 (17)	0.0031
Median (range)	62 (18, 91)	58 (19, 90)	65 (18, 91)	0.0005
<65	203 (60)	109 (63)	94 (50)	
65–75	76 (21)	42 (24)	34 (18)	<0.0001
≥75	84 (23)	23 (13)	61 (32)	
Gender, N (%)				
Female	175 (48)	70 (40)	105 (56)	0.0035
Male	188 (52)	104 (60)	84 (44)	
BMI, N (%)				
Mean (SD)	28.1 (6.3)	28.5 (5.9)	27.8 (6.8)	0.2742
Median (range)	26.8 (15.4, 52.1)	27.5 (17.1, 49.5)	26.4 (15.4, 52.1)	0.0624
Underweight	6 (2)	3 (2)	3 (2)	
Normal weight	104 (31)	43 (25)	61 (37)	
Overweight	126 (37)	70 (40)	56 (34)	0.1270
Obese	103 (30)	57 (33)	46 (28)	
Missing	24	1	23	
Stage at diagnosis*, N (%)				
I	19 (8)	12 (10)	7 (6)	
II	19 (8)	9 (7)	10 (9)	
III	56 (24)	35 (29)	21 (18)	0.1253
IV	142 (60)	65 (54)	77 (67)	
Missing	127	53	74	
Cell morphology, N (%)				
Leiomyosarcoma	104 (29)	50 (29)	54 (29)	
Liposarcoma	40 (11)	20 (11)	20 (11)	
Synovial Sarcoma	12 (3)	9 (5)	3 (2)	
Other STS**	207 (57)	95 (55)	112 (59)	
Tumor grade, N (%)				
1	24 (12)	11 (10)	13 (13)	
2	33 (16)	19 (18)	14 (14)	
3	142 (69)	74 (69)	68 (69)	0.8523
4+	8 (4)	4 (4)	4 (4)	
Missing	156	66	90	
Tumor type, N (%)				
Resectable	105 (61)	51 (50)	54 (61)	
Unresectable	68 (39)	34 (40)	34 (39)	0.8543
Missing	190	89	101	
Baseline ECOG, N (%)				
0	59 (20)	30 (22)	29 (18)	
1	153 (52)	79 (49)	74 (47)	0.0034
2+	84 (28)	25 (19)	59 (36)	
Missing	67	40	27	
ECOG after first-line treatment, N (%)				
0	17 (15)	17 (15)		
1	69 (59)	69 (59)		
2+	30 (26)	30 (26)		
Missing	58	58		

Table 1: Continued.

Characteristic	Total (N = 363)	Treated patients (N = 174)	Untreated patients (N = 189)	P
Primary site†				
Head and neck		14 (8)		
Lung		9 (5)		
Liver		3 (2)		
Trunk and viscera		25 (14)		
Retroperitoneal		33 (19)		
Extremity		58 (33)		
Other		29 (17)		
Missing		3 (2)		

SD: standard deviation, BMI: body mass index, and ECOG: Eastern Cooperative Oncology Group Performance Status. P: significance value by Chi-square test.
*The stage of disease for each patient is consistent with the descriptions of the AJCC7 classifications of disease.
**Other STS include angiosarcoma of soft tissue, alveolar rhabdomyosarcoma, alveolar soft part sarcoma, fibrosarcoma, Kaposi sarcoma, PNET, pleomorphic rhabdomyosarcoma, clear-cell sarcoma of soft tissue, malignant fibrous histiocytoma, myxofibrosarcoma, malignant phyllodes cystosarcoma, embryonal rhabdomyosarcoma, extraskeletal Ewing tumor, extraskeletal myxoid chondrosarcoma, osteosarcoma, malignant ossifying fibromyxoid tumor, malignant peripheral nerve sheet tumor, hemangiopericytoma, and sarcoma NOS.
†Primary sites were captured through chart reviews for the treated patient cohort (N = 174) only. Chart reviews were not conducted for the untreated patient cohort (N = 189).

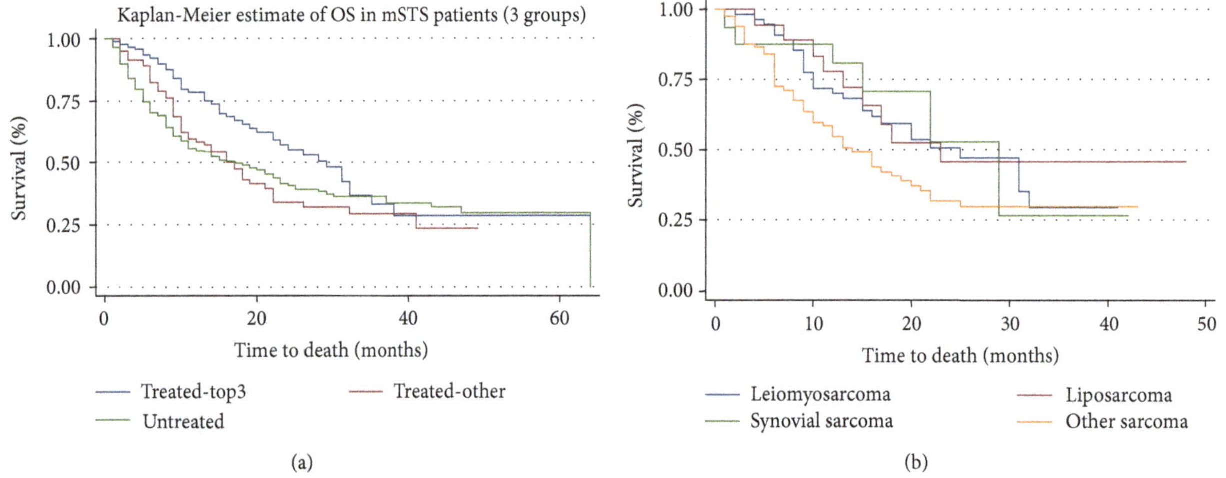

Figure 1: Kaplan-Meier estimates of overall survival in untreated and treated metastatic STS patients. (a) Treated patients were stratified according to histologic subtype. The top three histology subtypes were pooled into one group (treated-top 3), and the remainder were classified as "treated-other." (b) Kaplan-Meier plots for the three most common STS subtypes (leiomyosarcoma, liposarcoma, and synovial sarcoma) in the study population and the remaining subtypes (other sarcoma).

the other STSs (65.5%) received combination chemotherapy (Supplementary Table 1).

Among the 50 individuals receiving first-line monotherapy, 28% completed therapy as scheduled, and early discontinuation of therapy was attributable to disease progression in 18% and drug toxicity in 16%. Among the 129 subjects receiving first-line combination therapy, the corresponding values were 35%, 16%, and 13%, respectively. Twelve subjects received second-line monotherapy, and of these 33% completed therapy, 25% discontinued therapy early because of disease progression, and 17% terminated therapy early because of drug toxicity; the corresponding proportions for the 30 patients who received second-line combination chemotherapy were 27%, 17%, and 7%, respectively.

3.3. OS and PFS: Unstratified Analyses. Approximately 40% of the treated and untreated patients died during follow-up. The median OS of treated patients was 22 (95% CI, 17 to 29) months whereas for the untreated patients it was 17 (95% CI, 11 to 23) months (Supplementary Table 2). The percent OS of treated patients at 6, 12, 24, and 36 months was 88%, 69%, 45%, and 32%, respectively, while that of untreated patients was 70%, 55%, 41%, and 34%, respectively (Supplementary Table 2).

The OS estimates of patients stratified by STS subtype are shown in Supplementary Table 3 and depicted in Figure 1. Figure 1(a) shows the Kaplan-Meier plots for the OS of two treated subgroups and untreated patients, and Figure 1(b) shows the Kaplan-Meier plots of OS for each of the top three histology subtypes and the other sarcomas. The Kaplan-Meier plots for the top three subtypes were not different from each other (Figure 1(b)) but were different from the other sarcomas and the untreated patients (Figures 1(a) and 1(b)). The median OS for the treated patients with the top three most common

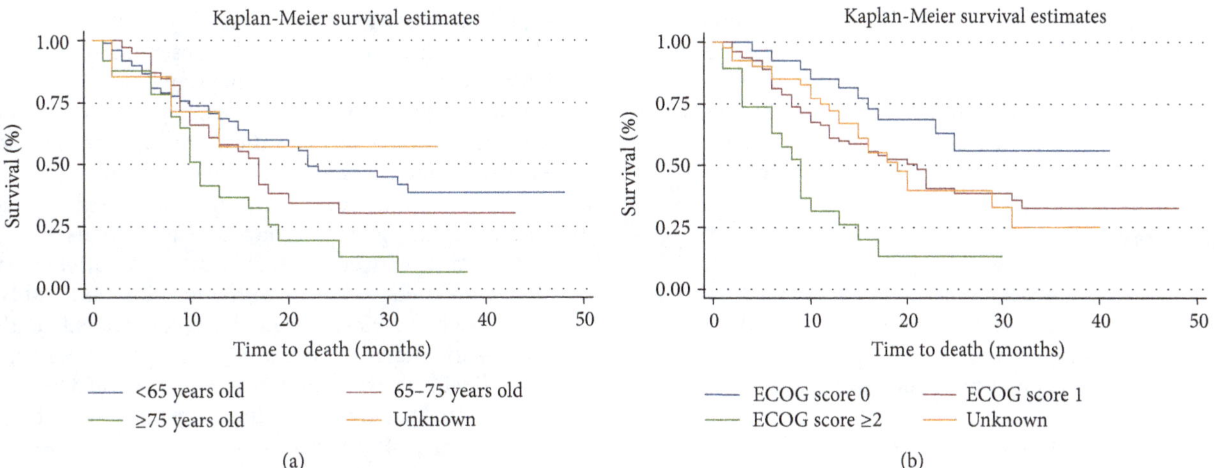

FIGURE 2: Overall survival by age and ECOG status among mSTS patients starting first-line therapy. (a) Kaplan-Meier plots by age group. (b) Kaplan-Meier plots by baseline ECOG status.

histologic subtypes was 29 (95% CI, 22 to 35) months. The median for the treated patients with the other histologic subtypes was 17 (95% CI, 11 to 22) months, similar to that observed in the untreated patients.

The PFS estimates of patients stratified by STS subtype are shown in Supplementary Table 4 and depicted in Supplementary Figure 2. The median overall PFS of treated patients was 11 (95% CI, 9 to 14) months. The median PFS for treated patients with leiomyosarcoma, liposarcoma, synovial sarcoma, or other sarcomas was 12, 18, 17, and 7 months, respectively (Supplementary Table 4).

3.4. OS and PFS: Stratified by Line of Therapy. The median OS of patients treated with first-line chemotherapy during the study period was 22 (95% CI, 17 to 28) months. The mean OS was 24 (95% CI, 24 to 24) months, and the 6-, 12-, 24-, and 36-month OS rates for first-line therapy were 88% (95% CI, 82% to 92%), 69% (95% CI, 62% to 76%), 45% (95% CI, 36% to 53%), and 33% (95% CI, 24% to 42%), respectively. The median OS of patients treated with second-line therapy was 11 (95% CI, 8 to 19) months, whereas the mean OS was 13 (95% CI, 12 to 13) months and the 6- and 12-month OS rates were 70% (95% CI, 54 to 82) and 44% (95% CI, 29 to 58%), respectively.

The median PFS of patients treated with first-line chemotherapy during the study period was 11 (95% CI, 9 to 14) months. The mean PFS was 15 (95% CI, 14 to 15) months, and the 6-, 12-, 24- and 36-month PFS rates for first-line therapy were 66% (95% CI, 58% to 72%), 46% (95% CI, 38% to 54%), 28% (95% CI, 20% to 36%), and 17% (95% CI, 10% to 26%), respectively (Supplementary Table 4). The median PFS of patients treated with second-line therapy was 9 (95% CI, 7 to 12) months, whereas the mean PFS was 11 (95% CI, 10 to 11) months, and the 6- and 12-month PFS rates were 64% (95% CI, 47% to 77%) and 35% (95% CI, 20% to 50%), respectively.

3.5. Overall Survival by Age. Among those receiving first-line therapy, 102 (58.9%), 39 (22.5%), and 25 (14.5%) were <65, 65–75, and ≥75 years old, respectively (age was unknown in 7 subjects (4.1%)), and the corresponding values for those receiving second-line therapy were 26 (61.9%), 9 (21.4%), and 3 (7.1%) (age was unknown in 4 (9.5%) subjects). Among those receiving first-line monotherapy ($n = 50$), 40%, 20%, and 36% were <65, 65–75, and ≥75 years old, respectively, and corresponding values for those receiving first-line combination therapy ($n = 129$) were 65.9%, 22.5%, and 7.8%, respectively. There was a similar age distribution by second-line monotherapy and combination chemotherapy.

The Kaplan-Meier analyses for OS by age at the start of first-line therapy are shown in Figure 2(a). The mean OS for those initiating first-line therapy at ages <65, 65 to 75, and >75 years was 21 (95% CI, 21 to 21), 16 (95% CI, 16 to 16), and 13 (95% CI, 13 to 14) months, respectively. The mean PFS for those initiating first-line therapy at ages <65, 65–75, and >75 years was 15 (95% CI, 15 to 15), 14 (95% CI, 14 to 15), and 12 (95% CI, 11 to 13) months, respectively (data not shown).

3.6. Overall Survival by ECOG Status. Among those receiving first-line therapy, 29 (16.7%), 83 (47.7%), and 19 (10.9%) had an ECOG status of 0, 1, and 2, respectively (ECOG status was unknown in 42 subjects (24.1%)). The Kaplan-Meier analyses of OS by baseline ECOG status are shown in Figure 2(b). The mean OS for those initiating first-line therapy by ECOG status of 0, 1, and ≥2 was 21 (95% CI, 20 to 21), 20 (95% CI, 20 to 20), and 9 (95% CI, 9 to 10) months, respectively. The corresponding mean PFS values were 17 (95% CI, 16 to 18), 15 (95% CI, 15 to 15), and 8 (95% CI, 7 to 8) months, respectively.

Among those receiving first-line monotherapy ($n = 50$), 6%, 50%, and 20% had ECOG scores of 0, 1, and ≥2, respectively, and the corresponding values for those receiving first-line combination therapy were 20.9%, 46.5%, and 6.9%, respectively. The relative distribution of ECOG scores by second-line monotherapy and combination chemotherapy was similar.

3.7. Overall Survival by Metastasis Site. Among subjects who initiated first-line therapy, the most common sites for metastasis were lung (36.9%), trunk and viscera (10.4%), retroperitoneal (8.6%), and multiple metastatic sites (8.6%). The mean OS in these patients was 15 (95% CI, 14 to 15), 16 (95% CI, 15 to 16), 17 (95% CI, 16 to 17), and 20 (95% CI, 20 to 21) months, respectively. The mean PFS was 10 (95% CI, 10 to 10), 14 (95% CI, 14 to 15), 14 (95% CI, 14 to 15), and 17 (95% CI, 17 to 18) months, respectively (data not shown).

4. Discussion

This retrospective observational study conducted in a large community oncology network yielded six key findings. First, STS histologic subtypes were similar between the treated and untreated subjects (i.e., tumor subtypes, stage, and grade). Leiomyosarcoma, liposarcoma, and synovial sarcoma were the top three most common histologic subtypes in this patient population, consistent with the previously reported distribution patterns [7, 15, 16]. Second, while tumor characteristics were similar, treated patients differed from untreated individuals in three respects: they were younger, a greater proportion was men, and they had lower ECOG scores.

Third, our study revealed insights into chemotherapy treatment patterns for mSTS in the community setting. Among patients receiving first-line chemotherapy, ~75% and ~25% received combination and monotherapy, respectively. Among patients with leiomyosarcoma, the most frequent form of mSTS in our study population, 84% received combination therapy. The most common combination regimens in the overall study population were doxorubicin plus ifosfamide (29%) and docetaxel plus gemcitabine (24%). This choice is expected based on prevailing clinical practice [18]. For example, gemcitabine with docetaxel has been found to be active in leiomyosarcoma of uterine and gastrointestinal origin: a phase 2 study reported a higher response rate in this subtype for combination docetaxel plus gemcitabine versus gemcitabine alone (32% versus 27%, resp.) and significantly improved progression-free survival (6.3 versus 3 months, resp.) [19]. Although the benefits of chemotherapy for mSTS and the use of combination versus single agent chemotherapy for mSTS are unclear, combination chemotherapy is generally an accepted practice standard in the USA [2, 3]. Further research is needed to determine the optimal dosing and tolerability of these regimens in these patients. Even though the primary focus of this study was the chemotherapy treatment patterns in the community setting, future research should also explore the effects of surgery and radiation on these patients.

Fourth, the median OS of treated and untreated patients prior to accounting for tumor subtype was 22 and 17 months, respectively. A retrospective analysis of seven clinical trials of chemotherapy-naïve patients with advanced STS revealed that the overall median survival time of the 2,185 patients in the therapy arms was 51 weeks [16]; similar data were observed in more recent clinical trials [15, 17]. The basis for the longer overall survival times in our study subjects treated in the community compared with results from clinical trials is unclear and needs further investigation. However, consistent with previous studies [15, 16], patients with the top three histologic subtypes had better outcomes than those with the other subtypes. Among patients with the top three histologic subtypes, the median overall survival was 29 months, with similar trends observed for PFS. This observation could relate to differences in the underlying biology of these three tumors, such that, compared to the heterogeneous group of STS that were pooled into one group (other), the top three histologic types may be more responsive to therapy and/or have less aggressive disease characteristics. Another possibility could be that a slightly greater proportion of patients with the top three subtypes were treated with combination therapy (78.3%) compared to those with the other STS subtypes (65.5%). Selection biases could have contributed to these differences in outcomes by histology subtype. However, this was less likely, as we found that ages and ECOG scores between treated patients were similar by histology subtype.

Fifth, consistent with prior studies [16], we also found that younger age and lower ECOG scores were associated with longer OS in treated patients. While there was a significant difference in mean age and baseline ECOG scores between treated and untreated patients, larger cohorts in future studies will be needed to properly control for the influence these factors may have on OS and PFS outcomes. Finally, lung was the most common site for metastasis, and those with lung metastasis had shorter OS and PFS compared to subjects with metastasis to other sites.

Due to the retrospective, observational design of this study, there are some limitations worth noting. While the use of a large geographically dispersed cohort of community-based patients provides confidence that our results may potentially be able to be generalized, patterns of care within the MSH/USON network may differ to some extent from community-based treatment patterns in general. This may be due to the encouragement given to oncologists by the MSH/USON network administration to base their therapy decisions on evidence-based treatment guidelines. Additional limitations of this study include the exclusion of patients from specific sites in the MSH/USON network from the study sample because only partial iKnowMed EHR capabilities were adopted at these sites; it is possible that patterns of care at these specific sites may differ to some extent from the remainder of the sites. Another limitation includes the lack of differentiation of STS subtypes. Our EHR and chart review did not capture the different variants of liposarcoma or other important subtypes. Selection bias of subtype variants may have influenced response and survival rates and should be considered in future research. Also, escalation in LOT was used as a proxy for disease progression. Since there may be some delay from disease progression to when patients received their next line of chemotherapy, the progression-free survival may be overestimated. In addition, the iKnowMed data are collected for clinical practice reasons and not for research purposes. This may limit the standardization of the data collection methods and instruments as well as the reporting practices of the physician. Finally, our study was not designed to compare the efficacy of monotherapy versus combination therapy or determine the factors that associate with poorer clinical outcomes in STS. Thus, the inferences of this observational study need confirmation in randomized, controlled trials of adequate size prospectively designed to address these questions.

5. Conclusions

To our knowledge, this is the first study to use a cancer-specific database to capture "realworld" clinical data on patients with mSTS in the community-based setting. The results of this study are strengthened by the large sample size and potentially greater diversity of care compared with clinical trial or tertiary care academic settings. Taken together, by examining a community-based, cancer-specific EHR, we provide new insights into the epidemiology, treatment patterns, and outcomes of patients with mSTS who received care outside of an academic or clinical trial setting in the USA and elaborate on their implications for future clinical research.

Acknowledgments

The research was supported by GlaxoSmithKline. The authors would like to thank Debra Rembert and Mark Yap for chart data extraction support and Brooke Middlebrook for editorial support.

References

[1] E. C. Borden, L. H. Baker, R. S. Bell et al., "Soft tissue sarcomas of adults: state of the translational science," *Clinical Cancer Research*, vol. 9, no. 6, pp. 1941–1956, 2003.

[2] G. D. Demetri, L. H. Baker, R. S. Benjamin et al., "Soft tissue sarcoma," *Journal of the National Comprehensive Cancer Network*, vol. 5, pp. 364–399, 2007.

[3] P. G. Casali, L. Jost, S. Sleijfer, J. Verweij, and J.-Y. Blay, "Soft tissue sarcomas: ESMO clinical recommendations for diagnosis, treatment and follow-up," *Annals of Oncology*, vol. 19, no. 2, pp. ii89–ii93, 2008.

[4] A. Jemal, R. Siegel, J. Xu, and E. Ward, "Cancer statistics, 2010," *CA: A Cancer Journal for Clinicians*, vol. 60, no. 5, pp. 277–300, 2010.

[5] N. H. Segal, P. Pavlidis, C. R. Antonescu et al., "Classification and subtype prediction of adult soft tissue sarcoma by functional genomics," *The American Journal of Pathology*, vol. 163, no. 2, pp. 691–700, 2003.

[6] M. A. Clark, C. Fisher, I. Judson, and J. Meirion Thomas, "Soft-tissue sarcomas in adults," *The New England Journal of Medicine*, vol. 353, no. 7, pp. 701–711, 2005.

[7] J. N. Cormier and R. E. Pollock, "Soft tissue sarcomas," *Ca: A Cancer Journal for Clinicians*, vol. 54, no. 2, pp. 94–109, 2004.

[8] S. A. Lietman, "Soft-tissue sarcomas: overview of management, with a focus on surgical treatment considerations," *Cleveland Clinic Journal of Medicine*, vol. 77, supplement 1, pp. S13–S17, 2010.

[9] T. F. DeLaney, L. Kepka, S. I. Goldberg et al., "Radiation therapy for control of soft-tissue sarcomas resected with positive margins," *International Journal of Radiation Oncology Biology Physics*, vol. 67, no. 5, pp. 1460–1469, 2007.

[10] R. Wesolowski and G. T. Budd, "Use of chemotherapy for patients with bone and soft-tissue sarcomas," *Cleveland Clinic Journal of Medicine*, vol. 77, supplement 1, pp. S23–S26, 2010.

[11] V. H. Bramwell, D. Anderson, and M. L. Charette, "Doxorubicin-based chemotherapy for the palliative treatment of adult patients with locally advanced or metastatic soft tissue sarcoma," *Cochrane Database of Systematic Reviews*, no. 3, Article ID CD003293, 2003.

[12] K. Antman, J. Crowley, S. P. Balcerzak et al., "An intergroup phase III randomized study of doxorubicin and dacarbazine with or without ifosfamide and mesna in advanced soft tissue and bone sarcomas," *Journal of Clinical Oncology*, vol. 11, no. 7, pp. 1276–1285, 1993.

[13] A. le Cesne, I. Judson, D. Crowther et al., "Randomized phase III study comparing conventional-dose doxorubicin plus ifosfamide versus high-dose doxorubicin plus infosfamide plus recombinant human granulocyte-macrophage colony- stimulating factor in advanced soft tissue sarcomas: a trial of the european organization for research and treatment of cancer/soft tissue and bone sarcoma group," *Journal of Clinical Oncology*, vol. 18, no. 14, pp. 2676–2684, 2000.

[14] S. Jelić, V. Kovčin, N. Milanović et al., "Randomised study of high-dose epirubicin versus high-dose epirubicin-cisplatin chemotherapy for advanced soft tissue sarcoma," *European Journal of Cancer Part A*, vol. 33, no. 2, pp. 220–225, 1997.

[15] B. L. Samuels, S. Chawla, S. Patel et al., "Clinical outcomes and safety with trabectedin therapy in patients with advanced soft tissue sarcomas following failure of prior chemotherapy: results of a worldwide expanded access program study," *Annals of Oncology*, vol. 24, pp. 1703–1709, 2013.

[16] M. van Glabbeke, A. T. van Oosterom, J. W. Oosterhuis et al., "Prognostic factors for the outcome of chemotherapy in advanced soft tissue sarcoma: an analysis of 2,185 patients treated with anthracycline- containing first-line regimens—a European organization for research and treatment of cancer soft tissue and bone sarcoma group study," *Journal of Clinical Oncology*, vol. 17, no. 1, pp. 150–157, 1999.

[17] W. T. van der Graaf, J. Y. Blay, S. P. Chawla et al., "Pazopanib for metastatic soft-tissue sarcoma (PALETTE): a randomised, double-blind, placebo-controlled phase 3 trial," *The Lancet*, vol. 379, pp. 1879–1886, 2012.

[18] R. G. Maki, "Gemcitabine and docetaxel in metastatic sarcoma: past, present, and future," *Oncologist*, vol. 12, no. 8, pp. 999–1006, 2007.

[19] R. G. Maki, J. K. Wathen, S. R. Patel et al., "Randomized phase II study of gemcitabine and docetaxel compared with gemcitabine alone in patients with metastatic soft tissue sarcomas: results of sarcoma alliance for research through collaboration study 002," *Journal of Clinical Oncology*, vol. 25, no. 19, pp. 2755–2763, 2007.

2

Clinical Features and Outcomes Differ between Skeletal and Extraskeletal Osteosarcoma

Sheila Thampi,[1] Katherine K. Matthay,[1] W. John Boscardin,[2] Robert Goldsby,[1] and Steven G. DuBois[1]

[1] *Department of Pediatrics, UCSF School of Medicine and UCSF Benioff Children's Hospital, 505 Parnassus Avenue M649, P.O. Box 0106, San Francisco, CA 94143, USA*
[2] *Department of Medicine and Epidemiology and Biostatistics, UCSF School of Medicine 505 Parnassus Avenue, San Francisco, CA 94143, USA*

Correspondence should be addressed to Steven G. DuBois; duboiss@peds.ucsf.edu

Academic Editor: Clement Trovik

Background. Extraskeletal osteosarcoma (ESOS) is a rare subtype of osteosarcoma. We investigated patient characteristics, overall survival, and prognostic factors in ESOS. *Methods.* We identified cases of high-grade osteosarcoma with known tissue of origin in the Surveillance, Epidemiology, and End Results database from 1973 to 2009. Demographics were compared using univariate tests. Overall survival was compared with log-rank tests and multivariate analysis using Cox proportional hazards methods. *Results.* 256/4,173 (6%) patients with high-grade osteosarcoma had ESOS. Patients with ESOS were older, were more likely to have an axial tumor and regional lymph node involvement, and were female. Multivariate analysis showed ESOS to be favorable after controlling for stage, age, tumor site, gender, and year of diagnosis [hazard ratio 0.75 (95% CI 0.62 to 0.90); $p = 0.002$]. There was an interaction between age and tissue of origin such that older patients with ESOS had superior outcomes compared to older patients with skeletal osteosarcoma. Adverse prognostic factors in ESOS included metastatic disease, larger tumor size, older age, and axial tumor site. *Conclusion.* Patients with ESOS have distinct clinical features but similar prognostic factors compared to skeletal osteosarcoma. Older patients with ESOS have superior outcomes compared to older patients with skeletal osteosarcoma.

1. Introduction

Extraskeletal osteosarcoma (ESOS) is a rare malignant soft tissue sarcoma with histologic similarities to primary bone osteosarcoma but without attachment to the bone or periosteum. ESOS accounts for 1% of all soft tissue sarcomas and 4% of osteogenic osteosarcomas [1]. Multiple case series ranging from 10 to 88 patients have described this rare and unique tumor, with distinct clinical features between ESOS and primary bone osteosarcoma [2, 3].

ESOS is a tumor primarily of older age with a mean age of 47.5 to 61 years [1]. The majority of case series describe a male predominance [1, 3–7]. An early report described an overall survival rate of 38% at 5 years [5]. However, more recent groups that have used multiagent chemotherapy and wide resection during surgical procedures have described overall survival rates of 66 to 77%, similar to skeletal osteosarcoma [7, 8]. Reported adverse prognostic factors include metastatic disease at presentation, large tumor size, and inability to achieve complete surgical resection [1, 4, 5, 7, 9].

In order to further characterize this rare malignancy and compare it statistically to primary skeletal osteosarcoma, we used a large registry to analyze the largest known cohort of patients with ESOS. We define patient and tumor characteristics, estimated overall survival rates, and prognostic factors specifically for patients with ESOS.

2. Methods

2.1. Patients. In this cohort study, the analytic cohort included patients with osteosarcoma of skeletal or extraskeletal origin reported to the US National Cancer Institute's SEER (Surveillance, Epidemiology, and End Results;

http://seer.cancer.gov/data/) system from 1973 to 2009. This registry captures clinical data and outcomes from approximately one-quarter of the US population. Data are collected from a variety of sources, including health providers, pathology reports, laboratories, autopsy reports, and death certificates. Standard data quality measures are employed.

We included a convenience sample of patients in SEER with histologically confirmed high-grade osteosarcoma of any age at time of diagnosis. Given their low metastatic potential, we excluded patients with low-grade osteosarcoma (e.g., parosteal and intraosseous subtypes). The SEER database included 4,178 cases of high-grade osteosarcoma. We excluded five patients with unknown tissue of origin, which resulted in an analytic cohort of the remaining 4,173 patients.

2.2. Predictor Variable. We evaluated patient characteristics and outcomes according to tissue of origin (skeletal versus extraskeletal). Primary site was identified in SEER based on ICD-O-3 topography codes, which was then used to code each patient as having a skeletal or extraskeletal primary tumor. As only tumors with the histology code for osteosarcoma were included, primary tumors reported to arise in a soft tissue site were defined as extraskeletal osteosarcoma. Imaging materials (scans and/or scan reports) were not available to confirm skeletal or extraskeletal tissue origin.

2.3. Outcome Variables. Patient characteristics and overall survival were evaluated based on extraskeletal versus skeletal disease. Analyzed variables included age at diagnosis (continuous variable and age categorized in tertiles with exclusion of the youngest patients, age ≤ 17 years), sex, year of diagnosis (in 10-year increments), race, primary tumor location (evaluated as distinct sites and also dichotomized with tumors of the head, neck, and trunk defined as axial versus tumors of the extremity defined as appendicular), presence of regional lymph nodes, histologic subtype, tumor size (dichotomized at 10 cm), use of radiation therapy, and stage of disease, defined as either localized or metastatic. Patients with only regional node involvement outside of the primary site of disease were determined to have localized disease.

To determine overall survival, we used total months of follow-up and patient vital status at the time of last follow-up. To determine competing events, we used the variables vital status and cause-specific death, which describes death related to cancer and noncancer causes.

2.4. Statistical Methods. We compared patient characteristics between groups with skeletal osteosarcoma or ESOS using chi-squared tests (for categorical variables) or Student's t-test (for continuous variables). Overall survival was estimated using Kaplan-Meier (KM) methods with 95% confidence intervals. Potential differences in overall survival between groups were evaluated with log-rank tests. The median follow-up time for the analytic cohort was 102 months.

We also performed competing risk analysis using the Fine-Gray proportional subhazard model to focus on death due to malignancy. Death due to causes other than osteosarcoma was coded as a competing event. If cause of death was unknown, then those patients were not included in the competing risk analysis.

Cox proportional hazard methods were used to determine the effect of extraskeletal disease on overall survival while controlling for other differences in patient characteristics between the groups. Time dependent covariates were used to test the proportional hazards assumption. The SEER database was accessed using SEER* Stat version 7.1.0.

3. Results

3.1. Patient Characteristics Differ between Extraskeletal and Skeletal Osteosarcoma. Of the 4,173 patients in the analytic cohort, 256 (6.1%) patients had ESOS. Table 1 provides patient characteristics according to tissue of origin. The mean age for patients with ESOS was 60.7 years compared to 31.4 years for those with skeletal osteosarcoma ($P < 0.0001$). Patients with extraskeletal involvement were more likely to be female (54.3% versus 44.5%, $P = 0.002$), have an axial tumor (61.1% versus 25.1%, $P < 0.0001$), and have regional lymph node involvement (7.7% versus 2.4%, $P < 0.0001$). There was a statistically significant difference in distribution in primary tumor sites ($P < 0.0001$), most notable in comparing the frequency of primary tumors arising in the lower extremity (32.7% for extraskeletal versus 62.6% for skeletal). Patients with extraskeletal tumors were more likely to receive radiation treatment than patients with skeletal tumors (25.3% versus 12.3%, $P < 0.0001$). Whether radiation was instituted prior to diagnosis of osteosarcoma is unknown. About 30% of ESOS were found in the thorax, which includes involvement of the chest wall, breast, heart, and soft tissue. However, 6 cases were primary lung lesions, 4 were primary pleural lesions, and all are without documented skeletal involvement. Almost all ESOS were reported to have conventional osteosarcoma histology, rather than other histologic subtypes of high-grade osteosarcoma. There were no statistically significant differences in patient race, tumor size, or stage of disease based upon tissue of origin.

3.2. Overall Survival Differs between Extraskeletal and Skeletal Osteosarcoma. On Kaplan-Meier testing of the entire analytic cohort, without accounting for competing risks, overall survival was inferior for patients with ESOS as compared to those with skeletal osteosarcoma (Figure 1(a)). The estimated five-year overall survival for those with extraskeletal disease was 37% (95% CI 30.6 to 43.3) compared to 50.8% (95%CI 49.1 to 52.5; $P < 0.0001$) for those with skeletal disease. Differential overall survival was also seen according to tissue of origin when looking exclusively at patients with localized disease, but a statistically significant difference in overall survival according to tissue of origin was not seen in the cohort of patients with metastatic disease (see Supplemental Figure available online at http://dx.doi.org/10.1155/2014/902620). Specifically, the estimated five-year overall survival for those with localized extraskeletal disease was 47% (95% CI 39.8 to 54.6) compared to 63% (95% CI 60.8 to 64.7) for patients with

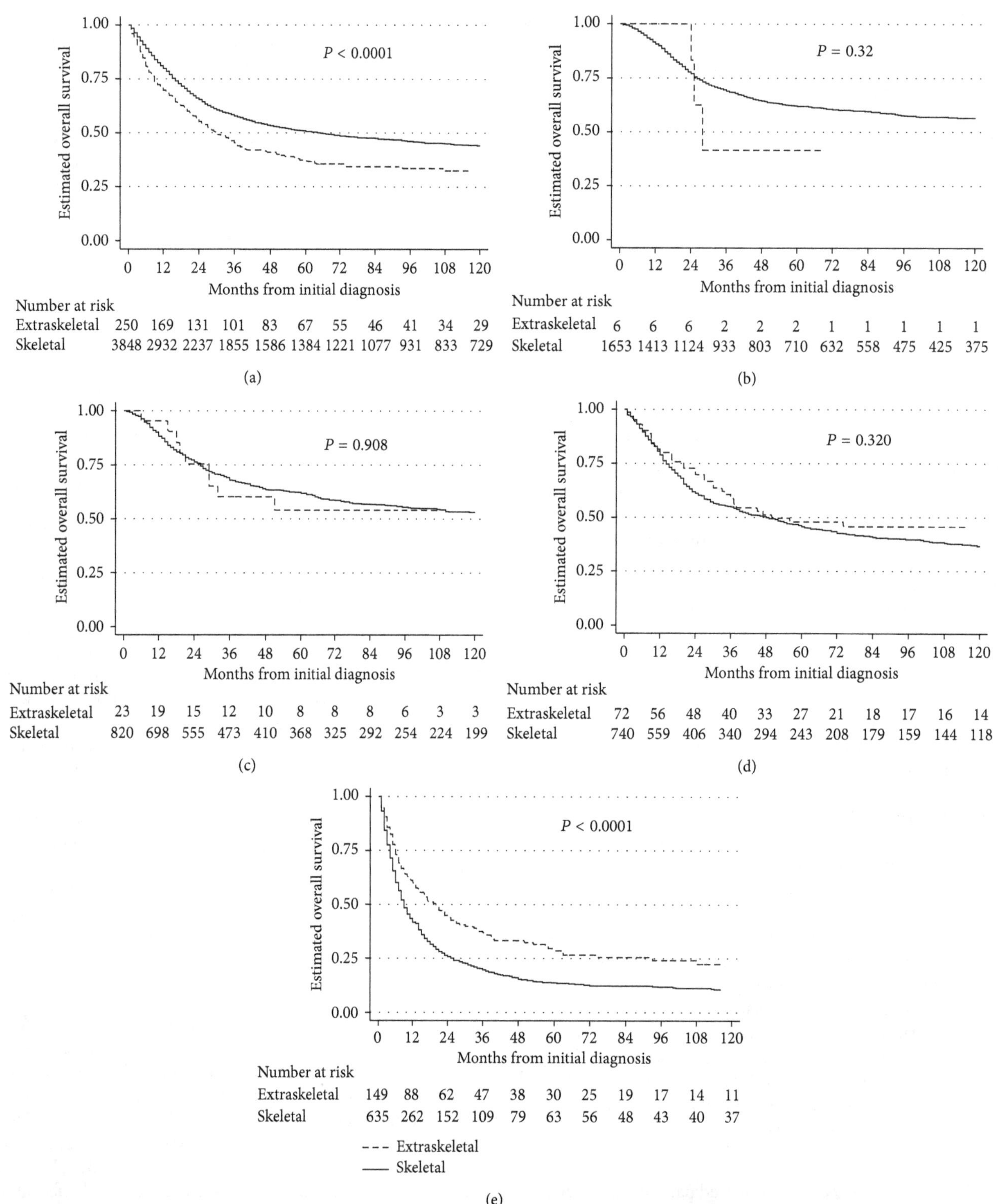

FIGURE 1: (a) Kaplan-Meier estimates of overall survival from the time of diagnosis according to tumor tissue of origin in all patients with high-grade osteosarcoma [n = 4,173 (256 with extraskeletal involvement and 3,917 with skeletal involvement)]. (b) Kaplan-Meier estimates of overall survival from the time of diagnosis according to tumor tissue of origin in patients aged from 0 to 17 years [n = 1,672 (6 with extraskeletal involvement and 1,666 with skeletal involvement)]. (c) Kaplan-Meier estimates of overall survival from the time of diagnosis according to tumor tissue of origin in patients aged from 18 to 32 years [n = 849 (24 with extraskeletal involvement and 825 with skeletal involvement)]. (d) Kaplan-Meier estimates of overall survival from the time of diagnosis according to tumor tissue of origin in patients aged from 33 to 59 years [n = 824 (72 with extraskeletal involvement and 752 with skeletal involvement)]. (e) Kaplan-Meier estimates of overall survival from the time of diagnosis according to tumor tissue of origin in patients aged from 60 to 99 years [n = 828 (154 with extraskeletal involvement and 674 with skeletal involvement)].

TABLE 1: Characteristics of 4,173 patients with osteosarcoma according to tissue of origin.

Characteristic	Skeletal osteosarcoma (N = 3,917)	ESOS (N = 256)	P value
Mean age (range)	31.4 years* (0–99 years)	60.7 years** (9–96 years)	<0.0001
Sex			
Male	2,175 (55.5%)	117 (45.7%)	0.002
Female	1,742 (44.5%)	139 (54.3%)	
Year of diagnosis			
1973–1979	395 (10.1%)	9 (3.5%)	
1980–1989	609 (15.5%)	21 (8.2%)	<0.0001
1990–1999	857 (21.9%)	64 (25%)	
2000–2009	2,056 (52.5%)	162 (63.3%)	
Race			
Caucasian	3,031 (77.8%)	212 (82.8%)	
African American	536 (13.8%)	30 (11.7%)	0.232
Asian	297 (7.6%)	12 (4.7%)	
Native American	32 (0.8%)	2 (0.8%)	
Primary site			
Lower extremity	2,392 (62.6%)	80 (32.7%)	
Upper extremity	467 (12.2%)	18 (7.3%)	
Head	398 (10.4%)	18 (7.3%)	
Spine	114 (3%)	1 (0.4%)	
Ribs/sternum	105 (2.8%)	0	<0.0001
Pelvis	343 (9%)	31 (12.7%)	
Thorax	0	70 (28.6%)	
Abdomen/retroperitoneum	0	27 (11%)	
Primary tumor location			
Axial	961 (25.1%)	154 (61.1%)	<0.0001
Appendicular	2,870 (74.9%)	98 (38.9%)	
Regional lymph node			
Present	61 (2.4%)	13 (7.7%)	<0.0001
Absent	2,519 (97.6%)	155 (92.3%)	
Stage			
Distant metastasis	794 (22.3%)	43 (18.6%)	0.188
No distant metastasis	2,763 (77.7%)	188 (81.4%)	
Tumor size			
<10 cm	1,252 (63.1%)	113 (58.9%)	0.241
≥10 cm	731 (36.9%)	79 (41.1%)	
Radiation use			
No	3,374 (87.7%)	186 (74.7%)	<0.0001
Yes	473 (12.3%)	63 (25.3%)	
Histologic type			
Osteosarcoma NOS	3,322 (84.8%)	239 (93.4%)	
Fibroblastic OS	263 (6.7%)	10 (3.9%)	
Telangiectatic OS	128 (3.3%)	3 (1.1%)	
OS in Paget's	79 (2%)	0	0.016
Small cell OS	30 (0.8%)	2 (0.8%)	
Central OS	42 (1.1%)	1 (0.4%)	
Periosteal OS	40 (1%)	0	
High grade surface OS	13 (0.3%)	1 (0.4%)	

OS: osteosarcoma; ESOS: extraskeletal osteosarcoma; NOS: not otherwise specified; totals for each variable may vary due to missing data but percentages reflect the represented data.

*Median age is 20 years. **Median age is 64 years.

localized skeletal osteosarcoma ($P < 0.0001$). The estimated five-year overall survival for those with metastatic ESOS was 10% (95% CI 2.7 to 23.3) compared to 19% (95% CI 16.4 to 22.4) for those with metastatic skeletal osteosarcoma ($P = 0.137$).

Due to the significantly older age of patients with ESOS, we performed a competing risk analysis to account for death due to other causes in the older population with extraskeletal tumors. Once we controlled for competing events, there was no difference in the cumulative incidence of death from osteosarcoma between patients with extraskeletal or skeletal disease.

Given that the majority of patients with ESOS were > 60 years of age, we compared overall survival of patients with ESOS versus skeletal osteosarcoma categorized by tertiles of age, with the youngest group (age ≤ 17 years) excluded due to too few patients with extraskeletal disease in this group ($n = 6$; Figure 1(b)). We observed that the oldest group of patients with osteosarcoma had inferior overall survival compared to younger age groups (Figures 1(b)–1(e)). However, within this older group, patients with ESOS had superior overall survival compared to patients with skeletal disease (Figure 1(e)). There was no difference in overall survival based on tissue of origin for the remaining two age tertiles (ages 18 to 32 and 33 to 59 years; Figures 1(c)-1(d)).

We constructed Cox proportional hazards models to assess the impact of extraskeletal disease on overall survival independent of potential confounders and again excluding patients ≤ 17 years of age from the analysis. Covariates included in our final model were tertiles of age and sex. Metastatic status, decade of diagnosis, and primary site did not satisfy the proportional hazard assumption; thus we stratified on these covariates in our final model to control for potential differences between groups. After controlling for these variables, extraskeletal disease was predictive of superior overall survival compared to skeletal disease (reference group). The hazard ratio for death for patients with extraskeletal disease was 0.75 (95% CI 0.62 to 0.90; $P = 0.002$) compared to patients with skeletal disease.

To better assess the interaction between age and impact of extraskeletal disease on overall survival, we formally tested for the presence of a statistical interaction by constructing a Cox model of overall survival that included tertiles of age, tissue of origin, and interaction term of these two variables. The P value associated with this interaction term was 0.043, confirming a statistically significant interaction between the age and the impact of tissue of origin on overall survival. We next constructed a multivariate Cox model stratified by age tertile in order to obtain tertile-specific estimates of the hazard ratio for death in each tertile according to tissue of origin. As above, this model also controlled for sex, metastatic status, decade of diagnosis, and primary tumor site. We observed that the hazard ratio for death associated with ESOS compared to skeletal osteosarcoma decreased with increasing tertile of age: 1.05 (95% CI 0.51–2.14) for 18–32 years of age; 0.97 (95% CI 0.69–1.37) for 33–59 years of age; and 0.65 (95% CI 0.52–0.82) for 60–99 years of age.

Data on tumor size were not available in 48% of patients. As such, this variable was omitted from the preceding multivariate models but we used this variable to perform a sensitivity analysis that was similar to the final model. Covariates included in this sensitivity analysis were tertiles of age, sex, tumor size, tumor site, and year of diagnosis. Metastatic status did not satisfy the proportional hazard assumption; thus we stratified on this variable. This model yielded a similar estimate of the impact of extraskeletal origin on overall survival compared to our preceding model that did not include tumor size (hazard ratio of 0.79; 95% CI 0.63 to 0.99 for patients with extraskeletal disease compared to patients with skeletal disease; $P = 0.039$).

3.3. Prognostic Factors Predictive of Overall Survival in Extraskeletal Osteosarcoma. We next evaluated potential prognostic factors exclusively in the entire cohort of patients with ESOS. On univariate analyses using Cox proportional hazards methods, distant metastatic disease, larger tumor (maximum diameter ≥ 10 cm), older age (age 60 to 99 years), axial tumor site, and regional node involvement were all associated with statistically significantly inferior overall survival (Table 2). Sex and year of diagnosis were not found to be prognostic. We next performed multivariate analysis using Cox proportional hazards models to identify independent adverse prognostic factors in this disease. We included the following significant variables from the above univariate analyses: metastatic status; tumor size; age; and tumor site. Each of these variables remained prognostic on multivariate analysis (Table 2).

We next evaluated potential prognostic factors exclusively in patients with localized ESOS. On univariate analyses using Cox proportional hazards methods, larger tumor size (maximum diameter ≥ 10 cm), axial tumor site, and regional node involvement were all associated with statistically significantly inferior overall survival (Table 3). Age, sex, and year of diagnosis were not found to be prognostic. We next performed multivariate analysis using Cox proportional hazards models to identify independent adverse prognostic factors in patients with localized ESOS. We included the significant variables from the above univariate analyses and both tumor size and axial tumor site remained prognostic on multivariate analysis (Table 3).

Due to limited numbers of patients with data available for both tumor size and regional node involvement, the independent prognostic impact of regional node involvement in this cohort was not assessed as this variable had the fewest patients with available data in our cohort.

4. Discussion

In this study of ESOS, we observed that patients with ESOS had significantly different clinical features from patients with skeletal osteosarcoma, including older age, propensity for axial tumors, and female preponderance. Although univariate analysis demonstrated inferior overall survival for patients with extraskeletal disease, once we controlled for competing events, we found that patients with ESOS had a similar cumulative incidence of death due to cancer as patients with skeletal osteosarcoma. Multivariate analysis revealed for the

TABLE 2: Univariate and multivariate prognostic factors for overall survival in a cohort of patients with extraskeletal osteosarcoma.

	Univariate hazard ratio (95% confidence interval)	Univariate P value	Multivariate hazard ratio (95% confidence interval)	Multivariate P value
Distant metastasis	3.16 (2.11–4.73)	<0.0001	2.39 (1.34–4.25)	0.003
Tumor size ≥10 cm	2.03 (1.40–2.95)	<0.0001	2.11 (1.41–3.17)	<0.0001
Axial tumor	1.98 (1.39–2.80)	<0.0001	1.65 (1.08–2.53)	0.021
Age				
18–32 years	Reference		Reference	
33–59 years	1.30 (0.63–2.70)	0.477	1.13 (0.45–2.79)	0.796
60–99 years	2.59 (1.31–5.12)	0.006	2.53 (1.08–5.90)	0.032
Regional lymph node present	2.09 (1.14–3.83)	0.017	Not tested	Not tested
Male gender	1.32 (0.96–1.80)	0.086	Not tested	Not tested
Year of diagnosis			Not tested	Not tested
1973–1979	1.80 (0.87–3.75)	0.115		
1980–1989	0.80 (0.44–1.45)	0.465		
1990–1999	0.85 (0.59–1.23)	0.390		
2000–2009	Reference			

TABLE 3: Univariate and multivariate prognostic factors for overall survival in a cohort of patients with localized extraskeletal osteosarcoma.

	Univariate hazard ratio (95% confidence interval)	Univariate P value	Multivariate hazard ratio (95% confidence interval)	Multivariate P value
Tumor size ≥10 cm	2.06 (1.36–3.14)	0.001	2.36 (1.53–3.62)	<0.0001
Axial tumor	2.04 (1.35–3.07)	0.001	2.01 (1.30–3.11)	0.002
Age			Not tested	Not tested
18–32 years	Reference			
33–59 years	1.28 (0.53–3.07)	0.580		
60–99 years	2.26 (0.98–5.20)	0.055		
Regional lymph node present	2.33 (1.23–4.41)	0.009	Not tested	Not tested
Male gender	1.27 (0.88–1.85)	0.204	Not tested	Not tested
Year of diagnosis			Not tested	Not tested
1973–1979	1.39 (0.49–3.91)	0.537		
1980–1989	0.69 (0.34–1.42)	0.316		
1990–1999	0.99 (0.65–1.51)	0.964		
2000–2009	Reference			

first time that extraskeletal disease was in fact favorable. This effect was driven by an interaction between the age and the impact of tissue of origin on overall survival, with the majority of patients with ESOS being older and with ESOS being favorable in older patients. Adverse prognostic factors previously described for patients with skeletal osteosarcoma were also shown to be prognostic among patients with ESOS.

As reported by other groups, patients with ESOS are significantly older than patients with skeletal osteosarcoma [1, 4–9]. Our cohort included only 6 patients with ESOS < 18 years/1672 (0.4%) patients < 18 years with osteosarcoma, accounting for 2.3% of all patients with ESOS. In contrast to previous reports, we observed a higher incidence of axial primary tumors in patients with ESOS. Regional lymph node involvement in osteosarcoma is a rare and unfavorable finding previously reported by our group [10]. We observed a female predominance for ESOS as did Choi et al., suggesting that gender distribution varies in each cohort due to chance [9]. Understanding the etiology for these clinical differences will likely require greater understanding of the cell of origin of ESOS. The increasing cases of osteosarcoma by year of diagnosis reflect the expanding SEER database in each decade which resulted in more cases being captured and not an increase in the incidence of disease.

Previous literature prior to multimodal therapy reported dismal overall survival for patients with ESOS, while recent groups report similar overall survival with skeletal osteosarcoma [3–9, 11]. Overall survival for our ESOS cohort was inferior but controlling for competing events resulted in similar incidence of death due to cancer. We also observed that the oldest group of patients had the poorest survival, but the presence of extraskeletal disease as compared to skeletal disease renders a more favorable outcome specifically in this age group that accounted for the majority of ESOS cases. This finding could relate to differences in the biology of the tumor with age or differential propensity to perform aggressive surgical resection of soft tissue versus bone tumors in an older population. Unfortunately, neither hypothesis is testable with the data available in SEER. We note that radiation treatment was more likely to be used in extraskeletal tumors, which might suggest a lower rate of aggressive surgical resection of these tumors, though this suggestion cannot be validated in SEER. We also note that although 2% of the patients had osteosarcoma in the setting of Paget's disease, this is not a groups.
high enough proportion to account for the difference between

Among patients with ESOS, we found that distant metastatic disease, larger tumor size (≥10 cm), axial tumor site, and older age are adverse prognostic factors. In patients with localized ESOS, axial tumor site and large tumor size were adverse prognostic factors. We confirmed previous reports that distant metastatic disease at diagnosis is an unfavorable prognostic factor in ESOS [1]. Ahmad et al. found that on univariate analysis there was a significant difference in disease specific survival for tumor size >10 cm, microscopically positive surgical margins, and TNM stage >2 [4]. However, none of these factors remained significant in multivariate analysis. In our larger analysis, we were able to confirm the adverse prognostic impact of large tumor size. Lee et al. found on univariate analysis that patients with ESOS with chondroblastic subtype survived longer than those with osteoblastic subtype [6]. Given the lack of histologic heterogeneity of cases of ESOS in SEER, we were not able to evaluate this finding. Goldstein-Jackson et al. found that complete surgical resection was the only statistically significant prognostic factor in their univariate analysis [7]. We note that data on surgical margin and extent of surgical resection were not available for the current analysis, though it seems reasonable to anticipate that these established patients with ESOS.
prognostic factors in osteosarcoma would likewise apply to

Use of the SEER database has provided us with a large cohort for this otherwise rare subgroup of osteosarcoma, which has allowed us to analyze potential prognostic factors predictive of overall survival with greater power than other smaller studies. Other strengths with this registry include long-term patient follow-up and diverse population as patients are registered from across the United States. However, use of a registry has limitations, particularly with regard to variables available for analysis. We recognize that tumor size is an important clinical predictor and was only available for 52% of our cohort. We were unable to perform central review of imaging or pathology. In order to obtain a large cohort with ESOS we captured patients over several decades during which treatment has evolved. We were unable to analyze overall survival based on treatment strategies since use of chemotherapy and details on surgical procedure (amputation versus limb sparing or presence of microscopic margins) are either not provided or only sparsely provided in SEER. We also were unable to determine the incidence of each type of recurrence (local versus distant) to confirm previous case series showing both high local and distant recurrent rates [1, 4, 6]. We also did not have access to the percent tumor necrosis after neoadjuvant chemotherapy, which is a known prognostic factor in skeletal osteosarcoma but has not been evaluated in ESOS thus far.

Our study reveals that the incidence of death from ESOS is similar to skeletal osteosarcoma in this cohort of patients and that overall survival varies by age such that the oldest patients have more favorable outcomes with extraskeletal disease as compared to skeletal osteosarcoma. Finally, further prospective research is needed to understand if there are biologic differences between extraskeletal and skeletal osteosarcoma as these differences may explain the variation in patient characteristics and overall survival between the two groups.

Acknowledgments

This work was supported by the Frank A. Campini Foundation; the National Institutes of Health [1K23CA154530-01 to S.D. and 5T32CA128583-05 to S.T.]; and the Mildred V. Strouss Chair in Translational Oncology (KM).

References

[1] G. Mc Auley, J. Jagannathan, K. O'Regan et al., "Extraskeletal osteosarcoma: spectrum of imaging findings," *American Journal of Roentgenology*, vol. 198, no. 1, pp. W31–W37, 2012.

[2] H. Wilson, "Extraskeletal ossifying tumors," *Annals of Surgery*, vol. 113, no. 1, pp. 95–112, 1941.

[3] E. B. Chung and F. M. Enzinger, "Extraskeletal osteosarcoma," *Cancer*, vol. 60, no. 5, pp. 1132–1142, 1987.

[4] S. A. Ahmad, S. R. Patel, M. T. Ballo et al., "Extraosseous osteosarcoma: response to treatment and long-term outcome," *Journal of Clinical Oncology*, vol. 20, no. 2, pp. 521–527, 2002.

[5] B. L. Bane, H. L. Evans, J. Y. Ro et al., "Extraskeletal osteosarcoma. A clinicopathologic review of 26 cases," *Cancer*, vol. 66, no. 22, pp. 2762–2770, 1990.

[6] J. S. Lee, J. F. Fetsch, D. A. Wasdhal, B. P. Lee, D. J. Pritchard, and A. G. Nascimento, "A Review of 40 Patients with extraskeletal osteosarcoma," *Cancer*, vol. 76, no. 11, pp. 2253–2259, 1995.

[7] S. Y. Goldstein-Jackson, G. Gosheger, G. Delling et al., "Extraskeletal osteosarcoma has a favourable prognosis when treated like conventional osteosarcoma," *Journal of Cancer Research and Clinical Oncology*, vol. 131, no. 8, pp. 520–526, 2005.

[8] T. Torigoe, Y. Yazawa, T. Takagi, A. Terakado, and H. Kurosawa, "Extraskeletal osteosarcoma in Japan: multiinstitutional study of 20 patients from the Japanese Musculoskeletal Oncology Group," *Journal of Orthopaedic Science*, vol. 12, no. 5, pp. 424–429, 2007.

[9] L. E. Choi, J. H. Healey, D. Kuk, and M. F. Brennan, "Analysis of outcomes in extraskeletal osteosarcoma: a review of fifty-three cases," *The Journal of Bone and Joint Surgery: American volume*, vol. 96, no. 1, article e2, 2014.

[10] S. Thampi, K. K. Matthay, R. Goldsby, and S. G. Dubois, "Adverse impact of regional lymph node involvement in osteosarcoma," *European Journal of Cancer*, vol. 49, no. 16, pp. 3471–3476, 2013.

[11] M. L. Jensen, B. Schumacher, O. M. Jensen, O. S. Nielsen, and J. Keller, "Extraskeletal osteosarcomas: a clinicopathologic study of 25 cases," *The American Journal of Surgical Pathology*, vol. 22, no. 5, pp. 588–594, 1998.

3

Wiki-Based Clinical Practice Guidelines for the Management of Adult Onset Sarcoma: A New Paradigm in Sarcoma Evidence

S. J. Neuhaus,[1] D. Thomas,[1] J. Desai,[1] C. Vuletich,[2] J. von Dincklage,[2] and I. Olver[2]

[1] *Australasian Sarcoma Study Group, Melbourne, VIC 3002, Australia*
[2] *Cancer Council Australia, Sydney, NSW 2000, Australia*

Correspondence should be addressed to S. J. Neuhaus; padrneuhaus@apsa.com.au

Academic Editor: Chandrajit Premanand Raut

In 2013 Australia introduced Wiki-based Clinical Practice Guidelines for the Management of Adult Onset Sarcoma. These guidelines utilized a customized MediaWiki software application for guideline development and are the first evidence-based guidelines for clinical management of sarcoma. This paper presents our experience with developing and implementing web-based interactive guidelines and reviews some of the challenges and lessons from adopting an evidence-based (rather than consensus-based) approach to clinical sarcoma guidelines. Digital guidelines can be easily updated with new evidence, continuously reviewed and widely disseminated. They provide an accessible method of enabling clinicians and consumers to access evidence-based clinical practice recommendations and, as evidenced by over 2000 views in the first four months after release, with 49% of those visits being from countries outside of Australia. The lessons learned have relevance to other rare cancers in addition to the international sarcoma community.

1. Introduction

Sarcomas are rare malignant tumours of bone and soft tissue [1]. They include a heterogeneous group of malignancies and involve many anatomical sites and subtypes. There are approximately 850 new cases of sarcoma each year in Australia [2].

The rarity of sarcoma and its subtypes makes it challenging to determine optimal treatment strategies. Multidisciplinary input, including specialist pathology and radiology expertise, is essential to providing best clinical practice outcomes [3]. However, there are significant gaps in the evidence base used to underpin clinical decision making for patients with sarcoma and significant geographic and site-specific treatment disparities.

2. Why Clinical Practice Guidelines?

Existing clinical practice guidelines for the management of sarcoma, such as those released by European Society of Medical Oncology (ESMO), National Institute for Health and Clinical Excellence (NICE), and National Comprehensive Cancer Network (NCCN), are consensus-based guidelines [4–7]. As such, although a useful point of reference, these guidelines are not optimized to address a number of features of the Australian environment.

Such differences include marked geographic disparity in sarcoma management. For example, the probability of radiotherapy as a primary (presurgical) modality in Australia is largely determined by centre-based preferences and access to sarcoma specialist centres. Similarly, availability as well as involvement of paediatric oncology expertise in treating patients in the Adult and Young Adolescent (AYA) age range varies by referral centre and co-location of paediatric and adult treatment centres and/or local networks. In addition, the mixture of private and public health funding models in Australia and national approval processes and funding for drugs have implications for Australian practice guidelines. For example, trabectedin is approved and reimbursed for the treatment of sarcomas in Europe, but not Australia.

Low levels of evidence often underpin clinical sarcoma practice. Balanced with this is a pragmatic requirement for clinicians to make decisions on the optimal management of their individual patients. Treatment algorithms rely heavily on individual clinician experience and consensus of the multidisciplinary team. As a consequence, variance in care between clinicians and centres is common. Similarly, access to clinical trials varies by geography and centre and translational research integration is often opportunistic, rather than nationally coordinated.

Increasingly, new prognostic factors and therapeutic approaches for sarcoma are being identified. The rapidly expanding knowledge base, particularly in areas of targeted therapy and molecular genetics, along with changes to pathological coding, new imaging modalities, and advances in surgery and radiotherapy, makes keeping up to date with the latest development in sarcoma management a challenge for all involved [8].

3. Promote Consistency in Decision Making through Provision of Best Evidence

The primary aim of the Sarcoma guidelines process was to bring together lead clinicians managing sarcoma, across a range of disciplines, to develop common shared understanding of the current evidence and to identify key research gaps in an Australasian setting. By promoting consistency in decision making through provision of best evidence, the development of pathways of care, both state and national, was identified as natural sequelae to this process.

4. Problem with Printed Guidelines

Traditional printed clinical practice guidelines are resource intensive and become out of date almost as soon as released, by virtue of new evidence constantly being published [9].

Wide stakeholder engagement and consultation is important in any guidelines process but adds to the delay. Nonautomatic electronic searching of bibliographic databases makes literature searches time consuming and expensive. In addition, there is a paucity of evidence demonstrating the impact on practice of printed guidelines [10].

Confronted with these challenges, the small size of the Australian sarcoma community and the pragmatic reality of "time poor" clinical practitioners, an innovative solution was required.

The Australian sarcoma community was fortunate to be able to utilize a relatively new and modern methodology for guidelines developed by Cancer Council Australia.

5. Wiki Platform

The sarcoma guidelines project was a collaborative project between the Australasian Sarcoma Study Group (ASSG) and Cancer Council Australia (CCA) which commenced in 2011 and utilized Cancer Council Australia's Wiki platform.

The term Wiki is derived from "swift" in Hawaiian and is a web application that allows the creation and editing of interlinked web pages via a web browser using simplified markup language to facilitate online collaboration [11].

CCA has modified and customized the MediaWiki, an open source Wiki software application, to facilitate the guideline development process.

The methodology and guideline development process has been translated into an online environment and adheres closely to that of traditional printed guidelines. The process is illustrated in Figure 1. The key difference is the ability to use the technological platform to provide continuous update of emerging literature as it becomes available [12]. In this way the Wiki sarcoma guidelines reflect the most recent, available, and up to date evidence base. CCA's Cancer Guidelines Wiki has access restrictions set in place, so that only authors can add content, but anyone can comment.

6. Methodology

A multidisciplinary working party including consumer representation was established in 2011. Expressions of interest were sought across the Australian sarcoma community, with the intent of providing both cross-discipline and geographic representation.

The working party comprised 42 members. The working party met at an initial "face to face" meeting to decide the clinical questions that were most relevant to their disciplines and determine the scope of the guidelines. The selected questions reflected the gaps in knowledge that impacted most on daily management decisions.

As an *ab initio* set of guidelines, the original scope of these guidelines was broad. The key areas covered have been refined to include

(i) diagnosis,

(ii) multidisciplinary treatment,

(iii) chemotherapy (systemic therapies),

(iv) radiotherapy,

(v) surgery,

(vi) follow-up.

Sarcomas affect children and adolescents, as well as adult members of the community. However, for reasons of pragmatism and resource, the scope of this first iteration is restricted to adult onset bone and soft tissue sarcoma. Gastrointestinal stromal tumours (GIST), Kaposi's sarcoma, and aggressive (desmoid) fibromatosis were excluded.

Childhood, adolescent (AYA), and gynaecological sarcomas are priorities for the next iteration of the guidelines.

Historically, clinical guidelines have been accompanied by a separate set of consumer guidelines. A decision was made not to do this with the clinical practice guidelines for adult onset sarcoma and reflects the availability of "online" consumer resources within Australia and the international community. The Wiki platform allows direct linkage to other relevant organisations' websites containing already available useful information for consumers. This has been integrated and linked to relevant sites from the guidelines table of contents page.

In addition, a number of external linkages have been embedded. These include links to the Australasian Sarcoma

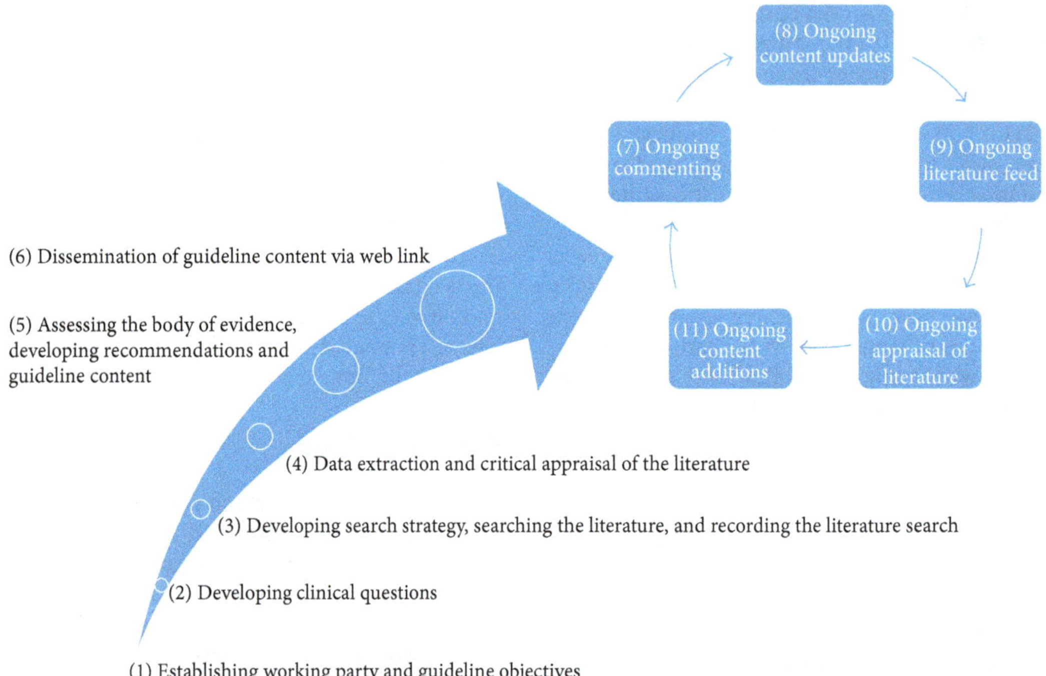

FIGURE 1: Developing guidelines on a Wiki platform.

Study Group, geographic sarcoma specialist expertise, and multidisciplinary centres across Australia and linkage to available clinical trials sites such as the National Health and Medical Research Council (NHMRC) trials registry and sites presenting detailed treatment protocols such as EviQ.

7. Process

As with traditional printed guidelines, following definition of the clinical questions and standardised PICO (patient/population; intervention; comparison; outcome) formats were developed online. The next step involved literature search retrieval and assessment. The use of online literature search tools facilitated this process. Systematic search strategies were developed for a range of databases, such as PubMed, Embase, Trip database, and others using predetermined search term fields and predefined inclusion/exclusion criteria. Retrieved literature was made available via the Wiki platform as designated to individual working party authors and reviewers to assess using the online critical appraisal form, providing a body of evidence from which guideline content development was undertaken [11]. Manuscript appraisals are available as part of the audit trail of how the guidelines were derived and can be viewed online [13]. In addition, each author had to record conflict of interests, which can be viewed online, to provide transparency through the process.

The online nature of the Wiki provides a uniquely interactive format, where chapter authors and others can easily view all recommendations via the summary of recommendations page (illustrated at Table 1) and more detailed content of each of the clinical question pages from the guideline's table of contents or landing page.

Each guideline question content page also contains the background methodological reports in the Appendices section. These Appendices, illustrated at Figure 2, provide transparency about the recommendation components, grading, and body of evidence used to generate the recommendation. Recommendation components include the grade, evidence base, evidence consistency, clinical impact, generalizability, and applicability to the Australian environment. In addition, users can view pending evidence, which has not yet been either assessed or incorporated into the body of evidence demonstrating at a glance the guideline's currency and allowing direct access via link to citations and abstracts. Users can also access individual critical appraisals of literature by navigating to the respective citation page.

The draft Clinical Practice Guidelines for Management of Adult Onset Sarcoma containing 54 recommendations and 35 practice points were released for initial public consultation for a 30-day period on 3 September 2013. The consultation process involved soliciting public comments by sending email alerts to recipients comprising relevant professional organisations, state and territory Cancer Councils, and individual clinical experts and consumer organisations in Australia and New Zealand. Organisations and individuals were invited to post comments on the Cancer Council Australia Cancer Guidelines Wiki. During the public consultation phase nine public comments (by five submitters) were received. The site received 488 visits (72% from Australia, 4% from New Zealand, 3% from United States, and remaining 21% from 37 other countries). These led to further edits, which were reviewed in detail by the working party.

TABLE 1: Excerpt of summary of recommendations.

(a)

Does referral to a specialist centre improve outcomes?	
+ Recommendation	Grade
Patients with suspected sarcoma to be referred to a specialist sarcoma unit prior to diagnosis in order to reduce the rates of incomplete excision, reoperation, and local recurrence and to improve survival.	C

(b)

Chemotherapy (systemic therapies) What is the role for adjuvant systemic therapy for adults with BSTT?	
+ Recommendation	Grade
Curative treatment of Ewing's sarcoma comprises a combination of chemotherapy and surgery and/or radiotherapy.	B
The use of postoperative chemotherapy in adult type soft tissue sarcomas is not the current standard of care.	D
Curative treatment of high-grade osteosarcoma comprises chemotherapy and surgery.	B

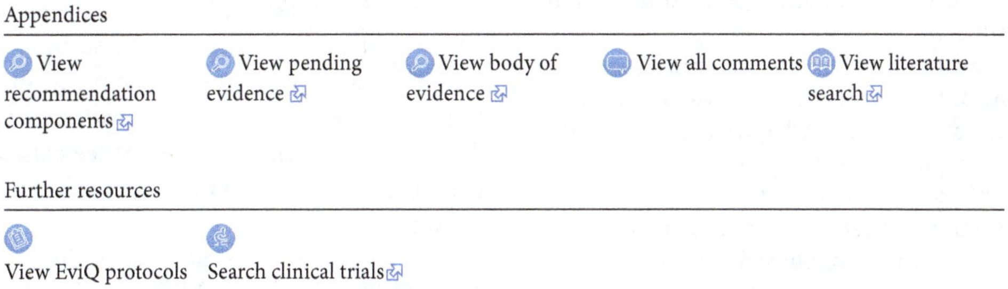

Appendices

View recommendation components | View pending evidence | View body of evidence | View all comments | View literature search

Further resources

View EviQ protocols | Search clinical trials

FIGURE 2: Appendices associated with each clinical question.

The guidelines were released nationally on 15 November 2013 and can be accessed at http://wiki.cancer.org.au/australia/Guidelines:Sarcoma. From release in November 2013 to May 15, 2014, the guidelines received 3,475 page views with 1,344 visits and an average of 2.6 pages per visit. Of these 52% of visits were from Australia, 8.9% from USA, 6% from United Kingdom, 6% from India, 2% from Singapore, 1.9% from Germany, and the remaining 25.3% from 39 additional countries.

The guidelines highlight the importance of early referral to multidisciplinary centers that specialize in treating sarcoma. Caseload and experience is associated with improved rates of functional limb preservation, lower rates of local recurrence, good rates of overall survival, and improved quality of life. These centers are usually involved in ongoing clinical trials, in which sarcoma patients' enrollment is highly encouraged.

The importance of the multidisciplinary team in initial assessment, diagnosis, and making decisions about treatment is strongly endorsed by the recommendations in the guidelines. A multidisciplinary approach (involving pathologists, radiologists, surgeons, radiation therapists, medical oncologists, and paediatric oncologists, with experience in sarcoma), or within reference networks sharing expertise and treating a high number of patients annually, is preferred.

It should be noted that participants in this guideline development process found challenges in assigning conventional levels of evidence for many recommendations. The heterogeneity and rarity of sarcomas, along with the increased molecular stratification of clinical trials, means that few studies reached what would be considered the "gold standard" in other diseases (multiple placebo-controlled double-blinded randomized controlled trials), including more common cancers. The absence of evidence, however, does not exonerate clinicians from the necessity to make clinical judgments in caring for patients with sarcomas. This raises questions about the need to develop standards of evidence that recognize the challenges of research in rare diseases, including sarcoma. Consequently these guidelines emphasise the need for increased participation in collaborative research and trials programs as a standard of care.

8. Next Steps

The Wiki platform provides the sarcoma guidelines with an iterative and constantly updating framework. Infrastructure is in place to automatically feed literature updates from PubMed and Embase to relevant question authors [14]. In addition, new or emerging evidence can be manually submitted by the experts at any time using the commenting and submit new evidence features embedded within each question page. The ability to appraise supporting evidence for new therapies in a timely manner is particularly important in Australia, to potentially decrease the lag time before these therapies, which may be available internationally, and can be brought into national clinical practice. Guidelines also promote evidence-based recommendations which may be helpful in lobbying for the funding of a new drug.

Expert working party authors will continue at regular intervals to assess new evidence and comments and update the content where necessary, ensuring that this remains an iterative and current guideline. We will work towards empowering small writing groups, to whom we will provide new literature as it is published, with the ability to update their section of the guidelines without requiring specific public consultation. While reliant on small working groups, any bias is mitigated by the design of the platform where the public and experts can post comments at any time. In addition to this, the larger working group will meet annually to review all updates.

The working party will meet in November 2014 as part of an annual process to review the content and updates and formulate the next generation of clinical questions (Paediatric/AYA). Gynaecological sarcoma questions will be incorporated in 2016.

Defining the "research gaps" in sarcoma care has been an important outcome of this process. In each section these are included in the form of future research questions that need to be addressed by good quality collaborative trials.

As a strategy for boosting implementation, Cancer Council Australia is developing educational modules to accompany each of the online guidelines established. This process will be managed by adopting spaced education (called Qstream) techniques for online education. Qstream utilises clinical scenarios presented in a short answer test question format [15]. Further information is provided in response to answers and wrong answers, thus presenting more data iteratively over several weeks. Experience with spaced education modules has been shown to increase knowledge and retention of guideline content and change clinical practices [16].

Education modules can be linked to key stakeholder groups such a radiology, pathology, primary care provider, and surgical colleges. Such web-based education resources provide a cost-effective way of engaging with health providers and consumers who may not otherwise have been able to access these opportunities and can be stratified by level of expertise (e.g., medical student versus specialist) and by resource availability.

These guidelines are intended to be a resource to help create awareness, for use in medical education and as a resource in multidisciplinary team meetings. Engagement from the breadth of the sarcoma community, both in Australia and internationally, via comments and submissions of new evidence, is actively encouraged [17].

Australia is situated within a region containing the largest growing population in the world: currently over 4.3 billion [18]. There is significant economic and resource disparity across the Asia-Pacific region, with rapid growth in socioeconomic status and rising expectations in health care for large countries such as India and China [19]. However, emerging Internet technology provides a cost-effective way to address engagement and education and engage with and connect previously isolated research teams and extend expertise and clinical collaboration across the region in new and innovative ways. Due to the online nature of the guidelines we can easily add new or emerging questions of relevance. Similarly, we can retire questions that become irrelevant for clinical practice.

We hope these guidelines will provide an accessible up-to-date platform for dissemination of current evidence in a rapidly changing landscape and assist in clinical management of adult onset sarcoma. In addition, the guidelines provide a national and regional resource for multidisciplinary sarcoma teams, individual clinicians, students, and consumers. Cancer Council Australia are developing a suite of Wiki based guidelines for other cancers including melanoma and lung cancer. Sharing our methodology with international guideline developers has allowed the sharing of literature searches. Such international collaboration and sharing is key to expanding the reach of the guidelines.

9. Conclusions

Advances in multidisciplinary care have improved the evaluation and care of patients with sarcoma. One of the key principles underlying the development of these guidelines was to address issues where the evidence was unclear, where divergent interpretations of evidence existed, or where particular issues unique to the Australian setting needed to be considered.

The Australian Clinical Practice Guidelines for the Management of Adult Onset Sarcoma are the first step towards more standardised care for patients with sarcoma across the nation and provides a framework to educate the community about referral pathways and develop more formal communications between sarcoma centres and clinicians, particularly in relation to current trials and access.

The Cancer Council Australia Cancer Guidelines Wiki platform used to develop these guidelines is unique. It enables iterative, ongoing, and interactive guideline development and revision processes and provides a cost-effective, efficient methodology and transparent assessment of the available evidence in sarcoma management. There are significant opportunities to leverage this platform for further international engagement and collaboration.

Key Message

Australian Clinical Practice Guidelines for the Management of Adult Onset Sarcoma were released in 2013. They constitute evidence-based guidelines in an accessible, interactive, and transparent format, which can be continuously reviewed and widely disseminated as new evidence becomes available.

Acknowledgments

(1) The authors thank *project team*: Professor Ian Olver, CEO, Cancer Council Australia, A/Professor Susan Neuhaus, Chair of the Sarcoma Guidelines Working Group, Christine Vuletich, Manager, Clinical Guidelines Network, CCA, Jutta von Dincklage, Product Manager, Wiki Development, and

Laura Holliday, Project Officer. (2) They also thank *all members of the working party*. (3) *Technical support* is provided by Andrew Garrett, Lead Developer, Redwerks (web design agency). Special thanks go to the Australasian Sarcoma Study Group for supporting the Guidelines.

References

[1] M. A. Clark, C. Fisher, I. Judson, and J. Meirion Thomas, "Soft-tissue sarcomas in adults," *The New England Journal of Medicine*, vol. 353, no. 7, pp. 701–711, 2005.

[2] J. A. Potter, R. Woods, T. Bessen, G. Farshid, D. Roder, and S. J. Neuhaus, "Incidence and reconstructive demand of sarcoma in Australia: first national data analysis," *ANZ Journal of Surgery*, vol. 84, supplement 1, pp. 140–165, 2014, abstract no. 21859.

[3] T. Ruhstaller, H. Roe, B. Thürlimann, and J. J. Nicoll, "The multidisciplinary meeting: an indispensable aid to communication between different specialities," *European Journal of Cancer*, vol. 42, no. 15, pp. 2459–2462, 2006.

[4] ESMO/European Sarcoma Network Working Group, "Bone sarcomas: ESMO clinical practice guidelines for diagnosis, treatment and follow-up," *Annals of Oncology*, vol. 23, supplement 7, pp. vii100–vii109, 2012.

[5] ESMO/European Sarcoma Network Working Group, "Soft tissue and visceral sarcomas: ESMO Clinical Practice Guidelines for diagnosis, treatment and follow-up," *Annals of Oncology*, vol. 23, supplement 7, pp. vii92–vii99, 2012.

[6] NICE, *Guidance on Cancer Studies. Improving Outcomes for People with Sarcoma*, National Institute for Health and Clinical Excellence, 2006.

[7] Clinical Practice Guidelines for Soft Tissue Sarcoma 2013, http://www.nccn.org/professionals/physician_gls/f_guidelines.asp.

[8] H. Bastian, P. Glasziou, and I. Chalmers, "Seventy-five trials and eleven systematic reviews a day: how will we ever keep up?" *PLoS Medicine*, vol. 7, no. 9, Article ID e1000326, 2010.

[9] I. N. Olver and J. J. von Dincklage, "It is time for clinical guidelines to enter the digital age," *The Medical Journal of Australia*, vol. 199, no. 9, pp. 569–570, 2013.

[10] A. L. Francke, M. C. Smit, A. J. E. de Veer, and P. Mistiaen, "Factors influencing the implementation of clinical guidelines for health care professionals: a systematic meta-review," *BMC Medical Informatics and Decision Making*, vol. 8, article 38, 2008.

[11] Cancer Council Australia Clinical Guidelines Network, *Development of Clinical Practice Guidelines Using Cancer Council Australia's Cancer Guidelines Wiki*, Handbook 2013 for Section Authors and the Guideline Working Party, Cancer Council Australia, 2013.

[12] J. L. Bender, L. A. O'Grady, A. Deshpande et al., "Collaborative authoring: a case study of the use of a wiki as a tool to keep systematic reviews up to date," *Open Medicine*, vol. 5, article e201, pp. 201–208, 2011.

[13] *Clinical Practice Guidelines for the Management of Adult Onset Sarcoma*, 2013, http://wiki.cancer.org.au/australia/Guidelines:Sarcoma.

[14] G. Tsafnat, A. Dunn, P. Glasziou, and E. Coiera, "The automation of systematic reviews," *British Medical Journal*, vol. 346, article f139, 2013.

[15] B. P. Kerfoot, M. C. Kearney, D. Connelly, and M. L. Ritchey, "Interactive spaced education to assess and improve knowledge of clinical practice guidelines: a randomized controlled trial," *Annals of Surgery*, vol. 249, no. 5, pp. 744–749, 2009.

[16] B. P. Kerfoot, E. V. Lawler, G. Sokolovskaya, D. Gagnon, and P. R. Conlin, "Durable improvements in prostate cancer screening from online spaced education: a randomized controlled trial," *American Journal of Preventive Medicine*, vol. 39, no. 5, pp. 472–478, 2010.

[17] A. Bleyer, M. Montello, T. Budd, and S. Saxman, "National survival trends of young adults with sarcoma: lack of progress is associated with lack of clinical trial participation," *Cancer*, vol. 103, no. 9, pp. 1891–1897, 2005.

[18] Central Intelligence Agency, *The World Factbook*, Central Intelligence Agency, Langley, Va, USA, 2013, https://www.cia.gov/library/publications/the-world-factbook/rankorder/2004rank.html.

[19] J. Lewin, A. Puri, R. Quek et al., "Management of sarcoma in the asia-pacific region: resource-stratified guidelines," *The Lancet Oncology*, vol. 14, no. 12, pp. e562–e570, 2013.

4

Management Strategies in Advanced Uterine Leiomyosarcoma: Focus on Trabectedin

Frédéric Amant,[1] Domenica Lorusso,[2] Alexander Mustea,[3] Florence Duffaud,[4] and Patricia Pautier[5]

[1]*Department of Obstetrics and Gynecology, UZ Gasthuisberg, Katholieke Universiteit Leuven, Herestraat 49, Box 7003, 3000 Leuven, Belgium*
[2]*Gynecologic Oncology Unit, Fondazione IRCCS National Cancer Institute, Via Venezian 1, 20133 Milan, Italy*
[3]*Department of Gynecology and Obstetrics, University Hospital Greifswald, Ferdinand-Sauerbruch-Strasse, 17475 Greifswald, Germany*
[4]*Department of Medical Oncology, La Timone University Hospital, 264 rue Saint Pierre, 13385 Marseille, France*
[5]*Département de Medecine, Institut Gustave-Roussy, 114 rue Edouard Vaillant, 94805 Villejuif Cedex, France*

Correspondence should be addressed to Frédéric Amant; frederic.amant@uzleuven.be

Academic Editor: Chandrajit Premanand Raut

The treatment of advanced uterine leiomyosarcomas (U-LMS) represents a considerable challenge. Radiological diagnosis prior to hysterectomy is difficult, with the diagnosis frequently made postoperatively. Whilst a total abdominal hysterectomy is the cornerstone of management of early disease, the role of routine adjuvant pelvic radiotherapy and adjuvant chemotherapy is less clear, since they may improve local tumor control in high risk patients but are not associated with an overall survival benefit. For recurrent or disseminated U-LMS, cytotoxic chemotherapy remains the mainstay of treatment. There have been few active chemotherapy drugs approved for advanced disease, although newer drugs such as trabectedin with its pleiotropic mechanism of actions represent an important addition to the standard front-line systemic therapy with doxorubicin and ifosfamide. In this review, we outline the therapeutic potential and in particular the emerging evidence-based strategy of therapy with trabectedin in patients with advanced U-LMS.

1. Introduction

Uterine leiomyosarcomas (U-LMS) are a group of rare and aggressive mesenchymal tumors, which comprise ~1% of all uterine malignancies and a third of uterine sarcomas [1, 2]. The incidence of U-LMS is about 0.55 cases per 100,000 women per year [3]. The diagnosis of uterine sarcomas is frequently discovered incidentally on histopathology review following hysterectomy. The most common uterine tumor, endometrial cancer, originates from the endometrial lining and results in early bleeding in its development. Therefore, early diagnosis is common since endometrial sampling yields malignant cells. In contrast, endometrial sampling for early U-LMS is likely to be negative and endometrial involvement resulting in vaginal bleeding only occurs when the tumor has reached a certain volume. In addition, for most cases, a confirmatory diagnosis cannot be made preoperatively, since there are no simple objective imaging characteristics that can objectively distinguish between benign and malignant mesenchymal growths [4]. Diagnosis of U-LMS commonly signifies an aggressive clinical course with a predilection for early hematogenous spread and development of lung metastases within two years of primary therapy [5]. Additionally, the metastatic recurrence rate even in patients diagnosed with localized early stage disease exceeds 50% according to the International Federation of Gynecology and Obstetrics (FIGO) [6, 7]. Therefore, optimal management of U-LMS is challenging and typically involves a multidisciplinary team whose approach generally depends on the disease spread (i.e., localized versus disseminated disease). Complete surgical resection is the mainstay of treatment for localized U-LMS. Indeed, the absence of primary surgery

[5] or incomplete cytoreduction [8] predicts poor survival. An "en-bloc" resection is highly recommended for U-LMS as morcellation of the tumor or uterus in total increases the rate of the abdominopelvic dissemination causing an iatrogenically advanced stage disease that translates to a worsened progression-free survival (PFS) and overall survival (OS) [9]. Usually, total abdominal hysterectomy (including removal of the cervix) with or without bilateral salpingoophorectomy (BSO) is performed [5, 10]. Noteworthily the incidence of occult ovarian (<4%) and lymph node metastases (<3%) in U-LMS is very low and is most commonly associated with extrauterine disease [11–14]. A large retrospective population study failed to demonstrate both a statistical difference in the 5-year disease-specific survival (DSS) for women who did or did not undergo BSO at the time of hysterectomy and comparable median OS for women who underwent or not lymphadenectomy [5]. Therefore, ovarian-sparing surgery may be considered in premenopausal women with early stage disease, while lymph node dissection should be reserved only for patients with clinically suspicious and enlarged lymph nodes without compromising outcome [5, 13, 14]. In metastatic disease the role of surgery and locally ablative therapies depends upon the patients' age and general condition, extent of disease, and the aims of treatment. Optimal metastasectomy, either pulmonary or extrapulmonary, has become a standard intervention in carefully selected patients [15, 16]. Pulmonary metastasectomy is the most widely studied and has been associated with 5-year survival rates ranging from 25% to 53% [16–19]. Patients with isolated, unilateral, or limited metastases, an excellent performance status, and a relatively prolonged disease-free interval may be considered as suitable candidates for metastasectomy. The principal predictors of improved outcome following metastasectomy include optimal complete resection of all detected lesions without significant surgical morbidity and prolonged time to first recurrence (>12 months) [15, 16].

Several retrospective, nonrandomized studies had suggested an improved local control without demonstrating a significant survival benefit in patients with resected U-LMS treated with adjuvant pelvic radiotherapy [20, 21]. To overcome the limitations of retrospective noncomparative studies, the European Organization for Research and Treatment of Cancer-Gynecological Cancer Group (EORTC-GCG) conducted the only prospective, randomized phase III study of radiotherapy in uterine sarcomas, comparing adjuvant pelvic radiation (51 Gy in 28 fractions over five weeks) with observation [22]. This study was opened in 1988 and ran over a 13-year period to accrue a total of 224 patients with completely resected FIGO Stage I and II uterine sarcomas, including 103 patients with U-LMS. For those with U-LMS there was no benefit for radiotherapy for either disease-free survival or OS. Based on these findings, the authors concluded that there was no evidence for the routine use of postoperative pelvic radiotherapy. Those results have been reinforced by the results of a much larger population-based study using the Surveillance, Epidemiology, and End Results (SEER) database that reported on outcomes of 1396 women treated for U-LMS, of whom 310 (23%) had undergone adjuvant postoperative radiotherapy, which reported that the addition of radiotherapy had no impact on 5-year DSS [5].

Similarly there is no good evidence for the routine use of adjuvant chemotherapy since all data to date have not conclusively proven adjuvant chemotherapy to be of clear benefit for patients with localized resectable disease [23–25]. A large meta-analysis of 14 studies of doxorubicin-based adjuvant chemotherapy for localized resectable soft tissue sarcoma (STS) in adults included 1568 patients of whom 264 had uterine sarcoma. Even though adjuvant chemotherapy appeared to significantly improve time to local and distant recurrence and overall recurrence-free survival, it had no significant impact on OS [26, 27]. Recently, the EORTC sarcoma group carried out the largest prospective randomized study of adjuvant chemotherapy in STS with the aim of finally answering the question of usefulness of such an approach [28]. In that study 351 patients with completely resected high grade STS were randomly assigned to receive either adjuvant chemotherapy (doxorubicin and ifosfamide with lenograstim) or no chemotherapy (control group). No benefit for adjuvant chemotherapy was found between groups neither for relapse-free survival nor for median OS and 5-year OS rate (chemotherapy group: 66.5% versus observation control group: 67.8%).

2. Treatment of Advanced Uterine Leiomyosarcoma

2.1. Chemotherapy. Despite adequate surgical resection of U-LMS, even in early stage, patients remain at high risk for local and distant recurrence [29]. Optimal treatment of advanced or unresectable disease generally involves palliative systemic chemotherapy regimens with poor prognosis demonstrating a median PFS of ~5 months and median OS of ~12 months, and 5-year DSS rates of less than 30% [5, 30]. In STS generally and in U-LMS specifically, chemotherapeutic options that achieve sustained responses remain limited [31]. Standard first-line chemotherapy has been largely unchanged for three decades and remains doxorubicin with or without ifosfamide (Table 1) [32–35]. Doxorubicin monotherapy has consistently demonstrated an objective response rate (ORR) of approximately 13–25% with response duration typically lasting less than 6 months and median OS of ~12 months [34, 35], whereas ifosfamide alone had a response rate of 17.2% with a median response duration of 3.8 months and median OS of 6 months [36]. Indeed, the use of doxorubicin (25–50 mg/m^2) in combination with ifosfamide (5–10 g/m^2) chemotherapy has resulted in higher ORR (doxorubicin 50 mg/m^2 and ifosfamide 5 g/m^2 showed an ORR of 30.3%; doxorubicin 75 mg/m^2 and ifosfamide 10 g/m^{2}showed an ORR of 48%), but this has been at the expense of increased treatment-related toxicities due to overlapping myelotoxicity and worsening in patients' quality of life and with no impact on OS (Table 1) [32, 37]. An open-label randomized phase II study that evaluated the efficacy of sequential high-dose doxorubicin and ifosfamide compared with standard-dose doxorubicin showed no advantage to sequentially adding ifosfamide to doxorubicin as compared to doxorubicin

TABLE 1: Summary of efficacy results of active chemotherapy regimens in uterine leiomyosarcoma (for trabectedin data see Table 2).

Drug(s)	Evaluable patients (n)	Trial design	Prior regimen(s)	ORR (%)	SD (%)	Median PFS (months)	Median OS (months)
Doxorubicin [35]	Uterine STS (72 with U-LMS)	Randomized phase III	0	16.3 (all) 25 (U-LMS)	NR	NR	12.1
Doxorubicin [34]	Uterine STS (38 with U-LMS)	Randomized phase III	0	19 (all) 13 (U-LMS)	54.0 (all) 70.0 (U-LMS)	5.1	NR
Ifosfamide [36]	35 U-LMS	Phase II	0	17.2	28.6	NR	6.0
Doxorubicin + ifosfamide [32]	34 U-LMS	Phase II	0	30.3	51.7	NR	9.6
Doxorubicin + ifosfamide [37]	Uterine STS (25 with U-LMS)	Phase I/II	0	49.0 (all) 48.0 (U-LMS)	30.0 (all)	NR	30.5 (all)
Gemcitabine [40]	42 U-LMS	Phase II	0-1	20.5	15.9	NR	NR
Gemcitabine + docetaxel [43]	39 U-LMS	Phase II	0	35.8	26.2	4.4	16.0+
Gemcitabine + docetaxel [42]	48 U-LMS	Phase II	1	27.0	50	6.7+	14.7
Gemcitabine + docetaxel [44]	LMS (29 with U-LMS)	Phase II	0–2	53.0	20.6	5.6	17.9
Gemcitabine + docetaxel [45]	Advanced STS (38 with U-LMS)	Randomized phase II	0–3	16.0 (all) 17.0 (U-LMS)	NR	6.2	17.9
Gemcitabine + docetaxel [47]	Advanced LMS (46 with U-LMS)	Randomized phase II	1	5.0 (LMS) 24.0 (U-LMS)	NR	3.4 (LMS) 4.7 (U-LMS)	13.0 (LMS) 23.0 (U-LMS)

NR: not reported; ORR: objective response rate; OS: overall survival; PFS: progression-free survival; SD: stable disease; STS: soft tissue sarcoma; U-LMS: uterine leiomyosarcoma.

alone in first-line treatment of advanced STS [38]. In that study patients were randomly assigned to either doxorubicin 75 mg/m^2 given as a bolus injection every three weeks (q3w) for six cycles (standard arm) or high-dose doxorubicin at 30 mg/m^2 per day for three days every two weeks for three cycles followed by ifosfamide at 12.5 g/m^2 as a continuous 5-day infusion, once q3w for three cycles with filgrastim or pegfilgrastim support. The ORR was 24.1% and 23.4% in the high-dose and the standard doxorubicin arm, respectively, and median PFS was shorter in the high-dose arm (24 weeks) compared with the standard arm (26 weeks). Febrile neutropenia (23% versus 7%) and study discontinuation due to drug-related toxicity (11% versus 1%) were more common in the high-dose sequential arm [38]. Recently, the results of a randomized, controlled phase III EORTC 62012 trial demonstrated that the combination of doxorubicin 75 mg/m^2 and ifosfamide 10 g/m^2 as first-line therapy for patients with advanced or metastatic STS ($n = 445$) failed to significantly improve OS (median OS: 14.3 months versus 12.8 months; $p = 0.076$) and was considerably more toxic than doxorubicin 75 mg/m^2 alone [39]. Moreover, all grade 3/4 toxicities were more common with doxorubicin and ifosfamide than with doxorubicin alone (leucopenia 43% versus 40%, neutropenia 42% versus 37%, febrile neutropenia 46% versus 13%, anemia 35% versus 5%, and thrombocytopenia 33% versus <1%).

Few chemotherapy agents or combinations have been demonstrated to be active in U-LMS that has progressed after doxorubicin-based treatment. A Gynecologic Oncology Group (GOG) phase II trial evaluated the antitumor activity and toxicity profile of gemcitabine (gemcitabine 1000 mg/m^2 on days 1, 8, and 15 of a 4-week cycle) as second-line chemotherapy in patients with recurrent or persistent U-LMS [40]. The schedule was well tolerated and an ORR of 20.5% (2.3% complete response and 18.2% partial response) was observed among 42 evaluable patients with the median duration of 4.9 months. In addition, seven (15.9%) patients achieved stable disease (SD). The combination of gemcitabine and docetaxel has recently emerged as a promising treatment for U-LMS, thus representing a valuable addition to doxorubicin and ifosfamide in the treatment of metastatic U-LMS (Table 1) [41]. In three prospective phase II studies the combination of gemcitabine and docetaxel has demonstrated efficacy as first- or second-line therapy for advanced U-LMS associated with a high ORR ranging from 27% to 53%, median PFS from 4.4 to 6.7 months, and median OS from 14.7 to 17.9 months [42–44]. However, for the combination of gemcitabine plus docetaxel as the second-line therapy, 50% of patients received red blood cell transfusions, 13% received platelet transfusion, and 8% of patients had pulmonary toxicity [42]. Similarly, in a randomized trial in patients with metastatic STS of multiple histologies, the combination of gemcitabine and docetaxel yielded superior ORR (16 versus 8%), median PFS (6.2 versus 3.0 months, $p = 0.02$), and median OS (17.9 versus 11.5 months, $p = 0.03$) to gemcitabine alone, but with increased toxicity [45]. Unfortunately, these encouraging efficacy results could not be confirmed in a subsequent French trial that included 133 patients with advanced STS as that observed an overall response with gemcitabine plus docetaxel combination of 18.4% and with no statistical difference between leiomyosarcomas and other histological subtypes (24.2% versus 10.4%; $p = 0.06$) [46]. The French Sarcoma Group recently completed a randomized multicenter phase II TAXOGEM study that aimed to evaluate the efficacy and toxicity of single-agent gemcitabine versus gemcitabine plus docetaxel as second-line therapy in patients with metastatic or unresectable uterine and nonuterine LMS [47]. A total of 90 patients (46 with U-LMS) received either single-agent gemcitabine (gemcitabine 1000 mg/m^2 on days 1, 8, and 15 of a 4-week cycle) or a combination of gemcitabine and docetaxel (gemcitabine 900 mg/m^2 i.v. on days 1 and 8, plus docetaxel 100 mg/m^2 i.v. for one hour on day 8 of a 3-week cycle with lenograstim). This study failed to show the superiority of gemcitabine plus docetaxel over gemcitabine alone since single-agent gemcitabine (ORR; 19%; median PFS: 5.5 months) yielded results similar to those of gemcitabine plus docetaxel (ORR: 24%; median PFS: 4.7 months) in this trial, but with less toxicity (one toxic death occurred in the gemcitabine plus docetaxel arm) [47]. In addition, the results of an analysis that pooled individual data from 12 patients with U-LMS from the SARC002 randomized phase II study and 40 patients from TAXOGEM study also showed no statistical difference between gemcitabine (ORR: 18%; median PFS: 4.9 months) and gemcitabine plus docetaxel (ORR: 23%; median PFS: 6 months) as mixed-line therapy (second-line therapy for >77% of patients) [48]. Therefore, the use of the combination of gemcitabine and docetaxel in U-LMS still remains controversial.

The preliminary results of a phase II prospective study of combination therapy with carboplatin and pegylated liposomal doxorubicin (PLD) in 40 patients with advanced or recurrent gynecologic sarcomas (14 with U-LMS) reported a high ORR and disease control rate (DCR; ORR plus SD) of the combination (ORR = 33.3%; DCR = 70.4%) and a 12-month PFS and OS rates of 32.5% and 77.0%, respectively, with the favorable safety profile [58]. A variety of other cytotoxic agents, including temozolomide [59–61], topotecan [62], thalidomide [59], paclitaxel [63], and cisplatin [64], have demonstrated very modest activity in U-LMS.

2.2. Other Approaches: Targeted and Hormonal Therapy

2.2.1. Targeted Agents. Sarcomas are vascular tumors with higher levels of vascular endothelial growth factor (VEGF) expression than most other solid tumors and this provides a potential target that could be exploited through inhibition of angiogenesis [10]. To date the only approved targeted therapy for patients with metastatic nonadipocytic STS after previous chemotherapy is pazopanib hydrochloride, a multi-targeted tyrosine kinase inhibitor, including VEGF-1, VEGF-2, and VEGF-3. In 2012, the European Medicines Agency and the U.S. Food and Drug Administration (FDA) have approved pazopanib based on the results of the pivotal, randomized, double-blind, placebo controlled, multicenter, phase III PALETTE study in 369 patients (165 with U-LMS), in which pazopanib significantly increased the time that patients remained progression-free compared with placebo (median PFS: 4.6 versus 1.6 months; $p < 0.001$) [65]. The 3-month improvement in PFS was observed despite only a 6% ORR in the pazopanib group, suggesting that the majority of patients benefited in the form of SD. However, the protocol-specified final analysis of OS showed that longer PFS with pazopanib did not translate into an improvement in OS (median OS: 12.5 versus 10.7 months; $p = 0.25$).

The role of bevacizumab, a monoclonal antibody directed against VEGF, in addition to fixed-dose-rate gemcitabine plus docetaxel (GD), has also been investigated as first-line treatment for metastatic U-LMS in a phase III, double-blind, placebo-controlled trial [66]. In that study 102 patients were randomly assigned to either gemcitabine (900 mg/m^2)/docetaxel (75 mg/m^2) plus bevacizumab (B; 15 mg/kg; $n = 50$) or GD plus placebo (P; $n = 52$). Unfortunately, the addition of bevacizumab to the combination of GD failed to improve PFS (GD + B: 4.1 months versus GD + P: 6.2 months), OS (GD + B: 23.3 months versus GD + P: 19.4 months), or ORR (GD + B: 32% versus GD + P: 36%) and worsened the overall toxicity profile. Formerly, a phase Ib study of the combination of docetaxel, gemcitabine, and bevacizumab in chemotherapy-naïve patients with advanced or recurrent STS reported the ORR of 31.4%, with five complete and six partial responses, and an additional 18 had SD lasting for a median of 6 months, similar to historical response rates with this cytotoxic combination alone [67]. Nevertheless, some concerning adverse events were attributed to bevacizumab as one patient died of a pulmonary embolism following surgery for a bowel perforation, one patient developed a grade 3 wound dehiscence, and another experienced a grade 3 tumor-related hemorrhage. Additionally, in a phase II study, the antitumor activity and tolerability of bevacizumab and doxorubicin were evaluated in 17 patients with metastatic STS (seven had U-LMS) who received up to one nonanthracycline prior therapy [68]. The ORR was lower than might be expected with single-agent doxorubicin in U-LMS, as there were only two partial responses (12%) and 11 disease stabilizations (65%). Of major concern, despite careful monitoring and the standard use of dexrazoxane, was the unexpected cardiac toxicity with the combination with a 35% incidence of grade 2 or worse cardiotoxicity.

Two other multitargeted protein tyrosine kinase inhibitors with activity against multiple VEGF isoforms, sunitinib and sorafenib, have also been evaluated in U-LMS with disappointing results as neither has met prespecified criteria to warrant further clinical development [69, 70]. Currently, an ongoing EORTC randomized double-blind phase II study (ClinicalTrials.gov Identifier: NCT01979393) evaluates the role of maintenance therapy with cabozantinib (XL184), an oral tyrosine kinase inhibitor, in high-grade undifferentiated uterine sarcoma (HGUS) following surgery and stabilization or response to doxorubicin ± ifosfamide or in patients with metastatic (HGUS) as first-line treatment.

2.2.2. Hormone Therapy. To date, the exact role of hormonal therapies in U-LMS is poorly defined despite some hints of efficacy due to lack of prospective validation with a control arm. The immunohistochemical expression of estrogen (ER) receptors (40–100%) and progesterone receptors in U-LMS (17–100%) is of relevance as it provides a possible therapeutic strategy for treatment [71–76]. It has been reported that hormone receptor positivity may have prognostic implications, with some studies relating hormonal expression to improved PFS and OS, particularly in cases with disease confined to the uterine body [72, 75, 77]. For instance, in a subset of patients with recurrent U-LMS with an indolent evolution, with a disease-free interval of ≥6 months, it is more likely to express hormonal receptors that may allow targeted treatment. Therefore, for those highly selected patients, with a less aggressive growth pattern, hormonal treatment or metastasectomy may be considered rather than a new line of chemotherapy [78, 79]. In a recent retrospective study of 54 patients (34 were ER positive) with uterine sarcoma they demonstrated improved OS when compared with ER negative patients (median OS: 36 versus 16 months, $p = 0.004$) [75]. On multivariate analysis, ER positivity retained significance as an independent predictor of survival, after controlling for stage, age, histology, and the use of pelvic radiotherapy ($p = 0.03$). Another retrospective study of patients with advanced or recurrent U-LMS treated with an aromatase inhibitor included 34 patients with measurable disease [76]. Best objective response was partial response in three patients (9%), all of whom were ER positive, and SD occurred in a further 11 (32%) patients. The median PFS was 2.9 months (95% confidence interval (CI): 1.8–5.1 months), with superior PFS rates for ER and progesterone-positive tumors as compared with patients whose tumors did not express hormone receptors who did not derive any benefit. While this study provides some evidence of efficacy, this data must be interpreted with caution since, in the absence of a no-treatment control group, the prolonged PFS cannot be attributed solely to the activity of the aromatase inhibitor treatment in this retrospective highly selected group of patients [76]. Therefore, prospective validation with a control arm is required. Only one prospective phase II study of aromatase inhibition with letrozole in estrogen and/or progesterone receptor-positive U-LMS has been reported [80]. The primary endpoint was the PFS at 12 weeks. Among 27 patients enrolled, no objective responses were observed and the best response was SD in 14 patients, but it reported a 12-week PFS rate of 50% with a median duration of treatment of 2.2 months. Overall, progestins and aromatase inhibitors seem to be a reasonable option in patients with estrogen receptor/progesterone receptor-positive, small volume, and/or slowly progressive disease and for whom neither resection nor cytotoxic chemotherapy is warranted.

2.3. Treatment Endpoints and Response Assessment in Advanced Uterine Leiomyosarcoma. The optimal treatment for women with U-LMS is developing in parallel with our understanding of the pathways and networks controlling tumorigenesis, cell signaling, proliferation, and cell death. However, decision-making strategies for optimal treatment of U-LMS are complex as the difficulty lies in knowing where new drugs or treatment regimens, such as monotherapy or combination, fit in the treatment algorithm. This also represents challenges in setting treatment expectations, optimal timing, and sequencing, particularly in the development of new clinical trials. The most controversial issue of the STS treatment in general surrounds the phenomenon of the observed clinical benefit in absence of objective response that has potentially important implications for the design of future studies [81, 82]. The inappropriateness of ORR according to the Response Evaluation Criteria in Solid Tumors (RECIST) criteria as a surrogate of clinical benefit appears to be particularly relevant in STS, since it has been shown that patients with STS may derive therapeutic benefit in the absence of tumor shrinkage qualifying for complete or partial response [83]. Therefore, the selection of clinically meaningful objectives and standardized study endpoints is critical. Now it seems largely recognized that disease stability and PFS are more relevant endpoints in STS than ORR [82]. PFS, a time-to-event endpoint that captures benefit from prolonged responses and disease stabilization, has become accepted as the most useful endpoint of efficacy in phase II studies in STS [84]. With this in mind, the EORTC, in an analysis of a large database of clinical trials with standard agents and various experimental drugs, has established 3- and 6-month PFS rates of at least 39% and 14%, respectively, as the thresholds criteria to define drug activity in pretreated STS [82]. Importantly, the occurrence of progression is the main cause of drug discontinuation in clinical practice and clinical studies. From the clinical perspective, the most important issue is not to discontinue the treatment on the basis of standardized assessment of tumor response for treatments which may have an atypical pattern of response, such as delayed responses to trabectedin in which shrinkage was not initially detected or even appeared after tumor increase [52]. This further underlines the importance of correct definition and interpretation of tumor progression in the decision-making strategy for treatment discontinuation. Upcoming research may also consider some new endpoints such as assessment based on density using contrast-enhancement sequences according to Choi assessment [85, 86] and the use of ^{18}fluorodeoxyglucose- (FDG-) positron emission tomography (PET-CT) imaging in assessing response to trabectedin treatment [87, 88], as well as evaluation of clinical or symptomatic benefit, which includes time to progression, the growth modulation index (GMI), progression arrest rate, and health-related QoL [89]. In particular, tumor assessment based on Choi criteria seems to be a useful tool for evaluation of response to trabectedin since atypical radiological patterns of response, such as massive central tumor necrosis or tumor calcification, associated with clinical improvement have been previously reported [90, 91].

3. Trabectedin

Trabectedin (Yondelis) is a tetrahydroisoquinoline alkaloid, originally isolated from the marine tunicate *Ecteinascidia turbinata* and currently produced synthetically. Trabectedin has a unique mechanism of action based on interaction with the minor groove of the DNA double helix, which triggers a cascade of events that interfere with several transcription factors, DNA binding proteins, and DNA repair pathways, resulting in G2-M cell cycle arrest and ultimately apoptosis [92]. Trabectedin cytotoxicity is influenced by the functional nucleotide excision repair (NER) and deficient homologous recombination repair (HRR) machinery [93]. Consequently, trabectedin shows decreased activity (from 2- to 8-fold) in NER-deficient cell lines, while cells deficient in HRR are approximately 100 times more sensitive to the drug, indicating that trabectedin causes DNA double-strand breaks [93–97].

Nevertheless, emerging evidence indicates that trabectedin has pleiotropic mechanisms of action, since, in addition to inducing direct growth inhibition, cell death, and differentiation of malignant cells, trabectedin at therapeutic concentrations has selective immunomodulatory properties as a result of the inhibition of production of factors that promote tumor growth, progression, and the inhibition of tumor-promoted angiogenesis [92]. Data suggest that trabectedin selectively targets monocytes and tumor associated macrophages (TAMs) and downregulates the production of inflammatory mediators, which induces changes in the tumor microenvironment contributing to its antitumor activity [92, 98–100]. The markedly reduced production of proinflammatory mediators, such as CCL2, interleukin-6 (IL-6), and the proangiogenic VEGF, may underlie the strong association between chronic inflammation and cancer progression [98–101]. Taken together, trabectedin is more than a cytotoxic drug given that it also has immunomodulatory and antiangiogenic properties which potentially contribute to a delayed response with a prolonged stabilization [102]. Consequently, the characteristic late and long-lasting responses reported with trabectedin have now gained greater theoretical support from the perspective of considering trabectedin as a multitarget drug with far more multifaceted activity than originally formulated [103, 104]. This is an active area of research both in preclinical and translational settings.

3.1. Trabectedin in Soft Tissue Sarcoma. The efficacy of trabectedin as salvage chemotherapy in adults with advanced, recurrent STS was assessed in three nonrandomized phase II trials [53, 54, 56] and in chemotherapy-naïve patients with unresectable advanced STS of multiple histologies [55]. A phase II randomized registration ET-743-STS-201 study (ClinicalTrials.gov Identifier: NCT00060944) in 270 patients with advanced liposarcoma (n = 93, 34.4%) and leiomyosarcoma (n = 177, 65.6%; 30 patients, 17% with U-LMS) after failure of prior conventional chemotherapy demonstrated a superior disease control of trabectedin 1.5 mg/m^2 given as a 24-hour i.v. infusion q3w compared with a weekly trabectedin regimen (0.58 mg/m^2; 3-hour i.v. infusion for three consecutive weeks in a 4-week cycle) in terms of longer time to progression (median TTP: 3.7 versus 2.3 months; $p = 0.0302$), median PFS (3.3 versus 2.3 months; $p = 0.0418$), and median OS (13.9 versus 11.8 months; $p = 0.1920$) [57]. These benefits from trabectedin therapy in patients treated using a 24 h infusion q3w were highlighted by PFS rate at 3 months (51.5%) and 6 months (35.5%), which surpassed the thresholds criteria established by the EORTC to define drug activity in pretreated STS [82]. Based on these results, in 2007, trabectedin was the first anticancer marine-derived drug to be approved in the European Union and in many other countries worldwide for the treatment of adult patients with advanced STS after failure of anthracyclines and ifosfamide or for those patients who are unsuitable to receive these agents [105].

Although the response rate to trabectedin in pretreated patients with STS is rather low (<18%), this drug has demonstrated prolonged disease control, with a DCR of 50–60%, and large median OS time that exceeds 12 months [15–18] with major benefits in liposarcoma and leiomyosarcoma compared to other STSs. Noteworthily delayed responses compared with other agents are observed with trabectedin (median time to observe an ORR = 5.3 months), which may account for the differences in clinical benefit, since an early and prolonged administration of trabectedin appears to be associated with improved efficacy outcomes when compared with short-term and later treatments [52, 53, 106]. Recent evidence have demonstrated that trabectedin, in addition to direct growth inhibition, has additional immunomodulatory effects, which exerts significant effects on the tumor microenvironment (see above) that may help to explain this phenomenon which commonly becomes apparent after several cycles of treatment. Thus, any decision to stop treatment with trabectedin should always be carefully evaluated by the clinician. Treatment duration with trabectedin as an important factor for long-term outcomes was reported in the French expanded access program [107]. In that study among the 56 patients who were not progressing after 6 cycles, the subgroup of 40 patients treated with seven or more cycles had a significantly longer median PFS (10.5 months versus 5.3 months, $p = 0.001$) that translated into a more than doubling of the median OS (33.4 versus 13.9 months, $p = 0.009$) as compared to patients who stopped after six initial cycles. The results of a large retrospective analysis of trabectedin in 885 patients with advanced STS further reinforce these observations reporting that patients with nonprogressive disease who received trabectedin until disease progression obtained a statistically significant superior median PFS (11.0 versus 7.2 months, $p < 0.003$) and median OS (25.1 versus 16.9 months, $p = 0.001$) compared to those who stopped the trabectedin treatment earlier [108]. Given that the retrospective nature of the study implies potential bias, these results reinforced the rationale for performing a prospective, randomized T-DIS study (ClinicalTrials.gov Identifier: NCT01303094) within the French Sarcoma Group to compare interruption versus continuation of trabectedin in responding patients after six cycles of treatment in 178 pretreated patients with advanced STS. The final result of T-DIS trial was recently reported at the 39th European Society for Medical Oncology (ESMO) congress and strongly supported continued long-term therapy with trabectedin in responding patients until intolerance/progression, since continuation of trabectedin beyond six cycles was well-tolerated and associated with a statistically significant improvement of median PFS (continuous treatment 7.2 months versus treatment interruption 4.0 months; $p = 0.03$) [109].

Noncumulative myelosuppression, with reversible neutropenia as the predominant component, and transient transaminase increases are the most common laboratory abnormalities seen with trabectedin, both of which are associated with a low incidence of relevant clinical consequences [110]. Premedication with 20 mg of dexamethasone i.v. 30 minutes prior to trabectedin provides hepatoprotective effects beyond its antiemetic effect [52, 110, 111]. In agreement with the safety profile of trabectedin the overall incidence and severity of these events decrease in frequency over cycles demonstrating no evidence of cumulative toxicity [110, 112, 113]. Common trabectedin-related adverse events reported in at least 20% of patients are nausea, fatigue, and vomiting, whereas only 3.7% and 5.7% of patients had alopecia and mucositis/stomatitis, respectively [110]. The safety profile of trabectedin, with a lack of end-organ cumulative toxic effects, compares favorably with those of other treatments for STS, especially compared to doxorubicin-induced cumulative cardiotoxicity which prevents prolonged treatment and retreatments in most cases [114]; renal toxicity and dose-limiting neutropenia have been largely associated with ifosfamide [115], and a high rate of severe myelosuppression and pulmonary toxicity are reported after the treatment with the combination of gemcitabine plus docetaxel [42, 45]. In contrast to this, trabectedin has an acceptable safety profile even in patients who remained on therapy for prolonged periods of time (i.e., up to 59 cycles), which potentially facilitates long-term treatment until disease progression or discontinuation for other reasons [57, 110].

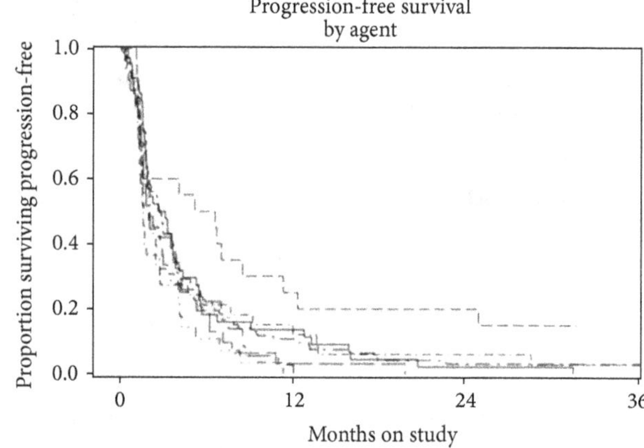

Agent		Events	Total	Median (mos)
—— 1: gemcitabine*	1	44	44	2.9
- - - 2: trabectedin	2	17	20	5.8
–·– 3: ifosfamide	3	91	93	2.8
— — 4: PLD**	4	31	31	2.1
--·-· 5: paclitaxel	5	33	33	1.6
— - 6: topotecan	6	36	36	1.8
-··– 7: VP-16	7	28	28	2.1

*In previously treated patients
**Pegylated liposomal doxorubicin

FIGURE 1: Kaplan–Meier plots demonstrating progression-free survival (PFS) for the 20 patients in the study population (GOG 87M) compared to other single agent studies in the GOG protocol 87 series studying cytotoxic agents. Reprinted from [49], with permission from Elsevier.

3.2. Trabectedin in Uterine Leiomyosarcoma. The GOG in the USA has conducted a prospective phase II study of trabectedin in chemotherapy-naïve patients with measurable advanced, persistent, or recurrent U-LMS with documented disease progression who were not previously exposed to chemotherapy and/or biological therapy [49]. Overall, 20 patients were enrolled and treated with trabectedin 1.5 mg/m^2 as a 24-hour infusion q3w. Two patients achieved partial responses (10%, 95% CI: 1.2%–31.7%) with response durations of 3.3 months and 5.7 months, respectively (Table 2). Disease stabilization was reported in an additional 10 patients (50%) giving a DCR of 60%. The median PFS was 5.8 months, while the median OS was 26.1+ months. The median PFS obtained with trabectedin was compared to that obtained with other single agents in the GOG 87 series of phase II studies among chemotherapy-naïve patients. A clinically relevant delay in progression associated with the use of trabectedin (median PFS = 5.8 moths) was the longest achieved in those GOG protocol series (Figure 1). Importantly, more than half the patients remained progression-free and without any evidence of treatment-ending toxicity for more than 10 cycles (>6 months). Regarding safety issues, the most common grade 3/4 was noncumulative neutropenia (16/20 patients) associated with infection in one patient. Even though trabectedin demonstrated modest response rate in this trial, the authors conclude that PFS rather than ORR would have been a better metric to assess activity of this drug in U-LMS.

The preclinical results prompted two phase I, dose-finding trials of trabectedin and doxorubicin in patients with recurrent or persistent STS to determine the dose of trabectedin plus doxorubicin with granulocyte colony-stimulating factor (G-CSF) support [116, 117]. The MTD of trabectedin and doxorubicin given in 3-week cycles was doxorubicin 60 mg/m^2 immediately followed by trabectedin 1.1 mg/m^2 given as a 3 h i.v. infusion. Results from a phase I study provided the rationale to evaluate the combination of trabectedin and doxorubicin for patients with advanced LMS. The French Sarcoma Group have recently presented the results of a phase II single-arm study of trabectedin in combination with doxorubicin as first-line treatment of locally advanced and/or metastatic leiomyosarcoma of the uterus

TABLE 2: Summary of efficacy results of trabectedin in advanced uterine leiomyosarcoma.

Study	Regimen	Evaluable patients (n)	Prior regimens Median (range)	ORR	DCR	Median PFS (months)	3-month PFS	6-month PFS	Median OS (months)	12-month OS	24-month OS
Phase II GOG study [49]	Trabectedin	20	0	10%	60%	5.8	NR	NR	26.1+	NR	NR
Phase II LMS-02 study [50]	Trabectedin/doxorubicin	47	0	59.6%	87.2%	8.2	87%	NR	20.2	NR	NR
Pooled analysis [51]	Trabectedin	62	2 (0–6)	17.7%	53.2%	2.5	46.4%	30.8%	12.1	51.6%	20.3%
Retrospective analysis [52]	Trabectedin	66	3 (1–5)	16%	51%	3.3	53%	33%	14.4	NR	NR

DCR: disease control rate; GOG: Gynecologic Oncology Group; NR: not reported; ORR: objective response rate; OS: overall survival; PFS: progression-free survival; U-LMS: uterine leiomyosarcoma.

(U-LMS) or soft tissue origin (ST-LMS) [50]. The patients were stratified by primary tumor location, so the U-LMS and ST-LMS cohorts were each considered to be independent phase II studies. A total of 108 patients were treated, 47 patients in the U-LMS cohort and 61 in the ST-LMS cohort. Patients received doxorubicin 60 mg/m^2 on day 1, followed by 3-hour intravenous infusion with trabectedin 1.1 mg/m^2 every three weeks for a maximum of six cycles of treatment. In the U-LMS group, 28 out of 47 evaluable patients achieved a partial response (59.6%) (Table 2). A further 13 patients (27.7%) had SD yielding a DCR of 87.2%. Median PFS was 8.2 months with 87% (95% CI: 75–94) of patients remaining progression-free at 3 months. With a median follow-up of 14.5 months, median OS was 20.2 months in the uterine cohort. These efficacy results compare very favorably with outcomes reported in other studies with combination regimens in the first-line treatment of U-LMS [32, 43]. The safety profile of trabectedin plus doxorubicin was similar in pattern with phase I dose-ranging study reporting neutropenia (45%), ALT increase (14%), and thrombocytopenia (17%) as the most common grade 3/4 treatment-emergent adverse events (AEs) [116]. This safety profile was considered potentially more acceptable than that of the doxorubicin plus ifosfamide and gemcitabine plus docetaxel combination given in the first-line setting [39, 43]. Overall, the findings in these homogeneous cohorts of patients consistently confirm that trabectedin in combination with doxorubicin as first-line chemotherapy is an active treatment that provides clinically meaningful benefits to patients with U-LMS with predicted and manageable toxicity.

In addition to the ET-743-STS-201 study, a number of other phase II clinical trials with trabectedin have enrolled pretreated patients with advanced U-LMS [53–57]. A retrospective pooled analysis was performed using data on 62 patients derived from five completed phase II trials with the aim to provide an overview of the efficacy and the safety of trabectedin in U-LMS [51] (Table 3). Most of the patients (91.9%) had been pretreated with a median of 2 prior chemotherapy regimens (range: 0–6; five patients were chemotherapy-naïve), 98.4% had undergone prior surgery, and 48.4% had prior radiotherapy. In all studies trabectedin 1.5 mg/m^2 was given as a 24-hour i.v. infusion q3w. Across trials, patients received a median of 3 cycles per patient, reaching up to 38 cycles with no signs of cumulative toxicities. According to investigators' assessment partial responses were observed in 11 patients (17.7%; 15% ≥6 months) and SD in 20 patients (32.3%; 13% ≥6 months) for a DCR of 53.2% (Table 2). For the entire patient population median PFS was 2.5 months (95% CI: 1.7–4.2) with 46.4% (95% CI: 33.7%–59.1%) and 30.8% (95% CI: 19.0%–42.7%) progression-free at 3 and 6 months, respectively. Median OS was 12.1 months (95% CI: 7.5–14.0), with 12- and 24-month OS rates of 51.6% (CI 95%: 39.2–64.1) and 20.3% (CI 95%: 10.1–30.4), respectively. The most common patient grade 3/4 adverse events were non-cumulative neutropenia (41.9%) and transient asymptomatic transaminase increases of ALT and AST observed in 43.5% and 30.6% of patients, respectively, without symptoms of hepatic failure. Thus, the results of phase II studies confirm

Table 3: Patients included in pooled analysis of five phase II studies.

Phase II studies	Reference	Evaluable patients (n) Total n = 62	1st line therapy
ET-B-005	Le Cesne et al. [53]	16	No
ET-B-008	Yovine et al. [54]	7	No
ET-B-016	Garcia-Carbonero et al. [55]	6	Yes
ET-B-017	Garcia-Carbonero et al. [56]	3	No
ET743-STS-201	Demetri et al. [57]	30	No

trabectedin as an efficacious single agent for the treatment of advanced U-LMS with the safety profile that favorably compares with those of other active drugs, including those who remained on therapy for prolonged periods of time [51].

An Italian phase II randomized, noncomparative, cross-over TAUL trial (EudraCT number 2009-016017-24) is currently assessing the activity of trabectedin and gemcitabine plus docetaxel in metastatic or locally relapsed uterine LMS pretreated with conventional chemotherapy.

The aforementioned results correspond to clinical studies which, by nature, are restrictive in the characteristics of the patients included. In the absence of large randomized studies, observational studies performed in clinical practice, although not as methodologically rigorous, can provide useful insights into the real-world efficacy, toxicity, and management of patients treated with trabectedin and show how results from clinical trials may translate in a "real-world" setting. Sanfilippo et al. carried out a retrospective analysis of all patients with advanced U-LMS treated with trabectedin from 2000 to 2010 at two European sarcoma reference centers (Istituto Nazionale Tumori, Milan, and Royal Marsden Hospital, London) [52]. Overall, 66 patients with metastatic U-LMS who had failed a median of three prior cytotoxic lines including anthracyclines with or without ifosfamide (100% of patients) and gemcitabine with or without docetaxel (87% of patients) were included in the analysis. Eleven patients achieved a partial response (16%) and an additional 23 (35%) achieved SD (three of them showing minor tumor shrinkage) for a DCR of 51%. Interestingly, two patients achieved a delayed response to treatment, showing a partial response (after a decrease in tumor density) and a minor response after 14 and 10 cycles, respectively. After a median follow-up of 22 months, the median PFS was 3.3 months (95% CI: 2.7–5) with 53% and 33% of patients progression-free at 3 and 6 months, respectively. The median OS was 14.4 months (95% CI: 8–20). Thus, the efficacy outcomes of this study in an unselected patient population representative of routine clinical practice were consistent with those seen in more selective populations enrolled in clinical trials.

4. Conclusions

Standard treatment for early U-LMS is hysterectomy with BSO. Adjuvant radiotherapy and chemotherapy are not administered since they do not result in a survival benefit. Treatment outcomes in U-LMS are far from being satisfactory, especially in patients with inoperable, locally advanced, and/or metastatic disease. Many patients with recurrent LMS receive multiple lines of therapy but the optimal sequencing of these drugs into the treatment algorithm for U-LMS has not been well defined. Available data from phase II studies and observational studies have demonstrated that trabectedin has significant activity in patients with advanced U-LMS with a high DCR ranging from 51% to 60% and an acceptable safety profile. In addition, trabectedin results in 30% PFS rate at 6 months with 12-month OS rate of more than 50% in pretreated patients with U-LMS. Taken together, the response rate, PFS, and OS with trabectedin are comparable with published outcomes on other single agents (doxorubicin, ifosfamide, and gemcitabine) in this indication [118].

Regarding safety, current treatment options for patients with U-LMS are frequently guided by safety considerations and convenience. Many of the currently available chemotherapeutics or combinations used in U-LMS are associated with cumulative, duration limiting, or irreversible toxicities that may jeopardize future long-term interventions. The safety profile of trabectedin compares favorably with that of other active drugs used in U-LMS, including those who remained on therapy for prolonged periods of time, as it allows patients to benefit from a longer-term treatment, with the potential for longer disease control.

Finally, the results from the GOG and the French Sarcoma Group phase II studies show very promising results of trabectedin as first-line therapy either as single agent or in combination with doxorubicin. Particularly, the findings of a phase II study of trabectedin in combination with doxorubicin demonstrated the feasibility of this combination reporting an encouraging synergistic and clinically meaningful response in patients with U-LMS with an acceptable and predictable tolerability profile. Noteworthily trabectedin plus doxorubicin yielded numerically higher response rate and superior survival compared with historical results of the two most active combination regimens (gemcitabine plus docetaxel and doxorubicin with or without ifosfamide) for advanced U-LMS. However, the difficulty lies in knowing where these regimens fit into the treatment algorithm for U-LMS given that there are no randomized comparisons of these regimens. Therefore, potential future combination of trabectedin with additional active agents should be further explored in patients with U-LMS as first- or second-line treatment.

Acknowledgment

The authors would like to acknowledge Adnan Tanović (PharmaMar, S.A.) for providing writing assistance for the paper.

References

[1] E. D'Angelo and J. Prat, "Uterine sarcomas: a review," *Gynecologic Oncology*, vol. 116, no. 1, pp. 131–139, 2010.

[2] F. Amant, P. Moerman, P. Neven, D. Timmerman, E. Van Limbergen, and I. Vergote, "Endometrial cancer," *The Lancet*, vol. 366, no. 9484, pp. 491–505, 2005.

[3] J. R. Toro, L. B. Travis, J. W. Hongyu, K. Zhu, C. D. M. Fletcher, and S. S. Devesa, "Incidence patterns of soft tissue sarcomas, regardless of primary site, in the Surveillance, Epidemiology and End Results program, 1978-2001: an analysis of 26,758 cases," *International Journal of Cancer*, vol. 119, no. 12, pp. 2922–2930, 2006.

[4] S. E. Rha, J. Y. Byun, S. E. Jung et al., "CT and MRI of uterine sarcomas and their mimickers," *American Journal of Roentgenology*, vol. 181, no. 5, pp. 1369–1374, 2003.

[5] D. S. Kapp, J. Y. Shin, and J. K. Chan, "Prognostic factors and survival in 1396 patients with uterine leiomyosarcomas: emphasis on impact of lymphadenectomy and oophorectomy," *Cancer*, vol. 112, no. 4, pp. 820–830, 2008.

[6] O. Zivanovic, L. M. Jacks, A. Iasonos et al., "A nomogram to predict postresection 5-year overall survival for patients with uterine leiomyosarcoma," *Cancer*, vol. 118, no. 3, pp. 660–669, 2012.

[7] A. Iasonos, E. Z. Keung, O. Zivanovic et al., "External validation of a prognostic nomogram for overall survival in women with uterine leiomyosarcoma," *Cancer*, vol. 119, no. 10, pp. 1816–1822, 2013.

[8] J.-Y. Park, D.-Y. Kim, D.-S. Suh et al., "Prognostic factors and treatment outcomes of patients with uterine sarcoma: analysis of 127 patients at a single institution, 1989–2007," *Journal of Cancer Research and Clinical Oncology*, vol. 134, no. 12, pp. 1277–1287, 2008.

[9] J.-Y. Park, S.-K. Park, D.-Y. Kim et al., "The impact of tumor morcellation during surgery on the prognosis of patients with apparently early uterine leiomyosarcoma," *Gynecologic Oncology*, vol. 122, no. 2, pp. 255–259, 2011.

[10] R. O'Cearbhaill and M. L. Hensley, "Optimal management of uterine leiomyosarcoma," *Expert Review of Anticancer Therapy*, vol. 10, no. 2, pp. 153–169, 2010.

[11] J. P. Shah, C. S. Bryant, S. Kumar, R. Ali-Fehmi, J. M. Malone, and R. T. Morris, "Lymphadenectomy and ovarian preservation in low-grade endometrial stromal sarcoma," *Obstetrics and Gynecology*, vol. 112, no. 5, pp. 1102–1108, 2008.

[12] J. K. Chan, N. M. Kawar, J. Y. Shin et al., "Endometrial stromal sarcoma: a population-based analysis," *British Journal of Cancer*, vol. 99, no. 8, pp. 1210–1215, 2008.

[13] M. M. Leitao, Y. Sonoda, M. F. Brennan, R. R. Barakat, and D. S. Chi, "Incidence of lymph node and ovarian metastases in leiomyosarcoma of the uterus," *Gynecologic Oncology*, vol. 91, no. 1, pp. 209–212, 2003.

[14] R. L. Giuntoli II, D. S. Metzinger, C. S. DiMarco et al., "Retrospective review of 208 patients with leiomyosarcoma of the uterus: prognostic indicators, surgical management, and adjuvant therapy," *Gynecologic Oncology*, vol. 89, no. 3, pp. 460–469, 2003.

[15] M. M. Leitao, M. F. Brennan, M. Hensley et al., "Surgical resection of pulmonary and extrapulmonary recurrences of uterine leiomyosarcoma," *Gynecologic Oncology*, vol. 87, no. 3, pp. 287–294, 2002.

[16] S. H. Blackmon, N. Shah, J. A. Roth et al., "Resection of pulmonary and extrapulmonary sarcomatous metastases is associated with long-term survival," *Annals of Thoracic Surgery*, vol. 88, no. 3, pp. 877–885, 2009.

[17] A. G. Casson, J. B. Putnam, G. Natarajan et al., "Five-year survival after pulmonary metastasectomy for adult soft tissue sarcoma," *Cancer*, vol. 69, no. 3, pp. 662–668, 1992.

[18] D. Gossot, C. Radu, P. Girard et al., "Resection of pulmonary metastases from sarcoma: can some patients benefit from a less invasive approach?" *Annals of Thoracic Surgery*, vol. 87, no. 1, pp. 238–243, 2009.

[19] A. Rehders, S. B. Hosch, P. Scheunemann, N. H. Stoecklein, W. T. Knoefel, and M. Peiper, "Benefit of surgical treatment of lung metastasis in soft tissue sarcoma," *Archives of Surgery*, vol. 142, no. 1, pp. 70–75, 2007.

[20] N. B. Hornback, G. Omura, and F. J. Major, "Observations on the use of adjuvant radiation therapy in patients with stage I and II uterine sarcoma," *International Journal of Radiation, Oncology, Biology, Physics*, vol. 12, no. 12, pp. 2127–2130, 1986.

[21] S. Sampath, T. E. Schultheiss, J. K. Ryu, and J. Y. Wong, "The role of adjuvant radiation in uterine sarcomas," *International Journal of Radiation Oncology, Biology, Physics*, vol. 76, no. 3, pp. 728–734, 2010.

[22] N. S. Reed, C. Mangioni, H. Malmström et al., "Phase III randomised study to evaluate the role of adjuvant pelvic radiotherapy in the treatment of uterine sarcomas stages I and II: an European Organisation for Research and Treatment of Cancer Gynaecological Cancer Group Study (protocol 55874)," *European Journal of Cancer*, vol. 44, no. 6, pp. 808–818, 2008.

[23] S. Ricci, R. L. Giuntoli II, E. Eisenhauer et al., "Does adjuvant chemotherapy improve survival for women with early-stage uterine leiomyosarcoma?" *Gynecologic Oncology*, vol. 131, no. 3, pp. 629–633, 2013.

[24] S. M. Schuetze and M. E. Ray, "Adjuvant therapy for soft tissue sarcoma," *Journal of the National Comprehensive Cancer Network*, vol. 3, no. 2, pp. 207–213, 2005.

[25] G. A. Omura, J. A. Blessing, F. Major et al., "A randomized clinical trial of adjuvant adriamycin in uterine sarcomas: a gynecologic oncology group study," *Journal of Clinical Oncology*, vol. 3, no. 9, pp. 1240–1245, 1985.

[26] "Adjuvant chemotherapy for localised resectable soft tissue sarcoma in adults. Sarcoma Meta-analysis Collaboration (SMAC)," *Cochrane Database of Systematic Reviews*, no. 2, Article ID CD001419, 2000.

[27] P. Pautier, A. Floquet, L. Gladieff et al., "A randomized clinical trial of adjuvant chemotherapy with doxorubicin, ifosfamide, and cisplatin followed by radiotherapy versus radiotherapy alone in patients with localized uterine sarcomas (SARCGYN study). A study of the French Sarcoma Group," *Annals of Oncology*, vol. 24, no. 4, pp. 1099–1104, 2013.

[28] P. J. Woll, P. Reichardt, A. le Cesne et al., "Adjuvant chemotherapy with doxorubicin, ifosfamide, and lenograstim for resected soft-tissue sarcoma (EORTC 62931): a multicentre randomised controlled trial," *The Lancet Oncology*, vol. 13, no. 10, pp. 1045–1054, 2012.

[29] T. A. Dinh, E. A. Oliva, A. F. Fuller Jr., H. Lee, and A. Goodman, "The treatment of uterine leiomyosarcoma. Results from a 10-year experience (1990–1999) at the Massachusetts General Hospital," *Gynecologic Oncology*, vol. 92, no. 2, pp. 648-652, 2004.

[30] O. Zivanovic, M. M. Leitao, A. Iasonos et al., "Stage-specific outcomes of patients with uterine leiomyosarcoma: a comparison of the international Federation of gynecology and obstetrics and american joint committee on cancer staging systems," *Journal of Clinical Oncology*, vol. 27, no. 12, pp. 2066–2072, 2009.

[31] S. Kanjeekal, A. Chambers, M. Fung Kee Fung, and S. Verma, "Systemic therapy for advanced uterine sarcoma: a systematic review of the literature," *Gynecologic Oncology*, vol. 97, no. 2, pp. 624–637, 2005.

[32] G. Sutton, J. A. Blessing, and J. H. Malfetano, "Ifosfamide and doxorubicin in the treatment of advanced leiomyosarcomas of the uterus: a Gynecologic Oncology Group study," *Gynecologic Oncology*, vol. 62, no. 2, pp. 226–229, 1996.

[33] S. Sleijfer, C. Seynaeve, and J. Verweij, "Using single-agent therapy in adult patients with advanced soft tissue sarcoma can still be considered standard care," *Oncologist*, vol. 10, no. 10, pp. 833–841, 2005.

[34] H. B. Muss, B. Bundy, P. J. DiSaia et al., "Treatment of recurrent or advanced uterine sarcoma. A randomized trial of doxorubicin versus doxorubicin and cyclophosphamide. (A phase III trial of the gynecologic oncology group)," *Cancer*, vol. 55, no. 8, pp. 1648–1653, 1985.

[35] G. A. Omura, F. J. Major, J. A. Blessing et al., "A randomized study of Adriamycin with and without dimethyl triazeoimidazole carboxamide in advanced uterine sarcomas," *Cancer*, vol. 52, no. 4, pp. 626–632, 1983.

[36] G. P. Sutton, J. A. Blessing, R. J. Barrett, and R. McGehee, "Phase II trial of ifosfamide and mesna in leiomyosarcoma of the uterus: a Gynecologic Oncology Group study," *The American Journal of Obstetrics and Gynecology*, vol. 166, no. 2, pp. 556–559, 1992.

[37] S. Leyvraz, M. Zweifel, G. Jundt et al., "Long-term results of a multicenter SAKK trial on high-dose ifosfamide and doxorubicin in advanced or metastatic gynecologic sarcomas," *Annals of Oncology*, vol. 17, no. 4, pp. 646–651, 2006.

[38] J. Maurel, A. López-Pousa, R. De Las Peñas et al., "Efficacy of sequential high-dose doxorubicin and ifosfamide compared with standard-dose doxorubicin in patients with advanced soft tissue sarcoma: an open-label randomized phase II study of the Spanish group for research on sarcomas," *Journal of Clinical Oncology*, vol. 27, no. 11, pp. 1893–1898, 2009.

[39] I. Judson, J. Verweij, H. Gelderblom et al., "Doxorubicin alone versus intensified doxorubicin plus ifosfamide for first-line treatment of advanced or metastatic soft-tissue sarcoma: a randomised controlled phase 3 trial," *The Lancet Oncology*, vol. 15, no. 4, pp. 415–423, 2014.

[40] K. Y. Look, A. Sandler, J. A. Blessing, J. A. Lucci III, and P. G. Rose, "Phase II trial of gemcitabine as second-line chemotherapy of uterine leiomyosarcoma: a Gynecologic Oncology Group (GOG) Study," *Gynecologic Oncology*, vol. 92, no. 2, pp. 644–647, 2004.

[41] M. L. Hensley, "Update on gemcitabine and docetaxel combination therapy for primary and metastatic sarcomas," *Current Opinion in Oncology*, vol. 22, no. 4, pp. 356–361, 2010.

[42] M. L. Hensley, J. A. Blessing, K. DeGeest, O. Abulafia, P. G. Rose, and H. D. Homesley, "Fixed-dose rate gemcitabine plus docetaxel as second-line therapy for metastatic uterine leiomyosarcoma: a Gynecologic Oncology Group phase II study," *Gynecologic Oncology*, vol. 109, no. 3, pp. 323–328, 2008.

[43] M. L. Hensley, J. A. Blessing, R. Mannel, and P. G. Rose, "Fixed-dose rate gemcitabine plus docetaxel as first-line therapy for

metastatic uterine leiomyosarcoma: a Gynecologic Oncology Group phase II trial," *Gynecologic Oncology*, vol. 109, no. 3, pp. 329–334, 2008.

[44] M. L. Hensley, R. Maki, E. Venkatraman et al., "Gemcitabine and docetaxel in patients with unresectable leiomyosarcoma: results of a phase II trial," *Journal of Clinical Oncology*, vol. 20, no. 12, pp. 2824–2831, 2002.

[45] R. G. Maki, J. K. Wathen, S. R. Patel et al., "Randomized phase II study of gemcitabine and docetaxel compared with gemcitabine alone in patients with metastatic soft tissue sarcomas: results of sarcoma alliance for research through collaboration study 002," *Journal of Clinical Oncology*, vol. 25, no. 19, pp. 2755–2763, 2007.

[46] J.-O. Bay, I. Ray-Coquard, J. Fayette et al., "Docetaxel and gemcitabine combination in 133 advanced soft-tissue sarcomas: a retrospective analysis," *International Journal of Cancer*, vol. 119, no. 3, pp. 706–711, 2006.

[47] P. Pautier, A. Floquet, N. Penel et al., "Randomized multicenter and stratified phase II study of gemcitabine alone versus gemcitabine and docetaxel in patients with metastatic or relapsed leiomyosarcomas: a fédération nationale des centres de lutte contre le cancer (FNCLCC) french sarcoma group study (TAXOGEM study)," *Oncologist*, vol. 17, no. 9, pp. 1213–1220, 2012.

[48] F. Duffaud, P. Pautier, B. Bui et al., "A pooled analysis of the final results of the two randomized phase II studies comparing gemcitabine (G) vs. gemcitabine + docetaxel (G+D) in patients (pts) with metastatic/relapsed leiomyosarcoma (LMS)," *Annals of Oncology*, vol. 21, supplement 8, pp. viii408–viii416, 2010, Proceedings of the 35th ESMO Congress, abstract 1345O, Milan, Italy, October 2010.

[49] B. J. Monk, J. A. Blessing, D. G. Street, C. Y. Muller, J. J. Burke, and M. L. Hensley, "A phase II evaluation of trabectedin in the treatment of advanced, persistent, or recurrent uterine leiomyosarcoma: a gynecologic oncology group study," *Gynecologic Oncology*, vol. 124, no. 1, pp. 48–52, 2012.

[50] P. Pautier, A. Floquet, D. Cupissol et al., "LMS-02: a phase II single-arm multicenter study of doxorubicin in combination with trabectedin as a first-line treatment of advanced uterine leiomyosarcoma (u-LMS) and soft tissue LMS (ST-LMS): first results in patients with u-LMS," *Journal of Clinical Oncology*, vol. 31, supplement, abstract 10505, 2013.

[51] I. R. Judson, J. Blay, S. P. Chawla et al., "Trabectedin (Tr) in the treatment of advanced uterine leiomyosarcomas (U-LMS): results of a pooled analysis of five single-agent phase II studies using the recommended dose," *Journal of Clinical Oncology*, vol. 28, no. 15s, supplement, abstract 10028, 2010.

[52] R. Sanfilippo, F. Grosso, R. L. Jones et al., "Trabectedin in advanced uterine leiomyosarcomas: a retrospective case series analysis from two reference centers," *Gynecologic Oncology*, vol. 123, no. 3, pp. 553–556, 2011.

[53] A. le Cesne, J. Y. Blay, I. Judson et al., "Phase II study of ET-743 in advanced soft tissue sarcomas: a European Organisation for the Research and Treatment of Cancer (EORTC) Soft Tissue and Bone Sarcoma Group trial," *Journal of Clinical Oncology*, vol. 23, no. 3, pp. 576–584, 2005.

[54] A. Yovine, M. Riofrio, J. Y. Blay et al., "Phase II study of ecteinascidin-743 in advanced pretreated soft tissue sarcoma patients," *Journal of Clinical Oncology*, vol. 22, no. 5, pp. 890–899, 2004.

[55] R. Garcia-Carbonero, J. G. Supko, R. G. Maki et al., "Ecteinascidin-743 (ET-743) for chemotherapy-naive patients with advanced soft tissue sarcomas: Multicenter phase II and pharmacokinetic study," *Journal of Clinical Oncology*, vol. 23, no. 24, pp. 5484–5492, 2005.

[56] R. Garcia-Carbonero, J. G. Supko, J. Manola et al., "Phase II and pharmacokinetic study of ecteinascidin 743 in patients with progressive sarcomas of soft tissues refractory to chemotherapy," *Journal of Clinical Oncology*, vol. 22, no. 8, pp. 1480–1490, 2004.

[57] G. D. Demetri, S. P. Chawla, M. von Mehren et al., "Efficacy and safety of trabectedin in patients with advanced or metastatic liposarcoma or leiomyosarcoma after failure of prior anthracyclines and ifosfamide: results of a randomized phase II study of two different schedules," *Journal of Clinical Oncology*, vol. 27, no. 25, pp. 4188–4196, 2009.

[58] P. Harter, U. Canzler, H. Lueck et al., "Pegylated liposomal doxorubicin and carboplatin in malignant mixed epithelial mesenchymal and mesenchymal gynecologic tumors: a phase II trial of the AGO study group," *Journal of Clinical Oncology*, vol. 29, supplement, abstract 5093, 2011.

[59] M. S. Boyar, M. Hesdorffer, M. L. Keohan, Z. Jin, and R. N. Taub, "Phase II study of temozolomide and thalidomide in patients with unresectable or metastatic leiomyosarcoma," *Sarcoma*, vol. 2008, Article ID 412503, 6 pages, 2008.

[60] S. Anderson and C. Aghajanian, "Temozolomide in uterine leiomyosarcomas," *Gynecologic Oncology*, vol. 98, no. 1, pp. 99–103, 2005.

[61] S. M. Talbot, M. L. Keohan, M. Hesdorffer et al., "A phase II trial of temozolomide in patients with unresectable or metastatic soft tissue sarcoma," *Cancer*, vol. 98, no. 9, pp. 1942–1946, 2003.

[62] D. S. Miller, J. A. Blessing, L. C. Kilgore, R. Mannel, and L. van Le, "Phase II trial of topotecan in patients with advanced, persistent, or recurrent uterine leiomyosarcomas: a Gynecologic Oncology Group study," *The American Journal of Clinical Oncology*, vol. 23, no. 4, pp. 355–357, 2000.

[63] D. G. Gallup, J. A. Blessing, W. Andersen, and M. A. Morgan, "Evaluation of paclitaxel in previously treated leiomyosarcoma of the uterus: a gynecologic oncology group study," *Gynecologic Oncology*, vol. 89, no. 1, pp. 48–51, 2003.

[64] J. T. Thigpen, J. A. Blessing, and G. D. Wilbanks, "Cisplatin as second-line chemotherapy in the treatment of advanced or recurrent leiomyosarcoma of the uterus. A Phase II trial of the Gynecologic Oncology Group," *American Journal of Clinical Oncology: Cancer Clinical Trials*, vol. 9, no. 1, pp. 18–20, 1986.

[65] W. T. A. van der Graaf, J.-Y. Blay, S. P. Chawla et al., "Pazopanib for metastatic soft-tissue sarcoma (PALETTE): a randomised, double-blind, placebo-controlled phase 3 trial," *The Lancet*, vol. 379, no. 9829, pp. 1879–1886, 2012.

[66] M. L. Hensley, A. Miller, D. O'Malley et al., "A randomized phase III trial of gemcitabine + docetaxel + bevacizumab or placebo as first-line treatment for metastatic uterine leiomyosarcoma (uLMS): a Gynecologic Oncology Group study," *Gynecologic Oncology*, vol. 133, supplement 1, p. 3, 2014.

[67] C. F. Verschraegen, H. Arias-pulido, S.-J. Lee et al., "Phase IB study of the combination of docetaxel, gemcitabine, and bevacizumab in patients with advanced or recurrent soft tissue sarcoma: the axtell regimen," *Annals of Oncology*, vol. 23, no. 3, pp. 785–790, 2012.

[68] D. R. D'Adamo, S. E. Anderson, K. Albritton et al., "Phase II study of doxorubicin and bevacizumab for patients with metastatic soft-tissue sarcomas," *Journal of Clinical Oncology*, vol. 23, no. 28, pp. 7135–7142, 2005.

[69] R. G. Maki, D. R. D'Adamo, M. L. Keohan et al., "Phase II study of sorafenib in patients with metastatic or recurrent sarcomas," *Journal of Clinical Oncology*, vol. 27, no. 19, pp. 3133–3140, 2009.

[70] M. L. Hensley, M. W. Sill, D. R. Scribner Jr. et al., "Sunitinib malate in the treatment of recurrent or persistent uterine leiomyosarcoma: a Gynecologic Oncology Group phase II study," *Gynecologic Oncology*, vol. 115, no. 3, pp. 460–465, 2009.

[71] B. M. Seddon and R. Davda, "Uterine sarcomas—recent progress and future challenges," *European Journal of Radiology*, vol. 78, no. 1, pp. 30–40, 2011.

[72] M. M. Leitao Jr., M. L. Hensley, R. R. Barakat et al., "Immunohistochemical expression of estrogen and progesterone receptors and outcomes in patients with newly diagnosed uterine leiomyosarcoma," *Gynecologic Oncology*, vol. 124, no. 3, pp. 558–562, 2012.

[73] K. Mittal and R. I. Demopoulos, "MIB-1 (Ki-67), p53, estrogen receptor, and progesterone receptor expression in uterine smooth muscle tumors," *Human Pathology*, vol. 32, no. 9, pp. 984–987, 2001.

[74] Y. L. Zhai, Y. Kobayashi, A. Mori et al., "Expression of steroid receptors, Ki-67, and p53 in uterine leiomyosarcomas," *International Journal of Gynecological Pathology*, vol. 18, no. 1, pp. 20–28, 1999.

[75] Y. J. Ioffe, A. J. Li, C. S. Walsh et al., "Hormone receptor expression in uterine sarcomas: prognostic and therapeutic roles," *Gynecologic Oncology*, vol. 115, no. 3, pp. 466–471, 2009.

[76] R. O'Cearbhaill, Q. Zhou, A. Iasonos et al., "Treatment of advanced uterine leiomyosarcoma with aromatase inhibitors," *Gynecologic Oncology*, vol. 116, no. 3, pp. 424–429, 2010.

[77] M. R. Raspollini, G. Amunni, A. Villanucci et al., "Estrogen and progesterone receptors expression in uterine malignant smooth muscle tumors: correlation with clinical outcome," *Journal of Chemotherapy*, vol. 15, no. 6, pp. 596–602, 2003.

[78] F. Amant, A. Coosemans, M. Debiec-Rychter, D. Timmerman, and I. Vergote, "Clinical management of uterine sarcomas," *The Lancet Oncology*, vol. 10, no. 12, pp. 1188–1198, 2009.

[79] R. L. Giuntoli II, E. Garrett-Mayer, R. E. Bristow, and B. S. Gostout, "Secondary cytoreduction in the management of recurrent uterine leiomyosarcoma," *Gynecologic Oncology*, vol. 106, no. 1, pp. 82–88, 2007.

[80] S. George, Y. Feng, J. Manola et al., "Phase 2 trial of aromatase inhibition with letrozole in patients with uterine leiomyosarcomas expressing estrogen and/or progesterone receptors," *Cancer*, vol. 120, no. 5, pp. 738–743, 2014.

[81] V. H. C. Bramwell, "Pazopanib and the treatment palette for soft-tissue sarcoma," *The Lancet*, vol. 379, no. 9829, pp. 1854–1856, 2012.

[82] M. van Glabbeke, J. Verweij, I. Judson, and O. S. Nielsen, "Progression-free rate as the principal end-point for phase II trials in soft-tissue sarcomas," *European Journal of Cancer*, vol. 38, no. 4, pp. 543–549, 2002.

[83] S. M. Schuetze, "Imaging and response in soft tissue sarcomas," *Hematology/Oncology Clinics of North America*, vol. 19, no. 3, pp. 471–487, 2005.

[84] J. Verweij, "Soft tissue sarcoma trials: one size no longer fits all," *Journal of Clinical Oncology*, vol. 27, no. 19, pp. 3085–3087, 2009.

[85] R. S. Benjamin, H. Choi, H. A. Macapinlac et al., "We should desist using RECIST, at least in GIST," *Journal of Clinical Oncology*, vol. 25, no. 13, pp. 1760–1764, 2007.

[86] H. Choi, C. Charnsangavej, S. C. Faria et al., "Correlation of computed tomography and positron emission tomography in patients with metastatic gastrointestinal stromal tumor treated at a single institution with imatinib mesylate: proposal of new computed tomography response criteria," *Journal of Clinical Oncology*, vol. 25, no. 13, pp. 1753–1759, 2007.

[87] M. J. Payne, R. E. Macpherson, K. M. Bradley, and A. B. Hassan, "Trabectedin in advanced high-grade uterine leiomyosarcoma: a case report illustrating the value of ^{18}FDG-PET-CT in assessing treatment response," *Case Reports in Oncology*, vol. 7, no. 1, pp. 132–138, 2014.

[88] B. Kasper, T. Schmitt, P. Wuchter, A. Dimitrakopoulou-Strauss, A. D. Ho, and G. Egerer, "The use of positron emission tomography in soft tissue sarcoma patients under therapy with trabectedin," *Marine Drugs*, vol. 7, no. 3, pp. 331–340, 2009.

[89] J. Verweij, "Other endpoints in screening studies for soft tissue sarcomas," *Oncologist*, vol. 13, no. 2, pp. 27–31, 2008.

[90] A. Hollebecque, A. Adenis, S. Taieb, C. Lebedinsky, and N. Penel, "Inadequacy of size-based response criteria to assess the efficacy of trabectedin among metastatic sarcoma patients," *Investigational New Drugs*, vol. 28, no. 4, pp. 529–530, 2010.

[91] A. Turpin, S. Taieb, and N. Penel, "Tumor calcification: a new response pattern of myxoid liposarcoma to trabectedin," *Case Reports in Oncology*, vol. 7, no. 1, pp. 204–209, 2014.

[92] M. D'Incalci and C. M. Galmarini, "A review of trabectedin (ET-743): a unique mechanism of action," *Molecular Cancer Therapeutics*, vol. 9, no. 8, pp. 2157–2163, 2010.

[93] P. Schoffski, P. Casali, M. Taron et al., "DNA repair functionality modulates the clinical outcome of patients with advanced sarcoma treated with trabectedin (ET-743)," *Journal of Clinical Oncology*, vol. 24, supplement 18, p. 9522, 2006.

[94] A. B. Herrero, C. Martín-Castellanos, E. Marco, F. Gago, and S. Moreno, "Cross-talk between nucleotide excision and homologous recombination DNA repair pathways in the mechanism of action of antitumor trabectedin," *Cancer Research*, vol. 66, no. 16, pp. 8155–8162, 2006.

[95] M. Tavecchio, M. Simone, E. Erba et al., "Role of homologous recombination in trabectedin-induced DNA damage," *European Journal of Cancer*, vol. 44, no. 4, pp. 609–618, 2008.

[96] Y. Takebayashi, P. Pourquier, D. B. Zimonjic et al., "Antiproliferative activity of ecteinascidin 743 is dependent upon transcription-coupled nucleotide-excision repair," *Nature Medicine*, vol. 7, no. 8, pp. 961–966, 2001.

[97] G. Damia, S. Silvestri, L. Carrassa et al., "Unique pattern of ET-743 activity in different cellular systems with defined deficiencies in DNA-repair pathways," *International Journal of Cancer*, vol. 92, no. 4, pp. 583–588, 2001.

[98] P. Allavena, M. Signorelli, M. Chieppa et al., "Anti-inflammatory properties of the novel antitumor agent yondelis (trabectedin): inhibition of macrophage differentiation and cytokine production," *Cancer Research*, vol. 65, no. 7, pp. 2964–2971, 2005.

[99] G. Germano, R. Frapolli, M. Simone et al., "Antitumor and anti-inflammatory effects of trabectedin on human myxoid liposarcoma cells," *Cancer Research*, vol. 70, no. 6, pp. 2235–2244, 2010.

[100] G. Germano, R. Frapolli, C. Belgiovine et al., "Role of macrophage targeting in the antitumor activity of trabectedin," *Cancer Cell*, vol. 23, no. 2, pp. 249–262, 2013.

[101] G. Germano, A. Mantovani, and P. Allavena, "Targeting of the innate immunity/inflammation as complementary anti-tumor therapies," *Annals of Medicine*, vol. 43, no. 8, pp. 581–593, 2011.

[102] R. Dossi, R. Frapolli, S. Di Giandomenico et al., "Antiangiogenic activity of trabectedin in myxoid liposarcoma: involvement of host TIMP-1 and TIMP-2 and tumor thrombospondin-1," *International Journal of Cancer*, vol. 136, no. 3, pp. 721–729, 2015.

[103] F. Grosso, G. D. Demetri, J. Y. Blay et al., "Patterns of tumor response to trabectedin (ET743) in myxoid liposarcomas," *Journal of Clinical Oncology*, vol. 24, no. 18, supplement 9511, 2006.

[104] F. Grosso, R. L. Jones, G. D. Demetri et al., "Efficacy of trabectedin (ecteinascidin-743) in advanced pretreated myxoid liposarcomas: a retrospective study," *The Lancet Oncology*, vol. 8, no. 7, pp. 595–602, 2007.

[105] European Medicines Agency (EMA), *Yondelis; Trabectedin*, 2010, http://www.ema.europa.eu/ema/index.jsp?curl=pages/medicines/human/medicines/000773/human_med_001165.jsp&murl=menus/medicines/medicines.jsp&jsenabled=true.

[106] P. G. Casali, R. Sanfilippo, and M. D'Incalci, "Trabectedin therapy for sarcomas," *Current Opinion in Oncology*, vol. 22, no. 4, pp. 342–346, 2010.

[107] J.-Y. Blay, A. Italiano, I. Ray-Coquard et al., "Long-term outcome and effect of maintenance therapy in patients with advanced sarcoma treated with trabectedin: an analysis of 181 patients of the French ATU compassionate use program," *BMC Cancer*, vol. 13, no. 1, article 64, 2013.

[108] A. Le Cesne, I. Ray-Coquard, F. Duffaud et al., "A large retrospective analysis of trabectedin in 885 patients with advanced soft tissue sarcoma," *Journal of Clinical Oncology*, vol. 31, supplement, abstract 10563, 2013.

[109] A. le Cesne, J. Blay, T. Ryckewaert et al., "Benefit of maintenance therapy with trabectedin (T) beyond the 6 first cycles: results of a prospective randomized phase II trial comparing interruption vs. continuation of T in patients (pts) with advanced soft tissue sarcoma (ASTS): an update," *Annals of Oncology*, vol. 25, supplement 4, Abstract 1414O, 2014.

[110] A. le Cesne, A. Yovine, J.-Y. Blay et al., "A retrospective pooled analysis of trabectedin safety in 1,132 patients with solid tumors treated in phase II clinical trials," *Investigational New Drugs*, vol. 30, no. 3, pp. 1193–1202, 2012.

[111] L. Paz-Ares, A. López-Pousa, A. Poveda et al., "Trabectedin in pre-treated patients with advanced or metastatic soft tissue sarcoma: a phase II study evaluating co-treatment with dexamethasone," *Investigational New Drugs*, vol. 30, no. 2, pp. 729–740, 2012.

[112] N. J. Carter and S. J. Keam, "Trabectedin: a review of its use in soft tissue sarcoma and ovarian cancer," *Drugs*, vol. 70, no. 3, pp. 355–376, 2010.

[113] P. Schöffski, P. Wolter, P. Clement et al., "Trabectedin (ET-743): evaluation of its use in advanced soft-tissue sarcoma," *Future Oncology*, vol. 3, no. 4, pp. 381–392, 2007.

[114] A. L. A. Ferreira, L. S. Matsubara, and B. B. Matsubara, "Anthracycline-induced cardiotoxicity," *Cardiovascular and Hematological Agents in Medicinal Chemistry*, vol. 6, no. 4, pp. 278–281, 2008.

[115] A. Le Cesne, E. Antoine, M. Spielmann et al., "High-dose ifosfamide: circumvention of resistance to standard-dose ifosfamide in advanced soft tissue sarcomas," *Journal of Clinical Oncology*, vol. 13, no. 7, pp. 1600–1608, 1995.

[116] J.-Y. Blay, M. Von Mehren, B. L. Samuels et al., "Phase I combination study of trabectedin and doxorubicin in patients with soft-tissue sarcoma," *Clinical Cancer Research*, vol. 14, no. 20, pp. 6656–6662, 2008.

[117] C. Sessa, A. Perotti, C. Noberasco et al., "Phase I clinical and pharmacokinetic study of trabectedin and doxorubicin in advanced soft tissue sarcoma and breast cancer," *European Journal of Cancer*, vol. 45, no. 7, pp. 1153–1161, 2009.

[118] A. Gadducci and M. E. Guerrieri, "Pharmacological treatment for uterine leiomyosarcomas," *Expert Opinion on Pharmacotherapy*, vol. 16, no. 3, pp. 335–346, 2015.

5

Identifying the Prevalence, Trajectory, and Determinants of Psychological Distress in Extremity Sarcoma

Melissa H. Tang, David J. Castle, and Peter F. M. Choong

St. Vincent's Hospital Melbourne, 35 Victoria Parade, Fitzroy, VIC 3065, Australia

Correspondence should be addressed to Melissa H. Tang; mel_tang2003@yahoo.com.au

Academic Editor: R. Lor Randall

Objective. Extremity sarcoma (ES) is a rare cancer that presents with unique challenges. This study was performed to identify the prevalence, trajectory, and determinants of distress and characterise sources of stress in this cohort. *Methods.* Consecutive patients with ES were prospectively recruited between May 2011 and December 2012. Questionnaires were administered during initial diagnosis and then six months and one year after surgery. *Results.* Distress was reported by about a third of our cohort and associated with poorer physical function, poorer quality of life, and pain. In addition to fears regarding mortality and life role changes, the most common sources of stress were centered on dissatisfaction with the healthcare system, such as frustrations with a lack of communication with the hospital regarding appointments and lack of education regarding management and outcomes. *Conclusions.* Psychological distress presents early in the cancer journey and persists up to one year after surgery. Distress is associated with negative outcomes. Active screening and effective interventions are necessary to improve outcomes. Sources of stress have been identified that may be amenable to targeted interventions.

1. Introduction

Psychological distress in cancer is associated with nonadherence to treatment recommendations, poorer satisfaction with care, poorer interpersonal relationships (resulting in poorer quality of relationships with both formal and informal social support sources and healthcare professionals), utilization of ineffective coping strategies (e.g., helplessness, passive coping, and risk taking behaviours), and poorer overall quality of life (QoL) [1–3]. The impact of psychological distress on people with extremity sarcoma (ES) has not been extensively studied.

Because of the rarity of sarcomas, homogeneous studies with large sample sizes may be difficult to obtain. Previous early studies exploring psychological distress and QoL in ES patients tended to be limited to cross-sectional, retrospective studies of survivors [4–10]. Most had small numbers of participants and few were prospectively designed with a baseline measure of QoL and mental health or controlled for the context of the timepoint of the cancer journey [11–15]. Compared to other cancers' patients, ES patients may represent a unique cohort with additional considerations. Compared to other cancers, ES is rare and affects people across all age groups and is associated with more physical disability than other cancer types [16]. These factors suggest that sarcomas require unique study and results from studies of other cancers cannot simply be extrapolated to represent ES patients.

In a systematic review of papers from 1972 to 2002, Massie [17] found that depressive symptoms were prevalent in 9% to 58% of cancer patients, which was highly dependent on the site of the primary. Lung and pancreatic cancers displayed the highest levels of distress (up to 57.6% and 52.2%, resp.), brain, head, and neck cancers displayed high levels of distress (up to 48.6%), and breast and prostate cancers displayed moderate levels of distress (up to 35.4% and 30.5%, resp.) [18, 19]. Prevalence was associated with prognosis of the cancer, the morbidity associated with the cancer (especially physical function and pain), and the effect the cancer or its treatment had on physical appearance and body image. In sarcoma-specific cohorts, the prevalence of depression ranged from 13.7% to 33.3% and the prevalence of anxiety disorders ranged from 11.8% to 47.2% [5, 7, 8, 14, 15], whilst the prevalence of psychological distress has been identified to be as high as 77% in one study [9].

Everyone's cancer journey is different. The experience is a continuum based on various hallmarks, which may include diagnosis and staging of cancer; treatment (surgery and/or radiation and chemotherapy); recovery and rehabilitation; follow-up and surveillance; and recurrence or terminal phase [14]. In general, levels of psychological distress reduce with time, with peak distress experienced in the initial month to one year after diagnosis and treatment, and may persist for a period of time following treatment [20–24].

Risk factors for psychological distress in the psychooncology population include previous psychiatric distress [15, 17, 25–29], high level of function impairment [2, 26, 30–32], pain [17, 25, 33–36], lower socioeconomic status [2, 19, 29, 37, 38], female gender [17, 39], younger age [17, 18, 40–42], and poor perceived social support [26, 29, 32].

This study was performed to address the following aims: (1) characterize the sources of stress preoperatively in this cohort; (2) identify the prevalence and trajectory of distress in people with ES from before surgery to one year after surgery; (3) compare distressed versus nondistressed participants; and (4) identify the determinants of distress one year after surgery.

2. Methods

All patients from the Australian states of Victoria and Tasmania with newly diagnosed ES who were referred to the Victorian Sarcoma Service (VSS) between May 30, 2011, and December 31, 2012, were screened for suitability for inclusion. The VSS is a dedicated multidisciplinary team of healthcare professionals managing patients above the age of fifteen years with sarcoma in both public and private hospital settings. Patients were eligible if they were diagnosed with an ES and surgery was planned to be part of their management. Ethics approval was acquired at all the relevant institutions. Patients were approached after their consultation with their healthcare professional immediately following the diagnosis of the ES by a member of the research team and invited to participate. Privately insured patients were approached in the private rooms of their healthcare professional and publically funded patients were approached at the hospital outpatient clinics. Participants completed their questionnaires within a week of their initial contact and questionnaires were returned within two weeks of initial contact via a reply paid envelope. This represented the first timepoint, $t = 0$, which was the preoperative, diagnosis phase. The second timepoint, $t = 1$, and third timepoint, $t = 2$, were at six months and twelve months after surgery, respectively. Participants were followed up through verbal contact and posting of the health questionnaires and returned within two weeks via a reply paid envelope.

3. Measures

3.1. Demographic and Health-Related Information. Medical information was gathered and verified through record linkage with secure medical records and consultation with pathologists, oncologists, radiation oncologists, radiologists, and surgeons. The Charlson Comorbidity Index (CCI), which is a measure of burden of disease due to medical comorbidities [43], was calculated for our participants (excluding the current sarcoma). Sociodemographic variables that were studied included gender, age, country of birth, SEIFA score (measure of relative socioeconomic status (SES) based on postcode of residence that is developed and updated by the Australian Bureau of Statistics based on five-yearly census data [44]), being in a partnered relationship, English not being a first language, having had to stop work or recreational activities because of the sarcoma, and the ability to work, drive, partake in leisure activities, and complete activities of daily living (ADL). Tumour-related variables included type of sarcoma, location of sarcoma, surgery, and whether the sarcoma was diagnosed unexpectedly or following a delay.

3.2. Psychological Distress and Cognitive Perceptions. The Depression Anxiety and Stress Scale 21 (DASS21) is a 21-item self-report quantitative measure encompassing three subscales of distress: *depression, anxiety,* and *stress* [46, 47]. The DASS21 does not assess somatic items and is therefore particularly useful in patients with medical conditions such as chronic pain and malignancies, such as head and neck cancers [27, 48]. Participants are asked to rate 21 items regarding distress according to a 4-point Likert scale (0–3). The final score for each subscale of stress, depression, and anxiety is the cumulative score multiplied by two. Cut-off scores have been developed for each subscale into five categories of severity with higher scores indicating a higher level of symptoms present. Where appropriate, the cohort was dichotomized into two groups according the severity labels from the DASS Manual [45]. The "distressed" group included participants who reported symptoms of distress that categorized them into moderate, severe, or extremely severe categories; the "nondistressed" group comprised patients that reported lower levels of symptoms (consistent with no or only mild distress).

Cancer-related stressors were assessed via free-text to the question "what has been the biggest source of stress, or frustration relating to the cancer journey so far?" with a follow-up telephone call to participants who required clarification of this item.

The Shame and Stigma Scale (SSS) was developed in 2013 by Kissane et al. [49] for use to assess the level of an individual's shame of their appearance, their sense of stigma, regret, and concerns with speech and social interactions. This was developed for use with oral squamous cell carcinoma patients. After discussion with the developer of the tool, a modified version of the SSS was used to assess shame of one's external appearance, following surgery for ES. Participants were asked to rate eight items regarding their attitudes towards the external appearance of their limb on a 5-point Likert scale (0–4). Three items were reverse-coded. The final score was derived by the sum of the five items and the sum of the three reverse-scored items, which was then scaled by conversion to a percentage. A higher SSS score represented a greater sense of disfigurement.

3.3. Activity Limitation. The Toronto Extremity Salvage Score (TESS) is an extremity-tumour-specific self-report measure of disability secondary to activity limitation [10]. Ease of completion of 29-30 everyday activities is assessed via a 5-point Likert scale with the option of indicating whether the specific task is not applicable to the respondent. The overall result is represented as a percentage with higher scores indicating better function. There are normative reference values that can be used as a base comparison with the general population [50]. In our study, items have been dichotomized according to difficulty in performing that particular activity, with "caseness" defined as moderate difficulty or harder. This dichotomy has also been used in other studies [51]. The physical function subscale of a non-extremity-tumour-specific QoL tool such as the EORTC QLQ C-30 is not able to discriminate functional status in this specific cancer cohort. As in other QoL studies in ES, QoL tools are therefore assessed in conjunction with a sarcoma-specific functional assessment tool.

3.4. Health-Related Quality of Life. The European Organisation for the Research and Treatment of Cancer Quality of Life Questionnaire Core Module 30 (EORTC QLQ C-30) is a cancer-specific, self-report QoL questionnaire. It comprises physical function, cancer symptom, and global health QoL subscales and also assesses financial difficulties. Compared to other global QoL assessment tools, such as the generic Short Form 36 (SF-36), it allows for assessment of symptoms such as nausea, vomiting, and bowel dysfunction [52]. In particular, subjective financial difficulties are assessed, which is especially important in working aged patients with ES. Each subscale ranges in score from 0 to 100; higher scores represent better global QoL and physical function but also higher levels of symptoms (e.g., pain) and more financial difficulties.

4. Statistics

The Statistical Package for the Social Sciences (SPSS) version 20.0 (SPSS Inc., Chicago, IL, USA) was used for all statistical analyses and a $P < 0.05$ was considered statistically significant.

Continuous data were expressed as means with standard deviations, percentages, and numbers.

In order to identify the trajectory of distress, we plotted the mean DASS21 scores, the proportion of participants with moderate to severe distress scores, and mean TESS scores at $t = 0, t = 1$, and $t = 2$.

A one-way repeated measured analysis of variance (ANOVA) was conducted to evaluate the null hypothesis that there was no change in participant's DASS21 scores when measured at $t = 0$, $t = 1$, and $t = 2$, using the Bonferroni correction to adjust for multiple comparisons.

In order to evaluate person-to-person differences in outcomes, we performed an exploratory data analysis via bivariate analyses. Phi coefficients were used to correlate dichotomized variables whilst Spearman rho correlations were assessed for ordinal and continuous data. Two-tailed values were calculated.

Independent t-tests were used to compare means of distressed with nondistressed groups for the null hypothesis that there were no differences in variables studied, including QoL, function, pain, and financial difficulties. We assumed that variances were equal if Levene's test for equality of variances were >0.10.

5. Results

5.1. Participants. During the recruitment period, 120 patients were referred to the VSS for management of a newly diagnosed ES. Participants were excluded from the study due to cognitive impairment ($n = 3$) and Non-English-speaking background ($n = 3$) or because surgery was not part of planned management (e.g., metastatic disease, palliation, or death) ($n = 12$). Five participants had undergone surgery prior to completing the questionnaires and six patients declined participation for time reasons. 91 participants were finally recruited for our study and completed our baseline questionnaires. Surgery on our participants was performed between August 9, 2011, and January 18, 2013.

76 participants completed the questionnaires at the final timepoint, one year after the index surgery (16.48% drop-out rate, $n = 15$). Six participants had deceased from disease, one participant died from intraoperative complications, one participant developed Alzheimer's disease, one participant moved overseas, and two participants were not contactable and were lost to follow-up. Four participants declined further participation due to time constraints, stating "they were not distressed and wouldn't be helping anybody with their responses anyway."

The data deviated slightly from a normal distribution; however, the skewness of the comparison groups followed the same directionality and, therefore, independent t-tests were carried out to assess between-group differences.

5.2. Sociodemographic Data. Characteristics of our cohort are summarised in Table 1. Out of the 76 participants, 40.8% were females ($n = 31$). The ages of our participants in our cohort ranged from sixteen to 86, with a mean of 55.1, a median of 57.0, and a standard deviation of 16.4. Outcome data for each timepoint is recorded in Table 2. Mean TESS scores were 77.40 ± 22.10, 68.83 ± 18.89, and 76.91 ± 18.95; mean DASS21 scores were 21.79 ± 18.60, 25.30 ± 25.62, and 24.09 ± 27.50 at $t = 0$, 1, and 2, respectively.

5.3. Objective 1: Source of Stress. Reported source(s) of stress at $t = 0$ are summarized in Table 1. Overall, 30.3% ($n = 23$) of our cohort reported that the disruption to life was the biggest source of stress, whilst 25.0% ($n = 19$) felt the healthcare system was the biggest source of frustration. 11.8% ($n = 9$) of the cohort reported that the loss of independence or change in life roles represented the major stressor and a similar proportion of the cohort worried about the unknown.

TABLE 1: Sociodemographic details.

Age (years)		16–86 (mean: 55.1 ± 16.4)
	$N = 76$	%
Demographic		
Gender		
Female	31	40.8
SEIFA stratification		
Low	17	22.4
Middle	35	46.1
High	24	31.6
Age group		
16–54	32	42.1
55–75	36	47.4
≥76	8	10.5
Country of birth		
Australia	60	78.9
Rurality		
Metropolitan	33	43.4
Regional	24	31.6
Rural	19	25.0
Non-Victorian resident		
Interstate	13	17.1
Education		
Primary	9	11.8
Secondary	36	47.4
Vocational	12	15.8
Tertiary/postgraduate	18	23.7
Social information		
Occupation		
Manager/admin/professional	23	30.3
Tradesperson	6	7.9
Sales/personnel/clerks	10	13.2
Machine operator/labourer	8	10.5
Home duties/student	4	5.2
Retired	25	32.9
Marital status		
Partnered: married/de facto	58	76.3
English 1st language		
Yes	69	90.8
Charlson Comorbidity Index		Mean: 2 ± 2.24
Health information		
Significant pain as a presenting feature		
Yes	26	34.2
Past history of depression and/or anxiety (no other psychiatric diagnoses listed)		
Depression	15	17.9
Anxiety	3	3.6
Depression and anxiety	1	1.2
Required psychological intervention for cancer diagnosis induced distress on diagnosis		
Yes	13	15.5

TABLE 1: Continued.

Age (years)		16–86 (mean: 55.1 ± 16.4)
Cancer characteristics		
Type of sarcoma		
Osteosarcoma, Ewing's sarcoma	9	11.9
Chondrosarcoma	7	9.2
Soft tissue sarcoma	60	78.9
Location of cancer (lower limb $n = 56$, 73.7%)		
Proximal upper limb	11	14.5
Distal upper limb	9	11.8
Proximal lower limb	39	51.3
Distal lower limb	17	22.4
Dominant upper limb involved (out of $n = 20$)		
Yes	9	45
Neoadjuvant therapy		
Radiation only	51	67.1
Chemotherapy	8	10.5
Sarcoma diagnosis delayed: for example, not thinking the lump was anything to worry about; doctor dismissed lump as not important		
Yes	37	48.7
Sarcoma diagnosis made from unplanned manipulation for misdiagnosed benign condition		
Yes	35	44.7
Surgery details		
Type of surgery		
Soft tissue resection	56	73.7
Limb-sparing surgery	12	15.8
Amputation	8	10.5
Perception of most significant source of stress at $t = 0$		
Mortality	2	2.6
Disruption to life/plans/goals, for example, career, school, and recreational/social interactions; financial implications	23	30.3
Change in life role(s), for instance, feeling useless, burden on family	9	11.8
Fear of the unknown	9	11.8
Loss of locus of control, for instance, having to wait for things to happen	2	2.6
Cosmetic related concerns	3	3.9
Let down by healthcare system	19	25.0
Other or cannot say	1	1.3
Not stressed/no complaint	8	10.6

Table 2: Prevalence of caseness for TESS, DASS21, and EORTC QLQ C-30.

	Diagnosis n (%)	6 months n (%)	12 months n (%)
TESS*			
Difficulty performing ADLs	25 (32.9)	34 (44.7)	21 (21.6)
Self-rate as disabled	11 (14.5)	22 (28.9)	16 (21.1)
DASS21**	22 (28.9)	28 (36.8)	24 (31.6)
Stress	13 (17.1)	18 (23.7)	19 (25.0)
Anxiety	17 (22.4)	16 (21.1)	15 (19.7)
Depression	10 (13.2)	21 (27.6)	21 (27.6)
EORTC QLQ C-30***			
QoL	20 (26.3)	21 (27.6)	19 (25.0)
PF	7 (9.2)	9 (11.8)	3 (3.9)
RF	18 (23.7)	27 (35.5)	14 (18.4)
EF	6 (7.9)	15 (19.7)	10 (13.2)
CF	4 (5.3)	6 (7.9)	6 (7.9)
SF	13 (51.3)	17 (22.4)	13 (17.1)
	39 (63.2)[1]	47 (61.8)[1]	35 (46.1)[1]
PA	22 (28.9)[2]	27 (35.5)[2]	23 (30.3)[2]
	16 (21.1)[3]	18 (23.7)[3]	15 (19.7)[3]
FI	20 (26.3)	21 (27.6)	14 (18.4)

*Caseness for TESS defined as moderate difficulty or harder.
**Caseness for DASS21 defined as being moderate to severe based on DASS Manual guidelines (S. H. Lovibond and P. F. Lovibond 1995 [45]).
***Caseness for EORTC QLQ C-30 subscales: QoL dichotomized at ≤4; other subscales dichotomized as quite a bit or more of difficulty or level of symptoms.
[1]Pain dichotomized at a little or more; [2]pain dichotomized at more than a little; [3]pain dichotomized at moderate to severe.

Table 3: (a) Paired sample t-test to compare baseline scores and scores twelve months after surgery. (b) Paired sample t-test to compare scores six months after surgery and twelve months after surgery.

(a)

	t
DASS21	−0.75
TESS	0.18
QoL	−0.92
PF	−0.03
RF	−0.66
EF	−1.47
CF	0.59
SF	0.71
PA	0.71
FI	−0.23

All not significantly different.

(b)

	t
DASS21	0.53
TESS	−5.43*
QoL	−1.88
PF	−5.21*
RF	−5.13*
EF	−1.71
CF	−0.34
SF	−1.38
PA	2.66*
FI	1.22

*$P < 0.01$ (2-tailed).

5.4. Objective 2: Prevalence and Trend of Distress. As summarized in Table 2, the overall prevalence of moderate to severe DASS21 scores for either of the subscales of stress, anxiety, and/or depression was 28.9% for our cohort of recently diagnosed, preoperative patients, 36.8% at six months after surgery, and 31.6% at twelve months after surgery. In terms of the trajectory of distress, of the three subscales of distress, anxiety was most prevalent at baseline (22.4%), but depression was most prevalent after surgery (27.6% at six months and at twelve months after surgery).

As shown in Figures 1 and 2, mean overall DASS21 scores peaked at six months but reduced at twelve months. Overall, the proportion of our cohort that reported moderate to severe stress and depression scores increased with time, whilst the proportion that reported moderate to severe anxiety scores reduced with time. Distress was most marked at six months. The prevalence of distress according to age showed that older adults were least likely to be distressed, compared to youths, working aged adults, and elderly people. Amongst people aged sixteen to 54 years, fifteen out of 32 (46.9%) were distressed; amongst those aged 55–75 years, only five out of 36 (13.9%) reported significant distress; and amongst those aged 76–86 years, half of the eight elderly people were distressed. TESS scores and ease of completing ADLs appeared to improve with time after surgery (mean TESS at six months was 68.8, which improved to 76.9 at twelve months after surgery) as shown in Figure 3.

Our paired sample t-tests showed that there were no significant differences between QoL, mental health, and physical function scores between baseline and twelve months after surgery. However, comparing scores between six months and twelve months after surgery, physical function, role function, and pain scores improved, whilst mental health, overall QoL, and social function scores remained relatively constant (Tables 3(a) and 3(b)).

The results of the ANOVA indicated that there were small and nonsignificant time effects for DASS21 and subscale scores between each of the timepoints. Also, $P > 0.05$, suggesting that DASS21 scores remained relatively stable.

There was a significant time effect for TESS scores, Wilks's Lambda = 0.69, $F(2, 74) = 17.03$, $P < 0.01$, and $\eta^2 = 0.32$. Thus, there was significant evidence to reject the null hypothesis. Follow-up comparisons indicated that there was a significant reduction in TESS scores between $t = 0$ and $t = 1$ and a significant improvement between $t = 1$ and $t = 2$ (both $P < 0.01$) (Figure 3). There was no significant difference

TABLE 4: Summary of DASS21, TESS, LOT-R, SSQ, SSS, and 12-month EORTC QLQ C-30 subscale scores (mean ± SD) by presence of distress at 12 months.

	Distress, $n = 24$ (M ± SD)	No distress, $n = 52$ (M ± SD)	Independent t-test
DASS21 at baseline	33.6 ± 20.1	16.4 ± 15.2	$t = -3.74^{**}$
DASS21 at 6 months	50.0 ± 26.7	13.9 ± 15.1	$t = -6.18^{***}$
TESS at baseline	69.9 ± 22.9	80.9 ± 21.1	$t = 2.05^{*}$
TESS at 6 months	59.9 ± 19.7	73.0 ± 17.2	$t = 2.95^{**}$
TESS at 12 months	66.6 ± 15.3	81.7 ± 18.7	$t = 3.46^{**}$
SSS	36.6 ± 21.7	16.8 ± 16.8	$t = -4.34^{***}$
Global QoL	57.6 ± 19.6	79.2 ± 18.2	$t = 4.68^{***}$
PF	66.9 ± 16.5	81.9 ± 20.4	$t = 3.15^{**}$
RF	50.0 ± 33.3	80.1 ± 23.1	$t = 4.01^{***}$
EF	46.9 ± 25.2	93.2 ± 10.3	$t = 8.67^{***}$
CF	68.1 ± 30.3	88.1 ± 16.9	$t = 3.04^{**}$
SF	43.8 ± 28.2	84.6 ± 21.4	$t = 6.32^{***}$
PA	47.9 ± 31.6	17.9 ± 25.7	$t = -4.39^{***}$
FI	56.9 ± 37.4	15.4 ± 20.3	$t = -5.11^{***}$

$^{*}P < 0.05$ (2-tailed).
$^{**}P < 0.01$ (2-tailed).
$^{***}P < 0.001$ (2-tailed).

between baseline TESS scores and $t = 2$ scores indicating that functional scores had returned to baseline at a year after surgery.

Pain scores displayed a small to medium, significant time effect, Wilks's Lambda = 0.91, $F(2, 74) = 3.61$, $P < 0.05$, and $\eta^2 = 0.09$, with pairwise comparison indicating that the difference was an improvement in pain scores from $t = 1$ to $t = 2$ ($P = 0.03$) (Figure 4).

5.5. Objective 3: Comparing Distressed and Nondistressed Participants. Distressed patients had poorer function (MSTS93, TESS) and QoL (from EORTC QLQ C-30) mean scores compared to nondistressed patients as presented in Table 4 and Figure 4. As shown in Figure 5, distressed participants reported worse scores for each domain assessed by the EORTC QLQ C-30.

5.6. Objective 4: Correlates of Distress

5.6.1. Baseline and Sociodemographic Variables. DASS21 score at diagnosis strongly correlated with distress twelve months after surgery ($\rho = 0.421$, $P < 0.01$). Reported QoL at baseline was moderately strongly and inversely correlated with distress ($\rho = -0.35$, $P < 0.01$). Being aged between 55 and 75 years was inversely correlated with distress ($\phi = -0.361$, $P < 0.01$) with moderate strength ($n = 37$, mean DASS21 score = 13.78) whilst being aged younger than 55 years was directly correlated with distress ($\phi = 0.28$, $P < 0.05$) ($n = 32$, mean DASS21 score = 32.03). DASS21 scores were significantly higher in the younger age group $t(48.18) = 2.87$, $P = 0.006$. Living in a postcode marked as middle SES was moderately strongly correlated with distress ($\phi = 0.34$, $P = 0.003$) ($n = 35$, mean DASS21 score = 32.14), whilst living in a postcode marked as low SES was weakly inversely correlated with distress ($\phi = -0.23$, $P < 0.05$) ($n = 17$, mean DASS21 score = 14.82). Distress was higher for people in middle SES compared to people in lower SES $t(44.22) = 2.46$, $P = 0.02$. There was no significant correlation between distress and living in a postcode marked as high SES. Significant pain as a presenting feature and having undergone chemotherapy were weakly correlated with distress ($\phi = 0.29$ and $\phi = 0.23$, resp., both $P < 0.05$). We did not find strong, significant correlations between distress and other tumour and demographic variables.

5.6.2. Outcome Variables at Twelve Months. Poor physical function was highly correlated with distress (TESS $\rho = -0.53$, PF $\rho = -0.49$, and RF $\rho = -0.54$). Social functioning and overall QoL were also highly correlated with distress ($\rho = -0.68$ and -0.62, resp.). Pain was also strongly correlated with distress ($\rho = 0.42$) as were financial difficulties ($\rho = 0.53$) and high shame and stigma scores ($\rho = 0.46$). The EF subscale and DASS21 scores were highly correlated ($\rho = -0.85$), indicating that they were both measuring psychological morbidity. All variables were significant at $P < 0.001$.

6. Discussion

We report on a cohort study of people with nonmetastatic ES, examining psychological distress up to one year after surgery. Our cohort was heterogeneous in terms of histological subtype and anatomical location of ES but homogeneous for timepoint of the cancer journey, as all participants represented prospectively recruited consecutive patients from an adult cancer institution, with a new diagnosis of ES. All patients received a standard protocol of treatment by a unified multidisciplinary sarcoma service (VSS).

Compared to other longitudinal psychosocial studies on adult ES patients, our cohort consisted of a relatively large sample size with 76 participants. Participants comprised people across a wide range of age groups. When compared to patients suffering from other cancers, a majority of our cohort were still of working age. Sarcoma is a nondiscriminatory cancer in terms of age and it has been reported that 60% of all sarcomas occur in people who are younger than 55 years [53].

6.1. Prevalence and Trend of Distress in People with Extremity Sarcoma. About a third of our cohort of people with recently diagnosed ES reported moderate to severe levels of psychological distress at any one point. This is comparable with previous reports on prevalence of distress in general cancer cohorts that included common primaries, including breast and prostate cancers [19, 25, 26, 30]. Our rates of distress appeared to be lower than the rate of distress in head, neck, lung, and pancreatic cancers [18, 19].

Paredes et al. [14] performed a cross-sectional study on sarcoma patients who were grouped according to phase of cancer journey: *diagnosis phase* ($n = 42$), *treatment phase* ($n = 37$), and *follow-up phase* ($n = 63$, mean time of 52.93 months after initial diagnosis). They found that moderate to severe anxiety was most prevalent in the diagnosis phase (29.3%), followed by treatment phase (25%) and follow-up phase (21%). They found that moderate to severe depression was most prevalent in the treatment phase (19.4%) followed by diagnosis phase (19%) and follow-up phase (6.5%). Females and older patients displayed higher levels of depression, whilst recurrence was associated with both anxiety and depression. Anxiety and depression scores reduced with time, reflecting that emotional distress is usually transitory and allows for adjustment.

In our cohort, although repeated measures ANOVA did not find a significant difference between DASS21 scores with time, a similar trend was found as shown in Figure 1. Mean overall distress, stress, and depression scores were most marked after the surgery (six months: 25.3, 11.24, and 8.62, resp.) and reduced with time (twelve months: 24.09, 10.84, and 8.28, resp.). The mean anxiety score was highest during diagnosis (5.61) and waned with time (six months: 5.45, twelve months: 4.97). Mean stress scores at twelve months (10.84) were higher than scores at baseline (10.05). The DASS Manual describes "stress" as being factorially distinct from depression and anxiety and a state that is characterized by nervous tension, difficulty relaxing, and irritability, which is similar to the DSM-IV diagnosis of generalized anxiety disorder (GAD) [45]. This was an interesting finding and perhaps reflected the accumulating incomplete tasks and responsibilities patients accrued that were unable to be fulfilled due to convalescing from the sarcoma and surgery. Rehabilitation following limb salvage surgery takes at least six to eight weeks to restore independent function and much longer if complications arise and if adjuvant therapy is required [54]. There are other possible explanations for the higher stress levels after surgery. It may reflect difficulty relaxing due to instructions on the need to protect the reconstructed limb, to prevent late complications, such as fracture, dislocation, or infection. Furthermore, survivors may report higher stress levels due to concerns about recurrence of their cancer. Unlike other cancers, the aetiology of sarcoma is usually sporadic. "Body betrayal" is the perceived notion that the body or a part of the body has betrayed the self because of illness, such as cancer or disability, despite living a life that did not involve lifestyle risk factors for disease (or, conversely, involved living a life that involved health-promoting behaviours) [55, 56]. This is associated with cancers that are not associated with lifestyle factors and with cancers that result in disabilities, such as breast cancer [57]. Body betrayal may be particularly relevant to ES survivors and may result in negative body image [58]. Survivors of ES may also feel anxious that they cannot do anything to reduce the likelihood of recurrence, which may contribute to a sense of helplessness regarding their future [59].

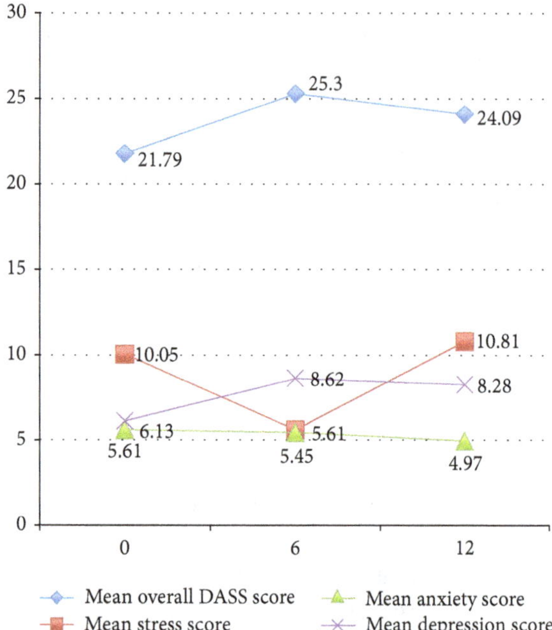

FIGURE 1: Mean DASS21 score with time

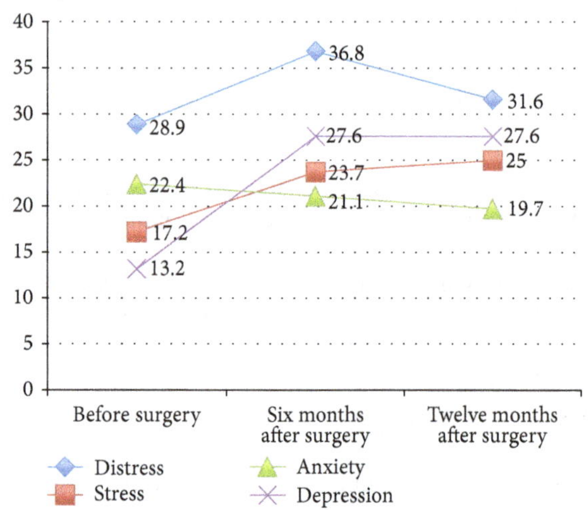

FIGURE 2: Proportion of moderately to severely distressed participants according to timeframe (based on Table 2).

It would be of interest for future investigations to follow up on the trend of stress and anxiety to evaluate the trend of stress levels further down the track, as well as to conduct a qualitative study exploring the sources of stress in survivors of ES.

6.2. Differences between Distressed and Nondistressed Participants and Correlates of Distress. Compared to nondistressed participants, people that were distressed displayed poorer physical function, higher levels of shame, and poorer QoL.

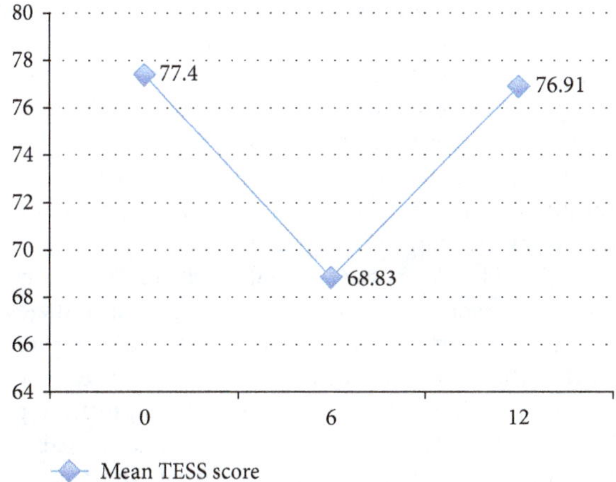

FIGURE 3: Mean TESS score with time (based on Table 2).

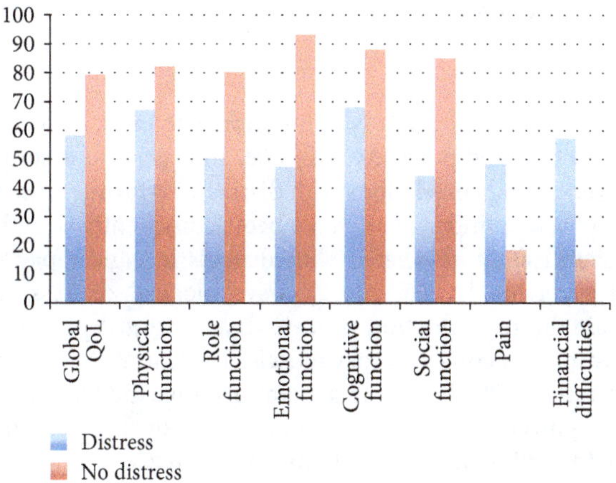

FIGURE 5: Summary of description of mean scores of EORTC QLQ C-30 (%) domains by presence of distress at 12 months.

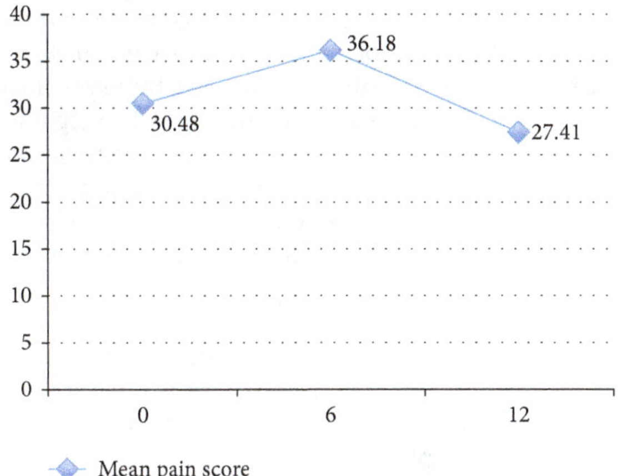

FIGURE 4: Mean pain score with time.

6.2.1. Sociodemographic Variables. Our study has found that AYAs and midlife adults (aged sixteen to 54 years) were more likely to be distressed at one year after surgery for ES compared to people aged 55 to 75 years. This could perhaps reflect that older adulthood is a relatively stable phase of life in terms of career and family responsibilities. Conversely, this could reflect the increased vulnerability of AYAs (defined as people between the ages of fifteen and 29 years) to psychological distress. Adolescence represents a period of developmental transitions, characterised by cognitive, biological, and socioeconomic challenges [60–62]. Health problems such as cancer, in this age group, are uncommon as cancer is predominantly a disease of the older population. Cancer occurring in AYAs represents a disruption in a phase of development, which includes increased responsibility for the self, autonomy in decision making, financial independence, and identity formation [61] and is associated with more psychological distress and lower self-esteem when compared to children and older adults with cancer [63]. It is also recognised that the prevalence of nonadherence to medical advice in the adolescent oncology population is higher than in nonadolescent populations [64]. Paediatric and adult cancer centres may not be adequately equipped to manage the unique demands of cancer patients in this age group [65]. Furthermore, research in other cancer types has shown an inverse relationship between age and unmet needs in the fact that young people with cancer have reported more unmet needs and less satisfaction with the care they received than older people with cancer [21, 66, 67].

Low income, lower educational attainment, and being from an ethnic minority have been found to be significant risk factors for depression and psychological distress in survivors of cancer [2, 19, 29, 37]. Low income is associated with unemployment and financial stress, which in turn is associated with lower QoL and distress [38]. Other risk factors for distress in the psychooncology population that have been described in the literature include female gender [17, 39], younger age [17, 18, 40–42], and poor perceived social support [26, 29, 32].

In our study, we found that financial stress was strongly correlated with distress. However, low educational attainment did not show a significant correlation with distress. Distress was higher for people living in a middle SES area compared to people in a lower SES area. There was no significant correlation between people in a high SES and distress. This may be attributed to people in a high SES having more resources available and having fewer stressors, whilst conversely people in a low SES may have fewer encumbrances, have lower expectations, or be identified as requiring more help and have more access to healthcare services and therefore were less likely to be distressed.

Tumour-related factors were not strongly correlated with distress at twelve months. In breast cancer cohorts, a similar finding of a lack of correlation between cancer variables, such as stage of cancer, and depression exists [29]. This perhaps suggests that a cancer diagnosis presents as an absolute threat to one's mortality and sense of self, which may affect mental health, as opposed to a relative threat based on the relative risk to mortality.

6.2.2. Physical Function. Poor function outcomes, such as low TESS scores and poor physical, role, and social functioning, showed strong correlations with distress. Performance status and physical impairment have been consistently found to be significantly associated with distress in cancer patients and survivors [2, 26, 30–32]. Psychological distress may impair the rehabilitation process that is critical postoperatively to train compensatory muscles to achieve effective gait restoration [68]. From the general orthopaedic literature, it is recognized that depression and anxiety during rehabilitation for orthopaedic conditions have a negative impact on recovery [69] and are associated with poor function and pain outcomes following joint arthroplasty in particular [70, 71]. Furthermore, psychosocial interventions have been shown to improve the effectiveness of rehabilitation after orthopaedic injuries [69]. Conversely, poor TESS scores may result in distress as mediated by poorer role and social functioning.

6.2.3. Shame. Body image is defined as the subjective concept of one's physical appearance based on self-observation and the reactions of others, which may be moderated by patient biological, psychological, and social/environmental factors [72]. Body image disturbance is associated with disfigurement [73], such as amputation, the presence of a visible scar, or an abnormal gait pattern. Maladaptation to a disturbed body image results in shame, which has been described as an affective state in which a sense of disgrace, dishonor, or humiliation may generate a desire to cover oneself [49]. Research on head and neck cancer patients suggests that body image disturbance is associated with mood disturbance, psychological distress, impaired social interactions, and poorer reported QoL [49, 72]. There is limited research regarding body image following ES surgery. Drawing from the research performed on traumatic amputees, poor physical function and pain were found to be associated with body image disturbance [74], which in turn was associated with psychological distress, low self-esteem, social avoidance, depression, and anxiety [74–77]. Adolescents with cancer may be particularly vulnerable to body image disturbance [73, 78] and there may also be a gender difference with regard to the perception of body image [72]. Preoperatively, only a minority of respondents indicated that cosmetic considerations were a major stressor. However, at one year after surgery, we found that higher modified SSS scores correlated strongly with distress, and participants that were distressed were more likely to report higher levels of shame towards their physical appearance compared to nondistressed participants. Negative self-perception of body image may be amenable to interventions that aim to promote resilience and improve self-esteem and social confidence such as through cognitive behavioural therapy and social skills training [77].

6.2.4. Quality of Life and Pain. Distressed participants were more likely than nondistressed cohorts to report poorer QoL in each subscale of the EORTC QLQ C-30, including poorer social functioning, lower cognitive functioning, higher subjective pain levels, and more financial difficulties.

The prevalence of pain in our cohort at twelve months after surgery was 46.1%, whilst the prevalence of moderate to severe pain at twelve months was 19.7%. This rate is consistent with other studies that have found the prevalence of pain in nonterminal and non-head-and-neck cancer patients (e.g., breast, nongynaecological urogenital and lung) to be around 30–50% [79–81]. A cross-sectional study on 149 sarcoma outpatients of varying histological subtypes and stages of disease and at varying timeframes of the cancer journey found that the prevalence of pain was 53% in their cohort. They found that 25% of the patients reported significant pain, 18.1% reported mild pain, 18.8% reported moderate pain, and 16.1% reported severe pain using the Visual Analogue Scale [82].

Distressed participants were more likely to report higher pain scores, and pain scores on the EORTC QLQ C-30 were strongly correlated with distress. Pain directly and indirectly negatively influences mental well-being and QoL [83] and is associated with decreased levels of social activities and social support [33]. Pain is complex and multidimensional in nature and the perception of pain is influenced by psychological distress [84]. It is well recognised that pain is a significant risk factor for psychiatric morbidity in the psychooncology population [17, 25, 33–36]. Malignant bone pain presents with a unique pain state that may be difficult to manage and require multimodal analgesics [85]. Effective pain management is therefore one of the designated goals of cancer care in the Victorian Cancer Action Plan [86]. Furthermore, clinical features of the cancer and adverse effects of treatment may overlap with symptoms of psychiatric distress. Severe persistent pain (more than three months after surgery) following elective joint arthroplasty occurs in about 7–20% and 2–8% of knee and hip replacement patients, respectively, and is predicted by the presence of depression [87]. Although the reason for pain in our cancer cohort was not assessed, it may be due to multifactorial reasons, such as surgical factors, previous tissue damage due to cancer or adjuvant therapy, ongoing tissue damage due to the cancer, and patient factors, such as depression. Pain acts as a stressor, contributing to psychological distress, and conversely being distressed negatively influences an individual's ability to cope with a noxious stimulus. It is clear that pain following ES surgery needs to be managed proactively via a multidisciplinary team, comprising pain specialists, oncologists, surgeons, and mental health professionals.

6.2.5. Distress at Baseline. There is consistent research to suggest that patients with high distress scores or poorer emotional functioning at baseline and those with a past history of a psychiatric disorder are at increased risk of persistent distress in the later parts of the cancer journey [15, 17, 25–29]. We found that distress at baseline was strongly correlated with distress at twelve months after surgery. However, we did not find a significant correlation between a past history of a mental health disorder (depression or anxiety) and distress at twelve months, suggesting that previous psychiatric morbidity per se may not be associated with an increased vulnerability to psychological distress in cancer.

6.3. Stressors. Almost a quarter of the cohort reported that the biggest source of stress was consequent upon their perceived frustration with the healthcare system. A mixed quantitative and qualitatively designed study on 295 mixed cancer patients throughout different phases of their cancer journey was performed in the United Kingdom, exploring the unmet needs of cancer patients [88]. They found that the majority of participants rated issues relating to the healthcare system as most important. These included issues relating to confidence in the health professionals, communication issues (such as taking the time to discuss issues with the individual honestly, sensitively, accurately, and respectfully), and easy and quick access to health professionals and health services. In our present study, this largely related to the perception that there was a lack of communication between auxiliary hospital staff (e.g., waiting times for imaging, biopsy, and follow-up appointments) and patients. This is an important area for clinical services to address.

Sarcoma is rare and the clinical features of soft tissue sarcoma may be insidious. Almost half of our cohort reported that their initial diagnosis was delayed due to being dismissed by themselves or a health practitioner, whilst a similar proportion had undergone surgery for a presumed benign condition prior to the diagnosis. Delayed diagnosis may result in tumour progression resulting in higher stage at time of diagnosis. Osteosarcomas that are diagnosed late or unexpectedly are more likely to have amputations and are associated with poorer survival and other worse oncological outcomes compared to osteosarcoma managed efficiently by a sarcoma service [89–91]. Unplanned manipulation of the affected limb such as through poorly planned biopsies and unintentional surgical excision due to misdiagnosis may result in contamination of compartments and require much bigger surgery, including amputation, to remove the tract as a site of seeding of the cancer [89, 92, 93].

This may have implications on the cosmetic outlook and physical function of the patients. This may also have implications on the patient's trust of medical professionals and result in reduced perception and expectation of the healthcare system and influence expectations of recovery. Increased education of primary healthcare physicians regarding identification of potential red flags for sarcoma is necessary in order to reduce the incidence of sarcomas that are diagnosed through unplanned manipulations.

Another commonly reported stressor was the fear of the unknown, in terms of both the logistic/practical aspects of their care and the unexpectedness of outcomes. Previous studies have found that clinical uncertainty is associated with hopelessness and consequent psychological distress [94]. Uncertain expectations have been found to be negatively associated with outcome following extremity sarcoma surgery [13]. Improved communication between hospital and patients may be necessary with a readily contactable liaison person in our integrated sarcoma service. There may also be a role for peer support and psychoeducational therapy to address uncertain expectations, in order to improve outcomes in ES management.

7. Implications for Further Research and Limitations of Our Study

Psychological distress is associated with poor outcomes such as poorer QoL and poorer physical function. Distress early on in the cancer journey predicts persistent distress at one year after surgery. Stressors have been identified that may be amenable to psychoeducational interventions. There is great scope for future research to investigate the role of early intervention to improve outcomes in people diagnosed with ES.

As we have discussed above, compared to other cancers, ES affects people of working age. Impaired social functioning and cognition may result in difficulties with work and employment, resulting in higher financial difficulties. Our study found that two-thirds of our cohort had reported that they had to modify or stop their work as a consequence of the sarcoma, and this change in employment status was instituted early on during the diagnosis. More than a quarter of our patients reported that they had persisting significant difficulties with performing their usual work one year after the surgery. Financial stress may be a stressor for distress. Clearly, further dedicated research into employment outcomes in people with ES would be of interest.

One of the limitations in our study included the use of the modified SSS, to assess shame, which is not validated for use in this cohort. As discussed above, body image is an important outcome of interest following ES surgery. Further studies may be required to develop an ES-specific tool to assess body image and to investigate the role of psychological interventions to target negative self-image. Furthermore, our analysis was limited by our sample size. Future studies with larger samples would improve sampling and reduce bias and variability and allow for more robust prediction analyses to be undertaken.

A large proportion of our cohort reported that their ES was either initially dismissed as benign and ignored or diagnosed through surgery for a presumed benign condition. As discussed above, this may be associated with greater morbidity and mortality. Increased education for primary care physicians and general and plastic surgeons, such as a protocol for management of large lumps, may reduce the incidence of unexpected and delayed diagnoses.

8. Conclusion

Almost a third of our cohort of recently diagnosed ES patients reported moderate, severe, or extremely severe stress, anxiety, or depression. From previous research, psychological distress is associated with negative outcomes in cancer and distress and may be amenable to management. In our cohort, distress was associated with poor QoL, financial difficulties, pain, and poor physical function. Patients with a past history of depression and/or anxiety and those that are distressed early in the diagnosis phase of the cancer journey may be especially vulnerable to persistent distress up to a year after surgery. In order to optimize outcomes in ES, it is important to actively screen and effectively manage psychological distress.

References

[1] L. Grassi, M. Indelli, M. Marzola et al., "Depressive symptoms and quality of life in home-care-assisted cancer patients," *Journal of Pain and Symptom Management*, vol. 12, no. 5, pp. 300–307, 1996.

[2] P. B. Jacobsen, K. A. Donovan, P. C. Trask et al., "Screening for psychologic distress in ambulatory cancer patients," *Cancer*, vol. 103, no. 7, pp. 1494–1502, 2005.

[3] M. Pinquart and P. R. Duberstein, "Depression and cancer mortality: a meta-analysis," *Psychological Medicine*, vol. 40, no. 11, pp. 1797–1810, 2010.

[4] C. Eiser, A.-S. E. Darlington, C. B. Stride, and R. Grimer, "Quality of life implications as a consequence of surgery: limb salvage, primary and secondary amputation," *Sarcoma*, vol. 5, no. 4, pp. 189–196, 2001.

[5] Y. Refaat, J. Gunnoe, F. J. Hornicek, and H. J. Mankin, "Comparison of quality of life after amputation or limb salvage," *Clinical Orthopaedics and Related Research*, no. 397, pp. 298–305, 2002.

[6] A. Zahlten-Hinguranage, L. Bernd, V. Ewerbeck, and D. Sabo, "Equal quality of life after limb-sparing or ablative surgery for lower extremity sarcomas," *British Journal of Cancer*, vol. 91, no. 6, pp. 1012–1014, 2004.

[7] P. K. Pardasaney, P. E. Sullivan, L. G. Portney, and H. J. Mankin, "Advantage of limb salvage over amputation for proximal lower extremity tumors," *Clinical Orthopaedics and Related Research*, no. 444, pp. 201–208, 2006.

[8] K. M. J. Thijssens, J. E. H. M. Hoekstra-Weebers, R. J. van Ginkel, and H. J. Hoekstra, "Quality of life after hyperthermic isolated limb perfusion for locally advanced extremity soft tissue sarcoma," *Annals of Surgical Oncology*, vol. 13, no. 6, pp. 864–871, 2006.

[9] L. Weiner, H. Battles, D. Bernstein et al., "Persistent psychological distress in long-term survivors of peditric sarcoma: the experience at a single institution," *Psycho-Oncology*, vol. 15, no. 10, pp. 898–910, 2006.

[10] L. H. Aksnes, H. C. F. Bauer, N. L. Jebsen et al., "Limb-sparing surgery preserves more function than amputation: a Scandinavian sarcoma group study of 118 patients," *Journal of Bone and Joint Surgery—Series B*, vol. 90, no. 6, pp. 786–794, 2008.

[11] A. M. Davis, B. O'Sullivan, R. S. Bell et al., "Function and health status outcomes in a randomized trial comparing preoperative and postoperative radiotherapy in extremity soft tissue sarcoma," *Journal of Clinical Oncology*, vol. 20, no. 22, pp. 4472–4477, 2002.

[12] D. Schreiber, R. S. Bell, J. S. Wunder et al., "Evaluating function and health related quality of life in patients treated for extremity soft tissue sarcoma," *Quality of Life Research*, vol. 15, no. 9, pp. 1439–1446, 2006.

[13] K. Davidge, R. Bell, P. Ferguson, R. Turcotte, J. Wunder, and A. M. Davis, "Patient expectations for surgical outcome in extremity soft tissue sarcoma," *Journal of Surgical Oncology*, vol. 100, no. 5, pp. 375–381, 2009.

[14] T. Paredes, M. C. Canavarro, and M. R. Simões, "Anxiety and depression in sarcoma patients: emotional adjustment and its determinants in the different phases of disease," *European Journal of Oncology Nursing*, vol. 15, no. 1, pp. 73–79, 2011.

[15] T. Paredes, M. Pereira, M. R. Simões, and M. C. Canavarro, "A longitudinal study on emotional adjustment of sarcoma patients: the determinant role of demographic, clinical and coping variables," *European Journal of Cancer Care*, vol. 21, no. 1, pp. 41–51, 2012.

[16] M. H. Tang, D. J. W. Pan, D. J. Castle, and P. F. M. Choong, "A systematic review of the recent quality of life studies in adult extremity sarcoma survivors," *Sarcoma*, vol. 2012, Article ID 171342, 15 pages, 2012.

[17] M. J. Massie, "Prevalence of depression in patients with cancer," *Journal of the National Cancer Institute: Monographs*, no. 32, pp. 57–71, 2004.

[18] J. Zabora, K. BrintzenhofeSzoc, B. Curbow, C. Hooker, and S. Piantadosi, "The prevalence of psychological distress by cancer site," *Psycho-Oncology*, vol. 10, no. 1, pp. 19–28, 2001.

[19] L. E. Carlson, M. Angen, J. Cullum et al., "High levels of untreated distress and fatigue in cancer patients," *British Journal of Cancer*, vol. 90, no. 12, pp. 2297–2304, 2004.

[20] I. Henselmans, V. S. Helgeson, H. Seltman, J. de Vries, R. Sanderman, and A. V. Ranchor, "Identification and prediction of distress trajectories in the first year after a breast cancer diagnosis," *Health Psychology*, vol. 29, no. 2, pp. 160–168, 2010.

[21] M. E. McDowell, S. Occhipinti, M. Ferguson, J. Dunn, and S. K. Chambers, "Predictors of change in unmet supportive care needs in cancer," *Psycho-Oncology*, vol. 19, no. 5, pp. 508–516, 2010.

[22] S. M. Spencer, C. S. Carver, and A. A. Price, "Psychological and social factors in adaptation," in *Psycho-Oncology*, J. C. Holland, Ed., pp. 211–222, Oxford University Press, New York, NY, USA, 1998.

[23] A. B. Kornblith, "Psychosocial adaptation of cancer survivors," in *Psycho-Oncology*, J. C. Holland, Ed., pp. 223–254, Oxford University Press, New York, NY, USA, 1998.

[24] M. Stommel, M. E. Kurtz, J. C. Kurtz, C. W. Given, and B. A. Given, "A longitudinal analysis of the course of depressive symptomatology in geriatric patients with cancer of the breast, colon, lung, or prostate," *Health Psychology*, vol. 23, no. 6, pp. 564–573, 2004.

[25] K. Bjordal and S. Kaasa, "Psychological distress in head and neck cancer patients 7–11 years after curative treatment," *British Journal of Cancer*, vol. 71, no. 3, pp. 592–597, 1995.

[26] L. Grassi, P. Malacarne, A. Maestri, and E. Ramelli, "Depression, psychosocial variables and occurrence of life events among patients with cancer," *Journal of Affective Disorders*, vol. 44, no. 1, pp. 21–30, 1997.

[27] K. A. Neilson, A. C. Pollard, A. M. Boonzaier et al., "Psychological distress (depression and anxiety) in people with head and neck cancers," *Medical Journal of Australia*, vol. 193, no. 5, pp. 48–51, 2010.

[28] T. Iwatani, A. Matsuda, H. Kawabata, D. Miura, and E. Matsushima, "Predictive factors for psychological distress related to diagnosis of breast cancer," *Psycho-Oncology*, vol. 22, no. 3, pp. 523–529, 2013.

[29] M. Reich, A. Lesur, and C. Perdrizet-Chevallier, "Depression, quality of life and breast cancer: a review of the literature," *Breast Cancer Research and Treatment*, vol. 110, no. 1, pp. 9–17, 2008.

[30] S. Pascoe, S. Edelman, and A. Kidman, "Prevalence of psychological distress and use of support services by cancer patients

at Sydney hospitals," *Australian & New Zealand Journal of Psychiatry*, vol. 34, no. 5, pp. 785–791, 2000.

[31] P. Hopwood and R. J. Stephens, "Depression in patients with lung cancer: prevalence and risk factors derived from quality-of-life data," *Journal of Clinical Oncology*, vol. 18, no. 4, pp. 893–903, 2000.

[32] W. A. Bardwell and L. Fiorentino, "Risk factors for depression in breast cancer survivors: an update," *International Journal of Clinical and Health Psychology*, vol. 12, no. 2, pp. 311–331, 2012.

[33] C. Zaza and N. Baine, "Cancer pain and psychosocial factors: a critical review of the literature," *Journal of Pain and Symptom Management*, vol. 24, no. 5, pp. 526–542, 2002.

[34] M. Vahdaninia, S. Omidvari, and A. Montazeri, "What do predict anxiety and depression in breast cancer patients? A follow-up study," *Social Psychiatry and Psychiatric Epidemiology*, vol. 45, no. 3, pp. 355–361, 2010.

[35] M.-L. Chen, H.-K. Chang, and C.-H. Yeh, "Anxiety and depression in Taiwanese cancer patients with and without pain," *Journal of Advanced Nursing*, vol. 32, no. 4, pp. 944–951, 2000.

[36] A. Ciaramella and P. Poli, "Assessment of depression among cancer patients: the role of pain, cancer type and treatment," *Psycho-Oncology*, vol. 10, no. 2, pp. 156–165, 2001.

[37] L. K. Zeltzer, Q. Lu, W. Leisenring et al., "Psychosocial outcomes and health-related quality of life in adult childhood cancer survivors: a report from the Childhood Cancer Survivor Study," *Cancer Epidemiology Biomarkers & Prevention*, vol. 17, no. 2, pp. 435–446, 2008.

[38] K. Ell, B. Xie, A. Wells, F. Nedjat-Haiem, P. J. Lee, and B. Vourlekis, "Economic stress among low-income women with cancer: effects on quality of life," *Cancer*, vol. 112, no. 3, pp. 616–625, 2008.

[39] E. E. Evan and L. K. Zeltzer, "Psychosocial dimensions of cancer in adolescents and young adults," *Cancer*, vol. 107, supplement 7, pp. 1663–1671, 2006.

[40] W. Linden, A. Vodermaier, R. MacKenzie, and D. Greig, "Anxiety and depression after cancer diagnosis: prevalence rates by cancer type, gender, and age," *Journal of Affective Disorders*, vol. 141, no. 2-3, pp. 343–351, 2012.

[41] A. Enns, A. Waller, S. L. Groff, B. D. Bultz, T. Fung, and L. E. Carlson, "Risk factors for continuous distress over a 12-month period in newly diagnosed cancer outpatients," *Journal of Psychosocial Oncology*, vol. 31, no. 5, pp. 489–506, 2013.

[42] C. Burgess, V. Cornelius, S. Love, J. Graham, M. Richards, and A. Ramirez, "Depression and anxiety in women with early breast cancer: five year observational cohort study," *British Medical Journal*, vol. 330, no. 7493, pp. 702–705, 2005.

[43] M. Charlson, T. P. Szatrowski, J. Peterson, and J. Gold, "Validation of a combined comorbidity index," *Journal of Clinical Epidemiology*, vol. 47, no. 11, pp. 1245–1251, 1994.

[44] ABS ABoS, "Census of population and housing: socio-economic indexes for areas (SEIFA). Australia, 2011," Catalogue Number 2033.0.55.001, Australian Bureau of Statistics, 2011.

[45] S. H. Lovibond and P. F. Lovibond, *Manual for the Depression Anxiety Stress Scales*, Psychology Foundation, Sydney, Australia, 2nd edition, 1995.

[46] P. F. Lovibond and S. H. Lovibond, "The structure of negative emotional states: comparison of the depression anxiety stress scales (DASS) with the Beck Depression and Anxiety Inventories," *Behaviour Research and Therapy*, vol. 33, no. 3, pp. 335–343, 1995.

[47] L. Parkitny and J. McAuley, "The depression anxiety stress scale (DASS)," *Journal of Physiotherapy*, vol. 56, no. 3, p. 204, 2010.

[48] M. K. Nicholas, C. M. Coulston, A. Asghari, and G. S. Malhi, "Depressive symptoms in patients with chronic pain," *Medical Journal of Australia*, vol. 190, no. 7, pp. S66–S70, 2009.

[49] D. W. Kissane, S. G. Patel, R. E. Baser et al., "Preliminary evaluation of the reliability and validity of the Shame and Stigma Scale in head and neck cancer," *Head & Neck*, vol. 35, no. 2, pp. 172–183, 2013.

[50] M. Clayer, S. Doyle, N. Sangha, and R. Grimer, "The toronto extremity salvage score in unoperated controls: an age, gender, and country comparison," *Sarcoma*, vol. 2012, Article ID 717213, 5 pages, 2012.

[51] R. Nagarajan, D. R. Clohisy, J. P. Neglia et al., "Function and quality-of-life of survivors of pelvic and lower extremity osteosarcoma and Ewing's sarcoma: the Childhood Cancer Survivor Study," *British Journal of Cancer*, vol. 91, no. 11, pp. 1858–1865, 2004.

[52] N. K. Aaronson, S. Ahinedzai, B. Bergman et al., "The European Organization for Research and Treatment of Cancer QLQ-C30: a quality-of-life instrument for use in international clinical trials in oncology," *Journal of the National Cancer Institute*, vol. 85, no. 5, pp. 365–376, 1993.

[53] B. A. Morrison, "Soft tissue sarcomas of the extremities," *Baylor University Medical Center Proceedings*, vol. 16, no. 3, p. 285, 2003.

[54] A. Shehadeh, M. E. Dahleh, A. Salem et al., "Standardization of rehabilitation after limb salvage surgery for sarcomas improves patients' outcome," *Hematology/Oncology and Stem Cell Therapy*, vol. 6, no. 3-4, pp. 105–111, 2013.

[55] S. A. Imes, P. R. Clance, A. T. Gailis, and E. Atkeson, "Mind's response to the body's betrayal: gestalt/existential therapy for clients with chronic or life-threatening illnesses," *Journal of Clinical Psychology*, vol. 58, no. 11, pp. 1361–1373, 2002.

[56] L. Palmer, S. Erickson, T. Shaffer, C. Koopman, M. Amylon, and H. Steiner, "Themes arising in group therapy for adolescents with cancer and their parents," *International Journal of Rehabilitation and Health*, vol. 5, no. 1, pp. 43–54, 1999.

[57] R. Thomas-MacLean, A. Towers, E. Quinlan et al., ""This is a kind of betrayal": a qualitative study of disability after breast cancer," *Current Oncology*, vol. 16, no. 3, pp. 26–32, 2009.

[58] C. Snöbohm, M. Friedrichsen, and S. Heiwe, "Experiencing one's body after a diagnosis of cancer—a phenomenological study of young adults," *Psycho-Oncology*, vol. 19, no. 8, pp. 863–869, 2010.

[59] D. K. Payne, J. C. Lundberg, M. F. Brennan, and J. C. Holland, "A psychosocial intervention for patients with soft tissue sarcoma," *Psycho-Oncology*, vol. 6, no. 1, pp. 65–71, 1997.

[60] AIHW AIoHaW, *Cancer in Adolescents and Young Adults in Australia*, AIHW, Canberra, Australia, 2011.

[61] K. M. Trevino, P. K. Maciejewski, K. Fasciano et al., "Coping and psychological distress in young adults with advanced cancer," *The Journal of Supportive Oncology*, vol. 10, no. 3, pp. 124–130, 2012.

[62] A. Rosen, K. A. Rodriguez-Wallberg, and L. Rosenzweig, Eds., *Psychosocial Distress in Young Cancer Survivors*, Elsevier, New York, NY, USA, 2009.

[63] M.-D. Tabone, C. Rodary, O. Oberlin, J.-C. Gentet, H. Pacquement, and C. Kalifa, "Quality of life of patients treated during childhood for a bone tumor: assessment by the Child Health Questionnaire," *Pediatric Blood and Cancer*, vol. 45, no. 2, pp. 207–211, 2005.

[64] B. D. Kennard, S. M. Stewart, R. Olvera et al., "Nonadherence in adolescent oncology patients: Preliminary data on psychological risk factors and relationships to outcome," *Journal of Clinical Psychology in Medical Settings*, vol. 11, no. 1, pp. 31–39, 2004.

[65] S. Palmer, "Improving care for AYA patients treated within adult hospitals: what can be done right now?" *Cancer Forum*, vol. 33, no. 1, pp. 22–25, 2009.

[66] A. Girgis, A. Boyes, R. W. Sanson-Fisher, and S. Burrows, "Perceived needs of women diagnosed with breast cancer: rural versus urban location," *Australian and New Zealand Journal of Public Health*, vol. 24, no. 2, pp. 166–173, 2000.

[67] L. Von Essen, G. Larsson, K. Oberg, and P. O. Sjödén, "'Satisfaction with care': associations with health-related quality of life and psychosocial function among Swedish patients with endocrine gastrointestinal tumours," *European Journal of Cancer Care*, vol. 11, no. 2, pp. 91–99, 2002.

[68] C. M. Custodio, "Barriers to rehabilitation of patients with extremity sarcomas," *Journal of Surgical Oncology*, vol. 95, no. 5, pp. 393–399, 2007.

[69] S. Ponzer, U. Molin, S.-E. Johansson, B. Bergman, and H. Törnkvist, "Psychosocial support in rehabilitation after orthopedic injuries," *The Journal of Trauma*, vol. 48, no. 2, pp. 273–279, 2000.

[70] M. G. Paulsen, M. M. Dowsey, D. Castle, and P. F. M. Choong, "Preoperative psychological distress and functional outcome after knee replacement," *ANZ Journal of Surgery*, vol. 81, no. 10, pp. 681–687, 2011.

[71] E. A. Lingard and D. L. Riddle, "Impact of psychological distress on pain and function following knee arthroplasty," *The Journal of Bone and Joint Surgery Series A*, vol. 89, no. 6, pp. 1161–1169, 2007.

[72] B. A. Rhoten, B. Murphy, and S. H. Ridner, "Body image in patients with head and neck cancer: a review of the literature," *Oral Oncology*, vol. 49, no. 8, pp. 753–760, 2013.

[73] S. S. Larouche and L. Chin-Peuckert, "Changes in body image experienced by adolescents with cancer," *Journal of Pediatric Oncology Nursing*, vol. 23, no. 4, pp. 200–209, 2006.

[74] C. D. Murray and J. Fox, "Body image and prosthesis satisfaction in the lower limb amputee," *Disability & Rehabilitation*, vol. 24, no. 17, pp. 925–931, 2002.

[75] B. Rybarczyk, D. L. Nyenhuis, J. J. Nicholas, S. M. Cash, and J. Kaiser, "Body image, perceived social stigma, and the prediction of psychosocial adjustment to leg amputation," *Rehabilitation Psychology*, vol. 40, no. 2, pp. 95–110, 1995.

[76] J. W. Breakey, "Body image: the lower-limb amputee," *Journal of Prosthetics and Orthotics*, vol. 9, no. 2, pp. 58–66, 1997.

[77] N. Rumsey and D. Harcourt, "Body image and disfigurement: issues and interventions," *Body Image*, vol. 1, no. 1, pp. 83–97, 2004.

[78] J. S. Pendley, L. M. Dahlquist, and Z. Dreyer, "Body image and psychosocial adjustment in adolescent cancer survivors," *Journal of Pediatric Psychology*, vol. 22, no. 1, pp. 29–43, 1997.

[79] M. H. J. van den Beuken-van Everdingen, J. M. de Rijke, A. G. Kessels, H. C. Schouten, M. van Kleef, and J. Patijn, "Prevalence of pain in patients with cancer: a systematic review of the past 40 years," *Annals of Oncology*, vol. 18, no. 9, pp. 1437–1449, 2007.

[80] R. K. Portenoy and P. Lesage, "Management of cancer pain," *The Lancet*, vol. 353, no. 9165, pp. 1695–1700, 1999.

[81] D. A. Marcus, "Epidemiology of cancer pain," *Current Pain and Headache Reports*, vol. 15, no. 4, pp. 231–234, 2011.

[82] P. Y. Kuo, J. T. C. Yen, G. M. Parker et al., "The prevalence of pain in patients attending sarcoma outpatient clinics," *Sarcoma*, vol. 2011, Article ID 813483, 6 pages, 2011.

[83] M. A. Morgan, B. J. Small, K. A. Donovan, J. Overcash, and S. McMillan, "Cancer patients with pain: the spouse/partner relationship and quality of life," *Cancer Nursing*, vol. 34, no. 1, pp. 13–23, 2011.

[84] P. A. McGrath, "Psychological aspects of pain perception," *Archives of Oral Biology*, vol. 39, pp. S55–S62, 1994.

[85] D. R. Clohisy and P. W. Mantyh, "Bone cancer pain," *Cancer*, vol. 97, supplement 3, pp. 866–873, 2003.

[86] "State Government V. Victoria's cancer action plan 2008–2011," in *Cancer Strategy and Development IC, Wellbeing, Integrated Care and Ageing*, Health Do, Ed., Victorian Government, Department of Human Services, Melbourne, Australia, 2012.

[87] V. Wylde, S. Hewlett, I. D. Learmonth, and P. Dieppe, "Persistent pain after joint replacement: prevalence, sensory qualities, and postoperative determinants," *Pain*, vol. 152, no. 3, pp. 566–572, 2011.

[88] K. Soothill, S. M. Morris, J. Harman, B. Francis, C. Thomas, and M. B. McIllmurray, "The significant unmet needs of cancer patients: probing psychosocial concerns," *Supportive Care in Cancer*, vol. 9, no. 8, pp. 597–605, 2001.

[89] M. A. Ayerza, D. L. Muscolo, L. A. Aponte-Tinao, and G. Farfalli, "Effect of erroneous surgical procedures on recurrence and survival rates for patients with osteosarcoma," *Clinical Orthopaedics and Related Research*, no. 452, pp. 231–235, 2006.

[90] M. S. Kim, S.-Y. Lee, W. H. Cho et al., "Prognostic effects of doctor-associated diagnostic delays in osteosarcoma," *Archives of Orthopaedic and Trauma Surgery*, vol. 129, no. 10, pp. 1421–1425, 2009.

[91] T. I. Wang, P. K. Wu, C. F. Chen et al., "The prognosis of patients with primary osteosarcoma who have undergone unplanned therapy," *Japanese Journal of Clinical Oncology*, vol. 41, no. 11, pp. 1244–1250, 2011.

[92] M. S. Kim, S.-Y. Lee, W. H. Cho et al., "Prognostic effect of inadvertent curettage without treatment delay in osteosarcoma," *Journal of Surgical Oncology*, vol. 100, no. 6, pp. 484–487, 2009.

[93] M. Ayvaz and N. Fabbri, "Musculoskeletal tumors and sports injuries," in *Sports Injuries: Prevention, Diagnosis, Treatment and Rehabilitation*, M. N. Doral, Ed., pp. 973–979, Springer, Heidelberg, Germany, 2012.

[94] NBCC and NCCI, *Clinical Practice Guidelines for the Psychosocial Care of Adults with Cancer*, Centre NBC, Ed., NHMRC, Camperdown, Australia, 2003.

Validation of the SF-6D Health State Utilities Measure in Lower Extremity Sarcoma

Kenneth R. Gundle, Amy M. Cizik, Stephanie E. W. Punt, Ernest U. Conrad III, and Darin J. Davidson

Department of Orthopaedics & Sports Medicine, University of Washington Medical Center, 1959 Pacific Street NE, Box 356500, Seattle, WA 98195, USA

Correspondence should be addressed to Kenneth R. Gundle; kgundle@u.washington.edu

Academic Editor: Charles Catton

Aim. Health state utilities measures are preference-weighted patient-reported outcome (PRO) instruments that facilitate comparative effectiveness research. One such measure, the SF-6D, is generated from the Short Form 36 (SF-36). This report describes a psychometric evaluation of the SF-6D in a cross-sectional population of lower extremity sarcoma patients. *Methods.* Patients with lower extremity sarcoma from a prospective database who had completed the SF-36 and Toronto Extremity Salvage Score (TESS) were eligible for inclusion. Computed SF-6D health states were given preference weights based on a prior valuation. The primary outcome was correlation between the SF-6D and TESS. *Results.* In 63 pairs of surveys in a lower extremity sarcoma population, the mean preference-weighted SF-6D score was 0.59 (95% CI 0.4–0.81). The distribution of SF-6D scores approximated a normal curve (skewness = 0.11). There was a positive correlation between the SF-6D and TESS ($r = 0.75$, $P < 0.01$). Respondents who reported walking aid use had lower SF-6D scores (0.53 versus 0.61, $P = 0.03$). Five respondents underwent amputation, with lower SF-6D scores that approached significance (0.48 versus 0.6, $P = 0.06$). *Conclusions.* The SF-6D health state utilities measure demonstrated convergent validity without evidence of ceiling or floor effects. The SF-6D is a health state utilities measure suitable for further research in sarcoma patients.

1. Introduction

The inclusion of patient-reported outcomes (PRO) is essential to the evaluation of interventions, in order to elucidate the impact of illness and treatments on the patient experience. PRO measures of health state utilities are tools to directly elicit health-related quality of life (HRQL), and they will be pivotal in the advancement of comparative effectiveness research (CER). A recent effectiveness guidance document by the Center for Medical Technology Policy (CMTP) on incorporating patient-reported outcomes in oncology research recommends the inclusion of PRO in prospective clinical CER studies in oncology, assessment of HRQL, and use of a measure that enables cost-utility analysis [1].

The majority of PRO instruments were not designed for use in economic or value-based evaluation. Without explicitly incorporated patient preferences into the scoring algorithm, measures such as the Short-Form 36 (SF-36) [2, 3] assume equal intervals between response choices and assume that each item is of equal importance. Without an understanding of how a population values one state of health in comparison to others, the relative utility of an intervention cannot be determined. The clinical relevance of the resulting nonpreference-based scores can be challenging to ascertain.

Health state utilities are a type of PRO that merge a respondent's health status with a preference for that health state, generating a single value that facilitates comparisons among interventions, as well as disparate conditions [4, 5]. These measures provide a score ranging between 0, representing death, and 1, representing perfect health. According to utility theory, the score represents an indifference to two treatment options, one associated with maintaining the current health state and the other improving from the current state to perfect health, but also risking immediate death with a probability of 1-p, where p represents the health state score. Furthermore, health state utilities scores can be combined with time intervals to calculate quality-adjusted life years (QALYs) and enable cost-utility analyses [6–8].

Due to these capabilities, health state utility measures are gaining importance in outcomes research. One such measure, the SF-6D, may be generated from the widely utilized SF-36 quality of life PRO measure [3, 5, 9]. From the SF-36, eleven questions were selected and mapped to a six-dimensional health state classification. The dimensions are physical functioning, role limitations, social functioning, pain, mental health, and vitality; each dimension has between two and six possible levels. A total of 18,000 health states can be uniquely defined [10]. Then, using a sample of the general public who ranked and valued a subset of the possible health states via a standard gamble technique, it is possible to compute a preference-weighted value for each of the possible states [11]. These values may range between zero (worst possible state) and 1.0 (no problems in any dimension).

Health state utility measures such as the SF-6D have the potential to fulfill the CMTP recommendations as a general measure to assess HRQL and facilitate CER [12]. Before widespread use, PRO measures should demonstrate validity, reliability, responsiveness, and feasibility in the population of interest. Although health state utilities have been evaluated in many conditions and populations, to our knowledge, there has been little use in sarcoma. The purpose of this study was to evaluate the SF-6D in a population of sarcoma patients.

2. Patients and Methods

As part of an ongoing prospective cohort with Institutional Review Board approval, a cross-sectional sample of lower extremity sarcoma patients at an academic institution completed the SF-36 and TESS (Toronto Extremity Salvage Score) [13] between 2011 and 2012 and were eligible for inclusion. SF-6D health states were computed from the SF-36 and given preference weights based on a Bayesian modeling of a prior standard gamble valuation, as previously described [11]. Descriptive statistics evaluated possible floor or ceiling effects and skewness.

The primary outcome was the correlation between the SF-6D and the TESS, as a measure of convergent validity. A power analysis determined that 40 responses would be necessary to have an 80% chance of finding at least a 0.6 correlation. Statistical analysis was performed using Stata 11.0 (College Station, TX). Respondents also reported the use of a walking aid, and the SF-6D scores among those with and without walking aids were compared as a measure of face validity. Continuous variables were compared with a Student's t-test. Pearson linear regression was used to test for associations.

3. Results

Between 2011 and 2012, 55 patients completed 63 pairs of surveys. All patients with lower extremity sarcoma who had completed both the SF-36 and TESS were included. Patient characteristics are listed in Table 1. This heterogeneous cross-sectional sample included short- and long-term follow-up, a variety of diagnoses, and several combinations of treatment modalities. The sample included eleven patients with metastatic disease. Time from surgery included negative values, indicating participants who completed the surveys at time of diagnosis, prior to neoadjuvant treatment and surgery.

Table 1: Characteristics of study participants.

Characteristic	
n	63
Female gender	40 (63)
Tissue type	
Bone	25 (40)
Soft tissue	38 (60)
Grade	
1	15 (24)
2	19 (30)
3	29 (46)
Surgery type	
Limb salvage	58 (92)
Amputation	5 (8)
Use of chemotherapy	34 (54)
Use of radiation therapy	37 (59)
Days from surgery	713
Mean (SD)	543 (713)
Median (range)	278 (−86–3281)

Data are presented as n (%) unless otherwise indicated.

The mean preference weighted SF-6D score was 0.59 (95% CI 0.4–0.81). With a skewness of 0.11, the SF-6D scores closely fit a normal distribution (Figure 1). There was no significant difference in SF-6D in patients with metastatic disease ($P = 0.88$).

SF-6D correlated significantly with the TESS ($r = 0.75$, $P < 0.01$, Figure 2). The SF-6D correlated with the physical component scale (PCS) of the SF36 ($r = 0.79$, $P < 0.01$) as well as the mental component scale (MCS, $r = 0.39$, $P < 0.01$). While the TESS was correlated with the PCS ($r = 0.83$, $P < 0.01$), it was not significantly correlated with the MCS ($r = 0.1$, $P = 0.44$).

The SF-6D of 17 patients who reported any use of a walking aid was 0.53 (95% CI 0.48–0.59), significantly lower than those who used no ambulatory aid ($n = 38$, SF-6D = 0.61, 95% CI 0.57–0.65, $P = 0.03$). The TESS was also lower in patients reporting a walking aid (mean 59 versus 77, $P < 0.01$). The SF-6D score of 58 patients treated with limb salvage (0.6, 95% CI 0.56–0.63) was greater than the 5 patients who underwent amputation (0.48, 95% CI 0.30–0.68) but this did not achieve significance ($P = 0.06$).

4. Conclusions

The purpose of this study was to evaluate the validity of the SF-6D health state utility measure in a population of lower extremity sarcoma patients. Preference-based measures such as the SF-6D have the potential to facilitate comparative effectiveness research, and it is critical to establish the validity

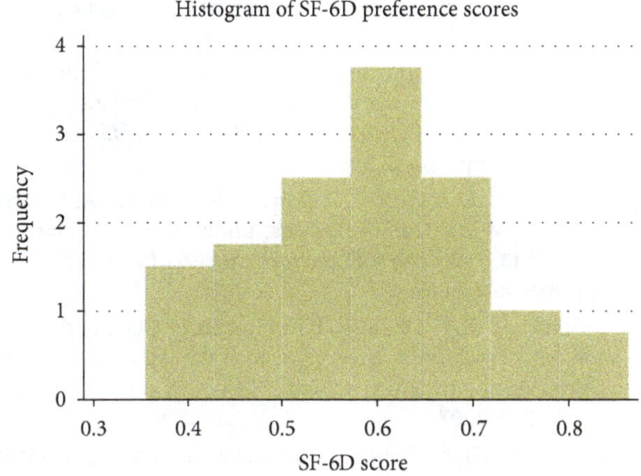

FIGURE 1: Histogram of SF-6D preference scores. Skewness = 0.11.

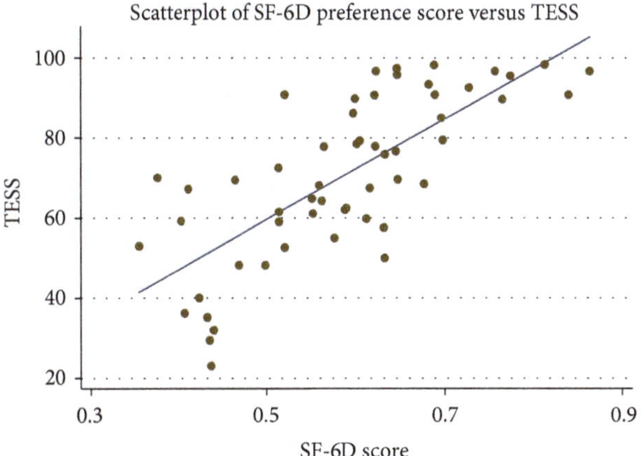

FIGURE 2: Plot of SF-6D preference scores versus TESS, with linear regression ($r = 0.75$, $P < 0.01$). TESS: Toronto Extremity Salvage Scale.

of PRO measures prior to their use in the population of interest.

In this population of lower extremity sarcoma patients, the SF-6D demonstrated convergent and face validity. The primary outcome was in correlation with the TESS, a widely used outcomes measure for extremity sarcoma. The significant positive correlation ($r = 0.75$, $P < 0.01$) between these measures is evidence of validity, as the SF-6D scores tracked appropriately across a range of TESS physical function scores. Low preference-weighted HRQL, as represented by the SF-6D results, were associated with lower physical function as represented by the TESS. And throughout the range of responses, as SF-6D scores rose so did the TESS. The TESS only assesses physical function in its content, and, unlike the SF-6D, the TESS did not correlate with the mental subscore of the SF-36. The ability to discriminate respondents with and without use of a walking aid also supports face validity of the SF-6D; this finding was convergent with the TESS. These results are consistent with the growing literature supporting the validity of the SF-6D in myriad conditions and populations [14–16].

Our finding of a close resemblance of SF-6D scores to a normal distribution in this population is important for its performance as an outcomes instrument. Significant floor or ceiling effects decrease the ability of a PRO to be sensitive to change during the course of a disease and following interventions. Previous studies have shown floor effects with the SF-6D [4, 16]. There was mild clustering at the lower end of the distribution in the present study, and patients with metastatic disease did not have a significant difference in SF-6D score. A larger sample that allows for meaningful analysis of comorbidities and burden of metastatic disease will be valuable to further assess potential floor effects of the SF-6D in this population. In contrast, the EuroQol Group's EQ-5D 3-level health state utilities measure [17] has demonstrated ceiling effects in several populations [18]. The EQ-5D has five questions, each representing a domain of health, and is scored between one and three, yielding 243 potential health states. For example, in populations with asthma or chronic obstructive pulmonary disease, over a quarter of respondents had a perfect utility score of 1.0 on the EQ-5D, while only 1 of 228 had a 1.0 utility score with the SF-6D [15]. In our study, no respondents had an SF-6D utility of 1.0, and the skewness of 0.11 reflects the near normal score distribution. High percentages of respondents scoring the top health state in the EQ-5D may also reflect insensitivity to less severe degrees of morbidity. In studies comparing these two health state utilities, there is a trend for EQ-5D scores to be higher than the SF-6D [16], and these differences can influence whether an intervention is considered cost-effective [19]. The more recently developed 5-level EQ-5D measure may be associated with fewer ceiling effects, but this has not yet been fully evaluated [20].

There are several limitations to consider. The cross-sectional, retrospective design includes a heterogeneous patient population in terms of time from surgery, type of sarcoma, and modes of treatment. This does, however, provide a sample that is representative of the different stages of treatment at which outcomes are determined. Furthermore, oncologic outcomes including recurrence and response to treatment were not assessed. While appropriate for an initial study investigating fundamental psychometric properties, no one study can establish validity. Important properties, including test-retest reliability, minimum clinically important difference, and magnitude of change, could not be established with the chosen design and require future study.

Assessing the HRQL impact of treatment decisions, such as limb salvage versus amputation, is central to the aims of reporting PRO measures. The present study had only 8% (5/63) patients treated with amputation, a subgroup too small for meaningful analysis. Further studies utilizing the SF-6D will likely contribute to this literature.

Health state utilities have the potential to facilitate comparative effectiveness research and economic modeling that incorporate patient experiences and preferences. PRO instruments with these capabilities are being recommended for all prospective oncology studies [1]. While the SF-6D can utilize the wealth of prior work and experience with the SF-36, no single health state utility measure has been convincingly proven superior [21]. This preliminary study supports the use of the SF-6D health state utilities measure in sarcoma patients, and further evaluation in a prospective cohort is warranted.

References

[1] E. Basch, A. P. Abernethy, C. D. Mullins et al., "Recommendations for incorporating patient-reported outcomes into clinical comparative effectiveness research in adult oncology," *Journal of Clinical Oncology*, vol. 30, no. 34, pp. 4249–4255, 2012.

[2] J. E. Ware, K. K. Snow, M. Kosinski, and B. Gandek, *New England Medical Center Hospital*, SF-36 Health Survey, Health Institute, Cambridge, Mass, USA, 1993.

[3] A. A. Patel, D. Donegan, and T. Albert, "The 36-item short form," *Journal of the American Academy of Orthopaedic Surgeons*, vol. 15, no. 2, pp. 126–134, 2007.

[4] J. A. Kopec and K. D. Willison, "A comparative review of four preference-weighted measures of health-related quality of life," *Journal of Clinical Epidemiology*, vol. 56, no. 4, pp. 317–325, 2003.

[5] J. W. Shaw, J. A. Johnson, and S. J. Coons, "US valuation of the EQ-5D health states: development and testing of the D1 valuation model," *Medical Care*, vol. 43, no. 3, pp. 203–220, 2005.

[6] G. W. Torrance, "Measurement of health state utilities for economic appraisal: a review," *Journal of Health Economics*, vol. 5, no. 1, pp. 1–30, 1986.

[7] A. Parthan, M. Kruse, N. Yurgin, J. Huang, H. N. Viswanathan, and D. Taylor, "Cost effectiveness of denosumab versus oral bisphosphonates for postmenopausal osteoporosis in the US," *Appl Health Econ Health Policy*, vol. 11, no. 5, pp. 485–497, 2013.

[8] D. H. Solomon, A. R. Patrick, J. Schousboe, and E. Losina, "The potential economic benefits of improved post-fracture care: a cost-effectiveness analysis of a fracture liaison service in the US health care system," *Journal of Bone and Mineral Research*, 2014.

[9] A. L. Stewart, R. D. Hays, and J. E. Ware Jr., "The MOS short-form general health survey. Reliability and validity in a patient population," *Medical Care*, vol. 26, no. 7, pp. 724–735, 1988.

[10] J. Brazier, J. Roberts, and M. Deverill, "The estimation of a preference-based measure of health from the SF-36," *Journal of Health Economics*, vol. 21, no. 2, pp. 271–292, 2002.

[11] S. A. Kharroubi, J. E. Brazier, J. Roberts, and A. O'Hagan, "Modelling SF-6D health state preference data using a nonparametric Bayesian method," *Journal of Health Economics*, vol. 26, no. 3, pp. 597–612, 2007.

[12] S. Bhinder, N. Chowdhury, J. Granton et al., "Feasibility of internet-based health-related quality of life data collection in a large patient cohort," *Journal of Medical Internet Research*, vol. 12, no. 3, p. e35, 2010.

[13] A. M. Davis, J. G. Wright, J. I. Williams, C. Bombardier, A. Griffin, and R. S. Bell, "Development of a measure of physical function for patients with bone and soft tissue sarcoma," *Quality of Life Research*, vol. 5, no. 5, pp. 508–516, 1996.

[14] I. Atroshi, C. Gummesson, S. J. McCabe, and E. Ornstein, "The SF-6D health utility index in carpal tunnel syndrome," *Journal of Hand Surgery*, vol. 32, no. 2, pp. 198–202, 2007.

[15] J. Tosh, J. Brazier, P. Evans, and L. Longworth, "A review of generic preference-based measures of health-related quality of life in visual disorders," *Value in Health*, vol. 15, no. 1, pp. 118–127, 2012.

[16] J. Brazier, J. Roberts, A. Tsuchiya, and J. Busschbach, "A comparison of the EQ-5D and SF-6D across seven patient groups," *Health Economics*, vol. 13, no. 9, pp. 873–884, 2004.

[17] R. Brooks and F. de Charro, "EuroQol: the current state of play," *Health Policy*, vol. 37, no. 1, pp. 53–72, 1996.

[18] A. Szende, N. K. Leidy, E. Ståhl, and K. Svensson, "Estimating health utilities in patients with asthma and COPD: evidence on the performance of EQ-5D and SF-6D," *Quality of Life Research*, vol. 18, no. 2, pp. 267–272, 2009.

[19] T. H. Sach, G. R. Barton, C. Jenkinson, M. Doherty, A. J. Avery, and K. R. Muir, "Comparing cost-utility estimates: does the choice of EQ-5D or SF-6D matter?" *Medical Care*, vol. 47, no. 8, pp. 889–894, 2009.

[20] A. S. Pickard, M. C. De Leon, T. Kohlmann, D. Cella, and S. Rosenbloom, "Psychometric comparison of the standard EQ-5D to a 5 level version in cancer patients," *Medical Care*, vol. 45, no. 3, pp. 259–263, 2007.

[21] D. G. T. Whitehurst, S. Bryan, and M. Lewis, "Systematic review and empirical comparison of contemporaneous EQ-5D and SF-6D group mean scores," *Medical Decision Making*, vol. 31, no. 6, pp. E34–E44, 2011.

7

Age, Tumor Characteristics, and Treatment Regimen as Event Predictors in Ewing: A Children's Oncology Group Report

Neyssa Marina,[1] Linda Granowetter,[2] Holcombe E. Grier,[3] Richard B. Womer,[4] R. Lor Randall,[5] Karen J. Marcus,[6] Elizabeth McIlvaine,[7,8] and Mark Krailo[7,8]

[1] *Department of Pediatrics, Stanford University and Lucile Packard Children's Hospital, 1000 Welch Road, Suite 300, Palo Alto, CA 94304-1812, USA*
[2] *Department of Pediatrics, New York University, Langone Medical Center, New York, NY 10016, USA*
[3] *Pediatric Hematology-Oncology, Dana Farber & Boston Children's Hospital, 44 Binney Street, Boston, MA 02115, USA*
[4] *Division of Oncology, Children's Hospital of Philadelphia, Philadelphia, PA 19104, USA*
[5] *Sarcoma Services, Huntsman Cancer Institute and Primary Children's Medical Center Department of Orthopaedics, University of Utah, Salt Lake City, UT 84112, USA*
[6] *Department of Radiation Oncology, Boston Children's Hospital/Dana Farber Cancer Institute Brigham and Women's Hospital, Harvard Medical School, Boston, MA 02115, USA*
[7] *Department of Preventive Medicine, University of Southern California, Los Angeles, CA 90027, USA*
[8] *Children's Oncology Group Statistics, Monrovia, CA 91016, USA*

Correspondence should be addressed to Neyssa Marina; nmarina@stanford.edu

Academic Editor: Akira Kawai

Purpose. To associate baseline patient characteristics and relapse across consecutive COG studies. *Methods.* We analyzed risk factors for LESFT patients in three randomized COG trials. We evaluated age at enrollment, primary site, gender, tumor size, and treatment (as randomized). We estimated event-free survival (EFS, Kaplan-Meier) and compared risk across groups (log-rank test). Characteristics were assessed by proportional hazards regression with the characteristic of interest as the only component. Confidence intervals (CI) for RR were derived. Factors related to outcome at level 0.05 were included in a multivariate regression model. *Results.* Between 12/1988 and 8/2005, 1444 patients were enrolled and data current to 2001, 2004, or 2008 were used. Patients were with a median age of 12 years (0–45), 55% male and 88% Caucasian. The 5-year EFS was 68.3% ± 1.3%. In univariate analysis age, treatment, and tumor location were identified for inclusion in the multivariate model, and all remained significant ($p < 0.01$). Since tumor size was not collected in the last study, the other two were reanalyzed. This model identified age, treatment, tumor location, and tumor size as significant predictors. *Conclusion.* Age > 18 years, pelvic tumor, size > 8 cms, and chemotherapy without ifosfamide/etoposide significantly predict worse outcome. AEWS0031 is NCT00006734, INT0091 and INT0054 designed before 1993 (unregistered).

1. Introduction

The 5-year event-free survival (EFS) for nonmetastatic Ewing sarcoma patients has improved to 60–70% [1–6], but 2-year survival for patients that relapse is 20–30% [7, 8]. Identifying factors predicting relapse may help develop new strategies for those patients. Other studies have consistently identified tumor location [3, 9–12] and age [9, 11–15] as EFS predictors. Factors less consistently identified include lactic dehydrogenase [9, 10, 13], histologic response [9, 13, 14, 16], tumor volume [3, 6, 13, 14, 16, 17], tumor size [12, 18], and surgical margins [19]. Histological response and surgical margin accurately predict risk of recurrence but because they can only be determined after chemotherapy and surgical resection, they cannot help identify potential new strategies for patients at the time of diagnosis.

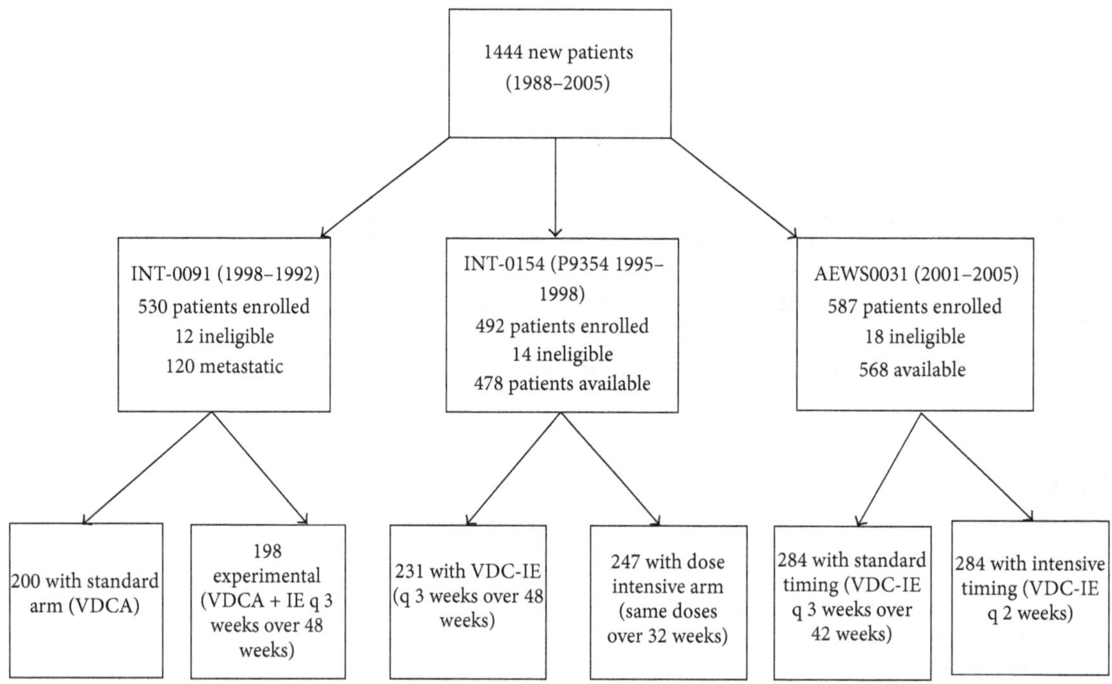

FIGURE 1: CONSORT diagram for 1444 patients enrolled in three consecutive COG studies. The arms to which patients were randomized are shown along with exclusion criteria and those patients who were thereby ineligible. CONSORT = Consolidated Standards of Reporting Trials; COG = Children's Oncology Group.

The Children's Oncology Group (COG) and its predecessors conducted three studies (1988–2005) for newly diagnosed localized Ewing sarcoma (ES) or peripheral primitive neuroectodermal tumor (PNET) of bone [1, 2, 5] and/or soft tissue. These studies included 1444 patients and used common chemotherapy agents. Most of the protocols' eligibility criteria overlapped and the schedule and evaluation methods were similar. They carried forward "standard" therapies for comparison. This series represents a group of patients who are homogeneous except for the patient/treatment factors examined in this analysis, reducing the likelihood that observed associations are attributable to historical changes in patients or evaluation methods.

We sought to pool the high-quality dataset represented by those COG trials [1, 2, 5] to identify (1) demographic (i.e., age and sex), (2) treatment-related (assigned chemotherapy), and (3) tumor-related factors (tumor size and location) associated with EFS.

2. Patients and Methods

2.1. Studies. We analysed selected factors at study enrolment for 1444 patients treated in three COG studies: (1) INT-0091 [1]; (2) INT-0154 [2]; and (3) AEWS0031 [5] (Figure 1). The INT-0091 study enrolled patients between 1988 and 1992 [1]; the INT-0154 enrolled patients between 1995 and 1998 [2]; while the most recent study (AEWS0031) enrolled patients between 2001 and 2005 [5]. Details of the three studies have been previously published [1, 2, 5].

Briefly, patients < 30 years of age with newly diagnosed, histologically confirmed primary ES or PNET were eligible for enrolment in INT-0091 [1]. Eligible patients were randomized to treatment with vincristine, doxorubicin, and cyclophosphamide (VDC), with or without ifosfamide and etoposide (IE). Although the study included patients with metastatic disease, those patients are not considered in our analysis. Patients < 30 years with newly diagnosed, histologically confirmed ES or peripheral PNET of bone or soft tissue were eligible for enrolment in INT-0154 and were randomized to dose-intensified or standard therapy (Figure 1) [2]. The dose-intensified arm of the study administered the same total doses of chemotherapy every 3 weeks over 32 rather than 48 weeks. Patients < 50 years with newly diagnosed, histologically confirmed ES or peripheral PNET of bone or soft tissue were eligible for enrollment in AEWS0031 and were randomized to receive the same chemotherapy doses every 2 weeks (dose-dense) or every 3 weeks (standard therapy) [5].

2.2. Treatment

2.2.1. Chemotherapy. The standard chemotherapy doses included the following: VCD—vincristine 2 mg/m^2 (2 mg maximum dose), doxorubicin 75 mg/m^2/dose (either as a single bolus, two daily boluses, or 48 h continuous infusion), and cyclophosphamide 1200 mg/m^2, followed by mesna uroprotection. Dactinomycin 1.25 mg/m^2/d was substituted for doxorubicin when a total doxorubicin dose of 375 mg/m^2 was reached in INT-0091. Courses of IE included ifosfamide

1800 mg/m^2/d for 5 days, given with mesna uroprotection and etoposide 100 mg/m^2/d over the same 5 days.

2.2.2. Local Control. The studies prescribed local control following 12 weeks of therapy, which in the first two studies [1, 2] and in the control arm of the third study included four cycles of chemotherapy but followed 6 cycles in the experimental arm (every-2-week treatment) of the third study [5]. Although the choice of local control was left up to the treating physician, all protocols provided guidelines [1, 2, 5]. The protocols allowed surgery for tumors deemed resectable. For radiotherapy alone, the initial tumor volume (soft-tissue and osseous tumor extent) with a 3 cm margin was treated with 4500 cGy, followed by reduction in treatment volume to the postchemotherapy, preradiotherapy tumor for 1080 cGy more (total dose 5580 cGy). A smaller margin was allowed to avoid radiation to the epiphysis. Patients with residual tumor after surgery were irradiated using the dose-volume guidelines for gross residual disease; for microscopic residual disease, irradiation was limited to 4500 cGy to the original volume with a 1 cm margin. No supplemental radiotherapy was administered to patients achieving a complete resection of the primary tumor with clear margins regardless of extent of necrosis or tumor size. For patients with extraosseous tumors and a complete response to induction chemotherapy, the initial tumor volume plus a 2 cm margin received 4500 cGy followed by a boost of 540 cGy with a 1 cm margin (total dose 5040 cGy).

2.3. Statistical Methods. We defined EFS as the time from study entry until the occurrence of an analytic event or date of last contact, whichever came first. An analytic event was defined as disease progression, diagnosis of second malignant neoplasm (SMN), or patient death prior to the development of disease progression or SMN. A patient who had not experienced an event by the date of last follow-up was censored.

Exploratory analysis was complicated by the fact that some data were not collected in all studies and even when intended to be collected some data were missing. The major sources and types of missing data were as follows: (1) INT-0091 excluded patients with extraosseous ES from enrollment; (2) in AEWS0031 tumor size was not collected; and (3) tumor size was not reported for 266 participants in the other two studies. We therefore excluded tumor size and soft-tissue ES from our first multivariate model. Participants whose data were truly missing (request for data present but not provided by the institutional investigators) were also eliminated from the analysis.

The distributions of EFS and overall survival were estimated by the method of Kaplan and Meier [20]. Risk of adverse event was compared across groups, defined by treatment or prognostic factors using the log-rank test. Comparisons involving the chemotherapy randomizations were conducted with patients' outcomes assigned to their randomized treatment arm at enrollment (intent-to-treat analyses). The prognostic significance and associated RR for various patient characteristics measured at study entry were assessed by a proportional hazards regression model with the characteristic of interest as the only component. Confidence intervals (CI) for RRs were derived from the proportional hazards regression model [21]. In addition, a likelihood ratio test was performed to confirm the homogeneity of model parameters across studies. The likelihood ratio test statistic was constructed by comparing the likelihood from the stratified Cox regression model fitting common risk coefficients stratified by study (assumes model parameters are not different across strata) with the likelihood of the Cox regression fitting study-specific risk coefficients.

Only potential prognostic factors measured at study enrollment were assessed in the dataset. In particular, the relationship between risks of an event and death and local control modalities were not analyzed. The potential prognostic factors considered included the following: (1) patient age at enrollment; (2) site of primary tumor; and (3) patient sex. Age at enrollment was categorized.

All the factors noted above were explored further to assess their relative prognostic effects when considered jointly. To determine whether tumor size had an impact on outcome using COG-directed therapy, we performed a second multivariate analysis including only patients enrolled in INT-0091 and INT-0154, where tumor size in two perpendicular dimensions was requested but not required for eligibility. This allowed us to determine whether tumor size was an independent predictor of EFS using US treatment (in COG). For this analysis, tumor size was categorized.

3. Results

A total of 1444 patients were enrolled in INT-0091, INT-0154, and AEWS0031 between December 1988 and August 2005 (Figure 1). The INT-0091 trial opened in December 1988 and closed in November 1992. Data current to August 2001 were used for our analysis, which included 395 eligible patients. The INT-0154 trial opened in March 1995 and closed in September 1998. Data current to December 2006 were used for our analysis, which included 477 eligible patients. The AEWS0031 trial opened in May 2001 and closed in August 2005. Data current to March 2009 were used for our analysis, which included 568 eligible patients. Baseline characteristics included a median age of 12 years (range, 0–45), and 55% of patients were male (see Table 1 for details).

The 5-year EFS for the 1444 patients enrolled in the three studies was 68.3% ± 1.3% (Figure 2). The 5-year EFS for INT-0091, INT-0054, and AEWS0031 was 61.5% ± 2.5%, 71% ± 2.1%, and 70% ± 2.6%, respectively. The risk for an EFS event differed significantly across studies ($p = 0.0071$). This is likely driven by the absence of IE in the control arm of INT-0091, since INT-0154 and AEWS0031 have very similar EFS.

As seen in Table 2, the RR of an event using the intensively timed treatment of AEWS0031 relative to the standard timing is 0.75 (0.5–1.01) confirming that intensively timed therapy reduced event risk compared to standard-dose-and-timing IE or non-IE containing treatment across the studies. In this pooled analysis, the confidence intervals cross 1 ($p = 0.061$) and are just outside conventional statistical significance.

TABLE 1: Characteristics of 1444 patients enrolled in COG studies.

Factor	Study			
	INT-0091	INT-0154 (P9354)	AEWS0031	Total
Number of patients	398	478	568	1444
Median age, years (range)	12 (0–28)	12 (0–30)	12 (0–45)	12 (0–45)
<9 years, n (%)	121 (30)	148 (31)	162 (28)	431 (29.9)
9–18 years	227 (57)	265 (55)	339 (60)	831 (57.6)
>18 years	50 (13)	65 (14)	67 (12)	182 (12.6)
Sex, %				
Men	57	55	54	55
Women	43	45	46	45
Primary sites, n (%)				
Appendicular	188 (47)	175 (36)	195 (34)	558 (39)
Thoracic	69 (17)	75 (16)	89 (16)	233 (16)
Pelvic	93 (23)	70 (15)	90 (16)	253 (18)
Other axial	48 (12)	57 (12)	75 (13)	180 (12)
Extraosseous	—	94 (20)	119 (21)	213 (15)
Missing	0 (0)	7 (1.5)	0 (0)	7 (0.48)
Tumor size, n (%)				
<8 cm	155 (30)	141 (29.5)	0 (0)	296 (10)
9–12 cm	113 (28)	98 (21)	0 (0)	211 (15)
>13 cm	64 (16)	39 (8.2)	0 (0)	93 (7)
Not reported	66 (17)	200 (42)	568 (100)	834 (57.8)

COG = Children's Oncology Group.

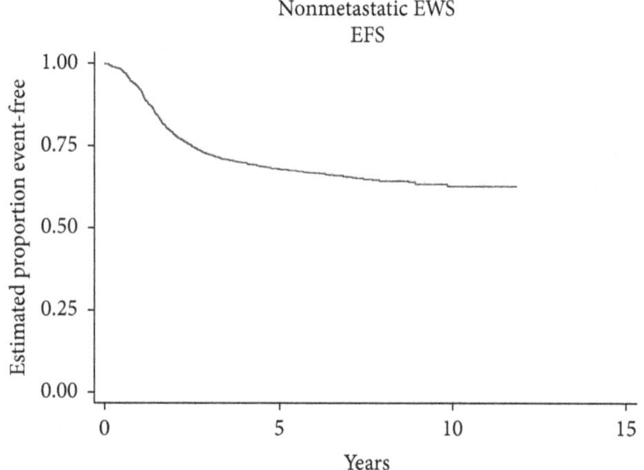

FIGURE 2: EFS for 1444 patients enrolled in consecutive COG trials. The 5-year EFS for the group was 68.32% ± 1.3%. EFS = event-free survival; COG = Children's Oncology Group.

Additionally, the RR of an event using the non-IE arm of INT-0091 relative to the standard timing arm of AEWS0031 is 1.5 (1.12–2). This confirms the inferiority of non-IE containing regimens as the risk of an event is 50% higher in those patients. The RRs are similar for patients in the standard timing IE treatments.

Univariate analysis identified three variables for consideration in assessing the relative values of prognostic factors measured at study enrollment (Table 3): (1) patient age at enrollment (≤9 years, 10–17 years, and ≥18 years); (2) assigned treatment (intensive-timing IE, standard timing IE, and non-IE); and (3) tumor location (pelvis, nonpelvic bone).

Table 4 presents the results of the multivariate analysis including the estimated risk coefficients and 95% confidence intervals. Patient age at enrollment remains a significant predictor of EFS, and patients ≥ 18 years have greater than a twofold increased risk of an event (RR 2.14 (CI 1.59–2.87, $p = 0.000$)) compared to patients ≤ 9 years.

Tumor location and assigned treatment also retain their role as significant predictors of EFS in the presence of one another. Patients with a pelvic tumor have a higher event risk RR 1.34 (1.07–1.67) than patients with nonpelvic tumors. Assigned treatment was also an important predictor of outcome and patients treated with non-IE containing treatment had an increased event risk RR 1.84 (1.33–2.53). In our multivariate analysis, risk of event was unrelated to patient sex. The estimates of the effects of age, tumor site, and treatment did not differ significantly between trials ($p = 0.2587$).

We also evaluated whether tumor size and tumor location were both predictive of outcome by performing a second multivariate analysis including only patients treated in INT-0091 and INT-0154. As shown in Table 5, age, tumor location, non-IE treatment, and tumor size were all significant predictors of EFS. In this analysis patients ≥ 18 years have a twofold event risk compared to younger patients (RR 1.97 (1.33–2.93)). Patients treated with a non-IE regimen have

TABLE 2: EFS risk by treatment arm relative to standard treatment in AEWS0031.

Treatment	Hazard ratio	Std. error	Z	$p > z$	Confidence intervals	
AEWS0031-ST	1.00					
AEWS0031-IT	0.7488	0.1157	−1.87	0.061	0.5532	1.0135
INT-0154-HD	0.8805	0.1339	−0.84	0.4020	0.6536	1.1861
INT-0154-SD	0.8034	0.1271	−1.38	0.1660	0.5891	1.0955
INT-0091-IE	0.9613	0.1527	−0.25	0.8040	0.7042	1.3123
INT-0091-Std.	1.5064	0.2212	2.79	0.0050	1.1296	2.0088

TABLE 3: Estimated risk coefficients on univariate analysis for 1444 patients treated in consecutive COG studies.

Factor	Characteristic	Relative risk	95% confidence interval	p value compared reference	Global p value
Age yrs. (ref. <9)					0.0000
	10–17	1.34	1.08–1.66	0.0090	
	18+	2.35	1.78–3.11	0.0000	
Primary site (ref. pelvis)					0.0002
	Nonpelvic tumor	0.70	0.52–0.93	0.0140	
	Extraosseous	0.52	0.37–0.72	0.0000	
Gender (ref. male)					0.3404
	Female	0.92	0.77–1.10	0.08	
Treatment (ref. standard timing)					0.0002
	Non-I/E	1.65	1.31–2.09	0.0000	
	Intensive timing	0.82	0.64–1.06	0.1260	
Tumor size, cm (ref. <8)					0.0002
	9–12 cm	1.26	0.96–1.65	0.0990	
	>13 cm	1.98	1.45–2.70	0.0000	

TABLE 4: Estimated risk coefficients for multivariate analysis excluding extraosseous patients ($N = 1231$).

Factor	Characteristic	Relative risk	95% confidence interval	p value compared to reference	Global p value
Age yrs. (ref. ≤9)					0.0000
	10–17	1.24	0.98–1.55	0.070	
	18+	2.14	1.59–2.87	0.000	
Primary site (ref. nonpelvic)					0.0110
	Pelvic tumor	1.34	1.07–1.67	0.009	
Treatment (ref. intensive timing)					0.0001
	Standard timing	1.13	0.86–1.48	0.384	
	Non-I/E	1.84	1.33–2.53	0.000	

TABLE 5: Estimated risk coefficients for patients treated in INT-0091 and INT-0154 (P9354) [excluding patients in AEWS0031] ($N = 716$).

Factor	Characteristic	Relative risk	95% confidence interval	p value compared reference	Global p value
Age yrs. (ref. ≤9)					0.0043
	10–17	1.27	0.93–1.72	0.130	
	18+	1.97	1.33–2.93	0.001	
Primary site (ref. nonpelvic)					0.0173
	Pelvic tumor	1.44	1.07–1.92	0.014	
Treatment (ref. standard timing)					0.0019
	Non-I/E	1.56	1.19–2.05	0.001	
Tumor size, cms (ref. <8)					0.0005
	9–12 cm	1.24	0.93–1.65	0.137	
	>13 cm	2.00	1.43–2.79	0.000	

a 56% higher event risk than those treated with IE regimens (RR 1.56 (1.19–2.05)). Importantly, both pelvic tumor location and tumor size are predictors of EFS in the presence of each other. Patients with pelvic tumors have a 44% increased risk of an event RR 1.44 (1.07–1.92) while patients with tumors > 13 cm have an event risk twofold higher than patients with tumors < 8 cm RR 2.00 (1.43–2.79).

4. Discussion

Previous studies have identified tumor location [3, 9–12] and age [9, 11–15] as consistent predictors of poor EFS. The two large series (>500 patients) [11, 13] assessing factors predicting relapse were both based on the European treatment approaches. The chemotherapy treatment and local control approaches in Europe differ from those in the United States. For instance, European investigators stratify patients based on tumor size [16, 17] and consider histological response to be the most important predictor of outcome [16, 22]. Therefore, we thought it important to evaluate demographic, treatment, and tumor characteristics for their impact on EFS using a large dataset of US treated patients.

Our study had several limitations related to its retrospective nature, including the fact that some patient characteristics were not missing at random. These included tumor size (not collected in AEWS0031) and patients with soft-tissue tumors (not included in INT-0091). We excluded these factors from our first multivariate model rather than employ methods to impute the missing information and adjust p values and confidence intervals accordingly. We also excluded any participants with missing data from our analysis. Our second multivariate analysis included only patients in INT-0091 and INT-0154 since tumor size was part of the data collection. This reduced dataset represents individuals where the initial data collection strategy included assessment of maximum tumor dimension. We consider this approach optimal for evaluating the relative importance of tumor size and tumor location in our studies.

We were able to confirm the importance of age ≥ 18 years as an independent predictor of worse EFS. Though older age has been consistently identified as predicting higher event rates in multiple series [9, 11, 13, 14], the age cutoff has varied from 12 to 15 years among those studies. This variability likely reflects the eligible patient population included in these studies. Additionally, a small study reported that older patients did as well as younger patients if treated with similar therapy [23]. Our analysis indicates that in the context of US-style therapy age ≥ 18 years is an important predictor of worse EFS. Our conclusions are limited by the small number of patients older than 25 years; therefore, continued enrollment of patients ≥ 18 years in randomized controlled trials will help further characterize the optimal age cutoff for predicting EFS.

Tumor location also predicted increased event risk; patients with pelvic primaries were particularly at high risk. This finding agrees with other studies of ES [1, 2, 11, 12, 15, 24] and is consistently used as a stratification factor in both European and North American studies. Determining whether the treatment of patients with pelvic tumors is better if they are treated with the combination of surgery and radiotherapy is difficult since randomization for this subset would not be feasible. European studies more frequently use a combination of surgery and radiotherapy for such patients. This strategy is one not frequently used in the United States, and EFS is similar suggesting that both approaches may be equivalent.

Assigned chemotherapy treatment was an important predictor of EFS in our study. As expected from results of our previous trials [1, 2], the EFS for patients treated with high- and standard-dose IE did not differ, but patients receiving non-IE containing therapy had a higher risk of an event with RR 1.63 (1.29–2.06). The use of IE with VDC has become part of the US standard treatment for patients with ES [1, 2, 5]. Additionally, in our analysis the RR of an event for patients treated with dose-dense therapy was 0.89 (0.67–1.16), consistent with a protective effect. However, this result does not achieve conventional statistical significance. The reference group (standard timing IE) is heterogeneous in that it included patients treated with increased doses of ifosfamide and cyclophosphamide. This is in contrast to the results of the COG randomized trial, which confirmed the importance of dose-dense therapy in improving EFS [5]. This phenomenon has been well documented in the literature and supports the contention that randomized controlled trials are the preferred method to evaluate the prognostic significance of interventions, where control can be exercised over factors that could confound the statistical comparison [25].

We were able to document the importance of tumor size in the context of tumor location in our second multivariate analysis (limited to INT-0091 and INT-0154), which revealed a twofold increased risk of an event for patients with tumors larger than 13 cm (RR 2.00 (1.44–2.79)). On average, patient risk appeared to increase with larger tumor size. The size of our population limited our sensitivity to these more subtle differences. Tumor size and/or volume have been identified in a number of studies as significant predictor of event risk [1, 3, 11–13, 16, 17] and have been incorporated into the current Euro-Ewing protocol where patients with estimated tumor volume greater than 200 mL [16, 17] are considered at high risk and are eligible for randomization to continuing standard chemotherapy versus intensification with the use of stem-cell transplant. The tumor cutoff of 200 mL used in European studies [13, 16, 17] is a smaller volume than the greater than 8 cm size used in North America (which corresponds to a 268 mL spherical tumor) [1, 12].

In conclusion, this is the largest series of US treated ES patients receiving a similar therapy backbone. We confirmed that primary tumor site (in the pelvis) and age ≥ 18 years are predictive of an increased event risk and should be considered at the time of treatment assignment. Patients ≥ 18 years and those with pelvic tumors might benefit from new treatment strategies. For example, chemoradiotherapy may allow resection for a larger number of pelvic tumors. Larger tumor size is also a predictor of worse EFS and should be included as a stratification factor in future US trials.

Disclosure

This work is presented in part at the Connective Tissue Oncology Society, October 2010, Paris, France.

Acknowledgments

This work is supported by Daniel P. Sullivan Fund (Rick Womer) and by the Children's Oncology Group Chair's Grant U10 CA98543 from the National Cancer Institute, National Institute of Health, Bethesda, MD, USA.

References

[1] H. E. Grier, M. D. Krailo, N. J. Tarbell et al., "Addition of ifosfamide and etoposide to standard chemotherapy for Ewing's sarcoma and primitive neuroectodermal tumor of bone," *The New England Journal of Medicine*, vol. 348, no. 8, pp. 694–701, 2003.

[2] L. Granowetter, R. Womer, M. Devidas et al., "Dose-intensified compared with standard chemotherapy for nonmetastatic Ewing sarcoma family of tumors: a children's oncology group study," *Journal of Clinical Oncology*, vol. 27, no. 15, pp. 2536–2541, 2009.

[3] H. Jurgens, V. Bier, J. Dunst, and et al, "The German Society of Pediatric Oncology Cooperative Ewing Sarcoma Studies CESS 81/86: report after 6 1/2 years," *Klinische Padiatrie*, vol. 200, no. 3, pp. 243–252, 1988.

[4] A. Craft, S. Cotterill, A. Malcolm et al., "Ifosfamide-containing chemotherapy in Ewing's sarcoma: the second United Kingdom Children's Cancer Study Group and the Medical Research Council Ewing's Tumor Study," *Journal of Clinical Oncology*, vol. 16, no. 11, pp. 3628–3633, 1998.

[5] R. B. Womer, D. C. West, M. D. Krailo et al., "Randomized controlled trial of interval-compressed chemotherapy for the treatment of localized ewing sarcoma: a report from the children's oncology group," *Journal of Clinical Oncology*, vol. 30, no. 33, pp. 4148–4154, 2012.

[6] H. Jurgens, U. Exner, H. Gadner et al., "Multidisciplinary treatment of primary Ewing's sarcoma of bone. A 6-year experience of a European Cooperative Trial," *Cancer*, vol. 61, no. 1, pp. 23–32, 1988.

[7] P. J. Leavey, L. Mascarenhas, N. Marina et al., "Prognostic factors for patients with Ewing sarcoma (EWS) at first recurrence following multi-modality therapy: a report from the children's oncology group," *Pediatric Blood and Cancer*, vol. 51, no. 3, pp. 334–338, 2008.

[8] C. Rodriguez-Galindo, C. A. Billups, L. E. Kun et al., "Survival after recurrence of Ewing tumors: the St. Jude children's research hospital experience, 1979–1999," *Cancer*, vol. 94, no. 2, pp. 561–569, 2002.

[9] G. Bacci, S. Ferrari, F. Bertoni et al., "Prognostic factors in nonmetastatic Ewing's sarcoma of bone treated with adjuvant chemotherapy: analysis of 359 patients at the Istituto Ortopedico Rizzoli," *Journal of Clinical Oncology*, vol. 18, no. 1, pp. 4–11, 2000.

[10] G. Bacci, S. Ferrari, A. Longhi et al., "Prognostic significance of serum LDH in Ewing's sarcoma of bone," *Oncology Reports*, vol. 6, no. 4, pp. 807–811, 1999.

[11] S. J. Cotterill, S. Ahrens, M. Paulussen et al., "Prognostic factors in Ewing's tumor of bone: analysis of 975 patients from the European Intergroup Cooperative Ewing's Sarcoma Study Group," *Journal of Clinical Oncology*, vol. 18, no. 17, pp. 3108–3114, 2000.

[12] C. Rodríguez-Galindo, T. Liu, M. J. Krasin et al., "Analysis of prognostic factors in Ewing sarcoma family of tumors: review of St. Jude Children's Research Hospital studies," *Cancer*, vol. 110, no. 2, pp. 375–384, 2007.

[13] G. Bacci, A. Longhi, S. Ferrari, M. Mercuri, M. Versari, and F. Bertoni, "Prognostic factors in non-metastatic Ewing's sarcoma tumor of bone: an analysis of 579 patients treated at a single institution with adjuvant or neoadjuvant chemotherapy between 1972 and 1998," *Acta Oncologica*, vol. 45, no. 4, pp. 469–475, 2006.

[14] R. D. Jenkin, I. Al-Fawaz, M. Al-Shabanah et al., "Localised Ewing sarcoma/PNET of bone—prognostic factors and international data comparison," *Medical and Pediatric Oncology*, vol. 39, no. 6, pp. 586–593, 2002.

[15] A. Argon, M. Basaran, F. Yaman et al., "Ewing's sarcoma of the axial system in patients older than 15 years: dismal prognosis despite intensive multiagent chemotherapy and aggressive local treatment," *Japanese Journal of Clinical Oncology*, vol. 34, no. 11, pp. 667–672, 2004.

[16] O. Oberlin, M. C. L. Deley, B. N. Bui et al., "Prognostic factors in localized Ewing's tumours and peripheral neuroectodermal tumours: the third study of the French Society of Paediatric Oncology (EW88 study)," *British Journal of Cancer*, vol. 85, no. 11, pp. 1646–1654, 2001.

[17] S. Ahrens, C. Hoffmann, S. Jabar et al., "Evaluation of prognostic factors in a tumor volume-adapted treatment strategy for localized Ewing Sarcoma of bone: the CESS 86 experience," *Medical & Pediatric Oncology*, vol. 32, no. 3, pp. 186–195, 1999.

[18] Y. Arai, L. E. Kun, M. T. Brooks et al., "Ewing's sarcoma: local tumor control and patterns of failure following limited-volume radiation therapy," *International Journal of Radiation Oncology, Biology, Physics*, vol. 21, no. 6, pp. 1501–1508, 1991.

[19] T. Ozaki, A. Hillmann, C. Hoffmann et al., "Significance of surgical margin on the prognosis of patients with Ewing's sarcoma. A report from the Cooperative Ewing's Sarcoma Study," *Cancer*, vol. 78, no. 4, pp. 892–900, 1996.

[20] E. L. Kaplan and P. Meier, "Nonparametric estimation from incomplete observations," *Journal of the American Statistical Association*, vol. 53, pp. 457–481, 1958.

[21] J. D. Kalbfleisch and R. L. Prentice, *The Statistical Analysis of Failure Time Data*, John Wiley & Sons, New York, NY, USA, 1980.

[22] P. Picci, T. Böhling, G. Bacci et al., "Chemotherapy-induced tumor necrosis as a prognostic factor in localized Ewing's sarcoma of the extremities," *Journal of Clinical Oncology*, vol. 15, no. 4, pp. 1553–1559, 1997.

[23] M. W. Verrill, I. R. Judson, C. L. Harmer, C. Fisher, J. M. Thomas, and E. Wiltshaw, "Ewing's sarcoma and primitive neuroectodermal tumor in adults: are they different from Ewing's sarcoma and primitive neuroectodermal tumor in children?" *Journal of Clinical Oncology*, vol. 15, no. 7, pp. 2611–2621, 1997.

[24] M. E. Nesbit Jr., E. A. Gehan, E. O. Burgert Jr. et al., "Multimodal therapy for the management of primary, nonmetastatic Ewing's Sarcoma of bone: a long-term follow-up of the first intergroup study," *Journal of Clinical Oncology*, vol. 8, no. 10, pp. 1664–1674, 1990.

[25] V. T. Farewell and G. J. D'Angio, "A simulated study of historical controls using real data," *Biometrics*, vol. 37, no. 1, pp. 169–176, 1981.

8

Cost Effectiveness of First-Line Treatment with Doxorubicin/Ifosfamide Compared to Trabectedin Monotherapy in the Management of Advanced Soft Tissue Sarcoma in Italy, Spain, and Sweden

Julian F. Guest,[1,2] Monica Panca,[1] Erikas Sladkevicius,[1] Nicholas Gough,[3] and Mark Linch[4]

[1] *Catalyst Health Economics Consultants, 34b High Street, Northwood, Middlesex HA6 1BN, UK*
[2] *School of Biomedical Sciences, King's College, London SE1 1UL, UK*
[3] *Palliative Care Department, Royal Marsden Hospital, London SW3 6JJ, UK*
[4] *Sarcoma Unit, Royal Marsden Hospital, London SW3 6JJ, UK*

Correspondence should be addressed to Julian F. Guest; julian.guest@catalyst-health.co.uk

Academic Editor: R. Pollock

Background. Doxorubicin/ifosfamide is a first-line systemic chemotherapy for the majority of advanced soft tissue sarcoma (ASTS) subtypes. Trabectedin is indicated for the treatment of ASTS after failure of anthracyclines and/or ifosfamide; however it is being increasingly used off-label as a first-line treatment. This study estimated the cost effectiveness of these two treatments in the first-line management of ASTS in Italy, Spain, and Sweden. *Methods.* A Markov model was constructed to estimate the cost effectiveness of doxorubicin/ifosfamide compared to trabectedin monotherapy, defined as the cost per QALY gained, in each country. *Results.* First-line treatment with doxorubicin/ifosfamide resulted in lower two-year healthcare costs and more QALYs than first-line treatment with trabectedin monotherapy in all three countries. Probabilistic sensitivity analysis showed that at a cost per QALY threshold of €35,000, >90% of a cohort would be cost effectively treated with doxorubicin/ifosfamide compared to trabectedin monotherapy in all three countries. *Conclusion.* Within the model's limitations, first-line treatment of patients with ASTS with doxorubicin/ifosfamide instead of trabectedin monotherapy affords a cost-effective use of publicly funded healthcare resources in Italy, Spain, and Sweden and is therefore the preferred treatment in all three countries. These findings support the recommendation that trabectedin should remain a second-line treatment.

1. Introduction

Soft tissue sarcomas are a heterogeneous group of rare malignant tumours originating from connective tissue [1, 2] which account for approximately 1% of all adult cancers [3]. Their incidence in the European population is 3 to 4 new cases per 100,000 which has remained stable over time [3]. The risk of developing soft tissue sarcoma increases with age and the disease mostly develops in people over 50 years [4]. Soft tissue sarcomas commonly occur in the extremities (50% of patients), trunk/retroperitoneum (40%), or the head and neck (10%) [5]; they generally develop without pain and can be difficult to diagnose. Prognosis depends on several factors, including patients' age and the size, depth, histologic grade, and stage of the tumour [2, 6]. Curative treatment largely consists of radical surgery and/or radiotherapy. However, these tumours are often aggressive and over 50% of soft tissue sarcoma patients develop metastases [7, 8].

Patients with advanced soft tissue sarcoma (ASTS) present with either locally advanced "inoperable" or metastatic disease [9]. With some exceptions, patients with ASTS are generally considered incurable and have poor long-term survival. Moreover, histological subtypes differ in their sensitivity to cytotoxic drugs [10]. Consequently, patient selection for an appropriate treatment strategy requires expert multidisciplinary team involvement [11, 12].

Palliative chemotherapy is the mainstay of treatment for ASTS where the aim is to establish disease control and improve both quantity and quality of life. Sarcomas have proved resistant to many conventional cytotoxic therapies with only doxorubicin and ifosfamide showing significant response rates when used alone or in combination as first-line treatments [13]. However, high-dose ifosfamide is associated with an increased risk of toxicity [14–16]. Consequently, many clinicians do not initiate chemotherapy with ifosfamide monotherapy. A standard dose combination of doxorubicin and ifosfamide leads to a higher response rate than when either is used as a single agent [17].

Trabectedin is a newly licensed chemotherapeutic agent for the treatment of ASTS, with demonstrable clinical response and an acceptable toxicity profile [18–20]. It is indicated for the treatment of adult patients with ASTS (1) after failure of anthracyclines and ifosfamide or (2) who are unsuited to receive these agents. However, trabectedin is being increasingly used off-label as a first-line treatment. Trabectedin has a relatively high acquisition cost compared to doxorubicin and ifosfamide. In the context of limited healthcare resources, pharmacoeconomic analyses are important in aiding policy makers and clinicians to make the most appropriate decisions about resource allocation and patient management. Against this background, the objective of this study was to estimate the cost effectiveness of doxorubicin/ifosfamide compared with trabectedin monotherapy in the first-line management of ASTS in Italy, Spain, and Sweden from the perspective of the publicly funded health service in each country.

2. Methods

2.1. Data Sources. A systematic literature search was performed using the search term of ASTS plus one of the following: incidence, prevalence, epidemiology, doxorubicin or Adriamycin and/or ifosfamide, liposomal doxorubicin or Caelyx, ifosfamide and epirubicin, trabectedin or ecteinascidin-743, gemcitabine and/or docetaxel, gemcitabine and dacarbazine, gemcitabine and vinorelbine, gemcitabine and paclitaxel, trofosfamide and/or etoposide, CYVADIC or cyclophosphamide and vincristine and Adriamycin and dacarbazine, utilities, quality of life, cost effectiveness, cost utility, resource utilisation, and economics and cost. The search strategy was not limited by year of publication; English, Italian, Spanish, and Swedish language papers were included. A manual literature search was also undertaken, based on citations in the published papers.

The search included studies published between 1988 and 2010 and included prospective and retrospective studies, randomised and nonrandomised studies, multicentre trials, single centre reports, and clinical reviews. Publications that only reported outcomes for specific subtypes of ASTS were excluded. The review yielded 53 different studies providing data on 2,977 patients. Analysis of the publications provided an estimate of

(i) the probability of patients achieving complete response (CR), partial response (PR), stable disease (SD), and progressive disease (PD),

(ii) the median duration of each type of response,

(iii) survival rates,

(iv) the incidence of grades 3-4 haematological complications including the incidence of anaemia, febrile neutropenia, neutropenia, and thrombocytopenia.

The literature search was unable to find any health economic studies on ASTS in Italy, Spain, or Sweden. Hence, estimates of healthcare resource use were obtained by interviewing six oncologists in each country who treated patients with sarcoma. The interviews used a structured questionnaire and focused on patient management and resource utilisation.

2.2. Economic Model. A Markov model was constructed depicting the management of a 65-year-old patient with ASTS (Figure 1). The model spans a period of 2 years and comprises the following health states: progressive disease, (PD), stable disease (SD), partial response (PR), complete response (CR), and death. The model comprises monthly cycles and the arrows depict the possible movement of patients between the different health states.

All patients enter the model with PD and receive treatment with either doxorubicin/ifosfamide or trabectedin. Within the model, following first-line chemotherapy, patients can remain in the PD health state, move into one of the other three health states (i.e., CR, PR, or SD), or die. Patients remain in the CR, PR, and SD health states for the median duration of response, before moving to the PD health state. The model assumed that patients who remain in the PD health state would be switched to a second-line chemotherapy after three cycles of their first-line treatment.

After second-line chemotherapy, patients can again remain in the PD health state, move into one of the other three health states, or they can die. The model only considered first- and second-line chemotherapies. Therefore, following failure of second-line chemotherapy, patients with disease progression were assumed to only receive palliative care alone.

Within the model, patients in any health state can die from age-related factors in accordance with the background death rate. Additionally, patients in the PD health state can die from ASTS-related factors.

2.2.1. Model Inputs: Resource Use. No publications were identified that quantified healthcare resource use for the management of ASTS in Italy, Spain, or Sweden. Therefore, this was estimated using information obtained from interviews with six oncologists in each country who managed ASTS and who collectively saw ~250, 300, and 200 patients with ASTS in Italy, Spain, or Sweden, respectively, at any one time.

Diagnosis. New cases of ASTS are generally diagnosed by oncologists, but patients are managed by a multidisciplinary team comprising oncologists, surgeons (general, orthopaedic, or thoracic depending on the site of the tumour), radiation oncologists, pathologists, and any other secondary care specialist depending on the sub-type of ASTS. Diagnosis of ASTS generally takes 2–6 weeks. However, the diagnosis can be delayed by up to 6 months due to unsuccessful biopsies.

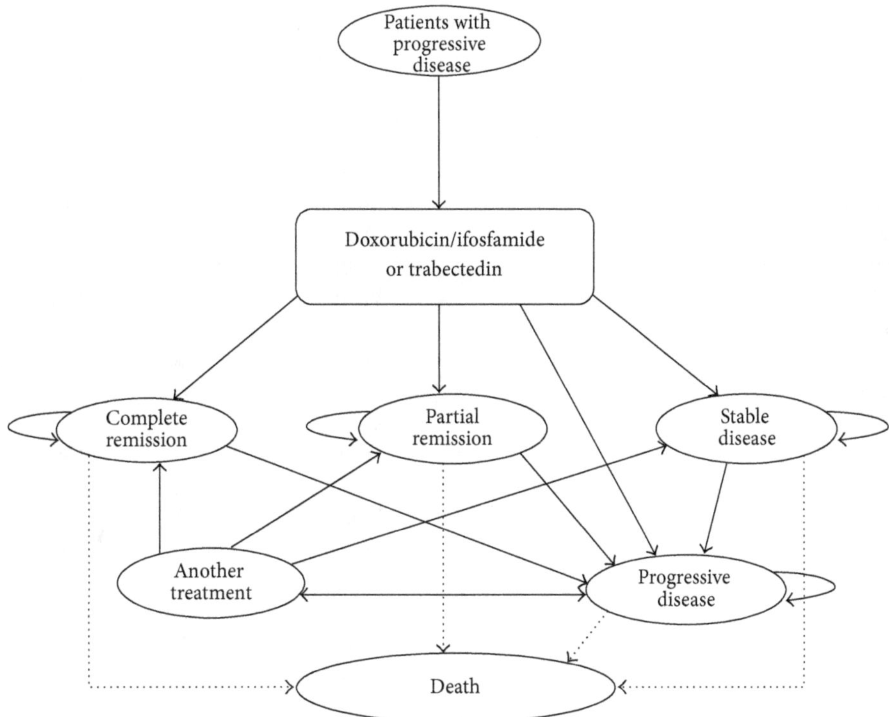

FIGURE 1: Markov model depicting the management of ASTS in Italy, Spain, and Sweden.

According to the interviewees, patients would be seen on an outpatient basis and would have a mean of 3 visits before a diagnosis of ASTS is confirmed. The tests and procedures performed during the diagnostic phase depend on the site of the disease and the histological sub-type of sarcoma. Nevertheless, all patients would have a full clinical examination and undergo the following diagnostic procedures: blood tests (100% of patients), other nonspecified pathological tests (100% of patients), biopsy (50–100% of patients), computerized tomography (CT scan; 75–100% of patients), magnetic resonance imaging (MRI; 40–80% of patients), positron emission tomography (PET scan; 5–35% of patients), chest X-ray (10–20% of patients), and ultrasound scan (5–50% of patients). Also, patients would be assessed for their performance status using the Eastern Cooperative Oncology Group (ECOG) scales and criteria, with regard to disease progression and its influence on patients' daily living abilities [21].

Treatment. Patients with ASTS often have widespread metastases and are therefore treated with systemic chemotherapy. Oncologists generally initiate chemotherapy at a mean of 2 weeks (range: 1–4 weeks) following a diagnosis of ASTS. Chemotherapy regimens are tailored according to the type of primary tumour since different sarcoma subtypes respond differently to different drugs. According to the interviewees, up to 75% of patients are expected to receive first-line doxorubicin/ifosfamide. The probabilities of receiving a second-line treatment following a lack of response or disease progression, as estimated by the interviewees and incorporated in the model, are summarised in Table 1.

It has to be noted that treatment patterns identified during the clinician interviews are only indicative, since a significant proportion of patients would be enrolled in clinical trials or only managed with palliative care following treatment failure.

There are no established third-line treatments for ASTS, and any chemotherapy drug that has not been used along the treatment pathway could be used as a third-line treatment and subsequently. Third-line treatments depend on many factors, including previous treatments, the patients' ECOG performance status, their preferences, the histological subtype of sarcoma, and the level of tolerable toxicity. Consequently, only second-line treatments have been modelled in the present study. Patients who remain alive following failure of a second-line treatment were assumed to only receive palliative care.

The characteristics of all the chemotherapy regimens utilised by the interviewees that have been incorporated in the model are summarised in Table 2.

Evaluation of Response to Chemotherapy. Patients generally receive 2–4 cycles of chemotherapy before evaluation of response. This would be ascertained using laboratory tests (100% of patients), CT scan (60–100% of patients), MRI scan (20–40% of patients), PET scan (5–15% of patients), ultrasound (10% of patients), and chest X-ray (8% of patients). Patients may also undergo other tests as needed. Patients not responding to treatment would be switched to a second-line treatment following the first response evaluation and they would be evaluated after another 2-3 cycles. Patients who respond to treatment would continue on it for a mean of 6 cycles or in some cases until disease progression.

Table 1: Probabilities of receiving second-line treatments.

Regimen	Probability of receiving second-line treatment in		
	Italy	Spain	Sweden
Following first-line treatment with doxorubicin/ifosfamide			
CYVADIC^	<0.01	<0.01	0.10
Gemcitabine/dacarbazine	<0.01	0.12	<0.01
Gemcitabine/docetaxel	0.18	0.20	0.48
Gemcitabine/paclitaxel	<0.01	0.10	<0.01
Gemcitabine/vinorelbine	<0.01	0.08	<0.01
Gemcitabine monotherapy	<0.01	0.12	<0.01
Ifosfamide monotherapy	0.20	0.12	<0.01
Liposomal doxorubicin	0.12	<0.01	<0.01
Trofosfamide	<0.01	<0.01	0.12
Trabectedin monotherapy	0.50	0.26	0.30
Following first-line treatment with trabectedin monotherapy			
Docetaxel monotherapy	0.26	<0.01	<0.01
Doxorubicin/ifosfamide	<0.01	<0.01	0.67
Doxorubicin monotherapy	<0.01	<0.01	<0.01
Gemcitabine/docetaxel	0.05	0.44	0.25
Ifosfamide/epirubicin	0.16	<0.01	<0.01
Ifosfamide monotherapy	0.53	0.56	<0.01
Trofosfamide/etoposide	<0.01	<0.01	0.08

^CYVADIC: cyclophosphamide, vincristine, adriamycin, and dacarbazine.

Table 2: Characteristics of chemotherapy regimens incorporated into the model.

Regimen	Mean dose per cycle	Admissions/outpatient clinic attendances per cycle
CYVADIC^	600 mg/m^2 cyclophosphamide 1 mg/m^2 vincristine 30 mg/m^2 doxorubicin 250 mg/m^2 dacarbazine	4 outpatient clinic attendances
Docetaxel	100 mg/m^2 docetaxel	1 outpatient clinic attendance
Doxorubicin	75 mg/m^2 doxorubicin	1 outpatient clinic attendance
Doxorubicin/ifosfamide	66 mg/m^2 doxorubicin 8.5 g/m^2 ifosfamide	3-4-day admission
Ifosfamide	12.5 g/m^2 ifosfamide	4-day admission or 2 outpatient clinic attendances
Ifosfamide/epirubicin	100 mg/m^2 epirubicin 5 g/m^2 ifosfamide	3-day admission
Gemcitabine	1,000 mg/m^2 gemcitabine	2 outpatient clinic attendances
Gemcitabine/dacarbazine	1,766 mg/m^2 gemcitabine 700 mg/m^2 dacarbazine	2 outpatient clinic attendances
Gemcitabine/docetaxel	1,000 mg/m^2 gemcitabine 75 mg/m^2 docetaxel	2 outpatient clinic attendances
Gemcitabine/paclitaxel	1,000 mg/m^2 gemcitabine 125 mg/m^2 paclitaxel	2 outpatient clinic attendances
Gemcitabine/vinorelbine	1,250 mg/m^2 gemcitabine 25 mg/m^2 vinorelbine	2 outpatient clinic attendances
Liposomal doxorubicin	50 mg/m^2 doxorubicin	1 outpatient clinic attendance
Trabectedin	1.3 mg/m^2 trabectedin	2-day admission
Trofosfamide	200 mg/m^2 trofosfamide	Oral administration over ~10 days, no hospital attendance
Trofosfamide/etoposide	150 mg/m^2 trofosfamide 25 mg/m^2 etoposide	Oral administration over ~10 days, no hospital attendance

^CYVADIC: cyclophosphamide, vincristine, adriamycin, and dacarbazine.

Nevertheless, an average patient would receive a mean of 6 cycles.

Pre- and Postchemotherapy Tests. All patients receiving chemotherapy would undergo haematological and renal function tests before each cycle of chemotherapy. Additionally, patients receiving doxorubicin-containing regimens would usually require functional cardiac assessment with an echocardiography (ECHO)/multiple gated acquisition scan (MUGA). Patients receiving trabectedin would also undergo liver function tests. Some clinicians would also perform a CT scan before each cycle of chemotherapy to monitor response. However, this would only be employed in selected patients and it is not a standard practice. Other tests may be performed before the administration of chemotherapy if toxicity is observed. The tests performed would depend on the type of toxicity present.

Approximately 6–30% of patients experiencing haematological toxicity require dose adjustments, which are very individual and depend on a patient's weight, their tolerance levels, and general performance status. Normally, the chemotherapy dose for the next cycle would be reduced by ~23% of a patient's initial chemotherapy dose (range: 18–28%). This applies to all regimens. Any dose reduction lasts for the rest of the treatment unless a patient's performance status significantly improves. According to the interviewees, dose reduction is most likely to be required at the end of a treatment.

Clinician Visits. During the period patients receive chemotherapy, an oncologist would see patients every 3-4 weeks. Patients experiencing haematological toxicity might need to be seen more than once during each cycle. Also, patients receiving a cycle over a few days may be seen on each day of the infusion. No other specialists would see patients during the treatment phase. However, other specialists may become involved if needed (e.g., gynaecological sarcomas would require the involvement of a gynaecologist).

Following completion of the chemotherapy phase, patients with complete or partial response would be seen every 3–6 months by oncologists and radiotherapists only. In some cases patients may require closer monitoring. Those with stable disease would be seen anywhere between every 3 weeks and every 3 months by oncologists and radiotherapists.

Follow-Up Tests and Procedures. After chemotherapy, patients who have responded would undergo the following procedures/tests during their follow-up: laboratory tests (100% of patients), CT scan (50–100% of patients), MRI scan (30–45% of patients), PET scan (10–15% of patients), chest X-ray (8% of patients), and ultrasound scan (<1% of patients). A range of other tests would be performed as needed. Follow-up procedures and tests would be performed every 3–6 months.

Pre- and Postchemotherapy Medications. Generally, all patients would receive medication before each chemotherapy administration with the aim of preventing haematological or nonhaematological toxicities. In Italy, patients would receive an antiemetic such as granisetron (3 mg; 50% of patients) or ondansetron (8 mg; 50% of patients) and a corticosteroid such as dexamethasone (4–16 mg; 100% of patients). In Spain, patients would receive palonosetron (1 mg; 20% of patients), aprepitant (125 mg; 100% of patients in most regimens except those containing trabectedin), granisetron (2 mg; 20% of patients), metoclopramide (30 mg; 20% of patients) or ondansetron (8–24 mg; 20% of patients), dexamethasone (4–20 mg; 100% of patients), and an antihistamine, such as diphenhydramine (150 mg; 100% of patients). Generally, an antihistamine would be only administered in regimens containing paclitaxel, docetaxel, and trabectedin. Patients receiving gemcitabine- and/or dacarbazine-containing regimens would be given a corticosteroid and an antiemetic. In Sweden, patients would receive corticosteroids such as betamethasone (4–8 mg; 100% of patients) and an antiemetic such as tropisetron (5 mg; 100% of patients) before administration of doxorubicin/ifosfamide and dexamethasone (8 mg; 100% of patients) before administration of trabectedin. Patients would receive antiemetics and laxatives for 2-3 days after chemotherapy.

In all three countries a granulocyte-colony-stimulating factor (G-CSF, filgrastim 6 mg) would be administered to prevent neutropenia in ~65% of patients receiving doxorubicin/ifosfamide and ~15% of patients receiving gemcitabine-containing regimens. Other patients would not receive prophylactic G-CSF but would receive it therapeutically when they experience haematological toxicities.

All patients receiving an ifosfamide-containing chemotherapy would also receive mesna. Typically, the dose of mesna administered would be the same as the ifosfamide dose.

Haematological Toxicities. According to the interviewed oncologists, the main complications associated with the aforementioned regimens are grades 3-4 haematological toxicities (i.e., anaemia, thrombocytopenia, neutropenia, and febrile neutropenia). Hence, the healthcare costs associated with managing these complications have been incorporated into the model.

Palliative Care. According to the interviewees, palliative care can be introduced at any stage along the treatment pathway. The necessity for palliative care is guided by a patient's performance status and could be introduced even before the initiation of chemotherapy. Frequently, palliative care units work in collaboration with oncology services and provide patient care when the disease is too advanced, when patients are unable to receive chemotherapy, when patients experience difficult to control symptoms, or when there is no active treatment that is effective. Accordingly, the costs associated with palliative care have been incorporated into the model.

2.2.2. Model Inputs: Clinical Outcomes. Clinical outcomes associated with the management of ASTS were estimated from the literature review. Published clinical outcomes analysed included the probability of achieving CR, PR, SD, and PD (Table 3), median duration of response (Table 3), cancer-related mortality stratified according to the regimens (Figures 2 and 3), and incidence of grades 3-4 haematological toxicities

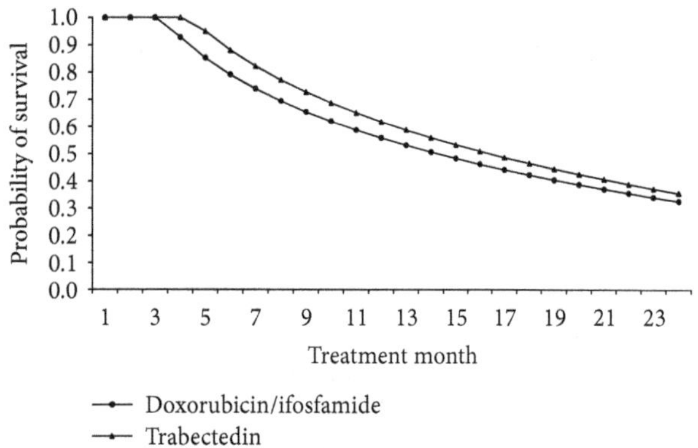

FIGURE 2: Survival rates associated with first-line treatment with doxorubicin/ifosfamide and trabectedin.

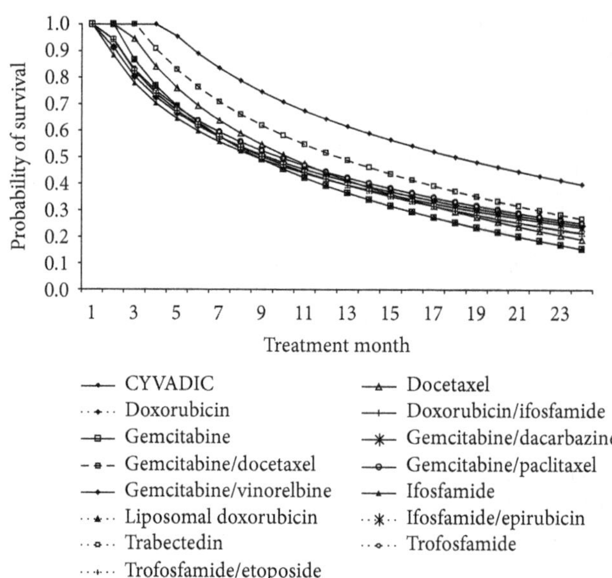

FIGURE 3: Survival rates associated with second-line treatments.

(Table 4). Where more than one publication was available, the mean rates were weighted according to the sample sizes.

The outcomes from studies in which doxorubicin/ifosfamide and trabectedin were used as first-line chemotherapies are shown separately from those studies in which these agents were used as second-line treatments. The literature review could not identify any publications reporting efficacy rates for second-line chemotherapy with CYVADIC (cyclophosphamide, vincristine, adriamycin, and dacarbazine), trofosfamide/etoposide, and gemcitabine/paclitaxel. Therefore, the efficacy rates for these cytotoxic agents were assumed to be the average of all the efficacy rates that were available for second-line chemotherapy (i.e., doxorubicin/ifosfamide, gemcitabine/docetaxel, and gemcitabine/dacarbazine). Also, efficacy rates for second-line chemotherapy with ifosfamide/epirubicin were assumed to be the same as those for doxorubicin/ifosfamide, as they were both ifosfamide-containing regimens, and the rates for liposomal doxorubicin were assumed to be the same as those for doxorubicin monotherapy since both are anthracyclines.

Median Duration of Response. Some publications reported only the overall median duration of response. Hence, the relationship between overall median duration of response and median duration associated with CR, PR, and SD derived from publications reporting stratified outcomes was used to estimate median duration of response for the missing response types.

The literature review could not identify any publications reporting median duration of response following second-line chemotherapy with doxorubicin/ifosfamide, doxorubicin monotherapy, ifosfamide/epirubicin, gemcitabine/docetaxel, gemcitabine/paclitaxel, trofosfamide, trofosfamide/etoposide, CYVADIC, and liposomal doxorubicin monotherapy. Hence, the reported average median duration of response associated with second-line ifosfamide monotherapy, gemcitabine/dacarbazine, and gemcitabine monotherapy was used to estimate the median duration of response associated with these regimens, since the median duration of response was only available for these second-line regimens. It was decided to exclude trabectedin's duration of response from this extrapolation since it was the only new generation chemotherapeutic agent.

Table 3 summarises the probabilities of achieving one of the health states and the duration of remaining in a health state following first- and second-line chemotherapies that have been incorporated in the model.

Mortality Rates. Age-related mortality was estimated using published mortality rates [84]. The literature review was used to estimate cancer-related mortality rates. Using a least squares regression methodology, lines of best fit were derived to estimate cancer-related mortality rates at various time points. The resulting mortality curves were adjusted to exclude age-related mortality for Italy [84], Spain [84], and Sweden [84]. Cancer-related mortality rates were available for all first-line treatments [17, 18, 23, 24, 28, 29] and some second-line treatments: gemcitabine monotherapy [40, 43, 46, 47], ifosfamide monotherapy [38, 57, 60], trabectedin monotherapy [19, 34, 61, 63–65, 67], gemcitabine/vinorelbine [56], and docetaxel monotherapy [35, 37]. Cancer-related mortality rates could not be identified for the following second-line regimens: doxorubicin monotherapy, doxorubicin/ifosfamide, ifosfamide/epirubicin, gemcitabine/dacarbazine, gemcitabine/paclitaxel, CYVADIC, trofosfamide/etoposide, trofosfamide, and liposomal doxorubicin monotherapy. Hence, cancer-related mortality rates for doxorubicin monotherapy and liposomal doxorubicin monotherapy were assumed to be the same as those for second-line ifosfamide monotherapy, because they appear comparable in clinical practice (Table 3). Cancer-related mortality rates for doxorubicin/ifosfamide and ifosfamide/epirubicin were assumed to be the average of those for second-line ifosfamide monotherapy and trabectedin monotherapy because of the reported similarities in the average median duration of response between the regimens. Also the interviewed clinicians considered that the mortality rates associated with these three

TABLE 3: Efficacy rates and duration of response associated with different chemotherapy regimens for ASTS.

	Probability of achieving:				Median duration of response (months) in:		
	Complete remission	Partial remission	Stable disease	Progressive disease	Complete remission	Partial remission	Stable disease
First-line treatments							
Doxorubicin/ifosfamide	0.06 [16, 17, 22–32]	0.21 [16, 17, 22–32]	0.38 [16, 17, 22–32]	0.35 [16, 17, 22–32]	15.44 [16, 17, 22, 24, 27, 28, 31, 33]	7.69 [16, 17, 22, 24, 27, 28, 31, 33]	6.41 [16, 17, 22, 24, 27, 28, 31, 33]
Trabectedin	0.03 [34]	0.11 [34]	0.14 [34]	0.72 [34]	17.74 [34]	8.75 [34]	7.48 [34]
Second-line treatments							
CYVADIC*^	0.03	0.19	0.39	0.39	12.13	6.57	5.75
Docetaxel	0.00 [35–37]	0.11 [35–37]	0.25 [35–37]	0.64 [35–37]	0.00 [35, 36]	6.60 [35, 36]	7.17 [35, 36]
Doxorubicin	0.02 [38, 39]	0.07 [38, 39]	0.31 [38, 39]	0.61 [38, 39]	12.13*	6.57*	5.75*
Doxorubicin/ifosfamide	0.05 [22, 38]	0.27 [22, 38]	0.37 [22, 38]	0.31 [22, 38]	12.13*	6.57*	5.75*
Gemcitabine	0.00 [40–45]	0.08 [40–45]	0.33 [40–45]	0.59 [40–45]	0.00 [43, 46, 47]	4.46 [43, 46, 47]	3.86 [43, 46, 47]
Gemcitabine/dacarbazine	0.01 [48–50]	0.10 [48–50]	0.39 [48–50]	0.51 [48–50]	10.48 [48]	6.50 [48]	5.79 [48]
Gemcitabine/docetaxel	0.05 [40, 51–54]	0.19 [40, 51–54]	0.41 [40, 51–54]	0.35 [40, 51–54]	12.13*	6.57*	5.75*
Gemcitabine/paclitaxel*	0.03	0.19	0.39	0.39	12.13	6.57	5.75
Gemcitabine/vinorelbine	0.02 [55, 56]	0.10 [55, 56]	0.10 [55, 56]	0.78 [55, 56]	16.10 [56]	16.10 [56]	9.60 [56]
Ifosfamide	0.02 [38, 57–60]	0.13 [38, 57–60]	0.24 [38, 57–60]	0.61 [38, 57–60]	13.77 [58, 60]	8.75 [58, 60]	7.61 [58, 60]
Ifosfamide/epirubicin*	0.05	0.27	0.37	0.31	12.13	6.57	5.75
Liposomal doxorubicin*	0.02	0.07	0.31	0.61	12.13	6.57	5.75
Trabectedin	<0.01 [19, 34, 61–67]	0.07 [19, 34, 61–67]	0.44 [19, 34, 61–67]	0.49 [19, 34, 61–67]	16.14 [19, 34, 61, 63–65]	10.25 [19, 34, 61, 63–65]	8.91 [19, 34, 61, 63–65]
Trofosfamide	0.00 [68–70]	0.03 [68–70]	0.19 [68–70]	0.79 [68–70]	12.13*	6.57*	5.75*
Trofosfamide/etoposide*	0.03	0.19	0.39	0.39	12.13	6.57	5.75

*Values were estimated. ^CYVADIC: cyclophosphamide, vincristine, adriamycin and dacarbazine.

TABLE 4: Probabilities of patients developing haematological toxicities stratified by chemotherapy regimen.

	Probability of developing			
	neutropenia	febrile neutropenia	thrombocytopenia	anaemia
First-line treatments				
Doxorubicin/ifosfamide	0.82 [23, 24, 26, 30]	0.12 [24, 26]	0.23 [17, 23, 24, 26, 30]	0.35 [23, 26, 30]
Trabectedin	0.33 [34]	0.00 [34]	0.00 [34]	0.03 [34]
Second-line treatments				
CYVADIC*^	0.52	0.19	0.17	0.16
Docetaxel	0.90 [36, 37]	0.12 [35, 37]	0.03 [35–37]	0.08 [35–37]
Doxorubicin	0.84 [39]	0.19 [39]	0.09 [39]	0.18*
Doxorubicin/ifosfamide*	0.52	0.19	0.17	0.18
Gemcitabine	0.18 [40, 41, 43, 47, 71]	0.07 [33, 40, 41, 43, 71]	0.18 [33, 40–43, 46, 71]	0.11 [40–43, 71]
Gemcitabine/dacarbazine	0.46 [49]	0.19*	0.12 [49]	0.23 [49]
Gemcitabine/docetaxel	0.31 [52, 54]	0.09 [52, 54]	0.33 [40, 52, 54]	0.18 [52, 54]
Gemcitabine/paclitaxel*	0.52	0.19	0.17	0.16
Gemcitabine/vinorelbine	0.38 [56]	0.08 [56]	0.10 [56]	0.05 [56]
Ifosfamide	0.82 [57–60]	0.39 [58, 59]	0.13 [57–60]	0.12 [57–59]
Ifosfamide/epirubicin*	0.52	0.19	0.17	0.18
Liposomal doxorubicin*	0.07	0.02	0.00	0.35
Trabectedin	0.50 [19, 34, 61, 64, 65, 67]	0.06 [19, 34, 61, 65]	0.16 [19, 34, 61, 64, 65, 67]	0.18 [19, 34, 61, 65]
Trofosfamide	0.52*	0.19*	0.17*	0.25 [70]
Trofosfamide/etoposide*	0.52	0.19	0.17	0.16

^CYVADIC: cyclophosphamide, vincristine, adriamycin, and dacarbazine.
*Values were estimated.

regimens were comparable in clinical practice. Cancer-related mortality rates for gemcitabine/paclitaxel, CYVADIC, trofosfamide, and trofosfamide/etoposide were assumed to be the average of those for second-line gemcitabine, ifosfamide, and trabectedin. This was based on the observed similarities in the average median duration of responses associated with the aforementioned regimens.

The estimated survival rates following first-line treatment with doxorubicin/ifosfamide and trabectedin monotherapy that have been incorporated in the model are shown in Figure 2. The estimated survival rates following second-line treatment after failing first-line treatment with doxorubicin/ifosfamide and trabectedin monotherapy that have been incorporated in the model are shown in Figure 3.

Incidence of Haematological Complications. According to the interviewees only grades 3-4 haematological complications would result in additional healthcare resource utilisation. The incidence of haematological complications was estimated from the literature review. However, the review could not identify any publications reporting the incidence of grades 3-4 haematological complications following second-line treatment with doxorubicin/ifosfamide, gemcitabine/paclitaxel, CYVADIC, trofosfamide/etoposide, and ifosfamide/epirubicin. Consequently, the average of the available incidence rates associated with the second-line combination regimens was used.

Also not reported was the incidence of grades 3-4 haematological complications following second-line treatment with liposomal doxorubicin monotherapy. The relationship between the incidence rates associated with first-line doxorubicin monotherapy and liposomal doxorubicin monotherapy was used to estimate the missing incidence rates. This assumption was made on the basis that liposomal doxorubicin monotherapy has equivalent activity to doxorubicin monotherapy treatment [97]. Also, not reported was the incidence of anaemia following second-line treatment with doxorubicin monotherapy. Therefore, the average of the rates of anaemia associated with other second-line treatments was used to interpolate missing values.

Table 4 summarises the incidence of grades 3-4 haematological toxicities following first- and second-line treatments that have been incorporated in the model.

2.2.3. Model Inputs: Utilities. Health state utilities for ASTS elicited from the general public using time trade-off methodology were assigned to the health states in our model [98]. The estimated utility values were as follows: complete response 0.60, partial response 0.51, stable disease 0.43, and progressive disease 0.30.

2.2.4. Model Outputs. By assigning unit costs in Euros at 2010/2011 prices (Table 5) to the resource use estimates in the different health states within the Markov model, the healthcare costs over two years after a patient initially received either doxorubicin/ifosfamide or trabectedin monotherapy were estimated. Unit costs that were only available for earlier periods were uprated to 2010/2011 prices using the relevant inflation index for each country.

The primary measure of clinical effectiveness in the model was the number of quality-adjusted life years (QALYs) two years after starting first-line treatment with doxorubicin/ifosfamide or trabectedin monotherapy. The model also estimated successful treatment at two years in terms of the proportion of patients achieving CR, PR, and SD.

In accordance with the guidelines for economic evaluations in Italy [99], Spain [100], and Sweden [101] healthcare costs and QALYs in the second year were each discounted at 3%.

2.3. Cost Effectiveness Analyses. The incremental cost effectiveness of doxorubicin/ifosfamide compared to trabectedin monotherapy was calculated as the difference between the expected discounted costs of the two treatment strategies over 2 years divided by the difference between the expected discounted number of QALYs of the two strategies over 2 years. Hence, the incremental cost effectiveness of doxorubicin/ifosfamide compared to trabectedin monotherapy was defined as the cost per QALY gained. If a treatment resulted in more QALYs for less cost, it was defined as a dominant treatment.

2.4. Sensitivity Analyses. Probabilistic sensitivity analyses (PSA) using Monte Carlo iterations (10,000 iterations of the model) were undertaken by simultaneously varying all the probabilities, utilities, unit costs, and resource use values within the model. The probabilities and utilities were varied randomly according to a beta distribution and the resource use estimates and unit costs were varied randomly according to a gamma distribution. Results from these analyses were used to construct cost effectiveness acceptability curves showing the probability of first-line treatment with doxorubicin/ifosfamide compared to trabectedin monotherapy to be cost effective at varying cost per QALY thresholds.

Deterministic sensitivity analyses were also performed to assess the impact of independently varying individual parameter values within the model. The parameter estimates were varied over plausible ranges by altering them to 20% below and 20% above the base case values.

3. Results

3.1. Expected Clinical Outcomes. The outcomes at two years following initial treatment with doxorubicin/ifosfamide or trabectedin are summarised in Table 6. Differences between the countries reflect the different second-line treatments that are used in Italy, Spain, and Sweden.

3.2. Expected Healthcare Costs. The expected costs at two years following initial treatment with doxorubicin/ifosfamide or trabectedin are summarised in Table 7. Differences between the countries reflect the different second-line treatments, different management algorithms, and different unit costs. Nevertheless, in all three countries, the expected two-year costs of starting treatment with doxorubicin/ifosfamide are between 4% and 10% less than those of starting treatment with trabectedin.

In Spain and Sweden the primary cost driver in patients starting chemotherapy with doxorubicin/ifosfamide was the cost of pre- and postchemotherapy medications. However, in Italy, the primary cost driver was the cost of second-line chemotherapy regimens. In all three countries, the primary cost driver in patients starting chemotherapy with trabectedin was the acquisition cost of this cytotoxic agent (Table 7).

3.3. Cost Effectiveness Analyses. Starting treatment with doxorubicin/ifosfamide instead of trabectedin monotherapy is expected to lead to a cost reduction of €1,710 in Italy, €3,497 in Spain, and €3,274 in Sweden. Additionally, starting treatment with doxorubicin/ifosfamide instead of trabectedin monotherapy is expected to lead to an improvement in health status at two years of 0.07 QALYs in Italy, 0.04 QALYs in Spain, and 0.02 QALYs in Sweden. Hence, doxorubicin/ifosfamide was found to be a dominant treatment relative to trabectedin in all three countries with a cost per QALY of −€26,308, −€87,423, and −€136,396 in Italy, Spain, and Sweden, respectively.

3.4. Probabilistic Sensitivity Analyses. Probabilistic sensitivity analyses highlighted the distribution in the incremental costs and QALYs at two years (Figure 4), from which it can be seen that the majority of the samples are located in the dominant (bottom right) quadrant (Figure 4). These analyses also showed that there is greater dispersion in Spain and Sweden than in Italy.

Cost effectiveness acceptability curves generated from the probabilistic sensitivity analyses showed the probability of doxorubicin/ifosfamide to be cost effective compared to trabectedin monotherapy across a wide range of cost per QALY thresholds (Figure 5). At a threshold of €35,000 per QALY, >90% of a cohort would be cost effectively treated with doxorubicin/ifosfamide compared to trabectedin monotherapy in all three countries.

TABLE 5: Unit resource costs (in Euros at 2010/2011 prices) used in the model.

Resource	Unit costs (in Euros at 2010/2011 prices)					
	Italy		Spain		Sweden	
Aprepitant (125 mg)			€90.9	[72]	€63.8	[73]
Betapred (4 mg)					€6.4	[73]
Betamethasone (8 mg)					€3.2	[73]
Biopsy	€129.1	[74]	€603.7	[75]	€314.1	[76]
Bone scintigraphy			€296.8	[77]		
Chest X-ray	€16.2	[78]	€6.5	[79]	€48.7	[76]
CT scan	€86.3	[74]	€87.5	[79]	€313.6	[76]
Cyclophosphamide (200 mg)					€4.1	[80]
Dacarbazine (1000 mg)			€21.7	[80]		
Dacarbazine (200 mg)					€8.9	[80]
Dexamethasone (0.75 mg, 10 tablets)	€1.1	[81]				
Dexamethasone (1 mg, 30 tablets)			€3.0	[72]		
Diphenhydramine (25 mg, 25 capsules)			€1.4	[72]		
Docetaxel (10 mg)	€84.4	[80]				
Docetaxel (100 mg)			€182.8	[80]		
Docetaxel (80 mg)					€403.1	[80]
Doxorubicin (50 mg)	€119.5	[80]	€4.1	[80]	€59.8	[80]
Echocardiography	€51.7	[74]	€18.2	[79]	€214.9	[76]
Electrocardiogram	€13.0	[78]	€13.5	[82]	€334.2	[76]
Epirubicin (50 mg)	€81.2	[80]				
Etoposide (100 mg)					€20.8	[80]
Filgrastim (300 mcg)			€94.8	[72]		
Filgrastim (6 mg)	€149.8	[81]				
Gemcitabine (1000 mg)	€113.2	[80]	€75.7	[80]	€104.6	[80]
General surgeon consultation					€230.3	[76]
Granisetron (1 mg, 10 tablets)	€133.9	[81]	€48.1	[72]		
Haematology tests	€3.7	[83]	€20.5	[82]	€5.2	[76]
Hospitalisation for chemotherapy infusion/day	€238.3	[84]	€212.9	[84]	€288.6	[84]
Ifosfamide (1 g)	€30.7	[80]	€19.7	[80]		
Ifosfamide (2 g)					€65.7	[80]
Lenograstim (1 vial)	€153.4	[81]				
Levocetirizine (5 mg, 20 tablets)	€10.5	[81]				
Liver function test	€9.2	[83]	€11.7	[79]		
Liposomal doxorubicin (2 mg)	€548.2	[80]				
Managing anaemia	€1,354.8	[85]	€900.0	[86]	€548.6	[87]
Managing febrile neutropenia	€3,305.0	[88]	€3829.5	[89]	€2,892.0	[90]
Managing neutropenia	€523.3	[85]	€2086.1	[91]		
Managing thrombocytopenia	€1,354.8	[85]	€900.0	[86]	€548.6	[87]
Mesna (3 g)			€13.2	[72]		
Mesna (6 g)	€25.7	[81]				
Mesna (5 g)					€192.2	[73]
Metoclopramide (250 mL)			€2.7	[72]		
MRI scan	€285.8	[83]	€168.0	[79]	€386.4	[76]
Multidisciplinary team assessment	€48.7	[74]	€61.3	[79]	€1,816.5	[76]
Nuclear medicine specialist consultation			€61.5	[79]		
Nurse home visit	€51.2	[92]	€56.5	[77]		

Table 5: Continued.

Resource	Unit costs (in Euros at 2010/2011 prices)					
	Italy		Spain		Sweden	
Oncologist consultation	€21.6	[83]	€61.5	[79]	€283.7	[76]
Ondansetron (4 mg, 6 tablets)	€57.8	[81]				
Ondansetron (4 mg, 15 tablets)			€36.3	[72]		
Orthopaedic surgeon consultation	€21.6	[83]	€61.5	[79]	€102.4	[76]
Outpatient attendance for chemotherapy	€122.8	[84]	€98.9	[84]	€288.6	[84]
Paclitaxel (30 mg)			€83.8	[80]		
Palliative care per patient	€3,265.0	[93]	€2167.7	[94]	€1,343.9	[95, 96]
Palonosetron (250 mcg)			€104.6	[72]		
Pathologist consultation	€21.6	[83]	€61.5	[79]		
Pegfilgrastim (1 syringe)			€1,062.6	[72]	€1,322.5	[73]
PET scan	€1,071.7	[74]	€500.0	[79]	€314.1	[76]
Radiologist consultation	€21.6	[83]	€61.5	[79]		
Radiotherapist consultation	€21.6	[83]	€61.5	[79]		
Renal function test	€5.0	[83]	€8.9	[79]		
Secondary care hospital specialist visit			€61.5	[79]		
Trabectedin (1 mg, 1 vial)	€2,970.1	[80]	€2,049.9	[80]	€1,913.3	[80]
Trofosfamide 50 mg/m^2					€1.4	[80]
Tropisetron (5 mg)					€20.5	[73]
Ultrasound scan	€17.6	[74]	€18.2	[79]		
Urine analysis	€6.1	[83]	€1.8	[79]	€20.9	[76]
Vincristine (1 mg)					€16.2	[80]
Vinorelbine (1 mL)			€24.1	[80]		

In Sweden unit costs were converted from Swedish Krona (SEK) to Euros at the rate of €1 = 9.55 SEK.

Table 6: Clinical outcomes at two years.

	Italy		Spain		Sweden	
	Doxorubicin/ ifosfamide	Trabectedin	Doxorubicin/ ifosfamide	Trabectedin	Doxorubicin/ ifosfamide	Trabectedin
Probability of						
complete response	0.01	<0.01	<0.01	<0.01	<0.01	0.01
partial response	0.01	<0.01	0.01	<0.01	0.01	0.01
stable disease	0.02	0.01	0.02	0.01	0.02	0.01
progressive disease	0.54	0.51	0.54	0.53	0.54	0.59
dying	0.43	0.47	0.42	0.45	0.42	0.39
Number of QALYs per patient	0.595 (0.593, 0.597)	0.530 (0.528, 0.533)	0.590 (0.587, 0.593)	0.550 (0.547, 0.553)	0.608 (0.606, 0.611)	0.584 (0.582, 0.587)

95% confidence intervals in parentheses.

3.5. Deterministic Sensitivity Analyses. Extensive deterministic sensitivity analyses (Table 8) showed that the model is robust to plausible changes in the model inputs. Varying the model inputs between 20% below and 20% above the base case values showed that doxorubicin/ifosfamide remained a dominant treatment in Spain and Sweden and a cost-effective treatment in Italy, across all the variables.

Additionally, doxorubicin/ifosfamide remained a dominant treatment when the use of second-line treatments was excluded from the patients' pathways, by assuming that those who do not respond to first-line chemotherapy, or those with disease progression, only receive palliative care. In these circumstances, starting chemotherapy with doxorubicin/ifosfamide or trabectedin is expected to lead to a two-year cost of

(i) €14,567 and €32,858 per patient, respectively, in Italy,

(ii) €18,085 and €26,198 per patient, respectively, in Spain,

(iii) €21,385 and €23,410 per patient, respectively, in Sweden.

Additionally, starting chemotherapy with doxorubicin/ifosfamide or trabectedin is expected to lead to 0.274 QALYs and

TABLE 7: Expected healthcare costs (at 2010/2011 prices) over 2 years following first-line treatment with doxorubicin/ifosfamide combination and trabectedin monotherapy.

Resource	Expected healthcare costs per patient (Euros at 2010/2011 prices) over 2 years following first-line treatment											
	Italy				Spain				Sweden			
	Doxorubicin/ifosfamide		Trabectedin		Doxorubicin/ifosfamide		Trabectedin		Doxorubicin/ifosfamide		Trabectedin	
Diagnosis	€634.4	(2%)	€634.4	(2%)	€1886.5	(6%)	€1886.5	(6%)	€2416.8	(7%)	€2416.8	(6%)
First-line cytotoxics	€2302.9	(6%)	€26885.4	(66%)	€1491.8	(5%)	€18432.1	(54%)	€3172.2	(9%)	€17934.5	(45%)
Second-line cytotoxics	€17007.3	(44%)	€2556.9	(6%)	€6524.1	(21%)	€1761.6	(5%)	€8469.5	(23%)	€3224.8	(8%)
Evaluations of response	€2025.7	(5%)	€1641.7	(4%)	€1280.4	(4%)	€1098.7	(3%)	€2758.0	(8%)	€2453.2	(6%)
Hospitalisations for chemotherapy infusion	€5093.0	(13%)	€3765.6	(9%)	€4704.7	(15%)	€3564.3	(10%)	€4326.8	(12%)	€3685.2	(9%)
Outpatient attendances for chemotherapy	€291.3	(<1%)	€338.0	(1%)	€560.9	(2%)	€423.4	(1%)	€998.6	(3%)	€439.0	(1%)
Tests before each cycle of chemotherapy	€212.5	(<1%)	€118.0	(<1%)	€266.2	(1%)	€197.9	(1%)	€244.3	(1%)	€217.0	(1%)
Pre- and postchemotherapy medication	€5706.9	(15%)	€1107.3	(3%)	€7621.1	(25%)	€1665.8	(5%)	€11732.4	(32%)	€7458.6	(19%)
Palliative care	€2918.9	(8%)	€1773.3	(4%)	€1942.7	(6%)	€1932.3	(6%)	€1200.9	(3%)	€1265.9	(3%)
Management of haematological toxicity	€2728.6	(7%)	€1811.1	(4%)	€4421.0	(14%)	€3233.7	(9%)	€1187.2	(3%)	€685.2	(2%)
Total	€38921.7	(100%)	€40631.7	(100%)	€30699.4	(100%)	€34196.3	(100%)	€36506.7	(100%)	€39780.2	(100%)

(Percentage of total expected cost is in parenthesis).

TABLE 8: Sensitivity analyses.

Scenario	Base case value in Italy	Base case value in Spain	Base case value in Sweden	Effect
Duration of partial remission following first-line treatment with doxorubicin/ifosfamide ranges from 6.1 to 9.2 months	7.7 months	7.7 months	7.7 months	Doxorubicin/ifosfamide remains a dominant treatment
Duration of stable disease following first-line treatment with doxorubicin/ifosfamide ranges from 5.1 to 7.7 months	6.4 months	6.4 months	6.4 months	Doxorubicin/ifosfamide remains a dominant treatment
Duration of partial remission following first-line treatment with trabectedin ranges from 7.0 to 10.6 months	8.8 months	8.8 months	8.8 months	Doxorubicin/ifosfamide remains a dominant treatment
Duration of stable disease following first-line treatment with trabectedin ranges from 6.0 to 9.0 months	7.5 months	7.5 months	7.5 months	Doxorubicin/ifosfamide remains a dominant treatment
Probability of being in stable disease after first-line doxorubicin/ifosfamide ranges from 0.3 to 0.5	0.38	0.38	0.38	Doxorubicin/ifosfamide remains a dominant treatment
Probability of being in stable disease after first-line trabectedin ranges from 0.1 to 0.2	0.14	0.14	0.14	Doxorubicin/ifosfamide remains a dominant treatment
Probability of being in stable disease after second-line trabectedin ranges from 0.35 to 0.50	0.44	0.44	0.44	Doxorubicin/ifosfamide remains a dominant treatment
Probability of switching to trabectedin after first-line doxorubicin/ifosfamide ranges from 80% below to 20% above the base case value	0.50	0.26	0.30	Doxorubicin/ifosfamide remains a dominant treatment except in Italy where its costeffectiveness ranges from being dominant to €21,500 per QALY, breaking even at a probability of 0.55
Length of hospital stay for doxorubicin/ifosfamide infusion ranges from 1 to 5 days	3 days	4 days	3 days	Doxorubicin/ifosfamide remains a dominant treatment except in Italy where its costeffectiveness ranges from being dominant to €16,400 per QALY, breaking even at 4 days
Unit cost of doxorubicin ranges from 80% below to 20% above the base case value	€119.50	€4.11	€59.79	Doxorubicin/ifosfamide remains a dominant treatment
Unit cost of ifosfamide ranges from 80% below to 20% above the base case value	€30.71	€19.71	€65.65	Doxorubicin/ifosfamide remains a dominant treatment
Unit cost of trabectedin ranges from 80% below to 20% above the base case value	€2,970.10	€2,049.91	€1,913.29	Doxorubicin/ifosfamide remains a dominant treatment except in Italy where its costeffectiveness ranges from €11,200 per QALY to being dominant, breaking even at €2,570
Cost of managing adverse events ranges from 80% below to 20% above the base case values				Doxorubicin/ifosfamide remains a dominant treatment
Cost of pre- and postchemotherapy medications ranges from 80% below to 20% above the base case values				Doxorubicin/ifosfamide remains a dominant treatment
Cost of palliative care ranges from 80% below to 20% above the base case values				Doxorubicin/ifosfamide remains a dominant treatment
Utility for progressive disease ranges from 0.24 to 0.36	0.30	0.30	0.30	Doxorubicin/ifosfamide remains a dominant treatment
Utility for stable disease ranges from 0.34 to 0.52	0.43	0.43	0.43	Doxorubicin/ifosfamide remains a dominant treatment
Difference in QALYs gained following the start of treatment with doxorubicin/ifosfamide and trabectedin ranges from 80% below and 20% above the base case value	0.07	0.04	0.02	Doxorubicin/ifosfamide remains a dominant treatment

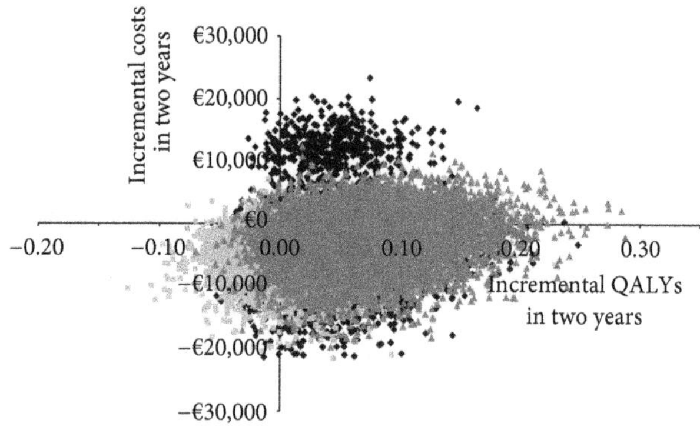

Figure 4: Scatterplot of the incremental cost effectiveness of doxorubicin/ifosfamide compared to trabectedin monotherapy (10,000 iterations of each model).

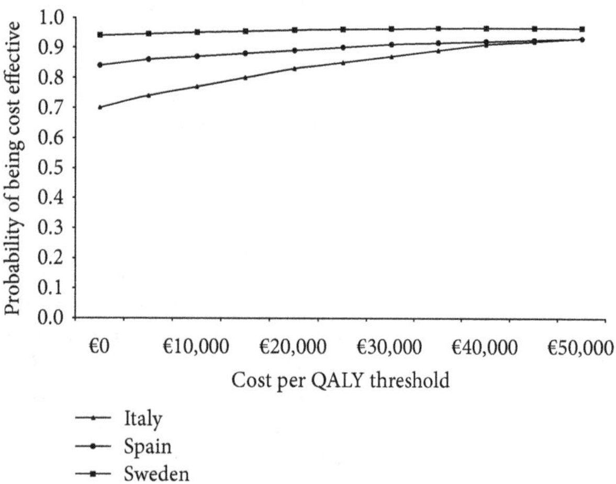

Figure 5: Acceptability curves.

0.178 QALYs per patient, respectively, at two years, irrespective of country.

4. Discussion

There have been several studies assessing the efficacy of first-line treatment of ASTS with trabectedin [18, 34]. Hence, the precedent had been set prior to performing this study to evaluate the cost effectiveness of doxorubicin/ifosfamide versus trabectedin as first-line treatment strategies for the management of this disease. Our literature search failed to find any health economic studies on ASTS in Italy, Spain, or Sweden. Consequently, using a range of published studies and estimates of resource use obtained from clinicians who manage sarcoma, a two-year Markov model was constructed to simulate the management of patients suffering from ASTS in each of these three countries. Due to the lack of published data, the time horizon of the model was limited to two years, by which time most patients would die. Markov models are suited to simulate the consequences of decisions when the timing of events is important and when events may happen more than once. Hence, they are appropriate for evaluating the consequences of decisions that are of a sequential or repetitive nature [102]. Since events such as response and relapse in ASTS recur over time, use of a Markov model was considered the most appropriate vehicle for performing this cost effectiveness analysis.

There are potential limitations with the model, mainly due to the combination of numerous sources and data assumptions. The clinical basis of the model was diverse studies that included patients with different types of ASTS, different severity of disease, different age of sufferers, different administration schedules, and prior treatments. Therefore, the patient populations may not be identical in all the studies. Consequently, the clinical outcomes observed in this study may not necessarily reflect those observed in clinical practice. Also, the Markov model was based on many assumptions pertaining to cancer-related mortality, chemotherapy efficacy rates, and duration of response. These assumptions were necessary due to the limited availability of data pertaining to some of the regimens employed by the interviewed oncologists. Nevertheless, these assumptions were tested using extensive deterministic and probabilistic sensitivity analyses and found to be robust to changes in the model inputs. Notwithstanding this, there is potential for confounding in this study due to the lack of any direct comparative evidence between the two first-line treatment regimens and some of the second-line treatment efficacy estimates are based on assumptions.

The literature search was unable to identify any published studies assessing healthcare resource utilisation and chemotherapy patterns for ASTS. Because of the low incidence of the disease, healthcare resource utilisation was not collected prospectively but was estimated from interviews with six oncologists in each country. Consequently, resource use for the "average clinician" throughout each country may not be the same as that for those clinicians who participated in this study.

The interviewees indicated that there are no treatment guidelines for the management of ASTS, and in Sweden, only ~20–30% of patients are covered by the Scandinavian Sarcoma Group protocol (SSG XX) [103]. Therefore, the chemotherapy patterns in this study reflect the individual judgment of the oncologists interviewed. Consequently, the levels of healthcare resource utilisation observed in the analysis might not be indicative for each country as a whole. Also, as a consequence, it is not known how the study results would generalise to patients treated in other oncology centres. Moreover, treatment of ASTS is very individual and the type of regimen chosen depends on (1) the histological sub-type of sarcoma and (2) the patient's characteristics. Also, following treatment failure, a proportion of patients would be enrolled into clinical trials or would only receive palliative care. Furthermore, treatment patterns are not very standardised. Hence, there may be other treatments that are used but have not been mentioned by the interviewees. Consequently, it was a very challenging task for the interviewees to provide generalised treatment patterns. Nevertheless, the chemotherapy patterns presented in this study provide an overview of current practice in all three countries. Moreover, according to the probabilistic sensitivity analyses, the conclusions reached are robust to changes in the distribution of the second-line treatments.

The model incorporated resource use and utility values for an "average patient" and did not take into account stage of disease and patients' characteristics such as age, gender, suitability of patients for different chemotherapy regimens, and other comorbidities. The model considered only direct healthcare costs borne by the secondary healthcare sector in each country and did not consider costs borne by the community. Moreover, the costs and consequences of managing patients who survive beyond two years are also excluded. Also, the study excluded costs incurred by patients, families, and/or their caregivers and indirect costs incurred by society as a result of patients taking time off work and/or not being able to lead productive lives, although the majority of patients are expected to have a mean age of 65 years. Consequently, inclusion of these costs may affect the study's results and need to be studied further in larger populations.

First-line treatment with doxorubicin/ifosfamide was found to be cost effective when compared to first-line trabectedin monotherapy in Italy, Spain, and Sweden. In this study, patients' health status, in terms of the number of QALYs at two years, is a reflection of the probability of being in different health states over the study period and the duration of being in each health state. According to the Markov model, first-line treatment with doxorubicin/ifosfamide yields more QALYs than with trabectedin monotherapy, irrespective of whether second-line chemotherapy is included in the analysis. Additionally, in all three countries use of doxorubicin/ifosfamide leads to lower two-year healthcare costs. Moreover, at a threshold of €35,000 per QALY, >90% of a cohort is expected to be cost effectively treated with doxorubicin/ifosfamide compared to trabectedin monotherapy in all three countries. The primary cost driver of managing patients in the trabectedin monotherapy group is the unit cost of this cytotoxic agent. Subsequent to completion of this study the results of the landmark EORTC62012 study comparing doxorubicin with doxorubicin/ifosfamide as first-line treatment for ASTS have been reported as an abstract [104]. This multi-institutional, phase III study recruited 455 patients and demonstrated an improved progression-free survival for the combination arm but significantly worse toxicity and no overall survival benefit. Many oncologists would therefore consider single agent doxorubicin to be the new standard of care, a treatment that would be expected to have lower acquisition and toxicity management costs than doxorubicin/ifosfamide. Hence, it is difficult to see how the high acquisition cost of trabectedin affords value for money to the publicly funded healthcare systems in Italy, Spain, and Sweden when used as a first-line treatment for ASTS. Consequently, trabectedin should be used following failure of doxorubicin and ifosfamide treatment in accordance with its indication.

In the absence of any published health economic studies assessing the cost effectiveness of treatments for the management of ASTS in any country, it is not known how the results of the present analysis would generalise to other settings and patient groups and whether all important factors for the decision under consideration have been taken into account. Nevertheless, within the limitations of the present study, doxorubicin/ifosfamide (or single agent doxorubicin [104]) is expected to be a preferred first-line treatment strategy for the management of ASTS compared to trabectedin monotherapy in all three countries.

In conclusion, within the model's limitations, first-line treatment of patients with ASTS with doxorubicin/ifosfamide instead of trabectedin monotherapy affords a cost-effective use of publicly funded healthcare resources in Italy, Spain, and Sweden. These findings support the recommendation that trabectedin should remain a second/third-line treatment.

Acknowledgments

The authors wish to thank the following oncologists for their contributions to this study: Dr. R. Berardi, Azienda Ospedaliero, Universitaria Ospedali Riuniti Umberto I, Ancona, Italy; Dr. M. Berretta, Centro di Riferimento Oncologico, IRCCS, Aviano, Italy; Dr. A. Comandone, Gradenigo Hospital and Gruppo Piemontese Sarcomi, Torino, Italy; Dr. M. C. Deidda, Policlinico Universitario di Monserrato, Cagliari, Italy; Dr. L. Tomasello, National Cancer Research Institute, Genoa, Italy; Dr. B. Vincenzi, University Campus Bio-Medico, Rome, Italy; Dr. C. Balaña, Hospital Germans Trias i Pujol, Badalona, Spain; Dr. J. M. Broto, Hospital Universitario Son Dureta, Palma De Mallorca, Spain; Dr. J. F. Gonzalez, Grupo Hospitalario Quirón, Pozuelo de Alarcón, Spain; Dr. V. M. Marín, Hospital Universitario La Paz, Madrid, Spain; Dr. A. L. Pousa, Hospital De Sant Pau, Barcelona, Spain; Dr. J. I. Verdum, Clínica Corachan, Barcelona, Spain; Dr. E. Lidbrink, Karolinska Institute, Stockholm, Sweden; Professor H. Hagberg, University Hospital, Uppsala, Sweden; Dr. K. Engström, Sahlgrenska University Hospital, Gothenburg, Sweden; Dr. M. Erlanson, University Hospital, Umeå, Sweden; Dr. M. Jerkeman, University Hospital, Lund, Sweden; and Dr. N. Wall, University Hospital, Linköping, Sweden. This study was supported by Baxter Healthcare, Zurich, Switzerland. However, Baxter Healthcare did not have any control of the methodology, conduct, results, or conclusion of this study or editorial involvement in this paper. The authors have no other conflict of interests that is directly relevant to the content of this paper, which remains their sole responsibility.

References

[1] P. A. Cassier, S. I. Labidi-Galy, P. Heudel et al., "Therapeutic pipeline for soft-tissue sarcoma," *Expert Opinion on Pharmacotherapy*, vol. 12, no. 16, pp. 2479–2491, 2011.

[2] M. A. Clark, C. Fisher, I. Judson, and J. M. Thomas, "Soft-tissue sarcomas in adults," *The New England Journal of Medicine*, vol. 353, no. 7, pp. 701–711, 2005.

[3] N. Penel, C. Nisse, S. Feddal, and E. Lartigau, "Soft tissue sarcoma," *Presse Medicale*, vol. 30, no. 28, pp. 1405–1413, 2001.

[4] "Cancer Research UK," 2011, http://www.cancerresearchuk.org/home/.

[5] M. F. Brennan, E. S. Casper, and L. B. Harrison, "Soft tissue sarcoma," in *Cancer: Principles and Practice of Oncology*, V. T. deVita Jr., S. Hellman, and S. A. Rosenberg, Eds., pp. 1738–1788, Lippincott-Ravel Publishers, Philadelphia, Pa, USA, 5th edition, 1997.

[6] A. Misra, N. Mistry, R. Grimer, and F. Peart, "The management of soft tissue sarcoma," *Journal of Plastic, Reconstructive and Aesthetic Surgery*, vol. 62, no. 2, pp. 161–174, 2009.

[7] J. F. Abellan, J. M. Lamo de Espinosa, J. Duart et al., "Nonreferral of possible soft tissue sarcomas in adults: a dangerous omission in policy," *Sarcoma*, vol. 2009, Article ID 827912, 7 pages, 2009.

[8] J. M. Coindre, P. Terrier, L. Guillou et al., "Predictive value of grade for metastasis development in the main histologic types of adult soft tissue sarcomas: a study of 1240 patients from the French Federation of Cancer Centers Sarcoma Group," *Cancer*, vol. 91, no. 10, pp. 1914–1926, 2001.

[9] M. van Glabbeke, A. T. van Oosterom, J. W. Oosterhuis et al., "Prognostic factors for the outcome of chemotherapy in advanced soft tissue sarcoma: an analysis of 2,185 patients treated with anthracycline- containing first-line regimens—a European organization for research and treatment of Cancer Soft Tissue and Bone Sarcoma Group Study," *Journal of Clinical Oncology*, vol. 17, no. 1, pp. 150–157, 1999.

[10] A. Italiano, M. Toulmonde, and B. Bui-Nguyen, "Chemotherapy options for patients with advanced soft-tissue sarcoma beyond anthracyclines," *Bulletin du Cancer*, vol. 97, no. 6, pp. 679–686, 2010.

[11] K. Thornton, C. E. Pesce, and M. A. Choti, "Multidisciplinary management of metastatic sarcoma," *Surgical Clinics of North America*, vol. 88, no. 3, pp. 661–672, 2008.

[12] The ESMO/European Sarcoma Network Working Group, "Soft tissue and visceral sarcomas: ESMO clinical practice guidelines for diagnosis, treatment and follow-up," *Annals of Oncology*, vol. 23, supplement 7, pp. vii92–vii99, 2012.

[13] S. Verma and V. Bramwell, "Dose-intensive chemotherapy in advanced adult soft tissue sarcoma," *Expert Review of Anticancer Therapy*, vol. 2, no. 2, pp. 201–215, 2002.

[14] J. M. Buesa, A. López-Pousa, J. Martín et al., "Phase II trial of first-line high-dose ifosfamide in advanced soft tissue sarcomas of the adult: a study of the Spanish Group for Research on Sarcomas (GEIS)," *Annals of Oncology*, vol. 9, no. 8, pp. 871–876, 1998.

[15] J. Verweij and H. M. Pinedo, "Systemic treatment of advanced or metastatic soft tissue sarcoma," in *Soft Tissue Sarcomas: New Developments in the Multidisciplinary Approach to Treatment*, H. M. Pinedo, J. Verweij, and H. D. Suit, Eds., pp. 75–91, Kluwer Academic, Boston, Mass, USA, 1991.

[16] J. Schütte, R. Kellner, and S. Seeber, "Ifosfamide in the treatment of soft-tissue sarcomas: experience at the West German Tumor Center, Essen," *Cancer Chemotherapy and Pharmacology*, vol. 1, no. 2, pp. S194–S198, 1993.

[17] A. Santoro, T. Tursz, H. Mouridsen et al., "Doxorubicin versus CYVADIC versus doxorubicin plus ifosfamide in first- line treatment of advanced soft tissue sarcomas: a randomized study of the European Organization for Research and Treatment of Cancer Soft Tissue and Bone Sarcoma Group," *Journal of Clinical Oncology*, vol. 13, no. 7, pp. 1537–1545, 1995.

[18] R. Garcia-Carbonero, J. G. Supko, R. G. Maki et al., "Ecteinascidin-743 (ET-743) for chemotherapy-naive patients with advanced soft tissue sarcomas: multicenter phase II and pharmacokinetic study," *Journal of Clinical Oncology*, vol. 23, no. 24, pp. 5484–5492, 2005.

[19] A. L. Cesne, J. Y. Blay, I. Judson et al., "Phase II study of ET-743 in advanced soft tissue sarcomas: a European Organisation for the Research and Treatment of Cancer," *Journal of Clinical Oncology*, vol. 23, no. 3, pp. 576–584, 2005.

[20] J. Fayette, I. R. Coquard, L. Alberti, D. Ranchère, H. Boyle, and J.-Y. Blay, "ET-743: a novel agent with activity in soft tissue sarcomas," *Oncologist*, vol. 10, no. 10, pp. 827–832, 2005.

[21] M. M. Oken, R. H. Creech, and T. E. Davis, "Toxicology and response criteria of the Eastern Cooperative Oncology Group," *American Journal of Clinical Oncology*, vol. 5, no. 6, pp. 649–655, 1982.

[22] J. L. Mansi, C. Fisher, E. Wiltshaw, S. MacMillan, M. King, and R. Stuart-Harris, "A phase I-II study of ifosfamide in combination with adriamycin in the treatment of adult soft tissue sarcoma," *European Journal of Cancer and Clinical Oncology*, vol. 24, no. 9, pp. 1439–1443, 1988.

[23] F. P. Worden, J. M. G. Taylor, J. S. Biermann et al., "Randomized phase II evaluation of 6 g/m2 of ifosfamide plus doxorubicin and granulocyte colony-stimulating factor (G-CSF) compared with 12 g/m^2 of ifosfamide plus doxorubicin and G-CSF in the treatment of poor-prognosis soft tissue sarcoma," *Journal of Clinical Oncology*, vol. 23, no. 1, pp. 105–112, 2005.

[24] A. Le Cesne, I. Judson, D. Crowther et al., "Randomized phase III study comparing conventional-dose doxorubicin plus ifosfamide versus high-dose doxorubicin plus infosfamide plus recombinant human granulocyte-macrophage colony-stimulating factor in advanced soft tissue sarcomas: a trial of the European Organization for Research and Treatment of Cancer/Soft Tissue and Bone Sarcoma Group," *Journal of Clinical Oncology*, vol. 18, no. 14, pp. 2676–2684, 2000.

[25] C. Bokemeyer, A. Franzke, J. T. Hartmann et al., "A phase I/II study of sequential, dose-escalated, high dose ifosfamide plus doxorubicin with peripheral blood stem cell support for the treatment of patients with advanced soft tissue sarcomas," *Cancer*, vol. 80, no. 7, pp. 1221–1227, 1997.

[26] T. de Pas, F. de Braud, L. Orlando et al., "High-dose ifosfamide plus adriamycin in the treatment of adult advanced soft tissue sarcomas: is it feasible?" *Annals of Oncology*, vol. 9, no. 8, pp. 917–919, 1998.

[27] N. Wall and H. Starkhammar, "Chemotherapy of soft tissue sarcoma: a clinical evaluation of treatment over ten years," *Acta Oncologica*, vol. 42, no. 1, pp. 55–61, 2003.

[28] S. Leyvraz, M. Bacchi, T. Cerny et al., "Phase I multicenter study of combined high-dose ifosfamide and doxorubicin in the treatment of advanced sarcomas. Swiss Group for Clinical Research (SAKK)," *Annals of Oncology*, vol. 9, no. 8, pp. 877–884, 1998.

[29] J. Schütte, H. T. Mouridsen, W. Steward et al., "Ifosfamide plus doxorubicin in previously untreated patients with advanced soft-tissue sarcoma," *Cancer Chemotherapy and Pharmacology*, vol. 31, no. 2, pp. S204–S209, 1993.

[30] A. Comandone, S. Bretti, O. Bertetto, C. Oliva, P. Bergnolo, and C. Bumma, "Low dose adriamycin and ifosfamide in the treatment of advanced adult soft tissue sarcomas," *Anticancer Research B*, vol. 20, no. 3, pp. 2077–2080, 2000.

[31] I. Barişta, G. Tekuzman, S. Yalçin et al., "Treatment of advanced soft tissue sarcomas with ifosfamide and doxorubicin combination chemotherapy," *Journal of Surgical Oncology*, vol. 73, no. 1, pp. 12–16, 2000.

[32] R. E. Hawkins, E. Wiltshaw, and J. L. Mansi, "Ifosfamide with and without adriamycin in advanced uterine leiomyosarcoma,"

Cancer Chemotherapy and Pharmacology, vol. 26, pp. S26–S29, 1990.

[33] P. J. Loehrer Sr., G. W. Sledge Jr., C. Nicaise et al., "Ifosfamide plus doxorubicin in metastatic adult sarcomas: a multi-institutional phase II trial," *Journal of Clinical Oncology*, vol. 7, no. 11, pp. 1655–1659, 1989.

[34] G. D. Demetri, "ET-743: the US experience in sarcomas of soft tissues," *Anti-Cancer Drugs*, vol. 13, no. 1, pp. S7–S9, 2002.

[35] W. J. Köstler, T. Brodowicz, Y. Attems et al., "Docetaxel as rescue medication in anthracycline- and ifostamide-resistant locally advanced or metastatic soft tissue sarcoma: results of a phase II trial," *Annals of Oncology*, vol. 12, no. 9, pp. 1281–1288, 2001.

[36] Q. G. van Hoesel, J. Verweij, G. Catimel et al., "Phase II study with docetaxel (Taxotere) in advanced soft tissue sarcomas of the adult. EORTC Soft Tissue and Bone Sarcoma Group," *Annals of Oncology*, vol. 5, no. 6, pp. 539–542, 1994.

[37] A. Santoro, A. Romanini, A. Rosso et al., "Lack of activity of docetaxel in soft tissue sarcomas: results of a phase II study of the Italian Group on Rare Tumors," *Sarcoma*, vol. 3, no. 3-4, pp. 177–181, 1999.

[38] A. Minchom, R. L. Jones, C. Fisher et al., "Clinical benefit of second-line palliative chemotherapy in advanced soft-tissue sarcoma," *Sarcoma*, vol. 2010, Article ID 264360, 8 pages, 2010.

[39] J. Verweij, S. M. Lee, W. Ruka et al., "Randomized phase II study of docetaxel versus doxorubicin in first- and second-line chemotherapy for locally advanced or metastatic soft tissue sarcomas in adults: a study of the European Organization for Research and Treatment of Cancer Soft Tissue and Bone Sarcoma Group," *Journal of Clinical Oncology*, vol. 18, no. 10, pp. 2081–2086, 2000.

[40] R. G. Maki, J. K. Wathen, S. R. Patel et al., "Randomised phase II study of gemcitabine and docetaxel compared with gemcitabine alone in patients with metastatic soft tissue sarcomas: results of sarcoma alliance for research through collaboration study 002," *Journal of Clinical Oncology*, vol. 25, no. 19, pp. 2755–2763, 2007.

[41] A. Amodio, S. Carpano, C. Manfredi et al., "Gemcitabine in advanced stage soft tissue sarcoma: a phase II study," *Clinical Therapeutics*, vol. 150, no. 1, pp. 17–20, 1999.

[42] O. Merimsky, I. Meller, G. Flusser et al., "Gemcitabine in soft tissue or bone sarcoma resistant to standard chemotherapy: a phase II study," *Cancer Chemotherapy and Pharmacology*, vol. 45, no. 2, pp. 177–181, 2000.

[43] E. Späth-Schwalbe, I. Genvresse, A. Koschuth, A. Dietzmann, R. Grunewald, and K. Possinger, "Phase II trial of gemcitabine in patients with pretreated advanced soft tissue sarcomas," *Anti-Cancer Drugs*, vol. 11, no. 5, pp. 325–329, 2000.

[44] V. Ferraresi, M. Ciccarese, M. C. Cercato et al., "Gemcitabine at fixed dose-rate in patients with advanced soft tissue sarcomas: a mono-institutional phase II study," *Cancer Chemotherapy and Pharmacology*, vol. 63, no. 1, pp. 149–155, 2008.

[45] J. T. Hartmann, K. Oechsle, J. Huober et al., "An open label, non-comparative phase II study of gemcitabine as salvage treatment for patients with pretreated adult type soft tissue sarcoma," *Investigational New Drugs*, vol. 24, no. 3, pp. 249–253, 2006.

[46] S. Okuno, J. Edmonson, M. Mahoney, J. C. Buckner, S. Frytak, and E. Galanis, "Phase II trial of gemcitabine in advanced sarcomas," *Cancer*, vol. 94, no. 12, pp. 3225–3229, 2002.

[47] S. R. Patel, V. Gandhi, J. Jenkins et al., "Phase II clinical investigation of gemcitabine in advanced soft tissue sarcomas and window evaluation of dose rate on gemcitabine triphosphate accumulation," *Journal of Clinical Oncology*, vol. 19, no. 15, pp. 3483–3489, 2001.

[48] J. M. Buesa, R. Losa, A. Fernández et al., "Phase I clinical trial of fixed-dose rate infusional gemcitabine and dacarbazine in the treatment of advanced soft tissue sarcoma, with assessment of gemcitabine triphosphate accumulation," *Cancer*, vol. 101, no. 10, pp. 2261–2269, 2004.

[49] R. Losa, J. Fra, A. López-Pousa et al., "Phase II study with the combination of gemcitabine and DTIC in patients with advanced soft tissue sarcomas," *Cancer Chemotherapy and Pharmacology*, vol. 59, no. 2, pp. 251–259, 2007.

[50] X. García-del-Muro, A. López-Pousa, J. Maurel et al., "Randomized phase II study comparing gemcitabine plus dacarbazine versus dacarbazine alone in patients with previously treated soft tissue sarcoma: a Spanish Group for Research on Sarcomas Study," *Journal of Clinical Oncology*, vol. 29, no. 18, pp. 2528–2533, 2011.

[51] K. M. Leu, L. J. Ostruszka, D. Shewach et al., "Laboratory and clinical evidence of synergistic cytotoxicity of sequential treament with gemcitabine followed by docetaxel in the treatment of sarcoma," *Journal of Clinical Oncology*, vol. 22, no. 9, pp. 1706–1712, 2004.

[52] M. L. Hensley, R. Maki, E. Venkatraman et al., "Gemcitabine and docetaxel in patients with unresectable leiomyosarcoma: results of a phase II trial," *Journal of Clinical Oncology*, vol. 20, no. 12, pp. 2824–2831, 2002.

[53] P. Ebeling, L. Eisele, P. Schuett et al., "Docetaxel and gemcitabine in the treatment of soft tissue sarcoma—a single-center experience," *Onkologie*, vol. 31, no. 1-2, pp. 11–16, 2008.

[54] J.-O. Bay, I. Ray-Coquard, J. Fayette et al., "Docetaxel and gemcitabine combination in 133 advanced soft-tissue sarcomas: a retrospective analysis," *International Journal of Cancer*, vol. 119, no. 3, pp. 706–711, 2006.

[55] J. A. Morgan, S. George, J. Desai et al., "Phase II study of gemcitabine/vinorelbine (GV) as first or second line chemotherapy in patients with metastatic soft tissue sarcoma.," *Journal of Clinical Oncology*, vol. 22, no. 14S, pp. 9004–9009, 2004, ASCO Annual Meeting Proceedings.

[56] P. Dileo, J. A. Morgan, D. Zahrieh et al., "Gemcitabine and vinorelbine combination chemotherapy for patients with advanced soft tissue sarcomas: results of a phase II trial," *Cancer*, vol. 109, no. 9, pp. 1863–1869, 2007.

[57] A. T. van Oosterom, H. T. Mouridsen, O. S. Nielsen et al., "Results of randomised studies of the EORTC Soft Tissue and Bone Sarcoma Group (STBSG) with two different ifosfamide regimens in first- and second-line chemotherapy in advanced soft tissue sarcoma patients," *European Journal of Cancer*, vol. 38, no. 18, pp. 2397–2406, 2002.

[58] O. S. Nielsen, I. Judson, Q. van Hoesel et al., "Effect of high-dose ifosfamide in advanced soft tissue sarcomas. A multicentre phase II study of the EORTC Soft Tissue and Bone Sarcoma Group," *European Journal of Cancer*, vol. 36, no. 1, pp. 61–67, 2000.

[59] R. Coriat, O. Mir, S. Camps et al., "Ambulatory administration of 5-day infusion ifosfamide + mesna: a pilot study in sarcoma patients," *Cancer Chemotherapy and Pharmacology*, vol. 65, no. 3, pp. 491–495, 2010.

[60] T. Tursz, "High-dose ifosfamide in the treatment of advanced soft tissue sarcomas," *Seminars in Oncology*, vol. 23, supplement 7, no. 3, pp. 34–39, 1996.

[61] A. Le Cesne, G. Demetri, and L. Jean, "Impact of Yondelis in the natural history of patients with pretreated advanced soft tissue sarcomas: long-term follow-up results," in *Proceedings of*

the AACR-NCI-EORTC International Conference on Molecular Targets and Cancer Therapeutics, pp. 17–23, November 2003.

[62] E. G. C. Brain, "Safety and efficacy of ET-743: the French experience," *Anti-Cancer Drugs*, vol. 13, no. 1, pp. S11–S14, 2002.

[63] G. Huygh, P. M. J. Clement, H. Dumez et al., "Ecteinascidin-743: evidence of activity in advanced, pretreated soft tissue and bone sarcoma patients," *Sarcoma*, vol. 2006, Article ID 56282, 11 pages, 2006.

[64] S. Delaloge, A. Yovine, A. Taamma et al., "Ecteinascidin-743: a marine-derived compound in advanced, pretreated sarcoma patients - Preliminary evidence of activity," *Journal of Clinical Oncology*, vol. 19, no. 5, pp. 1248–1255, 2001.

[65] A. Yovine, M. Riofrio, J. Y. Blay et al., "Phase II study of ecteinascidin-743 in advanced pretreated soft tissue sarcoma patients," *Journal of Clinical Oncology*, vol. 22, no. 5, pp. 890–899, 2004.

[66] J. Blay, N. Penel, A. Italiano et al., "Trabectedin for advanced sarcomas failing doxorubicin: analysis of 189 unreported patients in a compassionate use program," *Sarcoma*, 2009, ASCO Annual Meeting Poster Presentation.

[67] J. Fayette, H. Boyle, S. Chabaud et al., "Efficacy of trabectedin for advanced sarcomas in clinical trials versus compassionate use programs: analysis of 92 patients treated in a single institution," *Anti-Cancer Drugs*, vol. 21, no. 1, pp. 113–119, 2010.

[68] J. T. Hartmann, K. Oechsle, F. Mayer, L. Kanz, and C. Bokemeyer, "Phase II trial of trofosfamide in patients with advanced pretreated soft tissue sarcomas," *Anticancer Research C*, vol. 23, no. 2, pp. 1899–1901, 2003.

[69] P. Reichardt, D. Pink, J. Tilgner, A. Kretzschmar, P. C. Thuss-Patience, and B. Dörken, "Oral trofosfamide: an active and well-tolerated maintenance therapy for adult patients with advanced bone and soft tissue sarcomas. Results of a retrospective analysis," *Onkologie*, vol. 25, no. 6, pp. 541–546, 2002.

[70] C. Kollmannsberger, W. Brugger, J. T. Hartmann et al., "Phase II study of oral trofosfamide as palliative therapy in pre-treated patients with metastatic soft-tissue sarcoma," *Anti-Cancer Drugs*, vol. 10, no. 5, pp. 453–456, 1999.

[71] L. Švancárová, J. Y. Blay, I. R. Judson et al., "Gemcitabine in advanced adult soft-tissue sarcomas. A phase II study of the EORTC Soft Tissue and Bone Sarcoma Group," *European Journal of Cancer*, vol. 38, no. 4, pp. 556–559, 2002.

[72] Database, "Consejo General de Colegios Oficiales de Farmaceuticos," October 2011, https://botplusweb.portalfarma.com/botplus.asp.

[73] "Läkemedelsportalen (Swedish national pharmaceuticals price list)," October 2011, http://www.fass.se/LIF/info/forstabesoket.jsp.

[74] "Nomenclatore Tariffario Regione Lazio, 2010," 2010, http://www.asl.ri.it/index.php.

[75] J. Branera, J. Puig, M. Gil, R. Bella, A. Darnell, and A. Malet, "Outpatient US-guided percutaneous liver biopsy: technique and complications," *Radiologia*, vol. 47, no. 1, pp. 32–36, 2005.

[76] Regionförbundet- regioner prislistor, October 2011, http://www.norrlandstingen.se/lankar_prislistor.htm.

[77] BOC-Numero 64. Precios de los servicios sanitarios, "en los centros hospitalarios, 2007," October 2011, http://www.fmdv.org.

[78] A. Ringborg, R. Nieuwlaat, P. Lindgren et al., "Costs of atrial fibrillation in five European countries: results from the Euro Heart Survey on atrial fibrillation," *Europace*, vol. 10, no. 4, pp. 403–411, 2008.

[79] "Interviews with clinicians".

[80] "Baxter Healthcare SA".

[81] "Italian Medicines Agency, 2010," 2011, http://www.agenziafarmaco.gov.it/en.

[82] M. Vera-Llonch, E. Dukes, J. Rejas, O. Sofrygin, M. Mychaskiw, and G. Oster, "Cost-effectiveness of pregabalin versus venlafaxine in the treatment of generalized anxiety disorder: findings from a Spanish perspective," *European Journal of Health Economics*, vol. 11, no. 1, pp. 35–44, 2010.

[83] J. F. Guest, D. Concolino, R. di Vito, C. Feliciani, R. Parini, and A. Zampetti, "Modelling the resource implications of managing adults with Fabry disease in Italy," *European Journal of Clinical Investigation*, vol. 41, no. 7, pp. 710–718, 2011.

[84] "World Health Organisation," 2010, http://www.who.int/en.

[85] G. Mickisch, M. Gore, B. Escudier, G. Procopio, S. Walzer, and M. Nuijten, "Costs of managing adverse events in the treatment of first-line metastatic renal cell carcinoma: bevacizumab in combination with interferon-α2a compared with sunitinib," *British Journal of Cancer*, vol. 102, no. 1, pp. 80–86, 2010.

[86] M. Ortega-Andreu, H. Pérez-Chrzanowska, R. Figueredo et al., "Blood loss control with two doses of tranexamic acid in a multimodal protocol for total knee arthroplasty," *The Open Orthopaedics Journal*, vol. 5, pp. 44–48, 2011.

[87] A. H. Glenngård and U. Persson, "En blodtransfusion i Sverige - Så mycket kostar den samhället," *Lakartidningen*, vol. 103, no. 38, pp. 2752–2756, 2006.

[88] M. Danova, S. Chiroli, G. Rosti, and Q. V. Doan, "Cost-effectiveness of pegfilgrastim versus six days of filgrastim for preventing febrile neutropenia in breast cancer patients," *Tumori*, vol. 95, no. 2, pp. 219–226, 2009.

[89] J. I. Mayordomo, A. López, N. Viñolas et al., "Retrospective cost analysis of management of febrile neutropenia in cancer patients in Spain," *Current Medical Research and Opinion*, vol. 25, no. 10, pp. 2533–2542, 2009.

[90] F. Kasteng, M. Erlanson, H. Hagberg, E. Kimby, T. Relander, and J. Lundkvist, "Cost-effectiveness of maintenance rituximab treatment after second line therapy in patients with follicular lymphoma in Sweden," *Acta Oncologica*, vol. 47, no. 6, pp. 1029–1036, 2008.

[91] Y. Asukai, A. Valladares, C. Camps et al., "Cost-effectiveness analysis of pemetrexed versus docetaxel in the second-line treatment of non-small cell lung cancer in Spain: results for the non-squamous histology population," *BMC Cancer*, vol. 10, article 26, 2010.

[92] M. Percudani, C. Barbui, J. Beecham, and M. Knapp, "Routine outcome monitoring in clinical practice: service and non-service costs of psychiatric patients attending a Community Mental Health Centre in Italy," *European Psychiatry*, vol. 19, no. 8, pp. 469–477, 2004.

[93] S. Mercadante, G. Intravaia, P. Villari et al., "Clinical and financial analysis of an acute palliative care unit in an oncological department," *Palliative Medicine*, vol. 22, no. 6, pp. 760–767, 2008.

[94] X. Gómez-Batiste, A. Tuca, E. Corrales et al., "Resource consumption and costs of palliative care services in Spain: a multicenter prospective study," *Journal of Pain and Symptom Management*, vol. 31, no. 6, pp. 522–532, 2006.

[95] L. Dahlberg, J. Lundkvist, and H. Lindman, "Health care costs for treatment of disseminated breast cancer," *European Journal of Cancer*, vol. 45, no. 11, pp. 1987–1991, 2009.

[96] J. Hjelmgren, J. Ceberg, U. Persson, and T. A. Alvegård, "The cost of treating pancreatic cancer: a cohort study based on

patients' records from four hospitals in Sweden," *Acta Oncologica*, vol. 42, no. 3, pp. 218–226, 2003.

[97] I. Judson, J. A. Radford, M. Harris et al., "Randomised phase II trial of pegylated liposomal doxorubicin (DOXIL/CAELYX) versus doxorubicin in the treatment of advanced or metastatic soft tissue sarcoma: a study by the EORTC Soft Tissue and Bone Sarcoma Group," *European Journal of Cancer*, vol. 37, no. 7, pp. 870–877, 2001.

[98] J. F. Guest, E. Sladkevicius, N. Gough, M. Linch, and R. Grimer, "Utility values for advanced soft tissue sarcoma health States from the general public in the United kingdom," *Sarcoma*, vol. 2013, Article ID 863056, 9 pages, 2013.

[99] S. Capri, A. Ceci, L. Terranova et al., "Guidelines for economic evaluations in Italy: recommendations from the Italian group of pharmacoeconomic studies," *Drug Information Journal*, vol. 35, no. 1, pp. 189–201, 2001.

[100] J. López-Bastida, J. Oliva, F. Antoñanzas et al., "Spanish recommendations on economic evaluation of health technologies," *The European Journal of Health Economics*, vol. 11, no. 5, pp. 513–520, 2010.

[101] F. Borgström, O. Johnell, J. A. Kanis, A. Oden, D. Sykes, and B. Jönsson, "Cost effectiveness of raloxifene in the treatment of osteoporosis in Sweden: an economic evaluation based on the MORE study," *PharmacoEconomics*, vol. 22, no. 17, pp. 1153–1165, 2004.

[102] A. M. Gray, P. M. Clarke, J. Wolstenholme et al., *Applied Methods of Cost-Effectiveness Analysis in Health Care*, Oxford University Press, New York, NY, USA, 2010.

[103] "SSG XX- A Scandinavian Sarcoma Group treatment protocol for adult patients with non-metastatic high-risk soft tissue sarcoma of the extremities and trunk wall," Scandinavian Sarcoma Group and Oncologic Center, Lund, Sweden, 2007.

[104] W. T. A. van der Graaf, I. Judson, J. Verweij et al., "Results of a randomised phase III trial (EORTC, 62012) of single agent doxorubicin versus doxorubicin plus ifosfamide as first line chemotherapy for patients with advanced or metastatic soft tissue sarcoma: a survival study by the EORTC soft tissue and bone sarcoma group," ESMO Congress. Abstract LBA7, October 2012, http://oncologypro.esmo.org/meeting-resources/meeting-abstracts/european-society-for-medical-oncology-esmo-2012/results-of-a-randomised-phase-iii-trial-2882.aspx.

9

DDIT3 Expression in Liposarcoma Development

Christina Kåbjörn Gustafsson,[1] Katarina Engström,[2] and Pierre Åman[1]

[1] *Sahlgrenska Cancer Center, Department of Pathology, Institute of Biomedicine, University of Gothenburg, P.O. Box 425, 40530 Gothenburg, Sweden*
[2] *Department of Oncology, Institute of Medical Sciences, University of Gothenburg, Gothenburg, Sweden*

Correspondence should be addressed to Pierre Åman; pierre.aman@gu.se

Academic Editor: Enrique de Alava

Liposarcomas are mesenchymal tumors containing variable numbers of lipoblasts or adipocytes. The most common entities, well differentiated/dedifferentiated liposarcoma (WDLS/DDLS) and myxoid/round cell liposarcoma (MLS/RCLS), are both characterized by genetic rearrangements that affect the expression of the transcription factor DDIT3. DDIT3 induces liposarcoma morphology when ectopically expressed in a human fibrosarcoma. The role of DDIT3 in lipomatous tumors is, however, unclear. We have analyzed the expression of DDIT3 in 37 cases of liposarcoma (WDLS/DDLS $n = 10$, MLS/RCLS $n = 16$, and pleomorphic liposarcomas (PLS) $n = 11$) and 11 cases of common benign lipomas. Major cell subpopulations of WDLS/DDLS and MLS/RCLS tumors were found to express DDIT3 or the derived fusion protein, whereas PLS cases showed only a few positive cells. The lipomas contained large subpopulations expressing DDIT3. No correlation between numbers of DDIT3 expressing cells and numbers of lipoblasts/adipocytes was found. In vitro adipogenic treatment of two DDIT3 expressing cell lines induced lipid accumulation in small subpopulations only. Our results suggest a dual, promoting and limiting, role for DDIT3 in the formation of lipoblasts and liposarcoma morphology.

1. Introduction

Adipocytic tumors are the most frequent types of soft tissue tumors occurring in humans. They also represent the largest single group of mesenchymal tumors [1] and are characterized by the more or less prominent presence of lipoblasts or adipocytes. Some of the adipocytic neoplasms are characterized by recurrent tumor type specific genetic rearrangements. Most WDLS/DDLS cases contain amplified segments of chromosome 12q13–15 carried as ring chromosomes or large marker chromosomes [2–4]. The amplified regions contain many tumor associated genes and among them *DDIT3*. MLS/RCLS carry a rearranged *DDIT3* fused to *FUS* or *EWSR1* [5, 6]. *DDIT3* is expressed and involved in the regulation of adipocyte development and we have previously shown that expression of *DDIT3* in a low differentiated fibrosarcoma cell line results in morphological conversion towards a liposarcoma phenotype [7]. These observations suggest that expression of DDIT3 protein could be a common phenotype determining factor for several types of lipomatous tumors. The aim of the present study was to test this hypothesis by investigating the expression of the DDIT3 protein in 3 different subtypes of liposarcoma and in common lipoma.

We further evaluated the role of DDIT3 expression by studying lipoblast formation in cultured liposarcoma cells treated with adipogenic factors. DDIT3 expression is tightly regulated at several levels including translation and protein degradation [8]. This makes expression analysis at protein level the most relevant approach.

2. Material and Methods

2.1. Immunohistochemistry. Paraffin embedded sections were obtained from our pathology department in conformity with Swedish legislation. The material consists of 11 lipomas, 11 PLS, 10 WDLS, and 16 MLS/RCLS.

Sections were prepared from routine paraffin embedded tumor tissue samples from 48 cases of lipomas and liposarcomas (Table 1). Immunohistochemistry (IHC) was performed

Table 1: Cases and DDIT3 expression.

Case	Age	Site		DDIT3 %		FUS/DDIT3 rearrangement	Histological diagnosis
				Nucleus	Cytoplasm		
1	72	im	Axilla	79	0	ND	WLDS
2	69	im	Thigh	34	0	ND	WLDS
3	77	im	Hip	82	0	ND	WLDS
4	71	other	Retroperitoneal	0	36	ND	DDLS
5	42	other	Abdomen	70	0	ND	DDLS
6	80	other	Abdomen	94	0	ND	DDLS
7	73	other	Inguinal	40	0	ND	WDLS
8	77	other	Peritoneal	84	0	ND	WDLS
9	60	other	Inguinal	69	0	ND	WDLS
10	67	im	Thigh	81	0	ND	WDLS/DDLS
11	80	im	Thigh	59	0	Yes	MLS
12	34	im	Thigh	61	0	Yes	MLS
13	49	im	Hip	46	0	Yes	MLS
14	46	im/sc	Hip/thigh	71	0	Yes	MLS
15	39	im	Thigh	24	0	Yes	MLS
16	17	im	Thigh	39	0	Nev	MLS
17	45	im	Thigh	58	0	Yes	MLS
18	76	sc	Back	44	0	Yes	MLS/RCLS
19	42	im	Abdomen	70	0	Yes	MLS/RCLS
20	33	other	Abdomen	50	0	Yes	MLS/RCLS
21	45	other	Abdomen	41	0	Nev	MLS/RCLS
22	73	im	Leg	49	0	Nev	MLS/RCLS
23	38	im	Thigh	64	0	Yes	MLS/RCLS
24	36	im	Thigh	73	0	Yes	MLS/RCLS
25	37	im	Thigh	50	0	Yes	MLS/RCLS
26	46	im	Hip	0	57	Yes	RCLS
27	84	im	Arm	0	9	ND	PLS
28	57	im	Iliopsoas	0	0	ND	PLS
29	89	im	Leg	9	0	ND	PLS
30	88	im	Thigh	2	0	ND	PLS
31	70	im	Thigh	18	0	ND	PLS
32	72	im	Neck	0	7	ND	PLS
33	81	im	Axilla	0	6	ND	PLS
34	69	im	Thigh	0	1	ND	PLS
35	61	im	Thigh	0	9	ND	PLS
36	51	im	Hip	0	0	ND	PLS
37	54	im	Hip	0	20	ND	PLS
38	44	sc	Inguinal	53	0	ND	Lipoma
39	44	sc	Shoulder	54	0	ND	Lipoma
40	51	sc	Shoulder	68	0	ND	Lipoma
41	56	sc	Neck	32	0	ND	Lipoma
42	40	sc	Hip	40	0	ND	Lipoma
43	41	sc	Neck	15	0	ND	Lipoma
44	72	sc	Thigh	38	0	ND	Lipoma
45	38	sc	Arm	73	0	ND	Lipoma
46	66	sc	Arm	71	0	ND	Lipoma
47	66	sc	Thigh	81	0	ND	Lipoma
48	47	sc	Back	75	0	ND	Lipoma

Clinical, diagnostic, and DDIT expression data on the investigated cases. DDIT3 expression is shown as percent positive cells.
Abbreviations: im: 0 intramuscular; sc: subcutaneous; ND: not analyzed; nev: not possible to evaluate.

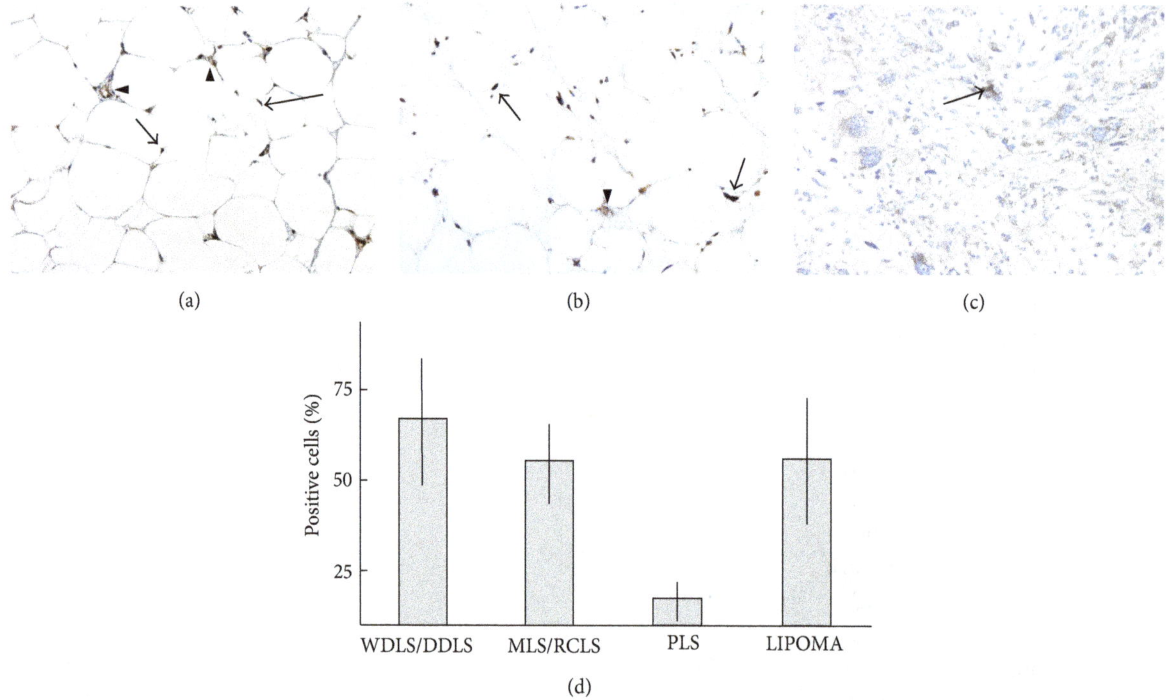

FIGURE 1: DDIT3 immunohistochemistry analysis of lipomatous tumors. (a) Lipoma, nuclear, and DDIT3 expression (arrow) and capillaries are indicated by arrowheads. (b) WDLS/DDLS, nuclear, and cytoplasmic DDIT3 expression (arrow). (c) PLS, nuclear, and cytoplasmic DDIT3 expression in lipoblasts (arrow). (d) Mean value and standard deviation of percent positively stained cells in 10 cases of WDLS/DDLS, 16 cases of MLS/RCLS, 11 cases of PLS, and 11 cases of lipoma.

as described previously [7] using the DDIT3 specific antibody Gadd153 R20 from Santa Cruz Biotechnology at a dilution of 1:200.

The histological specimens were examined and evaluated in a blinded fashion by two examiners. The proportion of stained tumor cells was counted at 200x magnification. Cells with nuclear and cytoplasmic expression were counted avoiding inflammatory cells, endothelial cells, and necrotic areas. Three different areas in each slide were counted and a mean value was calculated.

2.2. Fluorescence In Situ Hybridization Analysis. Interphase FISH analysis of formalin-fixed tumor tissue was performed on 1–4 μm paraffin sections. Three break-apart probes, DDIT3, FUS, and EWSR1 (Vysis, Inc., Downers Grove, IL), were used according to protocols supplied by the manufacturer. Nuclei were counterstained with 10 μL 4′,6′,-diamidino-2′-phenylindole dihydrochloride (DAPI). The sections were analyzed and reanalyzed by two independent reviewers. At least 100 nuclei per section were scored. The interpretation of intact, fusion, and split signals was based on guidelines recommended by the manufacturer and from other clinical laboratories using this method.

2.3. In Vitro Adipogenesis. The GOT3 cell line, established from a WDLS tumor [4], was used to study adipogenic differentiation. The cells were cultured in RPMI 1640 until 100% confluence, after which the medium was changed to adipogenesis induction medium (PT3004 containing human recombinant insulin, dexamethasone, indomethacin, and 3-isobutyl-l-methylxanthine (IBMX); Cambrex, East Rutherford, NJ) or maintenance medium (MM; RPMI 1640 containing 8% fetal calf serum). The cells were treated with adipogenesis induction medium for 3 days, followed by 1 to 3 days in MM. This was repeated three times. Control cultures were fed with only MM following the same schedule. After completed cycles, the cells were cultured for 7 more days in MM with replacement of the medium every 2 to 3 days. The cells were inspected using a microscope, and accumulation of fat was assessed by staining the cells with Oil Red O after fixation with 4% buffered formalin.

3. Results and Discussion

Clinical data, histological features, and DDIT3 protein expression are detailed in Table 1 and representative examples of IHC staining are shown in Figure 1. DDIT3 expression was detected in all but 2 of the 48 investigated cases.

In WDLS/DDLS tumors 40–94% of the cells expressed DDIT3 (Table 1). The constitutive DDIT3 expression in this tumor type could be explained by recurrent gene amplicons that carry the DDIT3 in this tumor type [2, 4]. There was no obvious difference in numbers of DDIT3 expressing cells between WDLS and DDLS in this small series of tumors.

In MLS/RCLS, DDIT3 is expressed as part of the FUS-DDIT3 or EWSR1-DDIT3 fusion oncoproteins [5, 9]. Transcription of the fusion oncogenes is regulated by the ubiquitously active promoters of the *FUS* or *EWSR1* partner genes

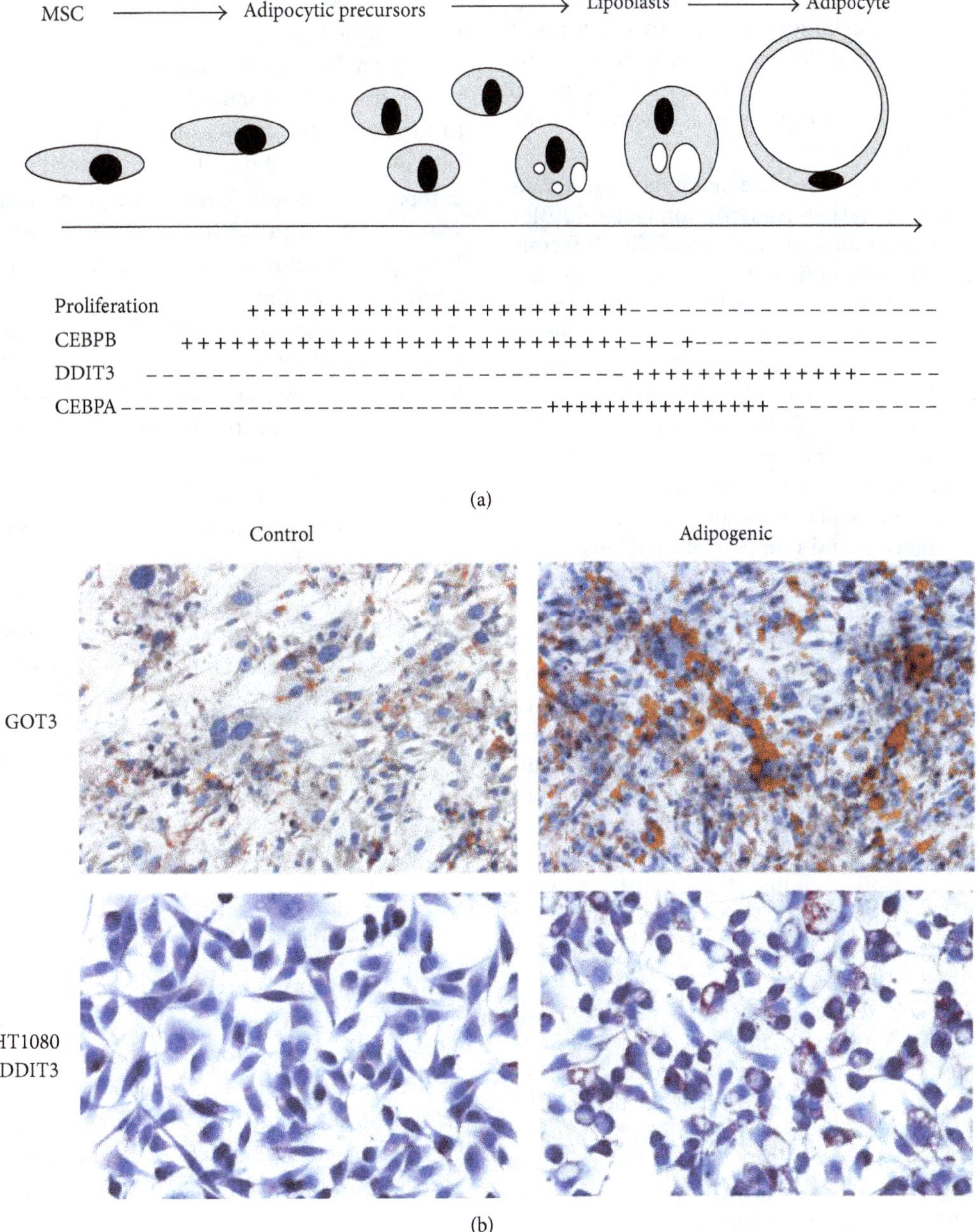

FIGURE 2: Adipocytic differentiation. (a) Schematic presentation of CEBPB, CEBPA, and DDIT3 expression in adipocyte differentiation. (b) Lipoblast formation and accumulation of lipids in GOT3 WDLS/DDLS derived cell line (top panels) and DDIT3 transfected HT1080 fibrosarcoma cell line (bottom panels) cultured in control or adipogenic medium. Oil Red O staining shows lipids in red.

[6]. The MLS/RCLS tumors contained 24–73% FUS-DDIT3 or EWSR1-DDIT3 positive cells (Table 1). The fact that the fusion proteins could be detected only in a subpopulation of the tumor cells indicates that the levels of fusion proteins are regulated also at posttranscriptional levels. There was no clear difference in numbers of positive cells between typical myxoid cases and those with round cell components.

A cytoplasmic DDIT3 staining pattern was seen in most PLS cases but only in a low percentage of the cells. Three tumors (cases 29, 30, and 31) showed a nuclear staining pattern of DDIT3 in a minority of the cells, mostly with bizarre nuclei. There are no reported recurrent genetic aberrations causing DDIT3 expression in PLS. Instead, stress induced expression may explain the presence of DDIT3 protein in these tumors. Cytoplasmic or nuclear DDIT3 expression may be induced as a response to various stress conditions such as DNA damage, hypoxia, and lack of nutrients [10–12]. Such conditions are common in tumor tissues and may thus lead to DDIT3 expression.

The highly differentiated common lipoma expressed DDIT3 in 15–81% of the cells (Figure 1). The DDIT3 protein was found both in univacuolated fat cells and surrounding spindle cells. *DDIT3* is not amplified or rearranged in lipomas. Instead, most of the cases carry a rearranged *HMGA2* gene that may promote adipocytic differentiation [13]. The DDIT3 expression found in lipoma cells may therefore result from a terminal adipocyte differentiation program in these tumor cells [14]. Thus, there is currently no reason to believe that aberrant DDIT3 expression is involved in the development of this tumor type.

DDIT3 is normally expressed late in adipocyte differentiation together with the related transcription factor CEBPA [14]. The timing of expression of DDIT3 and CEBP factors is crucial for normal differentiation (Figure 2). Premature or overexpression of DDIT3 in preadipocytes may block terminal differentiation [15–17]. In the context of liposarcoma development, aberrant DDIT3 or FUS-DDIT3 expression in primitive tumor cells may open an adipocytic differentiation pathway but block later stages of adipocyte development. We speculate that only a small minority of the tumor cells would make it through the block and differentiate to lipoblasts. This would also explain the lack of correlation between numbers of DDIT3 expressing cells and numbers of lipoblasts in the investigated tumors.

To test this hypothesis, the WDLS/DDLS derived cell line GOT3 was analyzed after adipogenic treatment. This cell line carries a large chromosome 12 derived amplicon including the DDIT3 gene and was found to express DDIT3 constitutively in almost all cells [4]. A limited accumulation of lipids in sporadic cells was seen under standard culture (Figure 2(b)). Transfer to adipogenic culture conditions resulted in lipid accumulation and lipoblast development but only in a minority of the cells. Similar results were obtained for a fibrosarcoma cell line stably transfected with EGFP tagged DDIT3 (Figure 2(b)). These results suggest that aberrant expression of DDIT3 can promote a liposarcoma phenotype in human primitive sarcoma cells [7].

FUS-DDIT3 transfected mouse mesenchymal stem cells cause MLS/RCLS like tumors when injected in mice and *FUS-DDIT3* transfection transforms 3T3 mouse fibroblasts [18, 19]. This shows that *FUS-DDIT3* is a powerful oncogene. The FUS-DDIT3 protein maintains the capacity of DDIT3 to form heterodimers with CEBPA and CEBPB and has been shown to modify or block the activity of its dimer partners [17, 19]. Blocking of CEBPA could inhibit terminal differentiation [17]. Since transcription of the fusion gene is driven by the ubiquitously active FUS promoter, failed expression timing of this abnormal variant of DDIT3 may also contribute to the oncogenic activity. The FUS part of FUS-DDIT3 was found to be necessary for transformation of 3T3 fibroblasts [19] and forced expression of FUS-DDIT3 failed to induce cell cycle arrest as reported for DDIT3.

In contrast to FUS-DDIT3, forced expression of the DDIT3 protein in mesenchymal cells or in transgenic mice gave no evidence of transformation or tumorigenic activity [20]. The normal DDIT3 protein thus cannot be considered a driving oncoprotein. DDIT3 expression may, however, halt proliferation [19, 21]. In WLDLS and DDLS it is overexpressed together with several other proto-oncogenes such as MDM2 and CDK4 that together may cause tumor development. Aberrantly expressed, DDIT3 may in this context act as a promoting or/and tumor-type directing factor by blocking or interfering with the adipocyte differentiation program and the associated growth termination.

Originally described as a nuclear DNA-binding transcription factor, stress induced DDIT3 has later been reported to localize in the cytoplasmic compartment [21]. Cytoplasmic DDIT3 was shown to induce partially distinct effects compared to nuclear DDIT3. One proposed mechanism was sequestration of its CEBP family dimerization partners [21]. In the present study we observed cytoplasmic DDIT3 primarily in PLS cells containing bizarre nuclei, thus supporting a stress related mechanism behind the expression in these cells. Stress induced DDIT3 expression is more likely temporary but could anyway trigger some of the low differentiated PLS cells into an adipocytic differentiation path explaining the presence of lipoblasts in this tumor type. As in WLDLS and DDLS, expression of DDIT3 may also contribute to tumor development by halting the adipocytic program and associated growth termination.

In summary, DDIT3 is expressed in subpopulations of tumor cells in all 4 investigated lipomatous tumor types. There was no obvious difference between the number of DDIT3 expressing cells in the more aggressive DDLS and RCLS compared to WDLS and MLS. Furthermore, DDIT3 was expressed at comparable levels in benign lipomas. Only a minority of DDIT3 expressing sarcoma cells responded to adipogenic conditions in vitro indicating a complex role for DDIT3 as a phenotype directing factor in lipomatous tumors.

Acknowledgments

This work was supported by grants from the Swedish Cancer Society, Assar Gabrielsson Research Foundation, Johan Jansson Foundation for Cancer Research, Socialstyrelsen, Swedish Society for Medical Research, Swedish Children's Cancer Society, BioCARE National Strategic Research Program at the University of Gothenburg, and Wilhelm and Martina Lundgren Foundation for Scientific Research.

References

[1] C. D. M. Fletcher, K. Krishnan Unni, and F. Mertens, *Tumors of Soft Tissue and Bone*, IARC Press, 2000.

[2] F. Pedeutour, A. Forus, J.M. Berner et al., "Structure of the supernumerary ring and giant rod chromosomes in adipose tissue tumors," *Genes, Chromosomes & Cancer*, vol. 24, no. 1, pp. 30–41, 1999.

[3] F. Pedeutour, R. F. Suijkerbuijk, A. Forus et al., "Complex composition and co-amplification of SAS and MDM2 in ring and giant rod marker chromosomes in well-differentiated liposarcoma," *Genes, Chromosomes & Cancer*, vol. 10, no. 2, pp. 85–94, 1994.

[4] F. Persson, A. Olofsson, H. Sjögren et al., "Characterization of the 12q amplicons by high-resolution, oligonucleotide array CGH and expression analyses of a novel liposarcoma cell line," *Cancer Letters*, vol. 260, no. 1-2, pp. 37–47, 2008.

[5] A. Crozat, P. Aman, N. Mandahl, and D. Ron, "Fusion of CHOP to a novel RNA-binding protein in human myxoid liposarcoma," *Nature*, vol. 363, no. 6430, pp. 640–644, 1993.

[6] P. Åman, I. Panagopoulos, C. Lassen et al., "Expression patterns of the human sarcoma-associated genes FUS and EWS and the genomic structure of FUS," *Genomics*, vol. 37, no. 1, pp. 1–8, 1996.

[7] K. Engström, H. Willén, C. Kåbjörn-Gustafsson et al., "The myxoid/round cell liposarcoma fusion oncogene FUS-DDIT3 and the normal DDIT3 induce a liposarcoma phenotype in transfected human fibrosarcoma cells," *American Journal of Pathology*, vol. 168, no. 5, pp. 1642–1653, 2006.

[8] C. Jousse, A. Bruhat, V. Carraro et al., "Inhibition of CHOP translation by a peptide encoded by an open reading frame localized in the chop 5′UTR," *Nucleic Acids Research*, vol. 29, no. 21, pp. 4341–4351, 2001.

[9] I. Panagopoulos, M. Höglund, F. Mertens, N. Mandahl, F. Mitelman, and P. Åman, "Fusion of the EWS and CHOP genes in myxoid liposarcoma," *Oncogene*, vol. 12, no. 3, pp. 489–494, 1996.

[10] A. Benavides, D. Pastor, P. Santos, P. Tranque, and S. Calvo, "CHOP plays a pivotal role in the astrocyte death induced by oxygen and glucose deprivation," *Glia*, vol. 52, no. 4, pp. 261–275, 2005.

[11] Y. Ma, J. W. Brewer, J. Alan Diehl, and L. M. Hendershot, "Two distinct stress signaling pathways converge upon the CHOP promoter during the mammalian unfolded protein response," *Journal of Molecular Biology*, vol. 318, no. 5, pp. 1351–1365, 2002.

[12] A. A. Welihinda, W. Tirasophon, and R. J. Kaufman, "The cellular response to protein misfolding in the endoplasmic reticulum," *Gene Expression*, vol. 7, no. 4–6, pp. 293–300, 1999.

[13] E. F. P. M. Schoenmakers, S. Wanschura, R. Mols, J. Bullerdiek, H. van den Berghe, and W. J. M. van de Ven, "Recurrent rearrangements in the high mobility group protein gene, HMGI-C, in benign mesenchymal tumours," *Nature Genetics*, vol. 10, no. 4, pp. 436–444, 1995.

[14] G. J. Darlington, S. E. Ross, and O. A. MacDougald, "The role of C/EBP genes in adipocyte differentiation," *The Journal of Biological Chemistry*, vol. 273, no. 46, pp. 30057–30060, 1998.

[15] G. Adelmant, J. D. Gilbert, and S. O. Freytag, "Human translocation liposarcoma-CCAAT/enhancer binding protein (C/EBP) homologous protein (TLS-CHOP) oncoprotein prevents adipocyte differentiation by directly interfering with C/EBPβ function," *The Journal of Biological Chemistry*, vol. 273, no. 25, pp. 15574–15581, 1998.

[16] N. Batchvarova, X.-Z. Wang, and D. Ron, "Inhibition of adipogenesis by the stress-induced protein CHOP (Gadd153)," *EMBO Journal*, vol. 14, no. 19, pp. 4654–4661, 1995.

[17] M. Kuroda, T. Ishida, M. Takanashi, M. Satoh, R. Machinami, and T. Watanabe, "Oncogenic transformation and inhibition of adipocytic conversion of preadipocytes by TLS/FUS-CHOP type II chimeric protein," *American Journal of Pathology*, vol. 151, no. 3, pp. 735–744, 1997.

[18] N. Riggi, L. Cironi, P. Provero et al., "Expression of the FUS-CHOP fusion protein in primary mesenchymal progenitor cells gives rise to a model of myxoid liposarcoma," *Cancer Research*, vol. 66, no. 14, pp. 7016–7023, 2006.

[19] H. Zinszner, R. Albalat, and D. Ron, "A novel effector domain from the RNA-binding protein TLS or EWS is required for oncogenic transformation by CHOP," *Genes and Development*, vol. 8, no. 21, pp. 2513–2526, 1994.

[20] J. Pérez-Losada, M. Sánchez-Martín, M. A. Rodríguez-García et al., "Liposarcoma initiated by FUS/TLS-CHOP: the FUS/TLS domain plays a critical role in the pathogenesis of liposarcoma," *Oncogene*, vol. 19, no. 52, pp. 6015–6022, 2000.

[21] A. Jauhiainen, C. Thomsen, L. Strömbom et al., "Distinct cytoplasmic and nuclear functions of the stress induced protein DDIT3/CHOP/GADD153," *PLoS ONE*, vol. 7, no. 4, Article ID e33208, 2012.

10

Analysis of Surgical Site Infection after Musculoskeletal Tumor Surgery: Risk Assessment using a New Scoring System

Satoshi Nagano,[1] Masahiro Yokouchi,[1] Takao Setoguchi,[2] Hiromi Sasaki,[1] Hirofumi Shimada,[1] Ichiro Kawamura,[1] Yasuhiro Ishidou,[3] Junichi Kamizono,[1] Takuya Yamamoto,[1] Hideki Kawamura,[4] and Setsuro Komiya[1]

[1] *Department of Orthopaedic Surgery, Graduate School of Medical and Dental Sciences, Kagoshima University, 8-35-1 Sakuragaoka, Kagoshima City, Kagoshima 890-8520, Japan*

[2] *The Near-Future Locomotor Organ Medicine Creation Course (Kusunoki Kai), Graduate School of Medical and Dental Sciences, Kagoshima University, 8-35-1 Sakuragaoka, Kagoshima City, Kagoshima 890-8520, Japan*

[3] *Department of Medical Joint Materials, Graduate School of Medical and Dental Sciences, Kagoshima University, 8-35-1 Sakuragaoka, Kagoshima City, Kagoshima 890-8520, Japan*

[4] *Infection Control Team, Kagoshima University Hospital, 8-35-1 Sakuragaoka, Kagoshima City, Kagoshima 890-8520, Japan*

Correspondence should be addressed to Satoshi Nagano; naga@m2.kufm.kagoshima-u.ac.jp

Academic Editor: Akira Kawai

Surgical site infection (SSI) has not been extensively studied in musculoskeletal tumors (MST) owing to the rarity of the disease. We analyzed incidence and risk factors of SSI in MST. SSI incidence was evaluated in consecutive 457 MST cases (benign, 310 cases and malignant, 147 cases) treated at our institution. A detailed analysis of the clinical background of the patients, pre- and postoperative hematological data, and other factors that might be associated with SSI incidence was performed for malignant MST cases. SSI occurred in 0.32% and 12.2% of benign and malignant MST cases, respectively. The duration of the surgery ($P = 0.0002$) and intraoperative blood loss ($P = 0.0005$) was significantly more in the SSI group than in the non-SSI group. We established the musculoskeletal oncological surgery invasiveness (MOSI) index by combining 4 risk factors (blood loss, operation duration, preoperative chemotherapy, and the use of artificial materials). The MOSI index (0–4 points) score significantly correlated with the risk of SSI, as demonstrated by an SSI incidence of 38.5% in the group with a high score (3-4 points). The MOSI index score and laboratory data at 1 week after surgery could facilitate risk evaluation and prompt diagnosis of SSI.

1. Introduction

Surgical site infection (SSI) is defined as an infection at the site of direct operative manipulation that develops within 30 days of operation if no artificial materials (implants) are used or within 1 year if artificial materials are used [1]. In general, the incidence of SSI following orthopaedic surgery has been reported to be 1% to 3% [2]. The incidence of SSI following orthopaedic surgery in Japan is 0.83% for cases of spinal canal stenosis, 0.28% for cases of disc herniation, 0.80% for cases of total hip arthroplasty (THA), and 0.96% for cases of total knee arthroplasty (TKA) [3]. This indicates that the incidence of SSI following surgery with the use of artificial materials is higher than that in cases without the use of artificial materials.

The incidence of SSI following surgical treatment for cancer is relatively high, with large variations observed depending on the type of cancer (breast cancer 5.2% [1], rectal cancer 10% [2], gastric cancer 13.8% [3], liver cancer 21% [4], and oral cancer 40.6% [5]). Surgery for malignant musculoskeletal tumors is performed in the aseptic osteoarticular area. However, the incidence of SSI following surgery for this kind of tumor is anticipated to be higher than the incidence following orthopaedic surgery in general and the reasons for this include the following: (1) patients with malignant tumors require preoperative/postoperative chemotherapy and/or radiotherapy and (2) tumor resection creates a dead space. The onset of SSI following surgery for malignant musculoskeletal tumors can delay the start of postoperative

Table 1: Incidence of SSI by tumor types.

	SSI	Deep/organ SSI
Benign tumor		
Benign bone tumor (n = 87)	0	
Benign soft tissue tumor (n = 223)	1 (0.4%)	1 (100%)
Malignant tumor		
Malignant bone tumor (n = 46)	6 (13.0%)	6 (100%)
Malignant soft tissue tumor (n = 102)	12 (11.8%)	8 (66.7%)

adjuvant therapy, possibly leading to poor prognosis. To date, the incidence of SSI following orthopaedic surgery in general and the precautions for preventing SSI following such surgery have been studied sufficiently, yielding guidelines concerning the timing and duration of antimicrobial medication, techniques for operative field hair disposal, and so forth [6].

Malignant musculoskeletal tumors are relatively rare. Currently, there is no set of guidelines specific to the prevention of SSI following surgery for this kind of tumor because this issue has not yet been discussed sufficiently. The present study was undertaken to analyze data from patients with musculoskeletal tumors surgically treated at our department and to identify risk factors for SSI following surgery for malignant musculoskeletal tumors.

2. Patients and Methods

The study included 310 patients with benign musculoskeletal tumors and 147 patients with malignant musculoskeletal tumors who underwent surgery at our department between 2007 and 2012. Among these 147 patients, there were 22 metastatic tumor cases (14.9%). The incidence of SSI among these malignant musculoskeletal tumor patients was analyzed. According to the Centers for Disease Control and Prevention (CDC) definition, SSIs are classified as either incisional or of organ/space origin [7]. Incisional SSIs are further subclassified into those involving only skin and subcutaneous tissue (superficial incisional SSI) and those involving deeper soft tissues (deep incisional SSI). Organ/space SSIs involve any part of the anatomy (e.g., organ or space) other than incised body wall layers that were opened or manipulated during a surgical procedure [7].

In addition, factors related to the onset of SSI were analyzed in patients with malignant musculoskeletal tumors (n = 147). We analyzed factors affecting the incidence of infection: background variables (age, body mass index, presence/absence of hypertension, presence/absence of ischemic heart disease, presence/absence of diabetes mellitus, and presence/absence of preoperative chemotherapy) and surgery-related factors (skin incision size, duration of the surgery, blood loss, use of artificial materials, requirement of reconstructive surgery, and applicability of temporary wound closure). "Artificial materials" include prostheses, metal implants (screw, plates, and nails), and surgical meshes. "Reconstructive surgery" includes plastic surgical procedures such as musculocutaneous flap reconstruction, local skin flap reconstruction, and skin grafting. To analyze, in detail, the clinical courses of SSI cases, case-specific information such as isolated bacteria, treatment, oncological outcome, and treatment duration was collected. In addition, to explore biomarkers for the prediction and diagnosis of SSI, we analyzed hematological data (white blood cell [WBC] count, hemoglobin level [Hb], total protein level [TP], and C-reactive protein [CRP] level before operation; WBC, Hb, and TP on the day following operation; WBC and CRP one week after operation).

The standard protocols at our institution for prevention of SSI are based on the guidelines by the CDC [7] and the Society for Healthcare Epidemiology of America [8]. Briefly, these include reducing glycosylated hemoglobin A1c levels to 7% before surgery in diabetes patients, recommending smoking cessation within 30 days before the procedure, and improving nutritional status. The extrinsic procedure-related strategy includes no hair removal unless the hair that will interfere with the operation; if hair removal is necessary, it should be removed by clipping. The antimicrobial prophylaxis strategy includes administration within 1 hour before incision to maximize tissue concentration and withdrawal of prophylactic treatment within 24 hours after all procedures except cardiac surgery.

Statistical analysis was performed using Microsoft Excel. Statistical significance was analyzed using Student's t-test (one-tailed) or chi-square test, with $P < 0.05$ considered to indicate a significant difference. Odds ratio was used for analysis of risk factors.

To determine the musculoskeletal oncological surgery invasiveness (MOSI) index, 4 factors significantly associated with SSI development were chosen: operation duration, blood loss, preoperative chemotherapy, and use of artificial materials. To set a numerical cutoff for operation duration and blood loss, receiver operating characteristic (ROC) analysis was performed using Microsoft Excel. The point on the ROC curve closest to (0, 1) was selected as the optimal threshold (cutoff value) [9].

3. Results

The incidence of SSI was 0.4% (1/223) for cases of benign soft tissue tumors, 0% (0/87) for those of benign bone tumors, 11.8% (12/102) for those of malignant soft tissue tumors, and 13.0% (6/46) for those of malignant bone tumors, with the overall incidence of SSI being 12.2% for cases of malignant musculoskeletal tumors. Of the patients with malignant soft tissue tumors who developed SSI after surgery, 66.7% (8/12) had deep incision or organ/space SSI (Table 1). Among the patients with malignant bone tumor who developed SSI following surgery, 100% (6/6) had deep incision or organ/space SSI (Table 1).

TABLE 2: Analysis of risk factors for surgical site infection in malignant bone and soft tissue tumors.

	Non-SSI (n = 129)	SSI (n = 18)	Odds ratio	95% CI	P value
Age	57.6 ± 18.4	58.7 ± 17.6			0.40
Aged case (>60 y)	73 (53.3%)	12 (66.7%)	1.62	0.57–4.57	0.36
Gender (male/female)	66/63	6/12	0.48	0.16–1.35	0.16
BMI (kg/m^2)	23.0 ± 3.8	23.8 ± 3.1			0.20
Overweight (>25)	40 (31.0%)	7 (38.9%)	1.41	0.51–3.92	0.50
Hypertension	32 (25%)	6 (33.0%)	1.51	0.53–4.37	0.44
Ischemic heart disease	4 (3.1%)	4 (22.2%)	10.4	2.31–47.0	0.001
Diabetes	15 (11.6%)	2 (11.1%)	0.95	0.19–4.54	0.95
Tumor location (Trunk/Extremity)	14/111	4/14	1.76	0.52–5.95	0.36
Primary/metastatic tumor	110/19	15/3	1.15	0.30–4.38	0.99
Preoperative chemotherapy	12 (9.3%)	6 (33.3%)	4.87	1.55–15.3	0.003
Skin incision (cm)	21.3 ± 12.0	23.1 ± 9.3			0.04
Large skin incision (>25 cm)	41 (31.8%)	10 (55.6%)	2.68	0.68–5.0	0.047
Use of artificial materials	34 (26.4%)	10 (55.6%)	3.49	1.27–9.58	0.01
Reconstructive procedure	42 (32.6%)	6 (33.3%)	1.04	0.37–2.95	0.95
Secondary wound closure	25 (19.4%)	3 (16.7%)	0.83	0.22–3.10	0.78
Duration of surgery (min)	265 ± 155	413 ± 202			0.0002
Prolonged surgery (≥355 min)	32 (24.8%)	12 (66.7%)	6.06	2.10–17.4	0.0003
Blood loss (g)	270 ± 431	726 ± 1053			0.0005
Massive blood loss (≥190 g)	23 (17.4%)	9 (50.0%)	4.39	1.47–13.0	0.005

Of the factors analyzed, ischemic heart disease (P = 0.001), preoperative chemotherapy (P = 0.003), skin incision length (P = 0.04), use of artificial materials (P = 0.01), duration of surgery (P = 0.0002), and blood loss (P = 0.0005) were significant risk factors for acquiring SSI (Table 2). Other factors analyzed in this study were not significantly associated with SSI (Table 2).

Results of the analysis of risk factor associations with SSI are presented in Table 2. The odds ratio (OR) was the highest for ischemic heart disease (OR: 10.4), followed by operation duration of ≥355 minutes (OR: 6.06), administration of preoperative chemotherapy (OR: 4.87), intraoperative blood loss of ≥190 g (OR: 4.39), and use of artificial materials (OR: 3.49).

Details of patients who developed SSI are presented in Table 3. The pathogens often identified were *Staphylococcus aureus* and coagulase-negative staphylococci. We also noted rare cases involving bacteria such as *Pseudomonas aeruginosa* and *Enterobacter* species as the pathogens of SSI. Of all cases of SSI, 7 cases (37%) required treatment for 1 year or longer, and 5 patients (28%) died after the onset of SSI (Table 3).

With regard to preoperative blood test data, the SSI and non-SSI groups did not differ significantly in terms of the WBC count, hemoglobin level, total protein level, or CRP level (Table 4). At 1 day after surgery as well, the WBC count and the hemoglobin and total protein levels did not differ significantly between the 2 groups (Table 4). With regard to the percent change at 1 day after surgery, the WBC count increased by 144% in the non-SSI group and by 154% in the SSI group relative to baseline values (preoperative level); however, these differences were not statistically significant (P = 0.44). The hemoglobin level decreased to 94% in the non-SSI group and to 88% in the SSI group relative to the baseline levels; these changes were not statistically significant either (P = 0.15). Further, the total protein level decreased to 82% in the non-SSI group and to 79% in the SSI group (P = 0.07). The levels of the 2 inflammation markers (WBC and CRP) at 1 week after surgery were significantly higher in the SSI group than in the non-SSI group (WBC P = 0.001 CRP $P < 0.001$) (Table 4).

ROC curve analysis revealed that the cutoff value for operation duration and blood loss was 355 minutes and 190 g, respectively. Therefore, the MOSI was calculated on the basis of each of these 4 factors (operation duration ≥355 m, blood loss ≥190 g, preoperative chemotherapy, and artificial material (Table 5)) using a 5-point scale (0–4). The average MOSI index of the SSI group (2.2 ± 0.3) was significantly higher than that of the non-SSI group (1.0 ± 0.1; $P < 0.0001$). The incidence of SSI was 38.5% when the MOSI index was 3-4 points and 7.1% at 0–2 points (Table 6).

4. Discussion

Limb-sparing surgery is a currently common procedure for the treatment of malignant musculoskeletal tumors. However, because tumors often develop at sites that are anatomically difficult to treat (e.g., around major nerves and blood

TABLE 3: Case-specific data of SSI patients of malignant musculoskeletal tumors.

	Age/sex	Diagnosis	Site	Surgical procedure	Reconstruction	Duration of surgery (min)	Blood loss (g)	Isolated bacteria from SSI	Treatment for SSI	Oncological outcome/SSI healing	Treatment duration for SSI (month)
1	62/F	Metastatic bone tumor	Sacrum	Marginal resection	Artificial mesh	355	978	MRSA	Antibiotics, HBOT, surgery	DOD/not healed	18
2	61/M	Chondrosarcoma	Femur	Wide resection	Pasteurized autograft, plate and screw	383	500	CNS	Antibiotics, HBOT, surgery	CDF/healed	12
3	62/M	Metastatic bone tumor (thyroid)	Humerus	Marginal resection	Tumor-prosthesis	397	270	MSSA	Antibiotics, HBOT, surgery	DOD/healed	5
4	13/M	Osteosarcoma	Tibia	Wide resection	Tumor-prosthesis Gastrocnemius muscle flap	445	470	MRSA	Antibiotics, HBOT, surgery	CDF/healed	9
5	35/M	Osteosarcoma	Pelvis	Hemipelvectomy	Liquid-nitrogen treated autograft, plate and screw, external fixator	890	4090	CNS	Antibiotics, HBOT, surgery	DOD/not healed	12
6	61/M	Metastatic bone tumor (kidney)	Femur	Wide resection	Tumor-prosthesis, Sartorius muscle flap	514	600	MSSA	Antibiotics, surgery (amputation)	AWD/healed	1
7	45/M	Myxoid liposarcoma	Thigh	Wide resection including Femur	Pasteurized autograft, plate and screw	680	1620	MRSA	Antibiotics, HBOT, surgery	DOD/not healed	18
8	79/F	MFH	Buttock	Wide resection	Gluteal artery perforator flap	145	50	MRSA	Antibiotics, HBOT	DOO/not healed	9
9	64/M	MFH	Thigh	Marginal resection	None	508	2505	*Pseudomonas aeruginosa*	Antibiotics, HBOT, surgery	DOD/not healed	9
10	82/M	Dedifferentiated liposarcoma	Thigh	Disarticulation of hip	None	391	220	*Enterobacter cloacae*	Antibiotics, surgery	CDF/healed	5
11	45/M	Myxoid liposarcoma	Thigh	Wide resection including Femur	Pasteurized autograft, plate and screw	550	470	CNS	Antibiotics, HBOT, surgery	CDF/healed	18
12	75/M	MFH	Lower leg	Wide resection including Tibia	Bone cement, intramedullary nail, Gastrocnemius muscle flap, FTSG	283	255	CNS	Antibiotics, HBOT, surgery (local flap)	CDF/not healed	21

Table 3: Continued.

	Age/sex	Diagnosis	Site	Surgical procedure	Reconstruction	Duration of surgery (min)	Blood loss (g)	Isolated bacteria from SSI	Treatment for SSI	Oncological outcome/SSI healing	Treatment duration for SSI (month)
13	30/M	MFH	Groin	Wide resection	None	250	105	*Pseudomonas aeruginosa*	Antibiotics, HBOT, surgery (rectus abdominis muscle flap)	CDF/not healed	3
14	70/F	MFH	Thigh	Marginal resection	Gastrocnemius muscle flap, FTSG	163	30	MSSA	Antibiotics, HBOT, NPWT	CDF/healed	3
15	59/M	MFH	Thigh	Wide resection	None	146	0	MSSA	Antibiotics, HBOT,	AWD/healed	1
16	73/F	Chondrosarcoma	Hand	Marginal resection including metatarsal bone	Iliac autograft, Kirschner wire	524	685	*Enterobacter cloacae*	Antibiotics, surgery (forearm flap)	CDF/healed	20
17	73/F	MFH	Thigh	Wide resection	Free latissimus dorsi flap, STSG	626	190	MRSA	Antibiotics, HBOT, surgery, NPWT	AWD/healed	3
18	68/F	Undifferentiated sarcoma	Thigh	Wide resection	STSG	189	30	MRSA	Antibiotics	CDF/healed	2

MFH: malignant fibrous histiocytoma (pleomorphic undifferentiated sarcoma); FTSG: full-thickness skin graft; STSG: split-thickness skin graft; MSSA: methicillin-sensitive *Staphylococcus aureus*; mRSA: Methicillin-resistant *Staphylococcus aureus*; CNS: coagulase-negative staphylococci; HBOT: hyperbaric oxygen therapy; NPWT: negative-pressure wound therapy; CDF: continuous disease free; DOD: died of disease; DOO: died of other cause (Case 8, uterine cervical cancer); AWD: alive with disease.

TABLE 4: Analysis of pre- and postoperative laboratory values.

	Non-SSI	SSI	P value
Preoperative values			
WBC (/m^3)	6,242 ± 278	6,016 ± 405	0.41
Hemoglobin (g/dL)	12.3 ± 0.2	12.3 ± 0.5	0.49
Total protein (g/dL)	6.9 ± 0.1	7.0 ± 0.1	0.32
CRP (mg/dL)	1.6 ± 0.3	1.4 ± 0.5	0.41
Postoperative (1 day) values			
WBC (/m^3)	8,959 ± 285	9,245 ± 602	0.36
Hemoglobin (g/dL)	11.3 ± 0.17	10.8 ± 0.4	0.17
Total protein (g/dL)	5.7 ± 0.7	5.5 ± 0.2	0.12
Postoperative (1 week) values			
WBC (/m^3)	6,528 ± 230	8,689 ± 993	0.001
CRP (mg/dL)	2.2 ± 0.3	8.8 ± 2.1	<0.0001

TABLE 5: Musculoskeletal oncological surgery invasiveness index (MOSI index).

Value	Points
Duration of surgery (min)	
<355	0
≥355	1
Blood loss (g)	
<190	0
≥190	1
Preoperative chemotherapy	
No	0
Yes	1
Artificial materials	
No	0
Yes	1

TABLE 6: Relationship between the incidence of SSI and the musculoskeletal oncological surgery invasiveness (MOSI) index.

MOSI index (points)	SSI (%)
3-4	38.5*
0–2	7.1

*$P < 0.0005$ versus cases of 0–2 points.

vessels), long operation times and high blood loss are common problems. Morii et al. reported that SSI developed in 7 (8.3%) of the 84 patients in their study after the surgical treatment of malignant soft tissue tumors, resulting in longer hospital stays [10]. In addition, they reported that intraoperative blood loss and tumor location (trunk) were significant risk factors for SSI and that the incidence of SSI did not differ according to age, tumor grade, use of preoperative chemotherapy, size of tumor, or the performance of accompanying plastic surgery [10]. For surgery in general, operation time [11, 12] and blood loss [4] have been reported as risk factors for SSI. These previous findings are consistent with the results of the present study. We considered that 4 factors (operation duration, blood loss, preoperative chemotherapy, and use of artificial materials) might reflect surgical invasiveness for the patients with malignant musculoskeletal tumors and would facilitate evaluation of the risk for SSI. However, operation duration and blood loss are sometimes correlated with each other. Therefore, we analyzed the statistical correlation of these 2 factors in our study. Pearson's correlation index was 0.542, which suggests that these 2 factors were not highly correlated in our study. One reason for this might be the difference between general orthopedic surgery and oncological surgery, in which we encounter massive blood loss in a short time period when dealing with hypervascular tumors. To test our hypothesis, the relationship between the MOSI index and the incidence of SSI was analyzed. As shown in Table 6, the MOSI index was significantly correlated with the incidence of SSI ($P < 0.0005$). These results suggest that the risk for SSI onset can be predicted to be very high (OR 8.82) in cases in which the MOSI index based on preoperatively estimated blood loss and operation time, and so forth, is 3 points or higher. A further study involving a larger number of patients is needed to verify the usefulness and validity of this index.

As a preoperative risk factor for SSI, preoperative chemotherapy was shown to elevate the incidence of SSI in a slight but statistically significant manner, suggesting that this factor affects the immune potentials of patients undergoing surgery. We analyzed blood data to determine the preoperative and postoperative condition (including immune function) of individual patients. None of the preoperative blood parameters analyzed was identified as a predictive factor for SSI. We hypothesized that the blood parameter data at 1 day after surgery would reflect the effects of surgery (bleeding, dehydration, inflammation, and malnutrition), possibly enabling prediction of SSI. In fact, however, there was no significant difference between the SSI group and the non-SSI group in terms of the WBC count, hemoglobin level, or total protein level. Next, we analyzed the differences in the percent changes in these 3 parameters at preoperative baseline and at 1 day after surgery. This analysis revealed a larger percent change in total protein levels in the SSI group (21% decrease) than in non-SSI group (18% decrease), but the difference was not significant ($P = 0.07$) possibly because of the limited number of subjects. Although blood loss was identified as a significant factor, postoperative hemoglobin levels did not differ between the 2 groups. This seems to reflect the influences of dehydration and blood transfusion.

Standard measures at our facility for the prevention of SSI include strict blood glucose control for diabetic patients and the use of antimicrobial agents (cephalosporins) before surgery until the day after surgery [7, 8]. The results of the present study indicate that the new measures to be adopted for the prevention of SSI should be careful observation of clinical symptoms (e.g., postoperative fever and local findings) and frequent blood tests in cases with an MOSI index of more than 2, so that early detection of SSI can be facilitated. It might be worthwhile to reconsider the use of antimicrobial agents in high-risk patients. Routine use of vancomycin is not recommended to prevent emergence of vancomycin-resistant microbials [7, 8]. However, the Society for Healthcare Epidemiology of America recommends the use of vancomycin in high-risk surgical procedures especially in procedures requiring the placement of implants [8]. Therefore, we could consider using vancomycin as an antimicrobial prophylactic agent in patients with MST who are at high risk for SSI.

Furthermore, in cases of patients with a high CRP level and WBC count at 1 week after surgery, SSI should be strongly suspected. In such cases, it is advisable to take preemptive measures such as performing diagnostic imaging studies (e.g., ultrasonography and computed tomography) and prompt exploration of the wound (puncture or opening). When dealing with patients with an elevated risk for SSI, we often administer hyperbaric oxygen therapy (HBOT). HBOT is considered to contribute to wound healing by stimulating neovascularization and oxygen tissue diffusion and thus improving oxygen transport to the wound [13]. The effects of HBOT on infection are based on several mechanisms, including reinforcement of the bacterial killing capacity of neutrophils [14], alleviation of inflammation and edema [15], and reinforcement of antimicrobial drug efficacy [16] (reviewed by Hopf and Holm [17]). We will clarify the effects of HBOT in the prevention and treatment of SSI in future separate studies. When performing surgery for musculoskeletal tumors for which no standard surgical-anatomical approach has been defined, the operation plan should be carefully drafted with discussion in preoperative case conferences, with goals set at shortening the operation time and reducing blood loss using measures specific to this kind of surgery. To this end, acquisition of good operative skill is needed, such as anatomical approach, handling of the vessels, or procedures of implant surgery. It may also be desirable to perform reconstruction simultaneously with tumor resection. As one such attempt, we have begun to incorporate preoperative simulation with a 3D-printer-created tumor model [18] and surgical training using the model. Preoperative embolization has been reported as a measure to be taken for hypervascular metastatic bone tumors [19] and it has also been reported to reduce blood loss when applied before surgery for sarcoma [20]. In our department, for some cases, embolization is performed on the basis of findings from angiograms taken on the day before surgery [21].

Although the use of artificial materials has been identified as a risk factor for infection, their use in surgery for malignant musculoskeletal tumors is often unavoidable. Gosheger et al. reported that failure due to infection occurred in 30 (12%) of the 250 patients undergoing musculoskeletal sarcoma resection and prosthetic joint reconstruction, thus demonstrating an incidence of failure higher than that associated with TKA and THA in general [22]. Some investigators reported that if the tumor-type joint prosthesis is positively combined with a flap, the postoperative complications can be reduced and the limb preservation rate can be increased [23]. Reconstructive surgery involving plastic surgery techniques is indispensable as a countermeasure for the dead cavity created after resection of giant soft tissue tumors [24]. We also use musculocutaneous flaps such as a rectus abdominis musculocutaneous flap, a sural musculocutaneous flap, and a latissimus dorsi musculocutaneous flap, sartorius to reconstruct the tissue defects. However, in the present study, the onset of SSI remained unaffected by the performance of plastic reconstructive surgery aimed at improving the coverage of the artificial materials and preventing the failure of wound healing. Prolonged duration of surgery resulting from adoption of complex reconstructive procedures is a dilemma we may continue to face. One possible option, which deserves discussion, may be to perform reconstruction as a two-stage operation so that the operation time can be shortened.

In the analysis of pathogens, *Staphylococcus* was isolated from 14 of the 18 cases, consistent with a past report [6, 10]. Methicillin-resistant *Staphylococcus aureus* (MRSA) was responsible for infection in 6 cases, including 3 cases in which the control of infection was not possible and the patient died without receiving appropriate postoperative chemotherapy (Table 4). Rao et al. reported that preoperative screening for *Staphylococcus aureus* within the nasal cavity and its eradication can reduce the incidence of *Staphylococcus aureus* SSI in patients undergoing orthopaedic surgery [25]. Similarly, at our facility, we make it a rule to perform bacterial screening of the nasal cavity in all cases and to perform bacterial eradication with mupirocin ointment in MRSA-positive cases. This practice is supported by a publication recommending the use of anti-MRSA drugs at the time of surgery instead of cefem family antibiotics for MRSA-positive patients [6]. In the present study, none of the 7 patients that developed SSI due to MRSA had been MRSA-positive preoperatively, suggesting that onset of SSI through endogenous MRSA infection was prevented in the present study. However, the fact that many patients developed SSI due to MRSA suggests that infection was due to MRSA transmission via healthcare workers or from the environment. It therefore seems necessary to review the current measures taken for the prevention of perioperative infection, including compliance with standard preventive measures (ensuring hand/finger cleanliness among healthcare workers), compliance with measures for the prevention of infection through contact with MRSA-positive patients, and appropriate use of antibacterial drugs to avoid selection of drug-resistant bacteria. This is particularly important when caring for patients with musculoskeletal tumors, which require more intense physical care than usual. In another recent study, we analyzed the MRSA genotype and biofilm-forming capability. We found that the biofilm-forming capability was increased in MRSA strains isolated from patients with SSI following surgery with the use of artificial materials [26]. In addition, the presence of the *agr*-2 gene was associated with biofilm-forming capability, indicating that biofilm-forming capability can be quickly evaluated by assaying for this gene. This is a potentially useful tool for the treatment and targeting of biofilms.

5. Conclusion

Blood loss, duration of surgery, skin incision size, and use of artificial materials were identified as risk factors associated with the onset of SSI after surgery for musculoskeletal tumors. Patient risk factors for SSI were preoperative chemotherapy and ischemic heart disease. Careful observation and early detection/treatment of SSI on the basis of the risk for SSI (estimated by the MOSI index) and inflammatory reactions at 1 week after surgery are important as countermeasures against SSI following surgery for musculoskeletal tumors, which can result in death as the worst outcome.

Authors' Contribution

Satoshi Nagano designed and performed analysis and written paper. Masahiro Yokouchi, Takao Setoguchi, Hiromi Sasaki, and Hirofumi Shimada participated in surgery and collection of the data. Ichiro Kawamura, Yasuhiro Ishidou, Junichi Kamizono, and Takuya Yamamoto performed data analysis and statistical analysis. Hideki Kawamura and Setsuro Komiya wrote and gave critical comments on the paper.

Acknowledgment

The authors thank Chihaya Koriyama for helpful discussion on the statistical analysis.

References

[1] M. A. Olsen, S. Chu-Ongsakul, K. E. Brandt, J. R. Dietz, J. Mayfield, and V. J. Fraser, "Hospital-associated costs due to surgical site infection after breast surgery," *Archives of Surgery*, vol. 143, no. 1, pp. 53–60, 2008.

[2] S. Biondo, E. Kreisler, D. Fraccalvieri, E. E. Basany, A. Codina-Cazador, and H. Ortiz, "Risk factors for surgical site infection after elective resection for rectal cancer. A multivariate analysis on 2131 patients," *Colorectal Disease*, vol. 14, no. 3, pp. e95–e102, 2012.

[3] E. Imai, M. Ueda, K. Kanao, K. Miyaki, T. Kubota, and M. Kitajima, "Surgical site infection surveillance after open gastrectomy and risk factors for surgical site infection," *Journal of Infection and Chemotherapy*, vol. 11, no. 3, pp. 141–145, 2005.

[4] T. Arikawa, T. Kurokawa, Y. Ohwa et al., "Risk factors for surgical site infection after hepatectomy for hepatocellular carcinoma," *Hepato-Gastroenterology*, vol. 58, no. 105, pp. 143–146, 2011.

[5] K. Karakida, T. Aoki, Y. Ota et al., "Analysis of risk factors for surgical-site infections in 276 oral cancer surgeries with microvascular free-flap reconstructions at a single university hospital," *Journal of Infection and Chemotherapy*, vol. 16, no. 5, pp. 334–339, 2010.

[6] P. M. Huddleston, T. A. Clyburn, R. P. Evans et al., "Surgical site infection prevention and control: an emerging paradigm," *Journal of Bone and Joint Surgery A*, vol. 91, supplement 6, pp. 2–9, 2009.

[7] A. J. Mangram, T. C. Horan, M. L. Pearson, L. C. Silver, and W. R. Jarvis, "Guideline for Prevention of Surgical Site Infection, 1999. Centers for Disease Control and Prevention (CDC) Hospital Infection Control Practices Advisory Committee," *American Journal of Infection Control*, vol. 27, no. 2, pp. 97–132, 1999.

[8] D. J. Anderson, K. S. Kaye, D. Classen et al., "Strategies to prevent surgical site infections in acute care hospitals," *Infection Control and Hospital Epidemiology*, vol. 29, supplement 1, pp. S51–S61, 2008.

[9] N. J. Perkins and E. F. Schisterman, "The inconsistency of "optimal" cutpoints obtained using two criteria based on the receiver operating characteristic curve," *American Journal of Epidemiology*, vol. 163, no. 7, pp. 670–675, 2006.

[10] T. Morii, K. Mochizuki, T. Tajima, S. Ichimura, and K. Satomi, "Surgical site infection in malignant soft tissue tumors," *Journal of Orthopaedic Science*, vol. 17, no. 1, pp. 51–57, 2012.

[11] M. Haridas and M. A. Malangoni, "Predictive factors for surgical site infection in general surgery," *Surgery*, vol. 144, no. 4, pp. 496–503, 2008.

[12] P. de Tarso Oliveira e Castro, A. L. Carvalho, S. V. Peres, M. M. Foschini, and A. D. C. Passos, "Surgical-site infection risk in oncologic digestive surgery," *Brazilian Journal of Infectious Diseases*, vol. 15, no. 2, pp. 109–115, 2011.

[13] G. B. Pitzer and K. G. Patel, "Proper care of early wounds to optimize healing and prevent complications," *Facial Plastic Surgery Clinics of North America*, vol. 19, no. 3, pp. 491–504, 2011.

[14] D. B. Allen, J. J. Maguire, M. Mahdavian et al., "Wound hypoxia and acidosis limit neutrophil bacterial killing mechanisms," *Archives of Surgery*, vol. 132, no. 9, pp. 991–996, 1997.

[15] G. Nylander, D. Lewis, H. Nordstrom, and J. Larsson, "Reduction of postischemic edema with hyperbaric oxygen," *Plastic and Reconstructive Surgery*, vol. 76, no. 4, pp. 596–603, 1985.

[16] J. T. Mader, M. E. Shirtliff, S. C. Bergquist, and J. Calhoun, "Antimicrobial treatment of chronic osteomyelitis," *Clinical Orthopaedics and Related Research*, no. 360, pp. 47–65, 1999.

[17] H. W. Hopf and J. Holm, "Hyperoxia and infection," *Best Practice and Research*, vol. 22, no. 3, pp. 553–569, 2008.

[18] F. Rengier, A. Mehndiratta, H. Von Tengg-Kobligk et al., "3D printing based on imaging data: review of medical applications," *International Journal of Computer Assisted Radiology and Surgery*, vol. 5, no. 4, pp. 335–341, 2010.

[19] R. J. T. Owen, "Embolization of musculoskeletal tumors," *Radiologic Clinics of North America*, vol. 46, no. 3, pp. 535–543, 2008.

[20] A. Hansch, R. Neumann, M. Gajda, I. Marintchev, A. Pfeil, and T. E. Mayer, "Transarterial catheter embolization of a sarcoma for preoperative conditioning," *Vasa*, vol. 39, no. 2, pp. 185–188, 2010.

[21] S. Nagano, M. Yokouchi, T. Yamamoto et al., "Castleman's disease in the retroperitoneal space mimicking a paraspinalschwannoma: a case report," *World Journal of Surgical Oncology*, vol. 11, article 108, 2013.

[22] G. Gosheger, C. Gebert, H. Ahrens, A. Streitbuerger, W. Winkelmann, and J. Hardes, "Endoprosthetic reconstruction in 250 patients with sarcoma," *Clinical Orthopaedics and Related Research*, vol. 450, pp. 164–171, 2006.

[23] D. P. Mastorakos, J. J. Disa, E. Athanasian, P. Boland, J. H. Healey, and P. G. Cordeiro, "Soft-tissue flap coverage maximizes limb salvage after allograft bone extremity reconstruction," *Plastic and Reconstructive Surgery*, vol. 109, no. 5, pp. 1567–1573, 2002.

[24] A. Moreira-Gonzalez, R. Djohan, and R. Lohman, "Considerations surrounding reconstruction after resection of musculoskeletal sarcomas," *Cleveland Clinic Journal of Medicine*, vol. 77, supplement 1, pp. S18–S22, 2010.

[25] N. Rao, B. Cannella, L. S. Crossett, A. J. Yates Jr., and R. McGough III, "A preoperative decolonization protocol for staphylococcus aureus prevents orthopaedic infections," *Clinical Orthopaedics and Related Research*, vol. 466, no. 6, pp. 1343–1348, 2008.

[26] H. Kawamura, J. Nishi, N. Imuta et al., "Quantitative analysis of biofilm formation of methicillin-resistant Staphylococcus aureus (MRSA) strains from patients with orthopaedic device-related infections," *FEMS Immunology and Medical Microbiology*, vol. 63, no. 1, pp. 10–15, 2011.

11

Rapid Screening of Novel Agents for Combination Therapy in Sarcomas

Christopher L. Cubitt,[1,2] Jiliana Menth,[2] Jana Dawson,[2] Gary V. Martinez,[3] Parastou Foroutan,[3] David L. Morse,[3] Marilyn M. Bui,[4,5] G. Douglas Letson,[4] Daniel M. Sullivan,[1] and Damon R. Reed[1,4]

[1] *Chemical Biology and Molecular Medicine, H. Lee Moffitt Cancer Center and Research Institute, 12902 Magnolia Drive, Tampa, FL 33612, USA*
[2] *Translational Research Lab, H. Lee Moffitt Cancer Center and Research Institute, 12902 Magnolia Drive, Tampa, FL 33612, USA*
[3] *Small Animal Imaging Lab, H. Lee Moffitt Cancer Center and Research Institute, 12902 Magnolia Drive, Tampa, FL 33612, USA*
[4] *Sarcoma Program, H. Lee Moffitt Cancer Center and Research Institute, 12902 Magnolia Drive, Tampa, FL 33612, USA*
[5] *Anatomic Pathology Department, H. Lee Moffitt Cancer Center and Research Institute, 12902 Magnolia Drive, Tampa, FL 33612, USA*

Correspondence should be addressed to Damon R. Reed; damon.reed@moffitt.org

Academic Editor: Chandrajit Premanand Raut

For patients with sarcoma, metastatic disease remains very difficult to cure, and outcomes remain less than optimal. Treatment options have not largely changed, although some promising gains have been made with single agents in specific subtypes with the use of targeted agents. Here, we developed a system to investigate synergy of combinations of targeted and cytotoxic agents in a panel of sarcoma cell lines. Agents were investigated alone and in combination with varying dose ratios. Dose-response curves were analyzed for synergy using methods derived from Chou and Talalay (1984). A promising combination, dasatinib and triciribine, was explored in a murine model using the A673 cell line, and tumors were evaluated by MRI and histology for therapy effect. We found that histone deacetylase inhibitors were synergistic with etoposide, dasatinib, and Akt inhibitors across cell lines. Sorafenib and topotecan demonstrated a mixed response. Our systematic drug screening method allowed us to screen a large number of combinations of sarcoma agents. This method can be easily modified to accommodate other cell line models, and confirmatory assays, such as animal experiments, can provide excellent preclinical data to inform clinical trials for these rare malignancies.

1. Introduction

Sarcomas account for 10% of pediatric diagnoses, 8% of cancers in the adolescent/young adult population, and 1% of adult cancers [1]. This diverse group of malignancies is often lethal in surgically unresectable, recurrent, or metastatic settings. Different subtypes predominate in different age groups, with rhabdomyosarcoma, osteosarcoma, and Ewing sarcoma predominating in children and young adults and leiomyosarcoma, liposarcoma, and other soft tissue sarcomas predominating in older adults. Chemotherapy has demonstrated clinical benefit in patients with advanced disease; however, for patients with advanced metastatic soft tissue sarcoma, the prognosis remains poor, with disease-free survival of 5 years or less than 25%; therefore, novel therapeutic strategies are needed.

Targeted therapy has shown promise in subtypes of sarcoma, with c-Kit mutant gastrointestinal stromal tumor demonstrating the most clinical efficacy to date [2]. Signaling pathways have long been known to be active in sarcomas, with Src being the first discovered oncogene. The success of single-agent targeted therapy in gastrointestinal stromal tumors has not been reproduced in other sarcomas, although investigations regarding targeted therapies with clinical benefit, particularly in combination, continue. Single agents or combinations that have demonstrated preclinical activity in sarcoma models are a rational choice for further clinical investigations. However, single agents tested at various dose levels over the years have shown a modest impact for relapsed and refractory sarcomas. In fact, the current clinical benchmark for activity in the second-line setting is a 40% 3-month progression-free survival [3]. This mark, demonstrating at least a promise for targeted therapies in patients with soft tissue sarcomas, was met by the targeted agent sunitinib in a phase II study at the Moffitt Cancer Center [4]. Other promising sarcoma agents include histone deacetylase (HDAC) inhibitors, tyrosine kinase inhibitors, and topoisomerase inhibitors.

Despite the promise shown by single-agent activity *in vitro*, clinical investigations have demonstrated that combinations of chemotherapy are often required to reliably induce responses and improve survival in sarcomas. Pediatric malignancies have traditionally seen improved response and cure rates with combinations of chemotherapies, with current standards of care employing 2–7 agents in the front-line setting for solid tumors. To this end, in this study, we explored combinations of cytotoxic and targeted agents in multiple sarcoma cell lines, including rhabdomyosarcoma, osteosarcoma, and Ewing sarcoma. In particular, we focused on topoisomerase inhibitors in combination with targeted agents, observing synergy across sarcoma cell lines in combination with selected tyrosine kinase inhibitors and HDAC inhibitors. We sought to establish a platform to allow for rapid determination of drug combination effects on tumor cell death and to assess for synergy, additivity, or antagonism across multiple sarcoma histologies.

2. Materials and Methods

2.1. Investigational Agents. Agents used included both cytotoxic and targeted agents. Many of these agents were obtained through the National Cancer Institute's Cancer Therapy Evaluation Program (see Table 1). Structures for all agents are publicly available. Combinations of investigational agents were all performed under material transfer agreements. All possible combinations of agents that were allowable were tested. Requests focused on tyrosine kinase inhibitors, HDAC inhibitors, though other agents with rationale were considered on a case by case basis.

2.2. Cell Culture. Sarcoma cell lines were obtained from the ATCC (Manassas, VA). Cells were maintained in RPMI or DMEM with 10% fetal bovine serum according to manufacturer recommendations. Cells were grown at 37°C and 5% CO_2. All cell lines tested free of mycoplasma every 3 months with MycoAlert tests (Lonza Rockland, Inc., Rockland, ME). Cell line identity was confirmed using StemElite ID system (Promega Corp., Madison, WI) using the manufacturer's instructions and the ATCC STR profile database.

2.3. Cell Viability Assays. The activity levels of drugs alone and in combination were determined by a high-throughput CellTiter-Blue (Promega Corp.) cell viability assay. Cells ($1.2–2 \times 10^3$) were plated in each well of 384-well plates using a Precision XS liquid handling station (Bio-Tek Instruments, Inc., Winooski, VT) and incubated overnight. A liquid handling station was used to serially dilute all drugs in media, and 5 μL was added to four replicate wells and an additional four control wells received a diluent control without drug. At the end of the incubation period with drugs, 5 μL of CellTiter-Blue reagent was added to each well. The fluorescence of the product of viable cells' bioreduction, resorufin (579 nm excitation/584 nm emission), was measured with a Synergy 4 microplate reader (Bio-Tek Instruments, Inc.). The fluorescence data were transferred to Microsoft Excel to calculate the percent viability. We determined IC50 values using a sigmoidal equilibrium model regression and XLfit version 5.2 (ID Business Solutions Ltd.). The IC50 values obtained from single-drug cell viability assays were used to design subsequent drug combination experiments.

2.4. Analysis of Additive and Synergistic Effects. For drug combination experiments, the cell viability assays were performed as described above, and the results were analyzed for synergistic, additive, or antagonistic effects using the combination index (CI) method developed by Chou and Talalay [5]. For the application of this method, the drug concentration dilutions were used at fixed dose molar ratios based on the IC50 levels of each drug obtained from preliminary experiments (e.g., 50 : 1, 2 : 5, and 1 : 250). Briefly, the dose-effect curve for each drug alone was determined based on experimental observations using the median-effect principle and then compared to the effect achieved with a combination of the two drugs to derive a CI value. This method involves plotting dose-effect curves, for each agent and their combination, using the median-effect equation: $f_a/f_u = (D/Dm)m$, where D is the dose of the drug, Dm is the dose required for a 50% effect (equivalent to IC50), f_a and f_u are the affected and unaffected fractions, respectively ($f_a = 1 - f_u$), and m is the exponent signifying the sigmoidicity of the dose-effect curve. XLfit software was used to calculate the values of Dm and m. The CI used for the analysis of the drug combinations was determined by the isobologram equation for mutually nonexclusive drugs that have different modes of action: $\text{CI} = (D)_1/(Dx)_1 + (D)_2/(Dx)_2 + (D)_1(D)_2/(Dx)_1(Dx)_2$, where $(Dx)_1$ and $(Dx)_2$ in the denominators are the doses (or concentrations) for *D1* (drug 1) and *D2* (drug 2) alone that gives x% inhibition, whereas $(D)_1$ and $(D)_2$ in the numerators are the doses of drug 1 and drug 2 in combination that also inhibited x% (i.e., isoeffective). CI < 1, CI $= 1$, and CI > 1 indicate synergism, additive effects, and antagonism, respectively. A confidence interval of <0.1 is represented as +++++ and indicates strong synergism by this method. Other CI symbols and description of effect of combinations are as follows: 0.1–0.3, ++++, strong synergism; 0.3–0.7, +++, synergism; 0.7–0.85, ++, moderate synergism; 0.85–0.90, +, slight synergism; 0.90–1.10, ±, nearly additive; 1.10–1.20, −, slight antagonism; 1.20–1.45, −−, moderate antagonism; 1.45–3.3, −−−, antagonism; 3.3–10, −−−−, strong antagonism; >10, −−−−−, very strong antagonism.

TABLE 1: Investigation, targeted agents used in study.

Agent	Mechanism of action	Source	Agreement
ABT-888	PARP inhibitor	AbbVie*	Single agent and with FDA approved
Dasatinib	Src, BCR-ABL inhibitor	BMS*	Single agent and with topoisomerase inhibitors or GX15-070
Etoposide	Topoisomerase II inhibitor	Commercial	FDA approved
GX15-070	BH3 mimetic	GeminX*	Single agent and with dasatinib or PXD101, and FDA approved
MK-2206	Akt inhibitor	Merck	Single agent and with dasatinib, MK-8669 or FDA approved
MK-8669	mTor inhibitor	Merck	Single agent and with dasatinib, MK-2206 or FDA approved
PXD101	HDAC inhibitor	CuraGen*	Single agent and with GX15-070
Saracatinib (AZD0530)	Src inhibitor	AstraZeneca*	Single agent and with saracatinib
Selumetinib (AZD6244, ARRY-142886)	MEK-1/2 inhibitor	AstraZeneca*	Single agent and with saracatinib and FDA approved
Sorafenib	VEGF, RAF inhibitor	Commercial	FDA approved
Topotecan	Topoisomerase I inhibitor	Commercial	FDA approved
Triciribine	AKT inhibitor, nucleoside	Commercial	FDA approved
Vorinostat	HDAC inhibitor	Merck*	FDA approved

*Obtained through CTEP N01-CM-62208.

Excess over the highest single agent (EOHSA) was calculated using MATLAB scripts provided by Brian Roberts of Merck & Co. For this method, the fraction unaffected was first calculated from dose-response data using a Michaelis-Menten model with Hill-type kinetics and incomplete inhibition. Specifically, EOHSA is calculated from the area between the measured combination and HSA response surfaces, where the "highest single agent" (HSA) is simply the higher of two single-agent effects at corresponding concentrations. The scripts were used to regress a best-fit CI value to a set of inhibitions yielded by two inhibitors, and predicted dose-response curves for a given CI were generated. Lastly, the area and a P value between the curves for actual data and HSA-predicted curves were calculated and averaged across replicate experiments.

2.5. Apoptosis Assay. Caspase 3/7 activation was measured using a 384-well plate based Caspase-Glo 3/7 (Promega) luminescent assay. Cells were treated for 24 hours with serial dilutions of each compound or a combination of two drugs.

2.6. Mouse Xenograft with A673 Ewing Sarcoma Cell Line. Animal experiments were carried out in strict accordance with recommendations in the Guide for the Care and Use of Laboratory Animals of the National Institutes of Health. The protocol was approved by the University of South Florida Institutional Animal Care and Use Committee (Application 2805).

Twenty-four, 3-month-old, male Balb/c Nu/Nu mice were injected subcutaneously with 10^6 cells on the right flank. The cells were mixed in a solution consisting of 50 μL PBS and 50 μL matrigel. Mice were separated into 4 groups: a control group, two groups receiving either dasatinib or triciribine, and a group receiving a combination of dasatinib and triciribine. Treated mice received dasatinib at 200 mg/kg daily, administered orally in a citrate solution, and/or triciribine at 2 mg/kg daily, given by intraperitoneal injection in a 40% DMSO solution with PBS equaling 100 μL. Both agents were given every 24 hours from Monday through Friday, every week starting one week after cells were injected. All mice were weighed daily, to the milligram. Caliper measurements in two directions of the tumors were taken daily to observe the growth. The tumors were allowed to grow to a diameter of 1.5–2.0 cm in either direction, with magnetic resonance imaging (MRI) performed at regular intervals, after which animals were sacrificed.

The tumor tissue was formalin fixed and paraffin embedded. Tumor was sectioned to 4 μm thick and stained with hematoxylin and eosin (H&E). We evaluated the therapy effect by examination under light microscopy; observed results were semiquantitatively analyzed by measuring percentage of viable tumor cells, necrosis, and fibrosis. The pathologist was blinded to the treatment.

2.7. MRI Methods. Mice were anesthetized with 1% isoflurane in O_2 and placed into a SWIFT insertion tube cradle fitted with a pressure-sensitive respiration pad beneath the animal. Body temperature was monitored with a fiber-optic rectal temperature probe and maintained at 37°C while being controlled using a small animal monitoring system (SA Instruments, Stony Brook, NY). All imaging was carried out at 7 Tesla using a horizontal bore Agilent ASR 310 MRI instrument (Agilent Technologies, Santa Clara, CA) equipped with actively shielded gradients capable of 400 mT/m gradient strength. Using a 35 mm inner diameter Litzcage coil (Doty Scientific, Inc.), we obtained T_2-weighted fast spin-echo images in axial planes that spanned the volume of the tumor. Imaging parameters for these images were repetition time (TR) = 2400 ms, elective echo time (TE_{eff}) = 72, echo spacing = 18 ms, echo train length (ETL) = 8, a field of view of $40 \times 40\,mm^2$, a matrix size of 128×128, 15 slices, a slice thickness of 1.25 mm, and an acquisition bandwidth of 100 kHz. To achieve fat suppression for each TR period, a 10 ms duration Gaussian saturation pulse was applied 1004 Hz upfield from water with a flip angle of 90°.

The data were analyzed using in-house scripts coded in Matlab (Mathworks, Inc., Natick, MA). Volumes were obtained from the fast spin-echo multislice images based on regions of interest drawn about the tumor in each slice.

3. Results

3.1. Demonstration of Synergistic Combinations. Many combinations of targeted agents and combinations of targeted and cytotoxic agents demonstrated synergy across multiple sarcoma cell lines. We used the EOHSA method to screen drug combination effects, as described in Materials and Methods. A representative volcano plot of synergy, expressed as EOHSA versus –log *P* value, is shown in Figure 1 (the average across all cell lines is shown in Supplementary any Material available online at http://dx.doi.org/10.1155/2013/365723 Figure S1). Combinations with promising synergy (i.e., higher EOHSA and –log *P* values) included mTOR inhibitors, HDAC inhibitors, and tyrosine kinase inhibitors, particularly those with Src and Akt activity. The complete combination effect data set for all 10 cell lines is shown in Supplementary any Material available online at http://dx.doi.org/10.1155/2013/365723 Tables S1 (concurrent treatment) and S2 (sequential treatment).

3.2. Histone Deacetylase Inhibitors and Topoisomerase II Inhibitors are Synergistic across a Variety of Sarcoma Cell Lines. Vorinostat (SAHA, suberoylanilide hydroxamic acid, Zolinza), a hydroxamate HDAC inhibitor, is particularly effective in inhibiting class I and II HDACs, more specifically HDAC1, HDAC2, HDAC3, and HDAC6 [6]. We found that vorinostat demonstrated single-agent activity in all 10 tested sarcoma cell lines. In pediatric-type cell lines, IC50 results ranged from 0.5 μM in the RD-ES cell line to 4.3 μM in the MNNG cell line, with a mean of 1.9 μM (Table 2). In the adult-type sarcoma cell lines, IC50 results were lowest in the SW-872 cell line (2.5 μM) and as high as 3.4 μM in SK-UT-1 cells, with a mean of 2.9 μM. These IC50 levels are within an order of magnitude of achievable levels in pediatric trials where the serum maximum concentration was 1 μM [7].

Topoisomerase II inhibitors such as etoposide also demonstrated broad activity. In the pediatric-type cell lines, IC50 results ranged from 0.5 μM in the SK-ES-1 cell line to 6.8 μM in the U2-OS cell line. In the adult-type sarcoma cell lines, IC50 results were lowest in the SK-UT-1 cell line at 2.5 μM and as high as 7.4 μM in HT-1080 cells (Table 2). Cells were also treated continuously with both agents for 72 hours at a constant 2 : 1 vorinostat: etoposide molar ratio. Using this combination, we found that 6 of 9 cell lines showed a synergistic interaction. The CI values for the pediatric cell lines ranged from 0.6 to 1.0 with a mean value of 0.8 (Table 2). The CI values for the adult-type cell lines ranged from 0.2 to 0.7 with a mean value of 0.5. The concurrent treatment of vorinostat and topotecan for 24 hours resulted in more than additive increases in caspase 3/7 activation, indicating that effects on viability are at least partially mediated through apoptosis (Figures 2(a) and 2(b)), as shown in the U2-OS cell line.

3.3. Tyrosine Kinases Have Varying Synergy with Topoisomerase I Inhibitors. Sorafenib is a multikinase inhibitor that affects specific targets involved in tumor cell proliferation [8]. Topotecan inhibits topoisomerase I and is currently being studied in a randomized controlled phase III study in Ewing sarcoma (ClinicalTrials.gov Identifier NCT01231906) with extensive use in a variety of pediatric tumors.

We found that sorafenib demonstrated single-agent activity in all 5 tested sarcoma cells. In the pediatric-type cell lines, IC50 ranged from 2.6 μM in the A-204 cell line to 8.0 μM in the MNNG cell line, with a mean of 5.8 μM (Table 2). Topotecan also demonstrated activity in all cell lines, with IC50 values ranging from 6.8 to 310 nM in pediatric sarcoma cell lines and from 73 to 400 nM in adult sarcoma cell lines (Table 2). Cells were also treated continuously with both sorafenib and topotecan for 72 hours in a 500 : 1 molar ratio, based on maximally achievable serum concentrations. This combination demonstrated a mix of additivity, synergy, and even some antagonism with the combination indices ranging from 0.53 in U2-OS cells to 1.7 in SK-ES-1 cells with an overall average of 1.05 (Table 2, Figures 2(c) and 2(d)).

3.4. Dasatinib and AKT Inhibitors Demonstrate Synergy across Many Sarcoma Cell Lines. Dasatinib is a targeted agent that inhibits multiple tyrosine kinases, including Src, Bcr-Abl, c-Kit, PDGFRβ, and FGFR-1, at submicromolar concentrations [9–11]. Triciribine (API2) is a tricyclic nucleoside analogue that inhibits AKT1, -2, and -3 by interfering with membrane integration, which has been shown to inhibit AKT *in vivo* [12, 13]. MK-2206 is an allosteric inhibitor of the AKT kinase family of proteins (at nanomolar levels) without additional kinase inhibitory activity in a panel of 256 kinases [14].

Here, we found that dasatinib demonstrated single-agent activity in all 10 sarcoma cell lines. In the pediatric-type cell lines, IC50 results ranged from 4.2 μM in the A-204 cell line to 12 μM in the RD-ES cell line, with a mean of 7.6 μM (Table 2). In the adult-type sarcomas, IC50 results were lowest in the SW-872 cell line at 4.6 μM and as high as 9.9 μM in SK-UT-1 cells, with a mean of 7.7 μM. MK-2206 was also tested and demonstrated broad activity as well, with IC50 results ranging from 4.3 μM in the SK-ES-1 cell line to 11 μM in the U2-0S cell line, with a mean of 7.8 μM (Table 2). In the adult-type sarcomas, IC50 results were lowest in the SK-LMS-1 cell line at 6.9 μM and as high as 11 μM in HT-1080 cells with a mean of 8.4 μM. Triciribine demonstrated activity as well, with IC50 results ranging from 6.3 μM in the RD-ES cell line to 69 μM in the MNNG cell line with a mean of 24 μM (Table 2). In the adult-type sarcomas, IC50 was lowest in the SK-LMS-1 cell line at 8.0 μM and as high as 30 μM in SK-UT-1 cells with a mean of 18 μM.

Cells were also treated continuously with dasatinib and MK-2206 for 72 hours at a constant 1 : 1 molar ratio. All 10 cell lines demonstrated a synergistic interaction. The CI values for

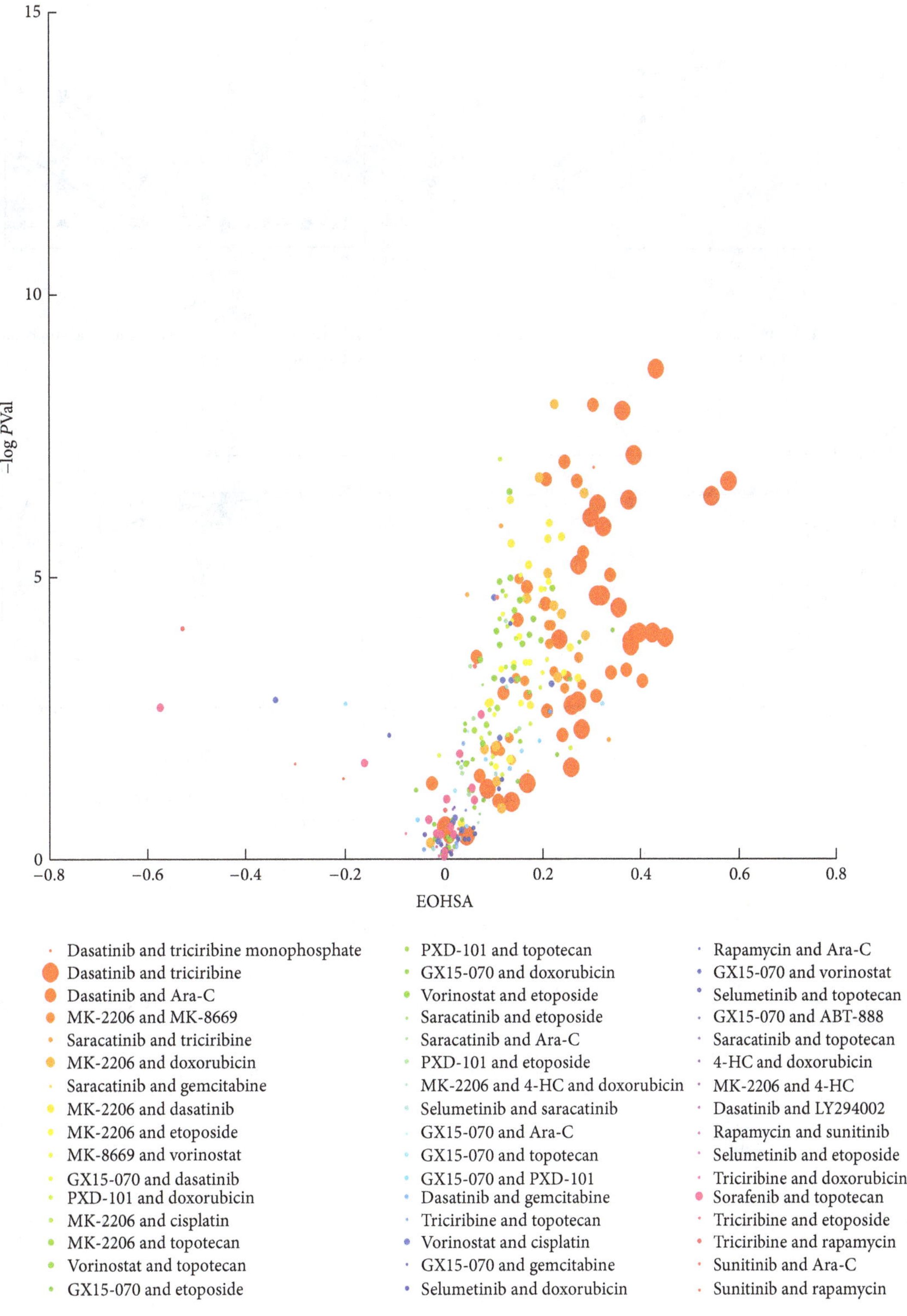

Figure 1: Mean excess over the highest single agent (EOHSA) versus P value for tested drug combinations in U2-OS osteosarcoma cells. EOHSA was calculated from cell viability assay dose response data for drug combinations and individual drugs for each combination. Results from combinations with potentially more significant synergy will show up in the upper right. Drug combinations are listed in the legend in order of the mean EOHSA value, with higher values appearing first. Symbol size represents the relative number of experiments included in the mean EOHSA value.

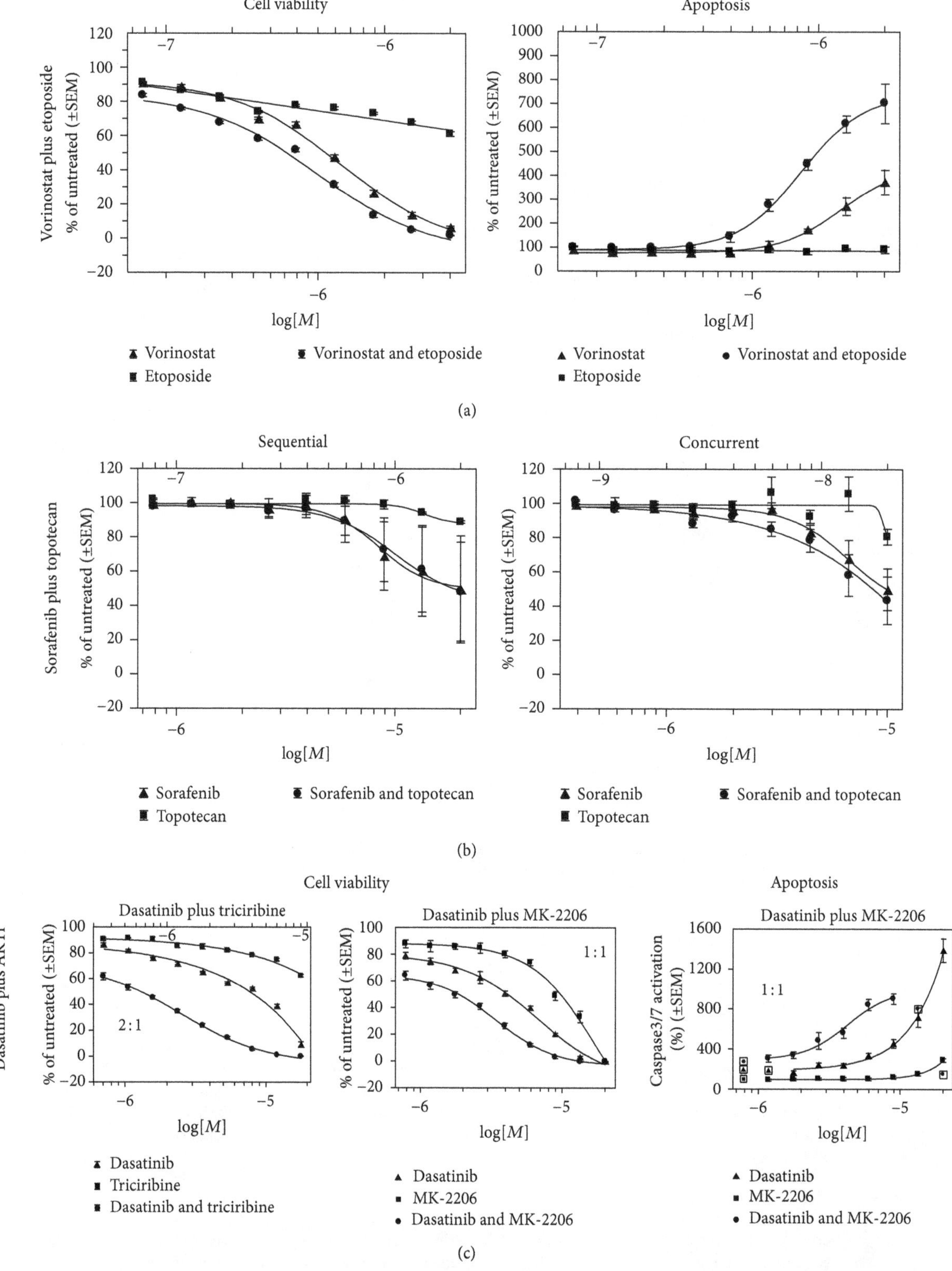

FIGURE 2: Drug combination effects in U2-OS osteosarcoma cells. The CellTiter-Blue assay was used to monitor viability in treated wells relative to untreated wells (% of untreated). Caspase 3/7 activation was measured after 24-hour concurrent treatments. (a) Vorinostat plus etoposide concurrent treatment. Cell viability was measured after 72-hour drug treatment. Vertical axis represents mean viability result for 5 independent experiments ($n = 5$). Apoptosis panel shows percent caspase 3/7 activation relative to untreated controls (100%). (b) Sorafenib plus topotecan concurrent and sequential drug treatment effects on cell viability. Sequential treatment consisted of a 24-hour pretreatment with sorafenib followed by the addition of topotecan. Cell viability was measured 48 hours after topotecan addition. (c) Dasatinib plus topotecan concurrent treatment. 72-hour cell viability assays were performed at constant drug ratios of 2 : 1 and 1 : 1. Caspase 3/7 activation was assayed after a 24-hour concurrent drug treatment (1 : 1 ratio) as in (a).

Table 2: Cell viability IC50 values and drug interaction measurements.

(a) Cell viability

Sarcoma type/cell line	Vorinostat			Etoposide			Sorafenib			Topotecan			Dasatinib			MK-2206			Triciribine		
	IC50 (μM)	SEM	n	IC50 (μM)	SEM	n	IC50 (μM)	SEM	n	IC50 (nM)	SEM	n	IC50 (μM)	SEM	n	IC50 (μM)	SEM	n	IC50 (μM)	SEM	n
Ewing																					
A-673	1.5	0.46	3	2.5	0.92	6				16	4.9	5	6.2	1.7	11				15	7.6	8
RD-ES	0.52		1	1.5	0.55	22	6.5	1.7	2	6.8	1.7	15	12	2.4	13	7.3	0.62	28	6.3	2.8	26
SK-ES-1	1.1	0.17	8	0.47	0.071	21	6.9	1.0	4	42	15	22	11	1.5	19	4.3	0.41	41	15	4.2	11
Osteosarcoma																					
MNNG HOS	4.3	1.2	4	5.6	2.0	15	8.0	0.71	3	310	140	20	5.8	0.77	22	9.2	0.55	40	69	27	3
U2-0S	1.6	0.25	8	6.8	1.1	14	4.9	0.75	2	190	56	7	6.4	0.76	19	11	0.72	29	19	5.0	11
Rhabdomyosarcoma																					
A-204	2.2	0.38	8	3.5	1.0	22	2.6	1.7	3	64	9.4	26	4.2	1.2	13	7.0	0.91	30	18	5.0	13
Fibrosarcoma																					
HT-1080	2.8	0.23	8	7.4	2.0	24				400	200	14	8.6	0.96	23	11	0.58	30	14	2.5	13
Leiomyosarcoma																					
SK-LMS-1	2.9	0.45	6	4.8	1.1	14				80	15	21	7.8	0.99	19	7.7	0.60	30	8.0	1.7	26
SK-UT-1	3.4	0.51	7	2.5	1.2	22				350	220	21	9.9	1.1	20	6.9	0.56	42	30	19	3
Liposarcoma																					
SW-872	2.5	0.41	7	2.9	0.84	21				73	27	21	4.6	0.72	23	7.9	0.57	41	18	3.6	7

(b) Drug interaction measurements

Sarcoma type/cell line	Vorinostat and etoposide							Sorafenib and topotecan						
	CI75	CI95	CI	SEM	n	EOHSA	neg log P Val	CI75	CI95	CI	SEM	n	EOHSA	neg log P Val
Ewing														
A-673														
RD-ES								1.00	1.19	1.10	0.07	2	0.046	1.12
SK-ES-1	1.10	0.93	1.01	0.10	3	0.10	1.67	1.58	1.75	1.66	0.35	3	0.076	2.24
Osteosarcoma														
MNNG HOS	0.78	0.95	0.86	0.27	3	0.08	1.62							
U2-OS	0.58	0.53	0.55	0.02	5	0.12	3.98	0.58	0.49	0.53	0.28	2	0.060	1.04
Rhabdoid														
A-204	0.85	1.20	0.99	0.20	5	0.09	2.58	0.61	1.29	0.91	0.32	3	0.088	2.41
Leiomyosarcoma														
SK-LMS-1	0.69	0.68	0.67	0.10	3	0.09	2.23							
SK-UT-1	0.73	0.68	0.70	0.17	3	0.11	5.39							
Liposarcoma														
SW-872	0.53	0.38	0.45	0.15	3	0.19	3.00							
Fibrosarcoma														
HT-1080	0.23	0.16	0.19	0.04	5	0.24	2.79							

Sarcoma type/cell line	Dasatinib and MK-2206							Dasatinib and triciribine						
	CI75	CI95	CI	SEM	n	EOHSA	neg log P Val	CI75	CI95	CI	SEM	n	EOHSA	neg log P Val
Ewing														
A-673								0.34	0.34	0.34	0.07	2	0.23	4.70
RD-ES	0.18	0.18	0.18	0.03	2	0.23	4.40	0.19	0.17	0.18	0.08	3	0.28	4.71
SK-ES-1	0.17	0.17	0.17	0.07	3	0.21	4.34	0.39	0.38	0.39	0.01	2	0.18	8.85
Osteosarcoma														
MNNG HOS	0.022	0.003	0.011		1	0.17	4.10							
U2-OS	0.38	0.54	0.46	0.05	3	0.18	3.72	0.10	0.03	0.06		1	0.36	7.94
Rhabdoid														
A-204	0.15	0.14	0.14		1	0.38	4.49							
Leiomyosarcoma														
SK-LMS-1	0.31	0.34	0.32	0.03	3	0.21	3.69	0.24	0.23	0.24	0.05	3	0.27	4.61
SK-UT-1	0.12	0.12	0.12	0.10	2	0.27	7.09	0.28	0.25	0.27		1	0.18	3.82
Liposarcoma														
SW-872	0.20	1.14	0.54	0.24	4	0.15	3.96							
Fibrosarcoma														
HT-1080	0.39	0.76	0.57	0.17	3	0.18	2.87							

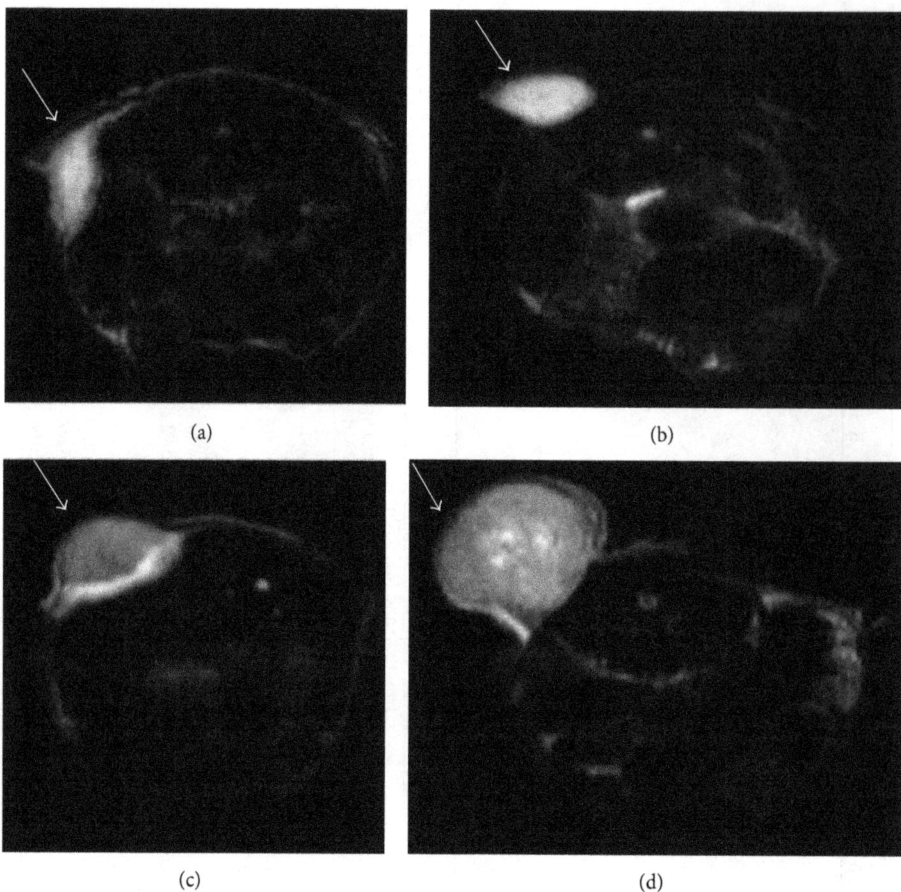

FIGURE 3: MRI imaging response to combination therapy in Ewing sarcoma. T2-weighted fast spin-echo images (TE/TR = 72/2400 ms) with a resolution of 312 mm demonstrating the tumor sizes in dasatinib (a), combination (b), triciribine (c), and untreated (d) at day 6. Representative datasets were chosen to reflect the overall trend of tumor size and growth. Lesions are indicated by arrows.

the pediatric cell lines ranged from 0.011 to 0.46 with a mean value of 0.19. The CI values for the adult-type cell lines ranged from 0.12 to 0.57 with a mean value of 0.39 (Table 2).

Cells were treated continuously with dasatinib and triciribine for 72 hours at a constant 2 : 1 molar ratio. All six tested cell lines indicated a synergistic interaction, with CI values for the pediatric cell lines ranging from 0.06 to 0.39 with a mean value of 0.24 (Table 2). The CI values for the two leiomyosarcoma cell lines were 0.24 and 0.27. The concurrent treatment of dasatinib with either MK-2206 or triciribine resulted in more than additive activity, and caspase 3/7 activation was also readily detected, indicating that effects on viability are at least partially mediated through apoptosis (Figure 3).

3.5. Dasatinib and Triciribine Have In Vivo Activity. Because of the robust synergy in the dasatinib and Akt inhibitor studies across sarcoma cell lines, we investigated the combination of dasatinib and triciribine *in vivo* using the A673 cell line. Tumors were evaluated for 3 weeks by caliper measurement and MRI.

As measured by MRI, the relative change in tumor volume demonstrated similar tumor growth rates for all animals initially (Figure 4(b)). On day 6, the untreated control group and the triciribine-treated mice showed notable increases in tumor growth versus that shown in the dasatinib and combination groups (Figures 4(a)–4(c)). In fact, after the fourth treatment on day 2, dasatinib demonstrated significantly smaller tumor volumes than triciribine at all time points throughout the course of the experiment. Similarly, the combination group also showed significantly lower tumor volumes following the treatment on day 6 versus that shown in the triciribine and control groups. By day 13, the dasatinib group appeared to display the smallest tumor volumes, whereas triciribine did not appear to affect tumor growth. These results also agree with the MRI volume results (Figure 4(b)) and the histology H&E stains (Figure 4(c)).

Semiquantitative histological analyses of tumor tissue stained with H&E demonstrated an overall higher amount of necrosis in the combination and dasatinib groups than in any of the other groups (Figure 4(c)). Meanwhile, the untreated control and the triciribine only treated tumors displayed an overall lower amount of necrosis, which reached statistical significance compared with the dasatinib and the combination groups. Corroborating the volumetric data, we also observed significantly higher cell viability in the untreated versus the combination group.

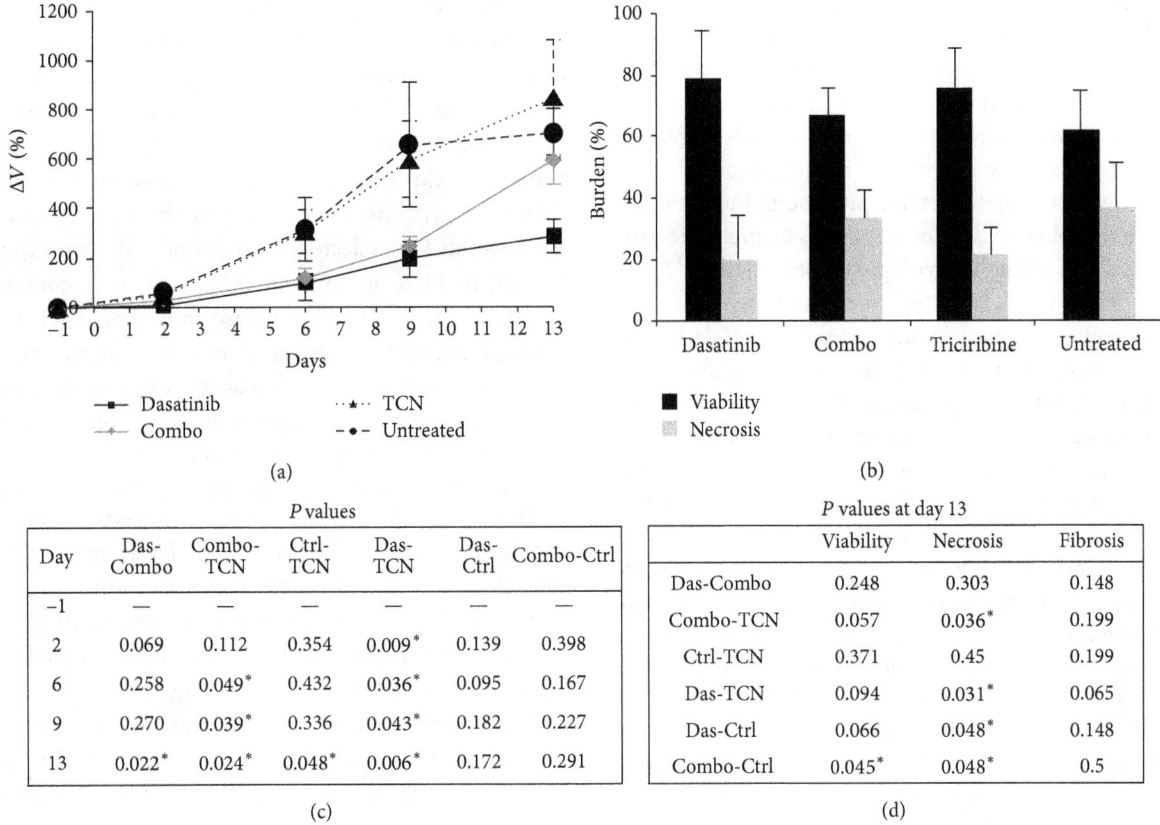

P values

Day	Das-Combo	Combo-TCN	Ctrl-TCN	Das-TCN	Das-Ctrl	Combo-Ctrl
−1	—	—	—	—	—	—
2	0.069	0.112	0.354	0.009*	0.139	0.398
6	0.258	0.049*	0.432	0.036*	0.095	0.167
9	0.270	0.039*	0.336	0.043*	0.182	0.227
13	0.022*	0.024*	0.048*	0.006*	0.172	0.291

(c)

P values at day 13

	Viability	Necrosis	Fibrosis
Das-Combo	0.248	0.303	0.148
Combo-TCN	0.057	0.036*	0.199
Ctrl-TCN	0.371	0.45	0.199
Das-TCN	0.094	0.031*	0.065
Das-Ctrl	0.066	0.048*	0.148
Combo-Ctrl	0.045*	0.048*	0.5

(d)

FIGURE 4: MRI tumor volume and pathologic response to combination therapy in Ewing sarcoma. (a) Region of interest analysis of T2-weighted MR datasets yielding the percent change in tumor size compared with that shown at initial value on day 0. (b) Quantitative histological results from H&E sections for viability, necrosis, and fibrosis at day 13. (c) *P* values comparing tumor volumes between treatment groups. (d) *P* values comparing pathologic determinants of response between treatment groups.

4. Discussion

In this study, we systematically investigated a large number of agents and combinations from many classes in a relatively high-throughput fashion to determine synergistic combinations of chemotherapies for sarcomas. Due to the rarity of sarcomas, clinical trials are difficult to conduct, increasing the need for strong preclinical data to inform clinical trials. In addition, clinical attempts to modify chemotherapy and to develop new agents in sarcomas have been slow.

The pediatric preclinical testing program (PPTP), a multi-institutional effort sponsored by the National Cancer Institute to evaluate new agents in pediatric malignancies using standardized *in vitro* and *in vivo* assays, has also tested agents across a variety of over 60 cell lines and xenografts [15, 16]. Through the PPTP, dasatinib, MK-2206, topotecan, sorafenib, and vorinostat have been tested [17–21], with results helping to inform single-agent, phase I pediatric studies. Our sarcoma cell line results were similar to the PPTP *in vitro* findings, with IC50 of >1 μM for dasatinib, 0.5–10 μM for vorinostat, around 10 μM for MK-2206, and under the 10 μM range for sorafenib [17, 18, 20, 21]. These micromolar IC50 levels are higher than the nanomolar IC50 for specific protein targets for tyrosine kinase inhibitors. Because of the manyfold higher concentrations leading to cell effects, the PPTP suggests off-target effects predominating [21]. The PPTP has demonstrated mostly low to intermediate *in vivo* activity of these compounds as single agents, although there was significant tumor growth delay in 4/5 tested osteosarcoma cells with sorafenib [18]. Topotecan had the most significant *in vivo* activity of the above compounds [19]. Importantly, although the PPTP has investigated combinations of drugs, the process is resource intensive [22].

The only FDA-approved agents for use in patients with front-line soft tissue sarcomas are doxorubicin and actinomycin D. Both have activity through topoisomerase II inhibition along with additional mechanisms of cellular toxicity. In this study, we tested additional topoisomerase I and II inhibitors, which may be given in select sarcomas and evaluated for synergy with a diverse collection of targeted agents. We also tested combinations of targeted agents and found multiple combinations that demonstrated synergy in our tested cell lines.

The antitumor effects of HDACs are largely thought to be related to effects on the 3-dimensional structure of DNA and effects on epigenetic modification of many genes; however, HDACs have other important roles in the cell, including roles in microtubule function, ubiquitination, and regulation of heat shock protein 90 [6]. Results from HDAC inhibitor and etoposide preclinical combination studies have contributed to a currently open pediatric phase I study (ClinicalTrials.gov Identifier NCI01294670) with vorinostat (SAHA) and etoposide. Since these data have been generated, there is increasing evidence of tolerability of HDACs in pediatric and adult patients. However, despite showing promise as a single agent, it has not led to phase II development, thus further validating the approach of looking for synergistic combinations [7, 23–25].

Other promising classes of compounds with demonstrated synergy are the tyrosine kinase inhibitors and topoisomerase inhibitors. As a class, tyrosine kinase inhibitors have an enormous variety in target specificity; thus it is not appropriate to consider them as one entity in terms of responses. In our study, dasatinib demonstrated synergy in most of our sarcoma models. Previous cell line experiments have shown that Src is activated in many sarcoma cells lines and that dasatinib can induce apoptosis and reduce cell migration [26, 27]. The dasatinib single-agent IC50 levels were more than an order of magnitude above achievable levels in pediatric trials, where the maximum concentration at the maximum tolerated dose was 0.3 μM [28]. Among other targeted pathways screened, inhibitors of the PTEN/PI3K/AKT/mTOR pathway demonstrated a strong signal of synergy with dasatinib. This pathway plays an important role in tumor growth and survival and is mutated in many human cancers, including a subset of leiomyosarcomas and osteosarcomas [29–31]. Expression levels of phosphorylated Akt have been shown to have prognostic implications in a small series of extremity soft tissue sarcomas [32]. In our mouse xenograft study in the A673 Ewing sarcoma cell line, we found that the *in vivo* synergy was not dramatic in the dasatinib and triciribine combination group; however, this method could be used to assess other promising drug combinations.

Sorafenib's targets include the serine/threonine kinases c-Raf and B-Raf, the receptor tyrosine kinases RET, Flt-3, and c-Kit, and receptor tyrosine kinases important in tumor angiogenesis, including the vascular endothelial growth factor receptor family (VEGFR1, -2, and -3) and platelet-derived growth factor-beta [8]. The antitumor activity of sorafenib *in vivo* is driven by its direct effects on tumor growth through its inhibition of the Raf/MEK/ERK pathway and on the antiangiogenic activity of the compound. Because sorafenib has a stromal mechanism of action through VEGF inhibition, it was not expected that this assay would reflect all possible mechanisms of antitumor activity of this combination. Topotecan has established efficacy as a single agent or as part of a combination in a variety of pediatric malignancies, including germ cell tumors, Wilm's tumor, neuroblastoma, acute lymphoblastic leukemia, CNS malignancies, and sarcomas [33–41]. It has been given in multiple combinations with conventional chemotherapeutic agents, including alkylators, topoisomerase II inhibitors, topoisomerase I inhibitors, and microtubule inhibitors [34, 39, 42, 43].

We are currently exploring a combination of sorafenib and topotecan in pediatric solid tumor patients, recognizing that sorafenib functions also as an angiogenesis inhibitor (ClinicalTrials.gov Identifier NCT01683149). Promising activity, a progression-free survival of 20 weeks versus 7 weeks in placebo control, of another angiogenesis-inhibiting tyrosine kinase, pazopanib, has recently been demonstrated in selected subtypes of soft tissue sarcoma, leading to FDA approval of this agent in sarcomas, only the third agent with this disease indication [44]. Efficacy through angiogenesis or stromal mechanisms cannot be readily assessed in our *in vitro* assay. A recent study showed more striking activity of a pazopanib and topotecan *in vivo* than *in vitro* in several sarcoma models [45].

We also found that dasatinib combined with Akt inhibitors MK-2206 or triciribine demonstrated significant synergy across our cell lines, albeit at levels that were higher than those readily achievable in patient serum [13, 46]. We investigated the combination with *in vivo* testing through our xenograft model. Although tumor measurements did not decrease dramatically, we investigated imaging changes in this sarcoma model by MRI and observed pathologic changes in the tumor after therapy. Although this specific combination may be difficult to translate into clinical benefit, it does establish a translational approach that can be explored with other promising combinations.

While we present data on many combinations, there are inherent difficulties and limitations towards translation. As was recently published, sorafenib is heavily protein bound *in vivo* and vorinostat has a short life that does not lead to sustained 24-hour *in vivo* dose levels [47]. We also report variation in effects between sarcoma subtypes and within histologic subtypes. We think this likely represents the inherent tumor variation between patients and tumor heterogeneity within patient samples currently being described in sequencing efforts [48]. Our focus was to describe the effect of the combinations, and we did not explore thus far biomarkers of resistance or sensitivity. These insights are being more fully explored and will be a focus of this methodology as it goes forward.

5. Conclusion

The methods presented here demonstrate a comprehensive, reproducible, and high-throughput method for exploring antitumor effects of combinations of therapies. Combinations of targeted, targeted and cytotoxic, or multiple cytotoxic agents can be explored with this methodology. Combining more than two agents is also possible but requires different methodology when evaluating for synergy. This important early preclinical data can serve as the basis for confirmatory assays, xenograft studies, and ultimately clinical trials. Results from these efforts have contributed to preclinical data informing two active clinical trials in pediatrics.

Acknowledgments

This study was generously supported by the Pediatric Cancer Foundation (http://fastercure.org/). This work has also been supported in part by the Clinical Trials Laboratory Core and Small Animal Imaging Laboratory at the H. Lee Moffitt Cancer Center and Research Institute, a NCI designated Comprehensive Cancer Center (P30-CA76292). The authors thank Rasa Hamilton (Moffitt Cancer Center) for editorial assistance, Shumin Zhang (Moffitt Cancer Center) for assistance with data analysis, and Brian Roberts (Merck & Co.) for providing MatLab scripts to calculate EoHSA (VHSA). The authors would also like to thank Laura Hall (Moffitt Molecular Genomics Core) for performing cell line identity testing and Dr. Jarret House for assisting in histology evaluation of tumor necrosis.

References

[1] D. Reed and S. Altiok, "Metastatic soft tissue sarcoma chemotherapy: an opportunity for personalized medicine," *Cancer Control*, vol. 18, no. 3, pp. 188–195, 2011.

[2] C. D. Blanke, C. Rankin, G. D. Demetri et al., "Phase III randomized, intergroup trial assessing imatinib mesylate at two dose levels in patients with unresectable or metastatic gastrointestinal stromal tumors expressing the kit receptor tyrosine kinase: S0033," *Journal of Clinical Oncology*, vol. 26, no. 4, pp. 626–632, 2008.

[3] M. Van Glabbeke, J. Verweij, I. Judson, and O. S. Nielsen, "Progression-free rate as the principal end-point for phase II trials in soft-tissue sarcomas," *European Journal of Cancer*, vol. 38, no. 4, pp. 543–549, 2002.

[4] S. Tariq Mahmood, S. Agresta, C. E. Vigil et al., "Phase II study of sunitinib malate, a multitargeted tyrosine kinase inhibitor in patients with relapsed or refractory soft tissue sarcomas. Focus on three prevalent histologies: Leiomyosarcoma, liposarcoma and malignant fibrous histiocytoma," *International Journal of Cancer*, vol. 129, no. 8, pp. 1963–1969, 2011.

[5] T.-C. Chou and P. Talalay, "Quantitative analysis of dose-effect relationships: the combined effects of multiple drugs or enzyme inhibitors," *Advances in Enzyme Regulation*, vol. 22, pp. 27–55, 1984.

[6] D. Siegel, M. Hussein, C. Belani et al., "Vorinostat in solid and hematologic malignancies," *Journal of Hematology and Oncology*, vol. 2, article 31, 2009.

[7] M. Fouladi, J. R. Park, C. F. Stewart et al., "Pediatric phase I trial and pharmacokinetic study of vorinostat: a children's oncology group phase I consortium report," *Journal of Clinical Oncology*, vol. 28, no. 22, pp. 3623–3629, 2010.

[8] S. M. Wilhelm, L. Adnane, P. Newell, A. Villanueva, J. M. Llovet, and M. Lynch, "Preclinical overview of sorafenib, a multikinase inhibitor that targets both Raf and VEGF and PDGF receptor tyrosine kinase signaling," *Molecular Cancer Therapeutics*, vol. 7, no. 10, pp. 3129–3140, 2008.

[9] L. J. Lombardo, F. Y. Lee, P. Chen et al., "Discovery of N-(2-chloro-6-methylphenyl)-2-(6-(4-(2-hydroxyethyl)-piperazin-1-yl)-2-methylpyrimidin-4-ylamino)thiazole-5-carboxamide (BMS-354825), a dual Src/Abl kinase inhibitor with potent antitumor activity in preclinical assays," *Journal of Medicinal Chemistry*, vol. 47, no. 27, pp. 6658–6661, 2004.

[10] O. Hantschel, U. Rix, and G. Superti-Furga, "Target spectrum of the BCR-ABL inhibitors imatinib, nilotinib and dasatinib," *Leukemia and Lymphoma*, vol. 49, no. 4, pp. 615–619, 2008.

[11] A. Olivieri and L. Manzione, "Dasatinib: a new step in molecular target therapy," *Annals of Oncology*, vol. 18, no. 6, pp. vi42–vi46, 2007.

[12] N. Berndt, H. Yang, B. Trinczek et al., "The Akt activation inhibitor TCN-P inhibits Akt phosphorylation by binding to the PH domain of Akt and blocking its recruitment to the plasma membrane," *Cell Death and Differentiation*, vol. 17, no. 11, pp. 1795–1804, 2010.

[13] C. R. Garrett, D. Coppola, R. M. Wenham et al., "Phase I pharmacokinetic and pharmacodynamic study of triciribine phosphate monohydrate, a small-molecule inhibitor of AKT phosphorylation, in adult subjects with solid tumors containing activated AKT," *Investigational new drugs*, vol. 29, no. 6, pp. 1381–1389, 2011.

[14] T. A. Yap, L. Yan, A. Patnaik et al., "First-in-man clinical trial of the oral pan-AKT inhibitor MK-206 in patients with advanced solid tumors," *Journal of Clinical Oncology*, vol. 29, no. 35, pp. 4688–4695, 2011.

[15] G. Neale, X. Su, C. L. Morton et al., "Molecular characterization of the pediatric preclinical testing panel," *Clinical Cancer Research*, vol. 14, no. 14, pp. 4572–4583, 2008.

[16] P. J. Houghton, C. L. Morton, C. Tucker et al., "The pediatric preclinical testing program: description of models and early testing results," *Pediatric Blood & Cancer*, vol. 49, no. 7, pp. 928–940, 2007.

[17] R. Gorlick, J. M. Maris, P. J. Houghton et al., "Testing of the Akt/PKB inhibitor MK-2206 by the pediatric preclinical testing program," *Pediatric Blood & Cancer*, vol. 59, no. 3, pp. 518–524, 2012.

[18] S. T. Keir, J. M. Maris, R. Lock et al., "Initial testing (stage 1) of the multi-targeted kinase inhibitor sorafenib by the pediatric preclinical testing program," *Pediatric Blood & Cancer*, vol. 55, no. 6, pp. 1126–1133, 2010.

[19] H. Carol, P. J. Houghton, C. L. Morton et al., "Initial testing of topotecan by the pediatric preclinical testing program," *Pediatric Blood & Cancer*, vol. 54, no. 5, pp. 707–715, 2010.

[20] N. Keshelava, P. J. Houghton, C. L. Morton et al., "Initial testing (stage 1) of vorinostat (SAHA) by the pediatric preclinical testing program," *Pediatric Blood & Cancer*, vol. 53, no. 3, pp. 505–508, 2009.

[21] E. A. Kolb, R. Gorlick, P. J. Houghton et al., "Initial testing of dasatinib by the pediatric preclinical testing program," *Pediatric Blood & Cancer*, vol. 50, no. 6, pp. 1198–1206, 2008.

[22] P. J. Houghton, C. L. Morton, R. Gorlick et al., "Stage 2 combination testing of rapamycin with cytotoxic agents by the pediatric preclinical testing program," *Molecular Cancer Therapeutics*, vol. 9, no. 1, pp. 101–112, 2010.

[23] R. Aplenc and C. Ahern, "Study ADVL0516 Progress Report," *Study Committee Progress Report—Children's Oncology Group*, August 2009.

[24] M. Fouladi, W. L. Furman, T. Chin et al., "Phase I study of depsipeptide in pediatric patients with refractory solid tumors: a children's oncology group report," *Journal of Clinical Oncology*, vol. 24, no. 22, pp. 3678–3685, 2006.

[25] J. Knipstein and L. Gore, "Entinostat for treatment of solid tumors and hematologic malignancies," *Expert Opinion on Investigational Drugs*, vol. 20, no. 10, pp. 1455–1467, 2011.

[26] J. Cortes, P. Rousselot, D.-W. Kim et al., "Dasatinib induces complete hematologic and cytogenetic responses in patients with imatinib-resistant or -intolerant chronic myeloid leukemia in blast crisis," *Blood*, vol. 109, no. 8, pp. 3207–3213, 2007.

[27] R. G. Maki, J. K. Wathen, S. R. Patel et al., "Randomized phase II study of gemcitabine and docetaxel compared with gemcitabine alone in patients with metastatic soft tissue sarcomas," *Journal of Clinical Oncology*, vol. 25, no. 19, pp. 2755–2763, 2007.

[28] R. Aplenc, S. M. Blaney, L. C. Strauss et al., "Pediatric phase I trial and pharmacokinetic study of dasatinib: a report from the children's oncology group phase I consortium," *Journal of Clinical Oncology*, vol. 29, no. 7, pp. 839–844, 2011.

[29] E. Choy, F. Hornicek, L. Macconaill et al., "High-throughput genotyping in osteosarcoma identifies multiple mutations in phosphoinositide-3-kinase and other oncogenes," *Cancer*, vol. 118, no. 11, pp. 2905–2914, 2011.

[30] E. Hernando, E. Charytonowicz, M. E. Dudas et al., "The AKT-mTOR pathway plays a critical role in the development of leiomyosarcomas," *Nature Medicine*, vol. 13, no. 6, pp. 748–753, 2007.

[31] I. Vivanco and C. L. Sawyers, "The phosphatidylinositol 3-kinase-AKT pathway in human cancer," *Nature Reviews Cancer*, vol. 2, no. 7, pp. 489–501, 2002.

[32] Y. Tomita, T. Morooka, Y. Hoshida et al., "Reassessment of the 1993 Osaka grading system for localized soft tissue sarcoma in Japan," *Anticancer Research*, vol. 26, no. 6C, pp. 4665–4669, 2006.

[33] R. Nitschke, J. Parkhurst, J. Sullivan, M. B. Harris, M. Bernstein, and C. Pratt, "Topotecan in pediatric patients with recurrent and progressive solid tumors: a pediatric oncology group phase II study," *Journal of Pediatric Hematology/Oncology*, vol. 20, no. 4, pp. 315–318, 1998.

[34] N. Hijiya, C. F. Stewart, Y. Zhou et al., "Phase II study of topotecan in combination with dexamethasone, asparaginase, and vincristine in pediatric patients with acute lymphoblastic leukemia in first relapse," *Cancer*, vol. 112, no. 9, pp. 1983–1991, 2008.

[35] M. L. Metzger, C. F. Stewart, B. B. Freeman III et al., "Topotecan is active against Wilms' tumor: results of a multi-institutional phase II study," *Journal of Clinical Oncology*, vol. 25, no. 21, pp. 3130–3136, 2007.

[36] J. Shamash, T. Powles, K. Mutsvangwa et al., "A phase II study using a topoisomerase I-based approach in patients with multiply relapsed germ-cell tumours," *Annals of Oncology*, vol. 18, no. 5, pp. 925–930, 2007.

[37] N. C. Daw, V. M. Santana, L. C. Iacono et al., "Phase I and pharmacokinetic study of topotecan administered orally once daily for 5 days for 2 consecutive weeks to pediatric patients with refractory solid tumors," *Journal of Clinical Oncology*, vol. 22, no. 5, pp. 829–837, 2004.

[38] D. O. Walterhouse, E. R. Lyden, P. P. Breitfeld, S. J. Qualman, M. D. Wharam, and W. H. Meyer, "Efficacy of topotecan and cyclophosphamide given in a phase II window trial in children with newly diagnosed metastatic rhabdomyosarcoma: a children's oncology group study," *Journal of Clinical Oncology*, vol. 22, no. 8, pp. 1398–1403, 2004.

[39] A. Garaventa, R. Luksch, S. Biasotti et al., "A phase II study of topotecan with vincristine and doxorubicin in children with recurrent/refractory neuroblastoma," *Cancer*, vol. 98, no. 11, pp. 2488–2494, 2003.

[40] K. Kramer, B. H. Kushner, and N.-K. V. Cheung, "Oral topotecan for refractory and relapsed neuroblastoma: a retrospective analysis," *Journal of Pediatric Hematology/Oncology*, vol. 25, no. 8, pp. 601–605, 2003.

[41] W. L. Furman, C. F. Stewart, M. Kirstein et al., "Protracted intermittent schedule of topotecan in children with refractory acute leukemia: a Pediatric Oncology Group study," *Journal of Clinical Oncology*, vol. 20, no. 6, pp. 1617–1624, 2002.

[42] H. Rubie, B. Geoerger, D. Frappaz et al., "Phase I study of topotecan in combination with temozolomide (TOTEM) in relapsed or refractory paediatric solid tumours," *European Journal of Cancer*, vol. 46, no. 15, pp. 2763–2770, 2010.

[43] C. Rodriguez-Galindo, K. R. Crews, C. F. Stewart et al., "Phase I study of the combination of topotecan and irinotecan in children with refractory solid tumors," *Cancer Chemotherapy and Pharmacology*, vol. 57, no. 1, pp. 15–24, 2006.

[44] W. T. van der Graaf, J. Y. Blay, S. P. Chawla et al., "Pazopanib for metastatic soft-tissue sarcoma (PALETTE): a randomised, double-blind, placebo-controlled phase 3 trial," *The Lancet*, vol. 379, no. 9829, pp. 1879–1886, 2012.

[45] S. Kumar, R. B. Mokhtari, R. Sheikh et al., "Metronomic oral topotecan with pazopanib is an active antiangiogenic regimen in mouse models of aggressive pediatric solid tumor," *Clinical Cancer Research*, vol. 17, no. 17, pp. 5656–5667, 2011.

[46] M. Talpaz, N. P. Shah, H. Kantarjian et al., "Dasatinib in imatinib-resistant Philadelphia chromosome-positive leukemias," *The New England Journal of Medicine*, vol. 354, no. 24, pp. 2531–2541, 2006.

[47] M. A. Smith and P. Houghton, "A proposal regarding reporting of in vitro testing results," *Clinical Cancer Research*, vol. 19, no. 11, pp. 2828–2833, 2013.

[48] M. Gerlinger, A. J. Rowan, S. Horswell et al., "Intratumor heterogeneity and branched evolution revealed by multiregion sequencing," *The New England Journal of Medicine*, vol. 366, no. 10, pp. 883–892, 2012.

12

The Discrepancy between Patient and Clinician Reported Function in Extremity Bone Metastases

Stein J. Janssen,[1] Eva A. J. van Rein,[1] Nuno Rui Paulino Pereira,[1] Kevin A. Raskin,[1] Marco L. Ferrone,[2] Francis J. Hornicek,[1] Santiago A. Lozano-Calderon,[1] and Joseph H. Schwab[1]

[1]*Department of Orthopaedic Surgery, Orthopaedic Oncology Service, Massachusetts General Hospital, Harvard Medical School, Boston, MA, USA*
[2]*Department of Orthopaedic Surgery, Orthopaedic Oncology Service, Brigham and Women's Hospital, Harvard Medical School, Boston, MA, USA*

Correspondence should be addressed to Stein J. Janssen; steinjanssen@gmail.com

Academic Editor: Fritz C. Eilber

Background. The Musculoskeletal Tumor Society (MSTS) scoring system measures function and is commonly used but criticized because it was developed to be completed by the clinician and not by the patient. We therefore evaluated if there is a difference between patient and clinician reported function using the MSTS score. *Methods.* 128 patients with bone metastasis of the lower ($n = 100$) and upper ($n = 28$) extremity completed the MSTS score. The MSTS score consists of six domains, scored on a 0 to 5 scale and transformed into an overall score ranging from 0 to 100% with a higher score indicating better function. The MSTS score was also derived from clinicians' reports in the medical record. *Results.* The median age was 63 years (interquartile range [IQR]: 55–71) and the study included 74 (58%) women. We found that the clinicians' MSTS score (median: 65, IQR: 49–83) overestimated the function as compared to the patient perceived score (median: 57, IQR: 40–70) by 8 points ($p < 0.001$). *Conclusion.* Clinician reports overestimate function as compared to the patient perceived score. This is important for acknowledging when informing patients about the expected outcome of treatment and for understanding patients' perceptions.

1. Introduction

Treatment for bone metastatic disease is often palliative and aims to maintain function and quality of life for the remaining life span [1, 2]. Traditionally, studies focused on oncological and surgical outcomes (e.g., survival and local recurrence), but more emphasis has been placed on measuring impairment and disability over the past decades [1, 3–5]. The Musculoskeletal Tumor Society (MSTS) recognized this and developed a system—the MSTS score—to evaluate function in patients with musculoskeletal tumors [3]. The validity and reliability of this tool were found to be acceptable when applied to a sample of patients with malignant musculoskeletal tumors [6]. The scoring system has been criticized because it was developed to be completed by a clinician, instead of measuring function as perceived by the patient [1, 7]; however, the MSTS score is still used because of its simplicity and brevity (it consists of six items) [8, 9]. Studies in other fields have demonstrated discrepancies between patient and physician assessment of physical and mental health [10–13]. It is unclear whether the clinician derived MSTS score is representative of the patients' perceived function. We therefore sought to evaluate if there is a difference between patient and clinician reported physical function using the MSTS score in a cohort of patients with bone metastases of the extremities. Secondarily, we compared MSTS domain scores and assessed agreement between the clinician and patient perceived scores.

2. Materials and Methods

2.1. Study Design. Our institutional review board approved secondary use of prospectively collected data for the purpose of this study, and a waiver of informed consent was obtained.

We included data from the first 128 patients who completed a set of physical function questionnaires for two prior studies. These studies compared physical function questionnaires in patients with lower ($n = 100$) and upper ($n = 28$) extremity bone metastases, myeloma, or lymphoma [14]. Only English-speaking patients aged 18 years or above who were able to provide informed consent were approached for these studies. Patients were enrolled between June 2014 and September 2015 from two orthopaedic oncology clinics. Patients were included regardless of previous treatment and disease stage [14]. Seventeen patients declined participation for the initial study, and three patients were excluded because of incomplete questionnaires.

An ante hoc sample size calculation determined that we would need a minimum of 128 patients to find an effect size of 0.25 with an alpha of 0.05 and power of 0.80 using a paired t-test comparing the clinician reported MSTS score with the patient perceived MSTS score.

2.2. Outcome Measures. Our primary outcome measure was the Musculoskeletal Tumor Society (MSTS) score, introduced in 1983 and modified in 1993 [3]. This scoring system was developed to be completed by a clinician—physician or physician extender—and it aims to assess physical function in patients with lower and upper extremity tumors. The modified version (1993) of the MSTS score consists of six domains, each scored on a scale from 0 to 5, with a higher score indicating better function. The total score, ranging from 0 to 30, can be transformed to a point scale of 0 to 100. There are two versions: one for lower extremity tumors and one for upper extremity tumors. These versions have three domains in common, pain, function, and emotional acceptance, and three region specific domains. The region specific domains for the lower extremity are use of supports, walking ability, and gait. The region specific domains for the upper extremity are hand-positioning, dexterity, and lifting ability. Patients completed one of the two versions based on the location of their most disabling bone metastasis.

In addition, patients completed questions about their level of education, marital status, presence of other disabling conditions, prior treatment, and other bone or visceral metastases. Prior treatment and presence of other metastases were also derived from medical records. We extracted age, sex, race, and location of bone metastasis from the medical records.

Two research fellows (SJ and EvR)—blinded to the patients' answers—independently completed the MSTS score based on the clinicians' report in the medical record of the patient; we used the report that was written at the time (or within a few days) of survey completion by the patient. Reports completed by the orthopaedic oncologist, medical oncologist, and physical therapist were used to complete the MSTS score. We averaged the scores assigned by the two researchers per domain and for the overall MSTS score. To assess reliability of extracting this data from medical records, we assessed difference in overall MSTS score and domain scores between researchers and assessed their interobserver agreement.

2.3. Statistical Analysis. We used frequencies with percentages to describe categorical variables and median with interquartile range for continuous variables as histograms suggested nonnormality.

The nonparametric Wilcoxon signed rank test was used to assess the difference between patient and clinician domain scores and overall MSTS scores as data was not normally distributed.

We assessed the relationship between the patient and clinician MSTS and domain scores using both Spearman rank correlation and intraclass correlation (ICC). Spearman rank correlation determines the relationship between two variables (range: −1 to 1): a score of 1 indicates a perfect correlation, 0 indicates no correlation, and −1 indicates a perfect inverse correlation. We used bootstrapping (number of resamples: 1,000) to calculate p values and 95% confidence intervals for the Spearman rank correlation coefficients. The intraclass correlation coefficient also assesses a relationship between two variables but accounts for discrepancy in measurements and therefore measures absolute agreement. We calculated the ICC through a two-way mixed-effects model with absolute agreement for the overall MSTS score and the domain scores. As with the Spearman rank correlation coefficient, an ICC of 1 reflects perfect agreement, whereas 0 reflects no agreement.

Additionally, we assessed difference in domain and total scores between the two researchers using the Wilcoxon signed rank test and assessed their interobserver agreement per domain and overall score using the ICC.

2.4. Patient Characteristics. The median age was 63 years (interquartile range [IQR]: 55 to 71) and the study included 74 (58%) women. The majority had a metastatic lesion in the lower extremity (78% [100/128]). Eighty (63%) patients had previous surgery, and 72 (56%) had previous radiotherapy (Table 1). Breast was the most common primary tumor type (26%) (Table 2).

3. Results

3.1. Patient Perceived Compared to Clinician MSTS Score. We found that the clinicians' MSTS score overestimated the physical function as compared to the patient perceived score. The median clinician MSTS score was 8 points higher (median: 65 and IQR: 49 to 83) as compared to the patient perceived score (median: 57 and IQR: 40 to 70) ($p < 0.001$) (Table 3). This difference also existed when analyzing the lower extremity and upper extremity versions separately (Table 3).

When comparing the three common domains, clinicians scored higher for function ($p < 0.001$) and emotional acceptance ($p < 0.001$) as compared to the patient perceived score; however, there was no difference in assessment of pain ($p = 0.076$). When comparing the three lower extremity specific domains, clinicians scored higher for use of supports ($p = 0.003$) and gait ($p = 0.006$) as compared to the patient perceived score, and there was no difference in assessment of walking ability ($p = 0.102$). When comparing the three

Table 1: Demographics (n = 128).

	Median (±interquartile range)
Age	63 (55–71)
	n (%)
Sex	
Women	74 (58)
Men	54 (42)
Race	
Caucasian	117 (91)
African American	10 (8)
Asian	1 (1)
Education	
High-school or less	41 (32)
College or Bachelor's degree	53 (41)
Graduate or professional degree	34 (27)
Marital status	
Married	84 (66)
Single	15 (12)
Widowed	15 (12)
Separated/divorced	9 (7)
Living with partner	5 (4)
Location of metastasis	
Upper extremity	28 (22)
Humerus	21 (16)
Scapula	5 (4)
Clavicule	1 (1)
Radius	1 (1)
Lower extremity	100 (78)
Femur	71 (55)
Acetabulum	14 (11)
Pelvis	12 (9)
Tibia	2 (2)
Fibula	1 (1)
Other disabling conditions	
Yes	37 (29)
No	90 (71)
Previous surgery for metastatic lesion	
Yes	80 (63)
No	48 (38)
Previous radiotherapy for metastatic lesion	
Yes	72 (56)
No	53 (41)
Unknown	3 (2)
Multiple bones affected	
Yes	61 (48)
No	55 (43)
Unknown	12 (9)
Visceral organs affected	
Yes	39 (30)
No	78 (61)
Unknown	11 (9)

Table 2: Tumor type (n = 128).

Bone metastases	
Breast	33 (26)
Renal cell	17 (13)
Prostate	11 (8.6)
Lung	11 (8.6)
Melanoma	7 (5.5)
Leiomyosarcoma	5 (3.9)
Bladder	3 (2.3)
Thyroid	3 (2.3)
Colorectal	2 (1.6)
Hepatocellular	2 (1.6)
Stomach	1 (0.8)
Esophageal	1 (0.8)
Neuroendocrine	1 (0.8)
Sarcoma	1 (0.8)
Primary bone tumors	
Myeloma	17 (13)
Lymphoma	13 (10)

upper extremity specific domains, clinicians scored higher for hand-positioning (p = 0.048) and lifting ability (p = 0.002) as compared to the patient perceived score, and there was no difference in assessment of dexterity (p = 0.890).

Agreement between the overall clinician score and the patient perceived score was substantial (ICC: 0.66, 95% CI 0.43–0.79, and p < 0.001) (Table 4). We found moderate agreement for assessment of the common domains: pain (ICC: 0.50) and function (ICC: 0.43), but no agreement for emotional acceptance (ICC: 0.08). Agreement was substantial for assessment of the lower extremity specific use of supports domain (ICC: 0.72) and moderate for walking ability (ICC: 0.47) and gait (ICC: 0.48). We found substantial agreement for the upper extremity specific hand-positioning domain (ICC: 0.61), moderate for dexterity (ICC: 0.51), and no agreement for lifting ability (ICC: 0.16). The Spearman rank correlation coefficients were higher than the intraclass correlation coefficients reflecting the discrepancy of scores between the clinician and patient (Table 4).

3.2. Assessing Reliability of Extracting the Clinician MSTS Score from Medical Records. We found no difference in overall clinician MSTS score derived from medical records between researchers (researcher 1: median: 67 and IQR: 48–90 and researcher 2: median: 63 and IQR: 50–82; p = 0.142), nor did we find a difference between researchers for deriving any of the medical record based domain scores. The interobserver agreement between researchers for the overall clinician MSTS score was substantial (ICC: 0.78, 95% CI 0.70–0.84, and p < 0.001). These analyses indicate substantial reliability for deriving the clinician MSTS score from the medical record.

4. Discussion

The MSTS scoring tool evaluates function in patients with extremity tumors and is developed to be completed by the

TABLE 3: MSTS score comparison.

	Patient score Median (±interquartile range)	Clinician score Median (±interquartile range)	p value
Overall MSTS score	57 (40–70)	65 (49–83)	**<0.001**
Lower extremity MSTS score	57 (37–70)	63 (48–84)	**<0.001**
Upper extremity MSTS score	63 (53–73)	74 (58–85)	**<0.001**
MSTS common domains			
Pain	4 (2–5)	3 (3-4)	0.076
Function	2 (2–4)	4 (3–5)	**<0.001**
Emotional acceptance	2 (1–3)	4 (3-4)	**<0.001**
Lower extremity specific domains			
Use of supports	1 (1–5)	3 (1–5)	**0.003**
Walking ability	4 (3-4)	3 (3-4)	0.102
Gait	3 (2–4)	4 (3–5)	**0.006**
Upper extremity specific domains			
Hand-positioning	4 (1–5)	4 (3-4)	**0.048**
Dexterity	5 (3–5)	4 (4-5)	0.890
Lifting ability	3 (1–4)	4 (3-4)	**0.002**

Bold indicates significant difference (two-tailed p value below 0.05).

TABLE 4: Comparison of interobserver reliability.

	Patient score compared with clinician score Spearman correlation coefficient (95% confidence interval)*	p value	Patient score compared with clinician score Intraclass correlation coefficient (95% confidence interval)	p value
Overall MSTS score	0.74 (0.64–0.83)	**<0.001**	0.66 (0.43–0.79)	**<0.001**
Lower extremity MSTS score	0.71 (0.59–0.82)	**<0.001**	0.64 (0.42–0.78)	**<0.001**
Upper extremity MSTS score	0.82 (0.68–0.97)	**<0.001**	0.74 (0.25–0.90)	**<0.001**
MSTS common domains				
Pain	0.50 (0.35–0.64)	**<0.001**	0.50 (0.36–0.62)	**<0.001**
Function	0.52 (0.38–0.66)	**<0.001**	0.43 (0.23–0.59)	**<0.001**
Emotional acceptance	0.16 (−0.02–0.35)	0.073	0.08 (−0.06–0.21)	0.105
Lower extremity specific domains				
Use of supports	0.74 (0.62–0.86)	**<0.001**	0.72 (0.60–0.81)	**<0.001**
Walking ability	0.54 (0.39–0.68)	**<0.001**	0.47 (0.30–0.61)	**<0.001**
Gait	0.49 (0.34–0.63)	**<0.001**	0.48 (0.29–0.62)	**<0.001**
Upper extremity specific domains				
Hand-positioning	0.84 (0.72–0.96)	**<0.001**	0.61 (0.29–0.81)	**<0.001**
Dexterity	0.51 (0.18–0.85)	**0.003**	0.51 (0.18–0.74)	**0.003**
Lifting ability	0.30 (−0.07–0.66)	0.110	0.16 (−0.12–0.46)	0.124

Bold indicates significant correlation (two-tailed p value below 0.05).
*95% confidence interval calculated through bootstrapping (1,000 resamples).

clinician [3]. It is unclear how this clinician-based score relates to the patients perceived function. We therefore compared the MSTS score as completed by the patient with a medical record based clinician reported MSTS score and assessed discrepancies and agreement. We found that the clinicians' MSTS score overestimated physical function as compared to the patient completed MSTS score. This discrepancy was the largest for the common overall function and emotional acceptance domains but was absent for the pain domain.

This study has limitations. First, we based the MSTS score on review of information provided by the clinician in the medical records; however, the MSTS score was developed to be completed by a clinician at time of the consultation.

We see this as an important limitation and explored its possible consequences by assessing discrepancies and interobserver agreement between two researchers who independently derived these data from medical records. There was no discrepancy between the researchers for the overall MSTS score and their interobserver agreement was substantial; this suggests reproducible assessment of the MSTS score based on the medical record. Previous studies used the same methodology to extract an MSTS score from information in the medical record [15–17]. In addition, the judgment of the two research fellows might have been different from the judgment of the attending surgeon. Future prospective study should therefore compare the patient completed MSTS score with an MSTS score completed by the clinician at time of the consultation. Second, patients might have misunderstood specific items or answer options as the scoring system is not developed to be completed by a patient and not validated in a patient sample. We considered this as a limitation but feel that this did not compromise our results, as we believe that erroneous answers would have occurred in both directions (i.e., better and worse). Third, the MSTS score is developed for evaluation of functional status in all musculoskeletal tumor types. Patient demographics differ per tumor type and we only studied a sample of patients with bone metastases; this limits the generalizability of our results to this specific population. Future study might help elucidate the discrepancy between patient and physician perceived function in primary bone tumors.

Previous studies in other fields also demonstrated an overestimation of patients' physical and mental health when estimated by a clinician as compared to the patients' perception [10, 13, 18]. Nelson et al. [10] demonstrated in 1,101 primary care patients that 12% rated major physical limitations in the preceding month, while only 4.4% of the patients were rated as such by their primary care physician. This study also demonstrated that 9% rated major emotional limitations, while only 5% were rated as such by their physician. Rosenberger et al. [18] demonstrated that physicians overestimated function and underestimated pain in 98 patients who underwent surgical anterior cruciate ligament reconstruction or meniscectomy. In line with these previous studies, we found the largest discrepancy for assessment of the function and emotional acceptance domains in our study. However, we found no difference for the pain domain. Pain level in the MSTS score is based on the amount of pain and the degree of disability it causes; this might explain why we did not find difference in pain score. Despite the discrepancies, clinicians' estimates do correlate reasonably well with patient scores for the overall MSTS score and domain scores, except for emotional acceptance and lifting ability. This means that clinicians recognize worse overall function as perceived by the patient; however, the clinician tends to underestimate its impact. Assessment of emotional acceptance by the clinician does not correlate with the patients' perception, which might be explained by the subjectivity and complexity of this measure. Lifting ability is a relatively objective measure and the absence of correlation between the patient and clinician score might have been a result of the small sample size (28 upper extremity patients).

The discrepancy between the clinicians' assessment and patients perception of health and symptoms can have several consequences. First, surgeons have an important role in counseling their patients regarding expected outcome after treatment. It is important for them to understand patients' perspectives about outcome to educate future patients. For example, patients might be less satisfied, if their expectations are not met or when recovery is slower than expected [18]. Second, patients might feel misunderstood or unheard by their physician. A previous study demonstrated that concordance (so called dyadic agreement) between the patients' and physicians' perceptions of health and symptoms are associated with higher patient satisfaction [19]. Another study demonstrated that dissatisfaction of the patient leads to less compliance with treatment recommendations and potentially jeopardizes patients' health and outcome [20]. A review of plaintiff depositions demonstrated that delivering information poorly and failure to empathize with the patients' or family's perspective are common causes of medical litigation [21, 22]. Third, a clinician might be biased towards certain treatments; this might compromise comparison of clinician reported outcomes across treatment options in prospective studies and nonblinded clinical trials. Fourth, overestimating outcomes tends to breed an attitude of complacency and inertia among clinicians which could preclude further improvement. Fifth, third-party payers may use reported (overestimated) outcomes to dissuade costly innovation and research.

Capturing patient reported outcome measures, questionnaires completed by the patient, using validated instruments for both research purposes and day-to-day clinical practice is key. Previous studies demonstrated that use of information from patient reported outcome measures leads to better communication and decision making between doctors and patients and improves satisfaction [11, 23, 24]. However, this does not mean that clinician measures are uninformative. Measuring pathophysiology and impairment (e.g., range of motion, strength, and stability), in addition to patient reported outcome measures (e.g., symptoms and disability), will help us to better understand patient perceptions and inform them about prognosis and outcome of different treatment options.

In conclusion, clinician reports overestimate function as compared to the patient perceived score. This is important to acknowledge when informing patients about the expected outcome of treatment and to understand patients' perceptions. Our study reinforces the need for obtaining patient reported outcomes using validated methods in orthopaedic oncology.

Disclosure

This work was performed at Massachusetts General Hospital, Boston, MA, USA.

Competing Interests

One author (Stein J. Janssen) certifies that he has received an amount less than USD 10,000 from the Anna Foundation (Oegstgeest, Netherlands), an amount less than USD

10,000 from the De Drie Lichten Foundation (Hilversum, Netherlands), an amount less than USD 10,000 from the KWF Kankerbestrijding (Amsterdam, Netherlands), and an amount less than USD 10,000 from the Michael van Vloten Foundation (Rotterdam, Netherlands).

References

[1] E. Y. Cheng, "Prospective quality of life research in bony metastatic disease," *Clinical Orthopaedics and Related Research*, no. 415, supplement, pp. S289–S297, 2003.

[2] R. H. Quinn, R. L. Randall, J. Benevenia, S. H. Berven, and K. A. Raskin, "Contemporary management of metastatic bone disease: tips and tools of the trade for general practitioners," *The Journal of Bone & Joint Surgery—American Volume*, vol. 95, no. 20, pp. 1887–1895, 2013.

[3] W. F. Enneking, W. Dunham, M. C. Gebhardt, M. Malawar, and D. J. Pritchard, "A system for the functional evaluation of reconstructive procedures after surgical treatment of tumors of the musculoskeletal system," *Clinical Orthopaedics and Related Research*, no. 286, pp. 241–246, 1993.

[4] M. Talbot, R. E. Turcotte, M. Isler, D. Normandin, D. Iannuzzi, and P. Downer, "Function and health status in surgically treated bone metastases," *Clinical Orthopaedics and Related Research*, no. 438, pp. 215–220, 2005.

[5] D. R. Clohisy, C. T. Le, E. Y. Cheng, D. C. Dykes, and R. C. Thompson Jr., "Evaluation of the feasibility of and results of measuring health-status changes in patients undergoing surgical treatment for skeletal metastases," *Journal of Orthopaedic Research*, vol. 18, no. 1, pp. 1–9, 2000.

[6] S. H. Lee, D. J. Kim, J. H. Oh, H. S. Han, K. H. Yoo, and H. S. Kim, "Validation of a functional evaluation system in patients with musculoskeletal tumors," *Clinical Orthopaedics and Related Research*, no. 411, pp. 217–226, 2003.

[7] A. M. Davis, J. G. Wright, J. I. Williams, C. Bombardier, A. Griffin, and R. S. Bell, "Development of a measure of physical function for patients with bone and soft tissue sarcoma," *Quality of Life Research*, vol. 5, no. 5, pp. 508–516, 1996.

[8] T. Wada, A. Kawai, K. Ihara et al., "Construct validity of the Enneking score for measuring function in patients with malignant or aggressive benign tumours of the upper limb," *The Journal of Bone & Joint Surgery—British Volume*, vol. 89, no. 5, pp. 659–663, 2007.

[9] D. C. S. Rebolledo, J. R. N. Vissoci, R. Pietrobon, O. P. De Camargo, and A. M. Baptista, "Validation of the Brazilian version of the musculoskeletal tumor society rating scale for lower extremity bone sarcoma tumor," *Clinical Orthopaedics and Related Research*, vol. 471, no. 12, pp. 4020–4026, 2013.

[10] E. Nelson, B. Conger, R. Douglass et al., "Functional health status levels of primary care patients," *The Journal of the American Medical Association*, vol. 249, no. 24, pp. 3331–3338, 1983.

[11] E. C. Nelson, E. Eftimovska, C. Lind, A. Hager, J. H. Wasson, and S. Lindblad, "Patient reported outcome measures in practice," *BMJ*, vol. 350, 2015.

[12] H. L. Richards, D. G. Fortune, A. Weidmann, S. K. T. Sweeney, and C. E. M. Griffiths, "Detection of psychological distress in patients with psoriasis: low consensus between dermatologist and patient," *British Journal of Dermatology*, vol. 151, no. 6, pp. 1227–1233, 2004.

[13] A. C. Justice, L. Rabeneck, R. D. Hays, A. W. Wu, and S. A. Bozzette, "Sensitivity, specificity, reliability, and clinical validity of provider-reported symptoms: a comparison with self-reported symptoms. Outcomes Committee of the AIDS Clinical Trials Group," *Journal of Acquired Immune Deficiency Syndromes*, vol. 21, no. 2, pp. 126–133, 1999.

[14] S. J. Janssen, N. R. Paulino Pereira, K. A. Raskin et al., "A comparison of questionnaires for assessing physical function in patients with lower extremity bone metastases," *Journal of Surgical Oncology*, 2016.

[15] C. P. Cannon, G. U. Paraliticci, P. P. Lin, V. O. Lewis, and A. W. Yasko, "Functional outcome following endoprosthetic reconstruction of the proximal humerus," *Journal of Shoulder and Elbow Surgery*, vol. 18, no. 5, pp. 705–710, 2009.

[16] M. T. Houdek, E. R. Wagner, A. A. Stans et al., "What is the outcome of allograft and intramedullary free fibula (Capanna Technique) in pediatric and adolescent patients with bone tumors?" *Clinical Orthopaedics and Related Research*, vol. 474, no. 3, pp. 660–668, 2016.

[17] Y. Mimata, J. Nishida, K. Sato, Y. Suzuki, and M. Doita, "Glenohumeral arthrodesis for malignant tumor of the shoulder girdle," *Journal of Shoulder and Elbow Surgery*, vol. 24, no. 2, pp. 174–178, 2015.

[18] P. H. Rosenberger, P. Jokl, A. Cameron, and J. R. Ickovics, "Shared decision making, preoperative expectations, and post-operative reality: differences in physician and patient predictions and ratings of knee surgery outcomes," *Arthroscopy*, vol. 21, no. 5, pp. 562–569, 2005.

[19] J. J. Coran, T. Koropeckyj-Cox, and C. L. Arnold, "Are physicians and patients in agreement? exploring dyadic concordance," *Health Education and Behavior*, vol. 40, no. 5, pp. 603–611, 2013.

[20] V. Francis, B. M. Korsch, and M. J. Morris, "Gaps in doctor-patient communication. Patients' response to medical advice," *The New England Journal of Medicine*, vol. 280, no. 10, pp. 535–540, 1969.

[21] H. P. Forster, J. Schwartz, and E. DeRenzo, "Reducing legal risk by practicing patient-centered medicine," *Archives of Internal Medicine*, vol. 162, no. 11, pp. 1217–1219, 2002.

[22] H. B. Beckman, K. M. Markakis, A. L. Suchman, and R. M. Frankel, "The doctor-patient relationship and malpractice: lessons from plaintiff depositions," *Archives of Internal Medicine*, vol. 154, no. 12, pp. 1365–1370, 1994.

[23] J. Chen, L. Ou, and S. J. Hollis, "A systematic review of the impact of routine collection of patient reported outcome measures on patients, providers and health organisations in an oncologic setting," *BMC Health Services Research*, vol. 13, no. 1, article 211, 2013.

[24] J. M. Valderas, A. Kotzeva, M. Espallargues et al., "The impact of measuring patient-reported outcomes in clinical practice: a systematic review of the literature," *Quality of Life Research*, vol. 17, no. 2, pp. 179–193, 2008.

13

MRI-Based Assessment of Safe Margins in Tumor Surgery

Laura Bellanova,[1] Thomas Schubert,[1] Olivier Cartiaux,[1] Frédéric Lecouvet,[2] Christine Galant,[3] Xavier Banse,[1] and Pierre-Louis Docquier[1]

[1] *Computer Assisted and Robotic Surgery (CARS), Institut de Recherche Expérimentale et Clinique (IREC), Université catholique de Louvain Tour Pasteur +4, Avenue Mounier, 53, 1200 Brussels, Belgium*
[2] *Département D'imagerie Médicale, Cliniques Universitaires Saint-Luc 10, Avenue Hippocrate, 1200 Brussels, Belgium*
[3] *Département de Pathologie, Cliniques Universitaires Saint-Luc 10, Avenue Hippocrate, 1200 Brussels, Belgium*

Correspondence should be addressed to Pierre-Louis Docquier; pierre-louis.docquier@uclouvain.be

Academic Editor: Luca Sangiorgi

Introduction. In surgical oncology, histological analysis of excised tumor specimen is the conventional method to assess the safety of the resection margins. We tested the feasibility of using MRI to assess the resection margins of freshly explanted tumor specimens in rats. *Materials and Methods.* Fourteen specimen of sarcoma were resected in rats and analysed both with MRI and histologically. Slicing of the specimen was identical for the two methods and corresponding slices were paired. 498 margins were measured in length and classified using the UICC classification (R0, R1, and R2). *Results.* The mean difference between the 498 margins measured both with histology and MRI was 0.3 mm (SD 1.0 mm). The agreement interval of the two measurement methods was [−1.7 mm; 2.2 mm]. In terms of the UICC classification, a strict correlation was observed between MRI- and histology-based classifications ($\kappa = 0.84$, $P < 0.05$). *Discussion.* This experimental study showed the feasibility to use MRI images of excised tumor specimen to assess the resection margins with the same degree of accuracy as the conventional histopathological analysis. When completed, MRI acquisition of resected tumors may alert the surgeon in case of inadequate margin and help advantageously the histopathological analysis.

1. Introduction

Limb-salvage surgery is nowadays the ideal treatment for bone and soft tissue sarcoma [1]. Although histological grade and tumor size are important prognostic factors, inadequate resection margins remain one of the most significant predictors of local recurrence for bone and soft tissue sarcomas, even in the presence of adjuvant therapies [2–4]. A local recurrence usually impairs limb preservation and functional outcomes, but it is also correlated with an increased risk of metastatic disease development [5, 6]. Identified causes of local recurrence are insufficient resection margins, undetected metastasis, for instance in the lymph nodes, and tumor venous emboli. While other causes cannot be treated by surgery alone and require adjuvant treatment, insufficient resection margins can be avoided with a careful dissection and safe resection margins [7, 8].

Gross extemporaneous macroscopical analysis of the excised tumor specimen by the surgeon, followed by delayed histopathological analysis, is the conventional method to evaluate the safety of the resection margins. In a histopathological study, Picci et al. correlated local recurrence with insufficient resection margins [9]. Histologic assessment of margin status was shown useful for predicting local recurrence of cutaneous malignant tumors in dogs and cats treated by means of excision alone [10]. Several prognostic classifications have been published to histologically evaluate surgical margins and identify high-/low-risk groups for local recurrence after limb salvage surgery. A standardized classification was created by the Union for International Cancer Control (UICC). It distinguishes R0 as *in sano* resection R1 as possible microscopic residuals (margin between 0 and 1 mm) and R2 as macroscopic residual disease [11].

Magnetic resonance imaging (MRI) is widely used for oncological diagnosis, disease extension assessment, surgical planning, and postoperative followup [12]. Current available resolution of preoperative MRI images enables accurate delineation of the tumor boundaries for surgical planning purposes [8, 13]. However, MRI has never been considered as a possible tool for assessing the safety of resection margins on the freshly explanted tumor specimen.

This experimental study, performed on rodent models, aimed at investigating the feasibility of using MRI to assess the resection margins of excised tumor specimen using the UICC classification and comparing MRI with the conventional extemporaneous histopathological method.

2. Materials and Methods

2.1. Animals and Tumor Induction. Experiments on animals were carried out in compliance with the Institutional Ethics Committee for Laboratory Animal Experimentation (CE Accred. number UCL/MD/2011/022). Animals were housed according to the guidelines of the Belgian Ministry of Agriculture and Animal Care. Seven 9-week-old male WAG/RijHsd rats (Harlan Laboratories, Boxmeer, The Netherlands) were used as recipients. Fragments from a syngeneic rhabdomyosarcoma [14] of approximately 1 mm^3 were grafted intramuscularly in both thighs under general anesthesia by Isoflurane inhalation (Forene, Abbott, Diegem, Belgium). The sarcoma was implanted bilaterally in the pelvic region/proximal thigh. Implanted tumor fragments grew within a 3- to 4-week delay to reach a gross volume of approximately 2 to 3 cm^3 at the time of imaging. No rat died nor showed any significant impairment in general status during the period of tumor growth.

Three to four weeks postimplantation, the rats were sacrificed by T61 (Intervet International GmbH, Germany) intracardiac injection under general anesthesia. In four rats (Rat1, Rat2, Rat3, and Rat4), the two tumors were explanted separately resulting in two resection specimens per rat. A wood stick was inserted in each specimen and considered as reference axis for the comparison between MRI-based and histological margin evaluation. For the three remaining rats (Rat5, Rat6, Rat7), "en-bloc" resection of the pelvis with both femurs was performed and the axis of the spine was used as reference axis during the evaluation process.

2.2. MRI Acquisition. MRI of the specimens was done after resection. The images were acquired using a 1.5-Tesla MRI unit (Gyroscan NT Intera T15; Philips Medical Systems, Bets, The Netherlands) with contiguous slices. Reference axis for slicing was the wood stick for the specimens excised from Rat1, Rat2, Rat3, and Rat4, and the spine axis for the specimens excised from Rat5, Rat6, and Rat7. The acquisition parameters used for the specimens were specified as follows: reconstruction matrix 176 × 176, repetition time 1500 ms, echo time 15 ms, section thickness 0.5 mm, and spacing between slices 0.5 mm. The specimens were scanned and the sequences saved in DICOM format prior to analysis with the picture archiving and communication system (PACS, Carestream, Health, NY, USA). The distance measurement tool of the PACS system was used to measure the resection margins as the distance (in mm) between the tumor boundary and the specimen edge.

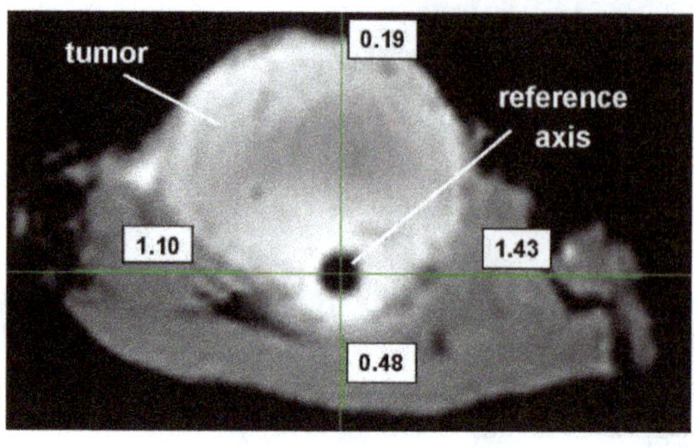

(a)

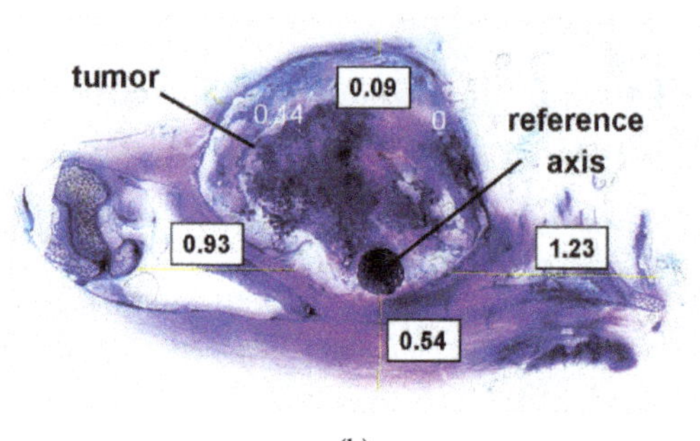

(b)

FIGURE 1: Example of a histological slice (b) associated with its corresponding MRI slice (a) of the same excised tumor specimen for the comparison of the two measurement methods. In this case, the reference axis for the measurements is the wood stick inserted in the excised specimen. Resection margins are measured in mm along the straight lines drawn manually by the operator.

2.3. Histology. After MRI acquisition, each excised specimen was fixed in methanol and methylmethacrylate (MMA) embedded. The polymerized blocks were sliced with 200-μm thickness with a diamond band saw (EXAKT, D-22581, Norderstedt, Germany) perpendicular to the same reference axis used in MRI slices (wood stick for the specimens excised from Rat1, Rat2, Rat3, and Rat4, and spine axis for the specimens excised from Rat5, Rat6, and Rat7). The slices were ground and polished up to 120 μm between two sheets of ground glass, stained with 1% Methylen Blue (85662, MERCK, Hohenbrunn, Germany) and 1% Fuchsin (B-2340, Sigma Aldrich, St-Louis, USA), and finally mounted on glass.

The histological slices were scanned with a flatbed scanner (Scanner Canon LiDE 210, Diegem, Belgium) and images were saved in "jpg" format. Evaluation of the resection margins was performed using ImageJ 1.43i software (ImageJ, Image Processing and Analysis in JAVA, National Institute of Health, Bethesda, MD, USA) and the built-in distance measurement tool.

2.4. Evaluation. Each histological slice was associated with its corresponding MRI slice (Figure 1). Eighty-six pairs of corresponding MRI and histological slices were available for the comparison between MRI-based and histological margin evaluation. On each pair of slices, the operator manually drew straight lines from the reference axis (wood stick or spine axis) to the slice boundary (Figure 1). Resection margins

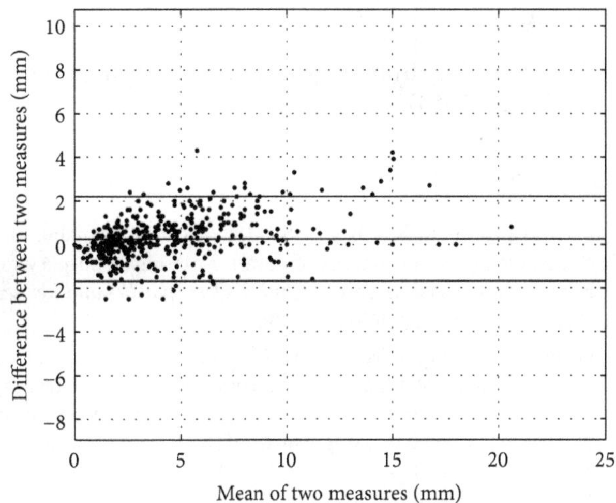

FIGURE 2: Bland and Altman plot of the two measurement methods (histology and MRI). The dashed line represents the mean value of the differences between the two measurement methods, and the lines above and below it represent the agreement interval.

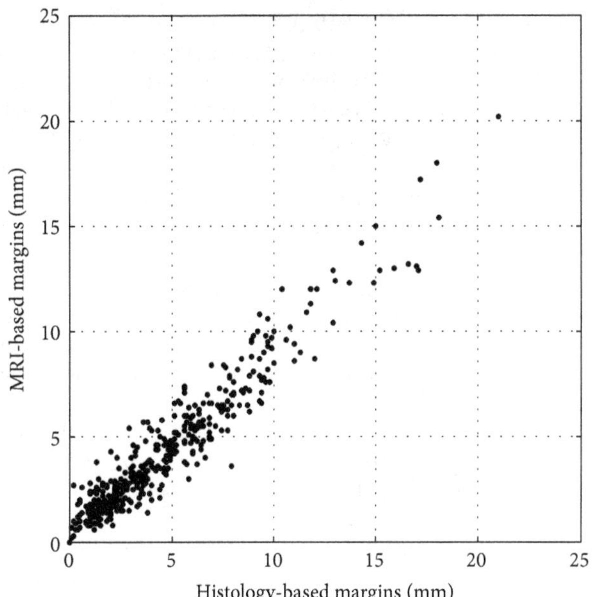

FIGURE 3: Correlation between the two measurement methods.

were measured in mm along the straight lines between the tumor boundary and the specimen boundary. In total, 498 measurements were performed on the histological slices and compared with the corresponding measurements on the MRI slices. The two series of 498 measured resection margins were also classified using the UICC classification as R0 (*in sano* if more than 1 mm), R1 (possible microscopic residuals if between 0 and 1 mm), and R2 (macroscopic residuals if 0).

2.5. Statistics. Statistical analyses were performed with PASW 19 (formerly SPSS, IBM, New York, NY, USA). The one-sample Kolmogorov-Smirnov test and Q-Q plots were used to assess normality of values. A Bland and Altman plot

TABLE 1: Cross tabulation of MRI-based classification by histology-based classification of the 498 measured resection margins.

Histology-based classification	MRI-based classification		
	R0	R1	R2
R0	404	7	0
R1	16	10	0
R2	0	0	61

(or difference plot) [15] was used to compare the two methods (MRI and histology) (Figure 2). In this plot, the differences between the two methods were plotted against the averages of the two methods. Horizontal lines were drawn at the mean difference and the limits of agreement (mean difference ±1.96 times standard deviation). The Pearson correlation was used to assess the linear relationship between the two methods. Statistical differences between groups were tested by Student's paired t-tests. A P value < 0.05 was considered significant. Results were expressed as mean and standard deviation (SD).

3. Results

The mean difference between the 498 margins measured both with histology and MRI was 0.3 mm (SD 1.0 mm) (Figure 2). Agreement interval of the two measurement methods was (−1.7 mm; 2.2 mm). A scatter plot showed the correlation between the two methods (Figure 3). The Pearson correlation coefficient was 0.97.

In terms of the UICC classification, 95.4% (475/498) of the resection margins were classified similarly by the two measurement methods (Table 1). In 3.2% (16/498), the resection margins were classified R1 using the histological measurements and R0 using the MRI measurements. On the contrary, 1.4% (7/498) were classified R1 with the MRI measurements and R0 with the histological measurements. R2 classification was fully identical with both methods. A strict correlation was observed between MRI- and histology-based classifications ($\kappa = 0.84$, $P < 0.05$).

4. Discussion

This experimental study showed the feasibility to use MRI imaging of excised tumor specimen to assess the resection margins with the same degree of accuracy than the conventional extemporaneous histopathological analysis. The Bland and Altman plot showed that the two measurement methods were concordant. Moreover, a good correlation coefficient was found. In terms of the UICC classification, good kappa coefficient was found, meaning a strict correlation. All cases with macroscopic residuals (R2) were concordant with the two methods and none was misinterpreted as R1 by one of the method. The only differing interpretations were between R0 and R1.

Magnetic resonance imaging remains the most accurate noninvasive tool for staging bone and soft-tissue extent of musculoskeletal sarcomas as it displays precisely the tumor, the compartmental spread, and the neurovascular and articular involvement [14]. Technological advances over the last years allowed significant improvement in tumor delineation and extension [15]. When the tumoral specimen is resected, it is available for MRI acquisition (in 30 minutes). Result of the MRI can be analysed by the surgeon before the end of the surgical procedure, allowing if needed further resection in case of inadequate margin. Nevertheless, MRI may not replace the anatomopathological specimen analysis as it gives no information about the local effect of chemotherapy, as expressed by percentage of tumor necrosis. The result of the thorough examination of the tumor specimen and of its resection margins will usually be available within the week.

Extemporaneous thorough examination of the entire specimen by the pathologist is not possible. MRI imaging of the entire specimen could on the contrary be quickly obtained and analysed by the surgeon or a radiologist and lead to immediate further resection. Serial histology of the specimen perpendicularly to the spine/marker allowed a good match between the MRI slices and the histological slides. A statistically significant high correlation was found between the anatomopathological and MRI findings. In 49.8% of the measures, larger resection margins were secondarily diagnosed by histology. This finding demonstrates the safety of the procedure. Only in a few cases, histologically R1 resections were found R0 by MRI (3.2%; 16/498).

MRI could also be used as additional tool to help the pathologist, by a preliminary investigation, to focus his attention on doubtful areas. This could be very effective in case of voluminous tumors where pathologic study of the whole resection specimen is difficult and time consuming.

One of the limitations of the MRI evaluation is the low resolution at the edge of the specimen. Additional studies have to improve the MRI analysis of the tumoral contour. MRI acquisition with the specimen in a formalin bath could increase the resolution at the specimen border. Moreover, extensive clinical trials in which both MRI and anatomopathology are undertaken together should be realized before one could however consider abandoning extemporaneous examination.

Another limitation of this study is the relatively small size of the resection specimens (rat limb). Clinical human specimens are generally larger and could be more difficult or complex to interpret.

Complementary animal and in vivo studies should be performed to fully validate the observed results in terms of accuracy, repeatability, and time.

5. Conclusion

When completed, intraoperative MRI acquisition of resected tumors may enable immediate assessment of surgical margins and help advantageously the histopathological analysis.

Funding

Funds were received from Belgian Foundation against Cancer (GrantSCIE2010-184).

References

[1] N. Kawaguchi, A. R. Ahmed, S. Matsumoto, J. Manabe, and Y. Matsushita, "The concept of curative margin in surgery for bone and soft tissue sarcoma," *Clinical Orthopaedics and Related Research*, no. 419, pp. 165–172, 2004.

[2] G. Bacci, A. Longhi, M. Versari, M. Mercuri, A. Briccoli, and P. Picci, "Prognostic factors for osteosarcoma of the extremity trerated with neoadjuvant chemotherapy: 15-year experience in 789 patients treated at a single institution," *Cancer*, vol. 106, no. 5, pp. 1154–1161, 2006.

[3] E. Arpaci, T. Yetisyigit, M. Seker, D. Uncu, U. Uyeturk, B. Oksuzoglu et al., "Prognostic factors and clinical outcome of patients with Ewing's sarcoma family of tumors in adults: multicentric study of the Anatolian Society of Medical Oncology," *Medical Oncology*, vol. 30, no. 1, p. 469, 2013.

[4] P. D. Stefanovski, E. Bidoli, A. De Paoli et al., "Prognostic factors in soft tissue sarcomas: a study of 395 patients," *European Journal of Surgical Oncology*, vol. 28, no. 2, pp. 153–164, 2002.

[5] A. Stojadinovic, D. H. Y. Leung, A. Hoos, D. P. Jaques, J. J. Lewis, and M. F. Brennan, "Analysis of the prognostic significance of microscopic margins in 2,084 localized primary adult soft tissue sarcomas," *Annals of Surgery*, vol. 235, no. 3, pp. 424–434, 2002.

[6] F. C. Eilber, G. Rosen, S. D. Nelson et al., "High-grade extremity soft tissue sarcomas: factors predictive of local recurrence and its effect on morbidity and mortality," *Annals of Surgery*, vol. 237, no. 2, pp. 218–226, 2003.

[7] G. K. Zagars, M. T. Ballo, P. W. T. Pisters, R. E. Pollock, S. R. Patel, and R. S. Benjamin, "Surgical margins and reresection in the management of patients with soft tissue sarcoma using conservative surgery and radiation therapy," *Cancer*, vol. 97, no. 10, pp. 2544–2553, 2003.

[8] L. Bellanova, L. Paul, and P.-L. Docquier, "Surgical guides (patient-specific instruments) for pediatric tibial bone sarcoma resection and allograft reconstruction," *Sarcoma*, vol. 2013, Article ID 787653, 7 pages, 2013.

[9] P. Picci, L. Sangiorgi, L. Bahamonde et al., "Risk factors for local recurrences after limb-salvage surgery for high- grade osteosarcoma of the extremities," *Annals of Oncology*, vol. 8, no. 9, pp. 899–903, 1997.

[10] F. Scarpa, S. Sabattini, L. Marconato, O. Capitani, M. Morini, and G. Bettini, "Use of histologic margin evaluation to predict recurrence of cutaneous malignant tumors in dogs and cats after surgical excision," *Journal of the American Veterinary Medical Association*, vol. 240, no. 10, pp. 1181–1187, 2012.

[11] C. Wittekind, C. C. Compton, F. L. Greene, and L. H. Sobin, "TNM residual tumor classification revisited," *Cancer*, vol. 94, no. 9, pp. 2511–2516, 2002.

[12] G. Colleran, J. Madewell, P. Foran, M. Shelly, and P. J. O'Sullivan, "Imaging of soft tissue and osseous sarcomas of the extremities," *Seminars in Ultrasound, CT and MRI*, vol. 32, no. 5, pp. 442–455, 2011.

[13] P.-L. Docquier, L. Paul, O. Cartiaux, C. Delloye, and X. Banse, "Computer-assisted resection and reconstruction of pelvic tumor sarcoma," *Sarcoma*, vol. 2010, Article ID 125162, 8 pages, 2010.

[14] D. Rommel, J. Abarca-Quinones, N. Christian et al., "Alginate moulding: an empirical method for magnetic resonance imaging/positron emission tomography co-registration in a tumor rat model," *Nuclear Medicine and Biology*, vol. 35, no. 5, pp. 571–577, 2008.

[15] J. M. Bland and D. G. Altman, "Measuring agreement in method comparison studies," *Statistical Methods in Medical Research*, vol. 8, no. 2, pp. 135–160, 1999.

14

Cured of Primary Bone Cancer, but at What Cost: A Qualitative Study of Functional Impairment and Lost Opportunities

Lena Fauske,[1] Oyvind S. Bruland,[1,2] Ellen Karine Grov,[3] and Hilde Bondevik[4]

[1] *Department of Oncology, Oslo University Hospital, Norwegian Radium Hospital, P.O. Box 5960, Nydalen, 0424 Oslo, Norway*
[2] *Institute of Clinical Medicine, University of Oslo, P.O. Box 1078, Blindern, 0316 Oslo, Norway*
[3] *Faculty of Health Sciences, Department of Nursing, Oslo and Akershus University College of Applied Sciences, St. Olavs plass, P.O. Box 4, 0130 Oslo, Norway*
[4] *Institute of Health and Society, Department of Health Sciences, University of Oslo, P.O. Box 1089, Blindern, 0317 Oslo, Norway*

Correspondence should be addressed to Lena Fauske; lena.fauske@ous-hf.no

Academic Editor: Peter C. Ferguson

Purpose. Our study aims to explore how former cancer patients experience physical and psychosocial late effects 3–7 years after they underwent treatment for primary bone sarcoma in the hip/pelvic region. A qualitative, phenomenological, and hermeneutic design was applied. *Methods.* Sarcoma survivors ($n = 10$) previously treated at Oslo University Hospital, Norwegian Radium Hospital were selected to participate. In-depth and semistructured interviews were conducted. The interviews were analysed using inductive thematic analysis. *Results.* The participants reported that the late effects had three core spheres of impact: "their current daily life," "their future opportunities," and "their identity." They expressed negative changes in activity, increased dependence on others, and exclusion from participation in different areas. Their daily life, work, sports activities, and social life were all affected. Several of their experiences are similar to those described by people with functional impairment or disability. *Conclusion.* Patients cured of bone cancer in the hip/pelvic region pay a significant price in terms of functional impairment, practical challenges, exclusion from important aspects of life, and loss of previous identity. It is important to appreciate this in order to help bone cancer survivors who struggle to reorient their life and build a secure new identity.

1. Introduction

Primary bone sarcomas are rare and represent less than 0.2% of all new cancers [1], with osteosarcoma, chondrosarcomas, and Ewing's sarcoma being the most common entities [2]. Whereas osteosarcoma and Ewing's sarcoma occur mainly in children and adolescents, chondrosarcoma is most commonly diagnosed in adults [3–5]. Cure of bone sarcomas in the hip/pelvic region may require extensive surgery, often in combination with chemotherapy and radiotherapy [2].

In general, former cancer patients frequently exhibit a poorer health status than those who have not had cancer. Studies show that the late effects of therapy may cause functional impairment, pain, and psychosocial challenges [6–12]. Fatigue and reduced cognitive function [13–15], changes in sexuality and reproduction [10, 16–18], changes in body image [19–23], and challenges in terms of educational and vocational life [24–27] as well as a negative impact on leisure activities and social life [10, 11] are all consequences that can affect former cancer patients' daily lives. These late effects can last for months or years after the patients are seemingly cured of cancer or may only occur many years later [7, 28]. This implies that former bone sarcoma patients may experience considerable health challenges and functional impairment as long lasting consequences of their treatment [29–31].

To our knowledge, no studies have addressed how the practical and psychosocial lives of former bone cancer patients who have undergone extensive surgery in the hip/pelvic region are perceived by the patients themselves several years after treatment. There are some functional [32, 33] and a few qualitative research publications concerning bone cancer in the lower limb [34, 35] as well as one on sacral cancers [36]. These studies show that functional impairment and fatigue affect activities in both daily living and social life, including an active outdoor life [35, 36] as well as the ability to have a vocational life [34, 37, 38]. Since many of the patients affected by bone sarcoma are young, any long-term effects of treatment can be expected to significantly impact their future opportunities. This has also been documented among children and adolescents cured of other cancers [10, 27, 39]. Drew states that children and adolescents, in particular, go through an extensive reorientation to life as part of their rehabilitation process [39]. Recovering from cancer does not necessarily mean that the patients are done with cancer but rather that they enter a new phase of life with different conditions than before. Drew's study illustrates how the original disease as well as the associated treatment influences each cancer survivor's long-term health, life-course experiences, and social interactions [39]. Parsons et al. report that their subjects, all of whom had been affected by bone cancer in the lower extremities, engaged in three types of "work" after getting their diagnosis: "illness work" when going through treatment and struggling with consequences, "identity work," and "vocational work." Importantly, participants in their study described an active process of "identity work," work that is characterised by "becoming other" through self-reflection and effort [34]. Despite the late effects and challenges experienced by former cancer patients, several studies also report positive growth and beneficial outcomes [40–43].

Cancer can be understood as a serious incident in life and as a biographical disruption [44–46] as well as a loss of self [47]. First of all, the cancer patient is a person for whom illness has broken into their daily life and changed their life experience. The old story of their life is broken as is their identity [44, 45, 48]. When affected by a serious disease and its consequences, people often have to reorient their life and construct a new story with their affected body as a new starting point. This helps to make sense, both in terms of understanding themselves and the world of illness and recognising new limitations in their lives [44, 49].

Our study is based on interpersonal encounters. The aim is to understand the experience of illness through qualitative methodology. We interviewed the vast majority of eligible former sarcoma patients who met the inclusion criteria. They were all treated at Oslo University Hospital, Norwegian Radium Hospital (OUS NRH). Their stories were analysed, highlighting how late effects have affected their current daily life as well as influencing their future possibilities and their identity.

2. Methods

To explore how former sarcoma patients experience life after cancer, we have applied phenomenological experience-based and hermeneutics interpretation-based perspectives on disease. In phenomenological research, the aim is to investigate individual human experience (phenomena) as manifested in daily life and in specific situations [46, 50–52]. Hermeneutics is about how to achieve understanding and how phenomena have to be interpreted in order to be understood. Here, comprehension develops through the entire process and is based on both participant's and researcher's preunderstanding and the historical and cultural context [53, 54]. This will impact on the questions raised, the interview process, its transcription, and the subsequent analysis [51, 53, 55]. Svenaeus, based on the philosophy of Heidegger [52], has developed a phenomenological approach to disease [45, 46]. He claims that serious illness forces people to reorient to life. Patients' ailments are multidimensional phenomena and, at the same time, meaningful on several levels [46]. We attempt to connect the biological concept of disease with patients' experiences as well as both the psychosocial and sociocultural aspects of illness.

2.1. Participants and Recruitment. Potential respondents were identified in the prospective clinical sarcoma database (MedInsight) at OUS NRH, which treats approximately 80% of patients with bone sarcomas in Norway [56]. Of the 12 eligible patients contacted, 10 agreed to participate.

Seven men and three women, aged between 18 and 60 years (see Table 1), who had been treated for bone sarcoma in the hip/pelvic region participated in this study. They represent a range of ages and have diverse backgrounds. They all write and speak Norwegian. All were treated with surgery: three had hip transposition, one saddle-prosthesis, one fibula-graft reconstruction, four only tumour resection without reconstruction, and one a proximal femur mutars-prosthesis. Seven participants received chemotherapy, while two had additional radiotherapy. One participant subsequently had an amputation with hemipelvectomy due to chronic infection. All participants were diagnosed between 2004 and 2009 (see Table 1) and were followed up at the oncological or orthopaedic surgical outpatient clinic at OUS NRH. None experienced a relapse of the disease for at least three and up to a maximum of seven years following primary diagnosis. Initial contact with the participants was made by the treating physician at OUS NRH. The first author then gave further details regarding the project before the participants provided informed consent. The interviews were conducted face-to-face by the first author in connection with a routine clinical follow-up appointment that took place at OUS NRH.

2.2. Procedure. This research is anchored in the fundamentals of the Helsinki declarations. Permission to conduct the interviews as well as to collect and store sensitive data was obtained both by our Institutional Review Board and the Regional Committee for Medical Research Ethics, REK South East. All information was stored confidentially. The analyses were carried out from anonymised transcripts.

The interviews had an average duration of 66 minutes (ranging from 31 minutes to 102 minutes) and were audiotaped and then transcribed verbatim by the first author (8) and a medical secretary at OUS NRH (2). Field notes were written following each interview in order to document observations made by the interviewer. The interview guide consisted of the following topics: how the participants experienced their cancer diagnosis and treatment; functional, practical, psychosocial, emotional, and vocational consequences of the disease and treatment; and whether the cancer experience has changed them as a person. In this

TABLE 1: Demographic data.

	Number
Gender	
Female	3
Male	7
Age	
18–25	3
26–35	3
36–50	2
51–60	2
Diagnosis	
Osteosarcoma	2
Ewing's sarcoma	5
Chondrosarcoma	3
Time of diagnosis	
3–5 years ago	5
6–10 years ago	5
Treatment	
Surgery	10
Chemotherapy	7
Radiation	2
Amputation	1

paper, we focus on how functional impairment, pain, and fatigue have influenced their lives. The interview guide was designed to allow the participants to tell their whole cancer story chronologically. The interview guide was, however, only loosely followed, so that the participants were able to highly influence the depth of the interview. Through this approach, structure and meaning are produced jointly by the participant and researcher [57]. As such, certain interpretations emerged during the interview from both sides. This enabled the confirmation or rejection of the interviewer's perceptions of what the participants expressed [51].

2.3. Data Analysis. The participants' accounts were analysed by hand by the first and last author using thematic analyses. The analysis took place in stages and followed an inductive strategy [58] within a contextualised framework [51]. First, the transcribed interviews were read through to gain an overall impression and to identify preliminary themes. Second, the entire data set was coded in detail and then organised into themes, and concepts were developed. The themes were reflected on in accordance with the study's objectives and were compared against the available literature and theory that highlights the interaction between cancer and the patient's life experiences.

3. Results

This study shows that both somatic consequences and psychosocial experiences present several challenges to former sarcoma patients. These effects are manifested in practical terms, in work and leisure times, and in their emotional and social life (see Table 2). The price paid for a cure leads to several changes, losses, and challenges; life is not the same as before. These survivors may be excluded from several contexts that were important in their lives before cancer. We have identified three main findings in this study: the impracticalities of daily life due to functional impairment, lost opportunities, and an identity change.

3.1. The Impracticalities of Daily Life. Despite previously being healthy and active, most participants now suffer different functional impairments that limit their daily lives. Several described how cancer has affected and changed their lives in fundamental ways and how they now require different kinds of support.

Six of the ten participants require technical aids to ambulate due to problems related to poor balance, decreased strength, or lack of mobility after the removal of their bone sarcoma, for one of the participants, an amputation. These six are dependent on crutches or a cane and two of them have to use a wheelchair. Stairs therefore pose a formidable challenge for many of them. P3 (participant #3), for example, has one leg 7 cm shorter than the other and with muscles removed. Hence, he has less strength in that leg and poor balance. As he expressed: *I use crutches to avoid pain and to be able to walk faster. I walk very slowly and with difficulty without crutches. [...] Of course, I cannot climb stairs without crutches.* Some participants also stated that poor balance and functional impairment prevent them from taking public transportation. They are now dependent on taxis or on having a car of their own. Most of them need a car with automatic transmission and a few require specially adapted vehicles. In Norway, snow and ice present severe challenges to getting around during several months of the year for those with poor balance and diminished strength. Most of the participants are afraid of falling because their prostheses can be damaged. Carrying bags or heavy things is difficult. P5 recounted how this is experienced: *It is obvious that I am more helpless; I need more help – definitely.* She also said that it has become challenging to go into the city alone. She prefers to have an arm to lean on in order to feel safe. The fear of being knocked over is real and it is difficult to carry anything. She also emphasises that the extent of her disability is not obvious to someone looking at her: *My functional impairment is, in fact, more than what people can see from watching me walk.* That makes it difficult for others to realise the challenges she faces and what they ought to therefore take into consideration.

When certain movements are limited or no longer possible, housework also presents formidable challenges. It may be impossible to do chores that involve bending over or accessing hard-to-reach places. Standing on a chair is difficult. Household chores may be not only painful and difficult but also time consuming. P10 stated: *I cannot get anything done (on crutches). [...] I cannot carry anything; I cannot take anything with me. I have to put everything in a rucksack. For example, making dinner on crutches and trying to carry hot pans is absolutely hopeless.* For him, the alternative is to perform most of the work he does at home from a wheelchair, which presents a whole new set of limitations. For many, this means that some housework is cumbersome and

TABLE 2: Key findings extracted from the individual stories.

	Participant									
	P1	P2	P3	P4	P5	P6	P7	P8	P9	P10
Age-group	>35	<35	<35	<35	>35	>35	<35	<35	>35	<35
Gender	M	M	M	M	F	F	F	M	M	M
Time since diagnosis (years)	5	7	8	4	6	3	4	8	5	7
Consequences										
Limping	x	x	x	x	x	x	x	x	x	x
Daily use of crutch/stick			x		x	x	x		x	x
Daily use of wheelchair									x	x
Problems with balance		x	x	x	x	x	x	x	x	x
Colostomy										x
Urostomy										x
Pain affecting daily life		x		x	x	x			x	x
Fatigue influencing daily life		x		x	x	x	x		x	x
Daily practical challenges		x	x	x	x	x	x		x	x
Impaired physical activity	x	x	x	x	x	x	x	x	x	x
Lost important hobby	x	x		x			x		x	
On disability benefit					x	x				x
Experienced positive growth		x	x	x			x	x		x

very strenuous to manage on their own. As a consequence, some work is postponed or not even done. Many of the participants have to ask others for help to get around in their daily lives.

Radical surgery on a bone sarcoma in the hip/pelvic region may result in stomata. P10 has both a colostomy and a urostomy. He pointed out that there are no merely practical challenges to having these, but also how stomata drain his energy when he is travelling or stays outside his home: *The urostomy is more difficult because there are often leaks and it is difficult to avoid them. [...] Then I have to find a lavatory and go in and change. I always carry a bag with extra equipment and clothes. [...] I never go out the door without it. That translates into a lot of bother, leading to delays and it wears me out as it takes a lot of energy.* For some of the participants, ordinary tasks like going to the bathroom or taking a shower can no longer be taken for granted. According to 4 out of the 10 participants, poor balance calls for armrests on the toilet or a special shower stool. As P9 explained: *The shower chair also has to be brought along if I am staying anywhere else than home.*

There did not seem to be any discrepancy between adolescents and adults in terms of the daily practical challenges faced.

3.2. Lost Opportunities and an Altered Future. One common denominator for many of the participants is that they were physically active before being diagnosed with cancer. Active lives, sports, and outdoors activities were important aspects of their lives. However, following treatment, it is no longer possible for several of them to engage in activities such as bicycling, jogging, skiing, playing football, tennis, outdoor life, or hunting. Accordingly, many feel cut off from an important part of their lives and from activities that previously helped fill their lives with content and meaning. Due to impairment, several participants have not had the possibility of getting involved in a new hobby involving physical activity. P2 was a semiprofessional athlete before getting sick: *I have no new hobby to replace the sport that was my passion.* At another place in the interview, he acknowledged: *One sits around and lives on the memories, even at the age of 30.* The study clearly found that those who had not had a physically demanding hobby before being diagnosed with cancer did not feel the same sense of being cut off from this part of their lives.

The participants' social lives are also affected when they are unable to participate in activities in the same way as before. Many of them state that they are left standing on the side-line or are left out. P4 was in his teens when he was diagnosed with cancer. He felt it was especially difficult to not be active along with other teenagers: *I cannot go skiing or play football. [...] I do feel it is sad.* P3 stated that he could have spent more time with others and participated in several activities if he had not been dependent on crutches: *Many times, I have felt that if I were without crutches, I could have walked normally and even run. Then I could have taken part in more activities and possibly even had more friends.* Other participants also recounted how reduced functionality, fatigue, and pain have impacted on their social lives. P6 stated explicitly that long-term consequences of her treatment have made her less social: *I spend less time with friends than I used to do. I feel sad about that. I feel it is the pain that is my biggest problem.*

The experience of loss and the feeling of uncertainty about the future are also linked to vocational life. For the majority of those included in this study, employment or studies account for a significant part of their lives. In our study, only two participants have had to give up working completely as a result of their cancer. When not employed, it is easy to become an outsider in many important aspects of life. P6 had to quit working in the restaurant industry as the job required physical mobility. Losing her job was the greatest change in her life after having cancer. She would still prefer to work, even though she cannot work full-time. Being outside the workforce makes her feel isolated and has posed challenges to her mental health: *I need something like work to go to, if not, anxiety will reappear.* She dreams of working for a few hours a week, but unpredictable health with pain and fatigue makes it difficult to get an employer to hire her.

P7 is a student at the moment and worries about her future job opportunities. She is on the threshold of adulthood, and she is training to work in tourism and dreams of a career in which she can use her education. Today she is dependent on crutches. As the situation is now, she does not feel very attractive for the labour market. As she reflected: *No one wants to hire anyone on crutches.* She hopes that having a leg extension will make her more mobile, but she also knows that the rehabilitation process can be both lengthy and difficult before she reaches her goal, if it is at all possible.

Both adolescents and adults expressed concerns about lost opportunities, although an altered future would arguably have the greatest impact on the youngest survivors.

3.3. I Am No Longer the Person I Once Was. The stories related in the interviews indicate that the participants' individual identities have been affected. The participants have gone from being healthy to being labelled by their disease, not as sick, but as disabled, not completely healthy or capable of functioning. As P3 articulated: *I am, of course, defined as being disabled.* In this study, the male participants' experience of themselves and their understanding of their own identities are expressed as the juxtaposition between what they say about sports, outdoor activities, work, and social relationships on the one hand and the young men's understanding of their own masculinity on the other. However, none of the female participants expressed that their gender identity was influenced as a consequence of being functionally impaired.

P2 was a semiprofessional athlete before being diagnosed with cancer. Today, he is not sufficiently functional to engage in sports, although he spends a lot of time working out at the fitness centre. This is essential for regaining functionality and strength after surgery. He does not try to hide that it has been mentally demanding to go from being an elite athlete to being physically impaired: *My identity was closely linked to being an athlete. [...] I have had to work really hard to carve out a new identity. [...] At least, I now feel as though I'm making a start. [...] And I understand that people like me even if I'm not playing sports.*

For generations of Norwegians, identity has been associated with skiing and an active outdoor life. No one can tell from looking at P4 that he can no longer go skiing. He has tried after recovering but has no control and so just falls. He is afraid that others will consider him lazy or not very sporty. This negative change in identity seems to bother him: *I'm embarrassed because I could do this before, but of course I cannot prove that now. This has something to do with identity – I feel a little less cool, less sporty and somewhat less of a man. [...] It is a kind of stupid, but it makes me focus on school to a much greater extent.* P4 stated that he has found a way to cope; he now does exceptionally well with his studies.

In P9's case, we see how important it is to get the opportunity to reorient to life after extensive cancer treatment. He eventually had a leg amputated involving a hemipelvectomy. Prior to that, he was sick for several years due to postsurgical infections. This prevented him from entering a new life as a cured and healthy person. He is today totally dependent on other people, especially his wife. Before the cancer, he spent a lot of time outdoors hunting and fishing. His life and identity were linked to being an active outdoorsman: *I am no longer an outdoorsman. [...] I have nothing, and I do nothing.* We recognise here that a prerequisite for imbuing new meaning in life after cancer is that one is sufficiently healthy to embark on this process. This is a process that calls for energy and spirit. In the case of P9, the adverse consequences of the cancer treatment were so extensive that he has not started on the process of reinventing himself. For him, life is still a struggle.

Before cancer struck, P10 was a young man who devoted all his spare time to organisational work and not sports. Despite now being nearly always confined to a wheelchair, he is still active in local organisations. With crutches, he can move over short distances, but this results in pain and exhaustion. Although a wheelchair is more practical, people's prejudices make him choose crutches more often than he would like. For him, it is important to be recognised as the positive resource he actually is and not as someone failing to contribute because he sits in a wheelchair. He dislikes how people give him an identity as a wheelchair user and not a person with strong resources and as an important contributor: *When joining meetings I use crutches because this give a completely different image [...] many have a theory that you have brain damage if you sit in a wheelchair. [...] They see the wheelchair and not the man.* He states that, if he had sufficient energy, he would have taken on the battle against people's prejudices.

The younger participants ($n = 6$) claim that experiences following their cancer diagnosis have also positively influenced them as human beings, despite all the physical challenges. P3 acknowledged that the cancer has given him an opportunity to reorient to life. Despite the fact that he sees himself as a person with disability, with all the challenges that are implied, the cancer has done more good for him than bad. He is young and feels he has become a totally different person, a more positive and grounded person: *Many aspects of my life have changed as a result of having cancer. I used to be lazy. I was more serious. [...] I was not very happy, took no joy in things, actually. Guess I felt that I was a bit boring. And I did not do much. I wasn't interested in much either. Not even curious. After having had cancer, I have become more positive, a little happier, and I have changed my opinion of myself. What I went through, and the fact that I was as strong as I was, gave me more zest for life. I am more appreciative of life. I sort of turned into a totally different person.* Four of the young participants were grateful for the positive experiences that the cancer had given them. Three of them went so far as to say their cancer has had more positive consequences than negative. As P10 stated: *Even though I sit in my wheelchair and have many bad days, I still believe that my cancer experience was ultimately beneficial for me.*

Several participants stated that staying in a job is important for their identity. P10 now holds 15% of an average full working week. However, to do that job, he actually has to be at work for at least twice that long: *Having a connection to work is important. It is not crucial for me to work full-time [...] but rather to have an affiliation to my employer. [...] Having a job makes a person feel like he or she is contributing to society. Then there is the question of what others think: Do you work or not? No, I am on disability benefits. I just cannot buy that at all.*

P5 received full disability benefits after a long career. She used to like her job and would have liked to continue with it, but fatigue, cognitive problems, reduced functions, and poor balance made it impossible: *My days are ups and downs, and I know that I tire quickly from things that never used to wear me out.* P5 also related that it was not possible for her to have a job and also to have enough energy for a social life. When she tried to work after having cancer, it took all of her energy. Today she has accepted that disability benefit is the best solution for her, although she is not comfortable with it. She wishes that she still had an identity as an employee.

The adolescents expressed more concerns than the adults about changes to their identity related to disability, sports, and masculinity. The exception to this was concerns about their work identity, which were expressed by several survivors regardless of age.

4. Discussion

In this study, we have addressed how the late effects of extensive treatment of bone sarcoma in the hip/pelvic area, especially surgery, have impacted former cancer patients cured of their disease three to seven years earlier. Besides both physical and functional impairments, most of the participants also reported changes and losses as well as lost future opportunities. Life is radically changed, with an impact on their vocational work, social life, and participation in leisure activities as well as their identity. Our findings are in line with other qualitative bone cancer researches [34–37]. Unlike many other cancer patients, our group expressed consequences and challenges that are similar to those experienced following traffic or sports accidents. They face barriers and challenging social structures that provide exclusion from activities they would have had access to without their cancer history. Below, we will discuss some of the implications of being a person with disabilities following bone cancer treatment.

In this study, several participants expressed alterations in terms of the experience and perception of who they are. The change from being healthy and employable to being functionally impaired emerged as important, in terms of both personal identity as well as practicalities. Among our participants, we observed changes in activity, dependence on others, and exclusion from participation in different arenas, similar to the experiences described by people with a disability [59]. In the scientific literature, disability is an umbrella term. On one side, functional impairment is referred to as a property of the individual, based on an individual and disease-related understanding. In the social model, however, the focus is not on disability as an individual defect but more on the interplay between subjective function and ambient requirements, social injustice, and changes in the social and physical environments. Disability comprises both the individual's reduced function with limitations in activity on one hand and limitations in participation in different arenas and in different life situations on the other [60]. In a society grounded on being healthy, a person with a functional impairment or disability could be banned from participating in certain activities or situations [61], as experienced by many of our participants.

Research indicates that having a functional impairment after cancer may lead to exclusion from the labour market in general or certain jobs in particular [37, 38]. In our study, some participants found that reduced mobility, pain, fatigue, and cognitive impairment decreased their ability to be fully or partially employed. Employment is one of the most important factors for social integration and contributes to defining people's social status and personal identity [62]. Research indicates that being excluded from employment as a result of cancer can affect people's everyday structure, a structure that is built around work and that gives life richness and meaning. Furthermore, this could also result in a reduced social life, in addition to a loss of identity [24]. A change from being employable to being totally or partially incapacitated from work can be a challenge in a country like Norway, where most of the adult population is in work and being employed constitutes the central norm. Being an outsider can be difficult to reconcile. For young people, the late effects of cancer could have an impact on their study and work opportunities in the future [27]. As one of our participants also noted, one is not necessarily as attractive as an employee after having undergone extensive bone cancer treatment [34].

Physical activity is important for both people's well-being and good health. Research indicates that physical activity has a positive effect on former cancer patients' life and health [63, 64]. Several of the participants in this study state that they are less physically active now. This may involve more than just inactivity. For some, this will lead to less social activities than before the cancer struck, in line with other publications [35, 36].

In particular, those participants in our study who had immersive sports or outdoor interests before getting cancer experienced a loss that profoundly influenced several aspects of their lives. For previously active young men, being cut off from participating in sports activities can make them feel less masculine. According to Connell [65], the ability to participate in sport is seen as an important aspect of masculinity. It is not just about the loss of a hobby and social environment; it is also about the loss of identity that says something about who you are and who you want to be. Illness can affect man's status in masculine hierarchies and create doubt about his own masculinity [66].

A change in social status from being healthy to being a person with a disability is a change in identity and might be perceived as a loss and so cause social challenges. This is due to how you see yourself and how others treat you [59]. Being disabled makes you deviate from the normal, which may be stigmatising [67]. Stigma in general means that a person is thought of as being "other." This can have many negative effects for those affected. They face prejudice and discrimination and are victims of stereotypes [68]. It is not uncommon to see people with disabilities as more dependent on others and as less intelligent [69]. One of our participants who uses a wheelchair faces such prejudices when he says that "they see the wheelchair and not the man." This makes him use crutches in specific situations even though he can hardly walk.

Although a former bone cancer patient may face many negative changes and losses, it may also involve positive growth. The hurdles such patients have overcome and their work adapting to the new challenges may also have impacted positively on their life and identity. In the literature, such positive changes are termed as posttraumatic growth and characterised as a changed sense of oneself, a changed sense of relationship with others, and a changed philosophy of life [70]. Studies report positive growth among former cancer patients, especially those who received their diagnosis a few years earlier, and among those who are young [40, 41]. Among cancer patients, higher growth, both with increasing time from diagnosis and a younger age [40, 41, 71], has been found. Thornton's review of benefit findings in the cancer experience reports that a "substantial proportion" of previous cancer patients link positive changes in life perspective and relation to others and to self to their cancer and illness experiences [72]. In some studies of former adolescent cancer patients, the majority report positive growth [42], including a study of long-term survivors of extremity osteosarcoma [43]. The last questions in the interview guide gave them an opportunity to reflect on their current situation. Here the participants also expressed experiences of positive growth, after we had talked mostly about their challenges following cancer treatment. Only the adolescents and young adults talked about the positive changes cancer has had for them as individuals. To our surprise, the two young participants who considered themselves to have experienced pronounced growth were among those who suffered the worst late effects and physical challenges. Our study was not designed to address the cause of such a paradox, although it would certainly be a worthwhile focus for subsequent study.

As mentioned before, being cured of cancer is not always about getting back to the life they had before but it also requires that they reorient themselves to a new life with an altered body. To construct such a new identity, one must complete illness work [34]. This presupposes having the energy to establish a new understanding of themselves where the new body and the new conditions are integrated as part of that new identity. Accepting changes and reconciling them can be crucial to achieve resilience or growth. We note that one of the participants in our study in particular is still struggling after years of complications from treatment, a challenge also previously reported [73]. Our participant was never given the opportunity to build a new life with the new conditions and his new identity as a disabled person. The result is that he today says he has "nothing." When all one's time and energy are devoted to cope with the complications of disease, it is difficult to shift focus and to reorient to life.

It is important to understand the challenges and struggles that this group of cancer survivors face. However, it is vital to not have a unilateral focus on negative late effects following treatment, as research shows that many cancer survivors, in addition to the aforementioned challenges, will find coping strategies that give them a good life despite the limitations they may have [74].

The small sample size may limit the generalizability of this study, although the majority of eligible participants did take part. However, in qualitative research, we are not looking for representative data but rather aim to illuminate the phenomena that the participants express. Nevertheless, when exploring cancer survivors' life experiences, we suggest using mixed methods to a greater extent. Qualitative and quantitative approaches together will gain a more complete picture of the consequences of cancer treatment. Another limitation is that we have only interviewed the participants once. Several interviews during a longer period from the time of diagnosis might have provided a more complete picture. In addition, prospective studies exploring how bone sarcoma survivors experience changes in sexuality and reproduction, as well as bodily deviations, are warranted.

5. Conclusions

Functional impairment that results in daily practical challenges, exclusion from important aspects of life, and loss of previous identity may be the price to pay for being cured of bone cancer in the hip/pelvic region. As osteosarcoma and Ewing's sarcoma particularly affect young people, a diverse range of life stages in which illness can affect and disrupt developmental milestones exists. It seems that such knowledge is important to help bone cancer survivors who struggle to reorient to life and build a new identity founded on their new situation in life. In order to advise the caregivers of those with sarcoma, the findings from this study suggest a systematic approach to long-term follow-up including provision of information, supervision and training regarding practical options, and social support. The assessment of each individual survivor's situation seems vital and so appropriate health services should be provided. Health personnel should therefore be available for ongoing surveillance (i.e., monitoring a life-long follow-up of the patient's medical, physical, and psychosocial health).

Acknowledgments

This work was supported by the Helse Sor Ost, Grant no. 2013032. The authors gratefully acknowledge the participating sarcoma survivors who willingly shared their life experiences with them.

References

[1] M. Hameed and H. Dorfman, "Primary malignant bone tumors—recent developments," *Seminars in Diagnostic Pathology*, vol. 28, no. 1, pp. 86–101, 2011.

[2] M. U. Jawad, A. A. Haleem, and S. P. Scully, "Malignant sarcoma of the pelvic bones: treatment outcomes and prognostic factors vary by histopathology," *Cancer*, vol. 117, no. 7, pp. 1529–1541, 2011.

[3] H. D. Dorfman and B. Czerniak, "Bone cancers," *Cancer*, vol. 75, no. 1, supplement, pp. 203–210, 1995.

[4] R. Eyre, R. G. Feltbower, E. Mubwandarikwa, T. O. B. Eden, and R. J. Q. McNally, "Epidemiology of bone tumours in children and young adults," *Pediatric Blood and Cancer*, vol. 53, no. 6, pp. 941-952, 2009.

[5] T. A. Damron, W. G. Ward, and A. Stewart, "Osteosarcoma, chondrosarcoma, and Ewing's sarcoma: National Cancer Data Base Report," *Clinical Orthopaedics and Related Research*, no. 459, pp. 40–47, 2007.

[6] J. Elliott, A. Fallows, L. Staetsky et al., "The health and well-being of cancer survivors in the UK: findings from a population-based survey," *British Journal of Cancer*, vol. 105, supplement 1, pp. S11–S20, 2011.

[7] C. Treanor, O. Santin, M. Mills, and M. Donnelly, "Cancer survivors with self-reported late effects: their health status, care needs and service utilisation," *Psycho-Oncology*, vol. 22, no. 11, pp. 2428–2435, 2013.

[8] C. Foster, D. Wright, H. Hill, J. Hopkinson, and L. Roffe, "Psychosocial implications of living 5 years or more following a cancer diagnosis: a systematic review of the research evidence," *European Journal of Cancer Care*, vol. 18, no. 3, pp. 223–247, 2009.

[9] M. Hewitt, J. H. Rowland, and R. Yancik, "Cancer survivors in the United States: age, health, and disability," *Journals of Gerontology Series A: Biological Sciences and Medical Sciences*, vol. 58, no. 1, pp. 82–91, 2003.

[10] V. Lehmann, H. Grönqvist, G. Engvall et al., "Negative and positive consequences of adolescent cancer 10 years after diagnosis: an interview-based longitudinal study in Sweden," *Psycho-Oncology*, vol. 23, no. 11, pp. 1229–1235, 2014.

[11] G. A. Curt, "The impact of fatigue on patients with cancer: overview of FATIGUE 1 and 2," *Oncologist*, vol. 5, supplement 2, pp. 9–12, 2000.

[12] N. Boykoff, M. Moieni, and S. K. Subramanian, "Confronting chemobrain: an in-depth look at survivors' reports of impact on work, social networks, and health care response," *Journal of Cancer Survivorship: Research and Practice*, vol. 3, no. 4, pp. 223–232, 2009.

[13] R. H. T. Koornstra, M. Peters, S. Donofrio, B. van den Borne, and F. A. de Jong, "Management of fatigue in patients with cancer—a practical overview," *Cancer Treatment Reviews*, vol. 40, no. 6, pp. 791–799, 2014.

[14] H. Knobel, J. H. Loge, E. Brenne, P. Fayers, M. J. Hjermstad, and S. Kaasa, "The validity of EORTC QLQ-C30 fatigue scale in advanced cancer patients and cancer survivors," *Palliative Medicine*, vol. 17, no. 8, pp. 664–672, 2003.

[15] T. Mitchell and P. Turton, "'Chemobrain': concentration and memory effects in people receiving chemotherapy—a descriptive phenomenological study," *European Journal of Cancer Care*, vol. 20, no. 4, pp. 539–548, 2011.

[16] A. Chapple, M. Salinas, S. Ziebland, A. McPherson, and A. Macfarlane, "Fertility issues: the perceptions and experiences of young men recently diagnosed and treated for cancer," *Journal of Adolescent Health*, vol. 40, no. 1, pp. 69–75, 2007.

[17] G. Dowswell, T. Ismail, S. Greenfield, S. Clifford, B. Hancock, and S. Wilson, "Men's experience of erectile dysfunction after treatment for colorectal cancer: qualitative interview study," *The British Medical Journal*, vol. 343, no. 1, Article ID d5824, 2011.

[18] K. Klaeson, K. Sandell, and C. M. Berterö, "Sexuality in the context of prostate cancer narratives," *Qualitative Health Research*, vol. 22, no. 9, pp. 1184–1194, 2012.

[19] D. M. Rasmussen, H. P. Hansen, and B. Elverdam, "How cancer survivors experience their changed body encountering others," *European Journal of Oncology Nursing*, vol. 14, no. 2, pp. 154–159, 2010.

[20] J. S. Pendley, L. M. Dahlquist, and Z. Dreyer, "Body image and psychosocial adjustment in adolescent cancer survivors," *Journal of Pediatric Psychology*, vol. 22, no. 1, pp. 29–43, 1997.

[21] S.-Y. Fan and C. Eiser, "Body image of children and adolescents with cancer: a systematic review," *Body Image*, vol. 6, no. 4, pp. 247–256, 2009.

[22] S. S. Larouche and L. Chin-Peuckert, "Changes in body image experienced by adolescents with cancer," *Journal of Pediatric Oncology Nursing*, vol. 23, no. 4, pp. 200–209, 2006.

[23] J. Brunet, C. M. Sabiston, and S. Burke, "Surviving breast cancer: women's experiences with their changed bodies," *Body Image*, vol. 10, no. 3, pp. 344–351, 2013.

[24] D. M. Rasmussen and B. Elverdam, "The meaning of work and working life after cancer: an interview study," *Psycho-Oncology*, vol. 17, no. 12, pp. 1232–1238, 2008.

[25] E. A. Grunfeld and A. F. Cooper, "A longitudinal qualitative study of the experience of working following treatment for gynaecological cancer," *Psycho-Oncology*, vol. 21, no. 1, pp. 82–89, 2012.

[26] J. Yarker, F. Munir, M. Bains, K. Kalawsky, and C. Haslam, "The role of communication and support in return to work following cancer-related absence," *Psycho-Oncology*, vol. 19, no. 10, pp. 1078–1085, 2010.

[27] E. E. Kent, C. Parry, M. J. Montoya, L. S. Sender, R. A. Morris, and H. Anton-Culver, "'You're too young for this': adolescent and young adults' perspectives on cancer survivorship," *Journal of Psychosocial Oncology*, vol. 30, no. 2, pp. 260–279, 2012.

[28] Macmillan Cancer Support, *Thorowing Light on the Consequences of Cancer and Its Treatment*, Macmillan, 2013.

[29] I. Han, Y. M. Lee, H. S. Cho, J. H. Oh, S. H. Lee, and H. S. Kim, "Outcome after surgical treatment of pelvic sarcomas," *Clinics in Orthopedic Surgery*, vol. 2, no. 3, pp. 160–166, 2010.

[30] F. Zeifang, M. Buchner, A. Zahlten-Hinguranage, L. Bernd, and D. Sabo, "Complications following operative treatment of primary malignant bone tumours in the pelvis," *European Journal of Surgical Oncology*, vol. 30, no. 8, pp. 893–899, 2004.

[31] L. H. Aksnes, H. C. F. Bauer, A. A. Dahl et al., "Health status at long-term follow-up in patients treated for extremity localized Ewing Sarcoma or osteosarcoma: a Scandinavian sarcoma group study," *Pediatric Blood and Cancer*, vol. 53, no. 1, pp. 84–89, 2009.

[32] A. M. Davis, S. Punniyamoorthy, A. M. Griffin, J. S. Wunder, and R. S. Bell, "Symptoms and their relationship to disability following treatment for lower extremity tumours," *Sarcoma*, vol. 3, no. 2, pp. 73–77, 1999.

[33] M. Malo, A. M. Davis, J. Wunder et al., "Functional evaluation in distal femoral endoprosthetic replacement for bone sarcoma," *Clinical Orthopaedics and Related Research*, no. 389, pp. 173–180, 2001.

[34] J. A. Parsons, J. M. Eakin, R. S. Bell, R.-L. Franche, and A. M. Davis, "'So, are you back to work yet?' Re-conceptualizing 'work' and 'return to work' in the context of primary bone cancer," *Social Science & Medicine*, vol. 67, no. 11, pp. 1826–1836, 2008.

[35] E. A. Earle, C. Eiser, and R. Grimer, "'He never liked sport anyway'—Mother's views of young people coping with a bone tumour in the lower limb," *Sarcoma*, vol. 9, no. 1-2, pp. 7–13, 2005.

[36] K. M. Davidge, C. Eskicioglu, J. Lipa, P. Ferguson, C. J. Swallow, and F. C. Wright, "Qualitative assessment of patient experiences following sacrectomy," *Journal of Surgical Oncology*, vol. 101, no. 6, pp. 447–450, 2010.

[37] A. Brown, J. A. Parsons, C. Martino et al., "Work status after distal femoral kotz reconstruction for malignant tumors of bone," *Archives of Physical Medicine and Rehabilitation*, vol. 84, no. 1, pp. 62–68, 2003.

[38] B. T. Rougraff, M. A. Simon, J. S. Kneisl, D. B. Greenberg, and H. J. Mankin, "Limb salvage compared with amputation for osteosarcoma of the distal end of the femur: a long-term oncological functional, and quality-of-life study," *The Journal of Bone & Joint Surgery—American Volume*, vol. 76, no. 5, pp. 649–656, 1994.

[39] S. Drew, "'Having cancer changed my life, and changed my life forever': survival, illness legacy and service provision following cancer in childhood," *Chronic Illness*, vol. 3, no. 4, pp. 278–295, 2007.

[40] S. C. Danhauer, G. B. Russell, R. G. Tedeschi et al., "A longitudinal investigation of posttraumatic growth in adult patients undergoing treatment for acute leukemia," *Journal of Clinical Psychology in Medical Settings*, vol. 20, no. 1, pp. 13–24, 2013.

[41] S. R. Sears, A. L. Stanton, and S. Danoff-Burg, "The yellow brick road and the emerald city: benefit finding, positive reappraisal coping and posttraumatic growth in women with early-stage breast cancer," *Health Psychology*, vol. 22, no. 5, pp. 487–497, 2003.

[42] L. P. Barakat, M. A. Alderfer, and A. E. Kazak, "Posttraumatic growth in adolescent survivors of cancer and their mothers and fathers," *Journal of Pediatric Psychology*, vol. 31, no. 4, pp. 413–419, 2006.

[43] T. Yonemoto, K. Kamibeppu, T. Ishii, S. Iwata, Y. Hagiwara, and S.-I. Tatezaki, "Psychosocial outcomes in long-term survivors of high-grade osteosarcoma: a Japanese single-center experience," *Anticancer Research*, vol. 29, no. 10, pp. 4287–4290, 2009.

[44] M. Bury, "Chronic illness as biographical disruption," *Sociology of Health and Illness*, vol. 4, no. 2, pp. 167–182, 1982.

[45] F. Svenaeus, "Illness as unhomelike being-in-the-world: heidegger and the phenomenology of medicine," *Medicine, Health Care and Philosophy*, vol. 14, no. 3, pp. 333–343, 2011.

[46] F. Svenaeus, "The body uncanny—further steps towards a phenomenology of illness," *Medicine, Health Care, and Philosophy*, vol. 3, no. 2, pp. 125–137, 2000.

[47] K. Charmaz, "Loss of self: a fundamental form of suffering in the chronically ill," *Sociology of Health & Illness*, vol. 5, no. 2, pp. 168–195, 1983.

[48] S. Sontag, *Illness as Metaphor*, Farrar, Straus and Giroux, New York, NY, USA, 1978.

[49] A. W. Frank, *The Wounded Storyteller: Body, Illness, and Ethics*, vol. 18, University of Chicago Press, Chicago, Ill, USA, 1995.

[50] M. Van Manen, *Researching Lived Experience : Human Science For An Action Sensitive Pedagogy*, State University of New York Press, Albany, NY, USA, 1990.

[51] S. Kvale and S. Brinkmann, *Interviews: Learning the Craft of Qualitative Research Interviewing*, Sage, Los Angeles, Calif, USA, 2009.

[52] M. Heidegger, *Being and Time*, Basil Blackwell, Oxford, UK, 1962.

[53] H.-G. Gadamer, *Truth and Method*, Continuum, London, UK, 2004.

[54] P. Ricœur, *Interpretation Theory: Discourse and the Surplus of Meaning*, Texas Christian University Press, Fort Worth, Tex, USA, 1976.

[55] C. G. Helman, *Culture, Health and Illness*, Hodder Arnold, London, UK, 2007.

[56] K. Berner, T. B. Johannesen, A. Berner et al., "Time-trends on incidence and survival in a nationwide and unselected cohort of patients with skeletal osteosarcoma," *Acta Oncologica*, vol. 54, no. 1, pp. 25–33, 2015.

[57] J. F. Gubrium, J. A. Holstein, A. B. Marvasti, and K. D. McKinney, *The SAGE Handbook of Interview Research: The Complexity of the Craft*, SAGE, Thousand Oaks, Calif, USA, 2012.

[58] V. Braun and V. Clarke, "Using thematic analysis in psychology," *Qualitative Research in Psychology*, vol. 3, no. 2, pp. 77–101, 2006.

[59] R. D. Galvin, "Researching the disabled identity: contextualising the identity transformations which accompany the onset of impairment," *Sociology of Health and Illness*, vol. 27, no. 3, pp. 393–413, 2005.

[60] T. Siebers, *Disability Theory*, The University of Michigan Press, Ann Arbor, Mich, USA, 2008.

[61] L. Barton, "Sociology, disability studies and education: some observations," in *The Disability Reader: Social Science Perspectives*, T. Shakespeare, Ed., p. 310, Cassell, London, UK, 1998.

[62] M. Jahoda, *Employment and Unemployment: A Social-Psychological Analysis*, Cambridge University Press, Cambridge, Mass, USA, 1982.

[63] R. M. Speck, K. S. Courneya, L. C. Mâsse, S. Duval, and K. H. Schmitz, "An update of controlled physical activity trials in cancer survivors: a systematic review and meta-analysis," *Journal of Cancer Survivorship*, vol. 4, no. 2, pp. 87–100, 2010.

[64] V. S. Conn, A. R. Hafdahl, D. C. Porock, R. McDaniel, and P. J. Nielsen, "A meta-analysis of exercise interventions among people treated for cancer," *Supportive Care in Cancer*, vol. 14, no. 7, pp. 699–712, 2006.

[65] R. W. Connell, *Masculinities*, University of California Press, Berkley, Calif, USA, 2005.

[66] K. Charmaz, "Identity dilemmas of chronically ill men," in *Men's Health and Illness: Gender, Power, and the Body*, D. Sabo and D. F. Gordon, Eds., Sage, 1995.

[67] P. Hunt, *A Critical Condition. Stigma*, edited by: P. Hunt, Geoffrey Chapman, London, UK, 1966.

[68] E. Goffman, *Stigma*, Penguin, Hammondsworth, UK, 1963.

[69] P. Hunt, *A Critical Condition. The Disability Reader: Social Science Perspectives*, edited by: T. Shakespeare, Continuum, London, UK, 1998.

[70] L. G. Calhoun and R. G. Tedeschi, *Handbook of Posttraumatic Growth: Research and Practice*, Lawrence Erlbaum, New York, NY, USA, 2006.

[71] M. J. Cordova, L. L. C. Cunningham, C. R. Carlson, and M. A. Andrykowski, "Posttraumatic growth following breast cancer: a controlled comparison study," *Health Psychology*, vol. 20, no. 3, pp. 176–185, 2001.

[72] A. A. Thornton, "Perceiving benefits in the cancer experience," *Journal of Clinical Psychology in Medical Settings*, vol. 9, no. 2, pp. 153–165, 2002.

[73] E. L. Masterson, A. M. Davis, J. S. Wunder, and R. S. Bell, "Hindquarter amputation for pelvic tumors: the importance of patient selection," *Clinical Orthopaedics and Related Research*, no. 350, pp. 187–194, 1998.

[74] R. Felder-Puig, A. K. Formann, A. Mildner et al., "Quality of life and psychosocial adjustment of young patients after treatment of bone cancer," *Cancer*, vol. 83, no. 1, pp. 69–75, 1998.

15

Fluorescence *In Situ* Hybridization for *MDM2* Amplification as a Routine Ancillary Diagnostic Tool for Suspected Well-Differentiated and Dedifferentiated Liposarcomas: Experience at a Tertiary Center

Khin Thway,[1] Jayson Wang,[2] John Swansbury,[3] Toon Min,[3] and Cyril Fisher[1]

[1] *Sarcoma Unit, Royal Marsden Hospital, London SW3 6JJ, UK*
[2] *Department of Histopathology, Royal Marsden Hospital, London SW3 6JJ, UK*
[3] *Clinical Cytogenetics, Royal Marsden Hospital, Sutton, Surrey SM2 5NG, UK*

Correspondence should be addressed to Khin Thway; khin.thway@rmh.nhs.uk

Academic Editor: Irene Andrulis

Background. The assessment of *MDM2* gene amplification by fluorescence *in situ* hybridization (FISH) has become a routine ancillary tool for diagnosing atypical lipomatous tumor (ALT)/well-differentiated liposarcoma and dedifferentiated liposarcoma (WDL/DDL) in specialist sarcoma units. We describe our experience of its utility at our tertiary institute. *Methods.* All routine histology samples in which *MDM2* amplification was assessed with FISH over a 2-year period were included, and FISH results were correlated with clinical and histologic findings. *Results.* 365 samples from 347 patients had FISH for *MDM2* gene amplification. 170 were positive (i.e., showed *MDM2* gene amplification), 192 were negative, and 3 were technically unsatisfactory. There were 122 histologically benign cases showing a histology:FISH concordance rate of 92.6%, 142 WDL/DDL (concordance 96.5%), and 34 cases histologically equivocal for WDL (concordance 50%). Of 64 spindle cell/pleomorphic neoplasms (in which DDL was a differential diagnosis), 21.9% showed *MDM2* amplification. Of the cases with discrepant histology and FISH, all but 3 had diagnoses amended following FISH results. For discrepancies of benign histology but positive FISH, lesions were on average larger, more frequently in "classical" (intra-abdominal or inguinal) sites for WDL/DDL and more frequently core biopsies. Discrepancies of malignant histology but negative FISH were smaller, less frequently in "classical" sites but again more frequently core biopsies. *Conclusions.* FISH has a high correlation rate with histology for cases with firm histologic diagnoses of lipoma or WDL/DDL. It is a useful ancillary diagnostic tool in histologically equivocal cases, particularly in WDL lacking significant histologic atypia or DDL without corresponding WDL component, especially in larger tumors, those from intra-abdominal or inguinal sites or core biopsies. There is a significant group of well-differentiated adipocytic neoplasms which are difficult to diagnose on morphology alone, in which FISH for *MDM2* amplification is diagnostically contributory.

1. Introduction

Adipocytic tumors are the commonest soft tissue neoplasms [1] and form a large group, which includes lipomas and their histological variants and liposarcomas (LPS). Of the latter, atypical lipomatous tumor (ALT)/well-differentiated liposarcoma (collectively referred to here as WDL) and dedifferentiated liposarcoma (DDL) form the largest subgroup and are considered to represent a morphological spectrum of the same disease entity [2, 3]. There is frequent histologic overlap between different subtypes of adipocytic neoplasm, including, importantly, between benign and malignant groups. The diagnosis of WDL depends on the presence of atypia within predominantly mature adipocytes or fibrous septa, but atypia can be focal or subtle, and distinguishing WDL from various benign adipocytic neoplasms, or even from normal fat, can be challenging, especially in the presence of additional factors such as fat necrosis [4, 5]. A further area of diagnostic difficulty is in distinguishing DDL from other soft tissue sarcomas. DDL is morphologically heterogeneous, usually with the appearance of undifferentiated spindle cell or pleomorphic sarcoma and can have heterologous differentiation towards other mesenchymal lineages [6]. Inflammatory DDL may resemble IgG4-associated sclerosing lesions or inflammatory myofibroblastic tumor [7], histologically low grade pattern DDL can mimic fibromatosis or low grade fibromyxoid sarcoma, and some patterns of WDL/DDL resemble pleomorphic or myxoid liposarcomatous subtypes [8, 9]. The accurate diagnosis of adipocytic neoplasms is crucial, as WDL is more prone to local recurrence than benign adipocytic tumors [10, 11] and has the potential to dedifferentiate, especially within the abdomen/retroperitoneum. The ability to diagnose DDL is useful prognostically, as it has a lower tendency to local recurrence and metastasis compared with both other liposarcomas and other morphologically similar sarcomas such as undifferentiated pleomorphic sarcoma (UPS) or leiomyosarcoma [12].

As several soft tissue sarcomas harbor characteristic genetic abnormalities, molecular genetic and molecular cytogenetic analyses are valuable ancillary diagnostic tools [13]. After early studies showing amplification of the chromosomal 12q13-15 region (which includes several genes such as *MDM2* and *CDK4*) in some sarcoma types including liposarcomas [14, 15], *MDM2* gene amplification, in the form of supernumerary ring and/or giant chromosomes, has been shown to be characteristic of WDL and DDL [16–18]. *MDM2* amplification is also associated with other sarcomas such as parosteal osteosarcoma and intimal sarcoma [19, 20], so while it is not entirely specific for WDL and DDL, its assessment by FISH has been developed as an adjunctive tool for their diagnosis [21]. We investigated the utility of assessment of *MDM2* amplification by FISH as an ancillary tool for the histological diagnosis of WDL and DDL and in distinguishing these tumors from other neoplasms in their differential diagnosis in routine diagnostic practice.

2. Methods

All cases were formalin fixed and paraffin embedded (FFPE) and comprised consecutive specimens from the routine surgical pathology workload that had fluorescence *in situ* hybridization (FISH) performed for *MDM2* amplification over a 2-year period from March 2011 to March 2013. Case numbers were retrieved from the molecular cytogenetics database (J. S.) and matched with the corresponding histopathological specimens from the electronic patient record. These were specimens in which well-differentiated or dedifferentiated liposarcoma was in the differential diagnosis and included (i) lipomatous tumors with atypical histological features for which a confirmatory positive FISH result was sought, (ii) histologically benign adipocytic neoplasms that were recurrent, large (>10 cm), or sited deeply, and (iii) spindle cell or pleomorphic sarcomas in which DDL was suspected or in the differential diagnosis, due to histologic features or anatomic site. Cases comprised both core biopsy and excision specimens of material biopsied or resected at our center and external cases which were sent for review or second opinion. All diagnoses had been previously made from morphology and immunohistochemistry by one or both of two specialist soft tissue pathologists (K. T. and C. F.). The histopathological reports, slides, and clinical histories were reviewed, and comparison was made between initial and final diagnoses. Clinical information included patient's age and sex and the site and size of lesions. For FISH, 2 μm thick FFPE sections were dewaxed overnight at 60°C, treated with hot buffer wash at 80°C (2-3 hrs) and then with proteolytic enzyme treatment at 37°C, and finally washed in distilled water and then an alcohol series before the addition of *MDM2* and chromosome 12 centromere (CEP12) DNA probes (Vysis *MDM2*/CEP 12 FISH Probe Kit, Abbott Laboratories Ltd., UK). Hybridization was performed overnight according to the manufacturer's protocols. Unless the entire tissue was involved, a stained slide was supplied with the area of interest marked, and this area was generally assessed first for FISH signal patterns. A normal result was of two *MDM2* and CEP12 signals. Signal loss, which is commonly found in thin sections, was ignored for the purposes of this study as being nondiagnostic. Occasional cells with an extra signal were also ignored. Cells with gains of roughly equal numbers of up to eight CEP12 and *MDM2* signals were deemed to be clonal with aneuploidy. The usual pattern of amplification was two to four CEP 12 signals with at least six extra *MDM2* signals. As well as being in greater number, the extra signals were usually smaller and were usually clustered. If no clear result was obtained, or if all the nuclei had a normal signal pattern, then the entire tissue section was screened. As far as possible, overlapping tumor nuclei were also excluded from evaluation. Each case was scored independently by two senior clinical cytogeneticists. If their findings did not match, or if they were suspicious of a low level abnormality, a third scientist was called in to provide an opinion. Representative images of the sections were captured using a cooled charged coupled device camera.

3. Results

365 FISH tests were performed in 347 patients in the 2-year period. Tests were repeated in 6 patients (3 due to initial technical failure and 3 on different blocks of the same tumor but with different morphologies). 11 patients had subsequent samples retested, while 1 had two separate lipomatous tumors tested (see FISH results).

3.1. Patient and Tumor Characteristics (Table 1). There were 214 males and 133 females (ratio 1.61 : 1), with median age at diagnosis of 59 years (range 12–95 years) and median tumor size 13.5 cm (range 2–109 cm). The commonest tumor sites were intra-abdominal/retroperitoneal (148), lower limb girdle/inguinal region (88), trunk (57), and upper limb/shoulder (35), with smaller numbers in head and neck (22), lower extremities (13), and thoracic cavity (3). 221 specimens were biopsied or excised in house, and 144 were referred from other hospitals. Where known, 174 cases were resection specimens and 82 were biopsies (most commonly needle core biopsies).

3.2. Histological Findings. All specimens had a provisional histological diagnosis made at our institute prior to FISH

Table 1: Patient and tumor characteristics.

Patient/tumor characteristics	Total
Male	214 (61.7%)
Female	133 (38.3%)
Median age	59 years (range 12–95 years)
Tumor size (where available from the gross specimen or cross-sectional imaging)	13.5 cm (range 2–109 cm)
Tumor site	
Intra-abdominal	148
Retroperitoneum	(113)
Bowel/mesentery	(25)
Pelvis	(10)
Inguinal/lower limb girdle	88
Thigh	(47)
Spermatic cord	(19)
Groin	(14)
Buttock/perineum	(8)
Trunk	57
Back	(22)
Chest wall	(17)
Abdominal wall	(14)
Breast	(4)
Upper limb/shoulder	35
Shoulder	(18)
Arm	(11)
Axilla	(4)
Hand	(1)
Head and neck	22
Neck	(14)
Mouth/jaw	(5)
Scalp/forehead	(2)
Ear	(1)
Lower extremities	13
Knee	(6)
Calf	(4)
Foot	(3)
Thoracic cavity (pleura, mediastinum, and lung)	3

analysis (Table 2). 122 were diagnosed as benign (most commonly lipomas, spindle cell/pleomorphic lipomas, and intramuscular lipomas). Of 209 cases diagnosed as malignant, there were 145 liposarcomas (73 WDL, 69 DDL, 1 myxoid LPS, and 2 pleomorphic LPS) and 64 other soft tissue neoplasms (most commonly UPS/spindle cell sarcomas), of which the majority were at intra-abdominal/retroperitoneal or inguinal sites ($n = 57$) (necessitating the need to exclude DDL), with small numbers in the abdominal wall, thorax/trunk, and leg. For 34 cases a conclusive histological diagnosis could not be made between a benign adipocytic lesion or WDL; in 19/34 a benign diagnosis was favored but WDL could not be excluded (due to occasional atypical cells, tumor site, or the fact that tumor was recurrent) while in 15/34, WDL had been strongly suspected, but a definite diagnosis was not made.

3.3. FISH Results. Of 362 technically successful tests, 170 were positive, that is, showing *MDM2* gene amplification, and 192 were negative, that is, not showing amplification. Of the negatives, 136 had the normal two *MDM2* and CEP12 signals while 56 showed abnormal CEP12 and *MDM2* signals (ranging from 1 to 10 copies of both CEP12 and *MDM2*), suggesting gain (or loss, in 2 cases) involving possibly the whole chromosome 12 (Table 2). These comprised a variety of neoplasms (both benign and malignant), including spindle cell and pleomorphic lipoma and UPS. Since there were equal numbers of CEP12 and *MDM2* signals in these cases and the *MDM2* signals were of usual sizes, there were no features to suggest specific amplification of the *MDM2* region. This implied possible aneuploidy involving chromosome 12, or even hyperploidy of all chromosomes in these neoplasms. In 3 patients, tests were repeated due to initial technical failure; all were external review cases, and the failures may have been due to fixation differences in other laboratories. The subsequent repeat samples were successful and were from material excised at our institute. One patient had 2 separate lipomatous neoplasms tested (1 positive for *MDM2* amplification, the other negative). 11 patients had retesting of the same tumor: 3 had 2 separate blocks from the same tumor tested (all 3 giving consistent results in separate blocks) and 8 had retesting on new samples (6 with core biopsies followed soon after by tumor resections and 2 instances of resampling after 2- and 3-year intervals). Of these 8, 4 were initially external review cases and 4 were internal biopsies. All 8 subsequent samples comprised internal material and of these retested samples, 2 tested positive on both first and second samples, 4 were negative in both, and 2 were initially *MDM2* amplification negative, but subsequently positive. These last 2 samples were initially core biopsies (both internal sampling), with subsequent resection specimens.

3.4. Correlation of FISH with Histology. Of the 122 lesions histologically diagnosed as benign, 113 showed no *MDM2* amplification (giving a 92.6% concordance rate between histology and FISH), but 9 showed *MDM2* amplification. These included 4 initially diagnosed as lipomas, 2 intramuscular lipomas, 2 pleomorphic lipomas, and 1 of fibroadipose tissue within scar at the site of previous retroperitoneal tumor. All but the last case were at extra-abdominal sites (extremity or trunk). In all 9 cases, the final diagnosis was amended according to the FISH results.

Of the 73 cases with histologic diagnoses of WDL, 71 showed *MDM2* amplification (giving a 97.3% histology:FISH concordance rate). Both of the 2 non-*MDM2* amplified histological WDL (1 from retroperitoneum, 1 from chest wall), as well as 2 amplified cases, showed abnormal CEP12 signals, with 4–6 copies of probe signals seen. For histologic DDL, 66/69 cases showed *MDM2* amplification (95.7% histology:FISH concordance rate), of which 15 showed additional CEP12 signals. The 3 negative cases all showed

TABLE 2: Comparison of histological tumor type and FISH results.

Histological diagnosis	Total	MDM+	MDM−	MDM2−, with multiple copies of CEP12 and *MDM2* signals
Benign	122	9	113	20
Lipoma	76	4	72	9
Intramuscular lipoma	12	2	10	0
Spindle cell lipoma	17	0	17	5
Pleomorphic lipoma	9	2	7	5
Fat necrosis	2	0	2	0
Lipoblastoma	2	0	2	0
Lipoleiomyoma	1	0	1	1
Hibernoma	1	0	1	0
Nevus lipomatosis	1	0	1	0
Fibroadipose tissue/scar	2	1	1	0
Liposarcoma	145	137	8	10
WDL	73	71	2	5
DDL	69	66	3	3
Myxoid LPS	2	0	2	0
Pleomorphic LPS	1	0	1	2
Equivocal cases	34 (including 1 technical fail)	10	23	0
Possible WDL/DDL	19	6	13	0
Probable/suspected WDL/DDL	15	4	10	0
Other soft tissue sarcomas/malignancies	64 (including 2 technical fails)	14	48	26
Undifferentiated pleomorphic sarcoma	28	5	21	14
Spindle cell sarcoma (NOS)	19	2	17	8
Rhabdomyosarcoma	5	3	2	2
Solitary fibrous tumor	3	1	2	1
Leiomyosarcoma	3	1	2	1
Malignant peripheral nerve sheath tumor	2	1	1	0
Osteosarcoma	1	1	0	0
Inflammatory myofibroblastic tumor	1	0	1	0
Poorly differentiated carcinoma	2	0	2	0

abnormal CEP12 signals, with 5–8 copies present. The 2 pleomorphic LPS and 1 myxoid LPS tested did not show *MDM2* amplification. Abnormal CEP12 signals were seen in the 2 pleomorphic LPS, but not the myxoid LPS (in keeping with pleomorphic LPS harboring complex karyotypes typical of other pleomorphic sarcomas and myxoid LPS having balanced translocations and not expected to exhibit aneuploidy). The overall concordance rate of histology with FISH for WDL/DDL was 96.5%. Of the 5 WDL/DDL negative for *MDM2* amplification, 4 had final diagnosis revised (2 presumed DDL revised to spindle cell sarcoma not otherwise specified (NOS), and 2 WDL revised to lipomas), while 1 (which was retroperitoneal, with adjacent unequivocal WDL components) had its histologic diagnosis of DDL retained.

Of the 19 cases where a benign diagnosis was favored histologically but WDL was a possibility, 13 were negative for *MDM2* amplification (68.4% concordance, i.e., 31.6% of histologically "possible WDL" were *MDM2* positive), with 1 of these showing abnormal CEP12 signals. The other 6 were positive for *MDM2* amplification, of which 4 had minor equivocal degrees of histologic atypia and 2 were suspected recurrences of WDL which morphologically resembled normal fat without atypia. All were extra-abdominal (from extremities). In all cases, the final diagnosis was amended according to FISH results.

In contrast, of the 15 cases where WDL was histologically favored, that is, histologically "probable WDL" but not conclusive, 1 failed technically, only 4 were positive for *MDM2* amplification (1 from retroperitoneum, 2 thigh, and 1 lower leg) (28.6% concordance), and 10 were negative (1 with abnormal CEP12 signals). 6/10 negative cases were from intra-abdominal (retroperitoneal) sites and 8/10 had their final diagnosis amended to lipoma variants (4 being classed as true retroperitoneal lipomas). However, in 2 retroperitoneal cases, the histologic features were such that the final report stated that WDL could not be excluded, with advice to monitor for recurrences.

Lastly, of the 64 histological soft tissue sarcomas (many of which were retroperitoneal/intra-abdominal and hence for which DDL was in the differential diagnosis) (sites: 30

TABLE 3: Comparison of patient and tumor characteristics in cases with concordance or discrepancies of histology and FISH.

Histological diagnosis	MDM2 amplified	Total	Sex of patients	Median age (years)	Median size of tumor (cm)	Classical sites for WDL/DDL (intra-abdominal or inguinal)	Review cases	Core biopsies	Resection specimens
Benign (definite/provisional)	−	126	84 M : 43 F	50.5	9	40 (31.5%)	60 (47.2%)	16 (21.6%)	58 (78.4%)
	+ (i.e., discrepant with histology)	15	8 M : 7 F	59	15	8 (53.3%)	5 (33.3%)	5 (45.5%)	6 (54.5%)
Liposarcoma (definite/provisional)	− (i.e., discrepant with histology)	15	5 M : 12 F	64	13.5	10 (66.7%)	2 (13.3%)	5 (38.5%)	8 (61.5%)
	+	142	92 M : 50 F	63	18	113 (79.6%)	27 (19.0%)	31 (29.2%)	75 (70.8%)

retroperitoneal, 16 intra-abdominal/mesenteric, 5 intrapelvic, 6 groin or spermatic cord, and 7 in abdominal wall, thorax/trunk, or leg), 14 (21.9%) (including 9/30 retroperitoneal tumors) showed *MDM2* amplification, with 8 also having abnormal *CEP12* signals. 9 of these 14 *MDM2* amplified tumors had their final diagnosis revised to DDL (3 showing heterologous differentiation). The diagnosis was not changed in 2 cases (1 rhabdomyosarcoma (RMS) and 1 malignant peripheral nerve sheath tumor in a patient with neurofibromatosis-1), and in the remaining 3 (2 retroperitoneal RMS and 1 solitary fibrous tumor in the thigh), the final conclusions remained equivocal. There were 48 cases without *MDM2* amplification, of which 31 showed abnormal CEP12 signals and 17 had normal *MDM2* and centromeric signals. However, in 2 (both core biopsies), FISH was repeated on subsequent resection specimens and produced positive results. 2 cases failed technically.

3.5. Analysis of Discordant Samples. Patient and tumor characteristics in the cases with discordant histology and FISH were compared (Table 3). For this, the 64 spindle cell neoplasms with a differential diagnosis of DDL (largely due to intra-abdominal/inguinal site but in which no conclusive evidence of DDL was present) were excluded, as were the 3 myxoid or pleomorphic LPS. The categories of "definite" and "probable" diagnoses were combined for each of benign and malignant diagnoses (benign adipocytic lesions and WDL/DDL groups). For benign histological diagnoses, 15/141 specimens were unexpectedly positive for *MDM2* amplification by FISH (10.6%). For histological WDL/DDL 15/157 were unexpectedly negative for *MDM2* amplification (9.6%).

For benign lesions, median tumor sizes for concordant and discordant cases were 9 cm and 15 cm, respectively. 31.5% of concordant cases were intra-abdominal or inguinal, compared with 53.3% of discordant. 21.6% of concordant cases and 45.5% of discordant cases were core biopsies. For malignant (WDL/DDL) cases, median tumor sizes were 18 cm and 13.5 cm for concordant and discordant cases. 79.6% of concordant cases and 66.7% of discordant cases were intra-abdominal or inguinal. 29.2% of concordant cases and 38.5% of discordant cases were core biopsies. Cases with discrepant "benign" histology but positive FISH were therefore on average larger, more frequently occurred intra-abdominally or inguinally and were core biopsy specimens. This is in keeping with the increased likelihood of larger neoplasms being malignant of intra-abdominally or inguinally sited neoplasms representing WDL/DDL and of core biopsies causing sampling error and erroneous "benign" histological interpretations. Cases with discrepant "malignant" histology but negative FISH were smaller, occurred less frequently intra-abdominally or inguinally but again occurred more frequently in cores. This is consistent with smaller, non-intra-abdominal/noninguinal tumors being more likely to represent simple lipoma subtypes, but also similarly subject to sampling error or morphologic distortion on core biopsy.

4. Discussion

The diagnosis of WDL and DDL can be challenging, particularly in core biopsy material where tissue is sparse, or where the histologic features are subtle. Particular areas of confusion include (a) distinguishing WDL (Figures 1(a)-1(b)) from benign mimics (e.g., lipomas including spindle cell/pleomorphic lipomas and fibrolipomas and fat necrosis (Figure 1(c)), (b) distinguishing DDL from other pleomorphic sarcomas in the absence of a well-differentiated component or antecedent history of WDL, and (c) differentiating morphologic variants of WDL/DDL (Figure 1(d)) from other (pleomorphic and myxoid) LPS (Figure 1(e)). These lead to differences in opinion even amongst soft tissue pathologists, and cases sent to tertiary referral centers often include lipomas that are reclassified as WDL and vice versa [4, 5].

Following early work showing *MDM2* amplification in LPS and some MFH [14, 15], *MDM2* amplification has been shown to be characteristic of WDL/DDL [16–18, 22–24] with similar genetic alterations demonstrated between paired well-differentiated and dedifferentiated components [25] (Figure 1(f)). While some earlier studies claimed 100% sensitivity and specificity in distinguishing lipomas from WDL (although also showing that up to 40% of high grade sarcomas harbored *MDM2* amplification) [21], others did not find *MDM2* amplification in all ALT/WDL [16, 26]. Differing results may be due to the use of different techniques in detecting *MDM2* gene amplification, including FISH, real time polymerase chain reaction (RT-PCR), and Southern blotting [16, 26–28], as well as differences in sampling of

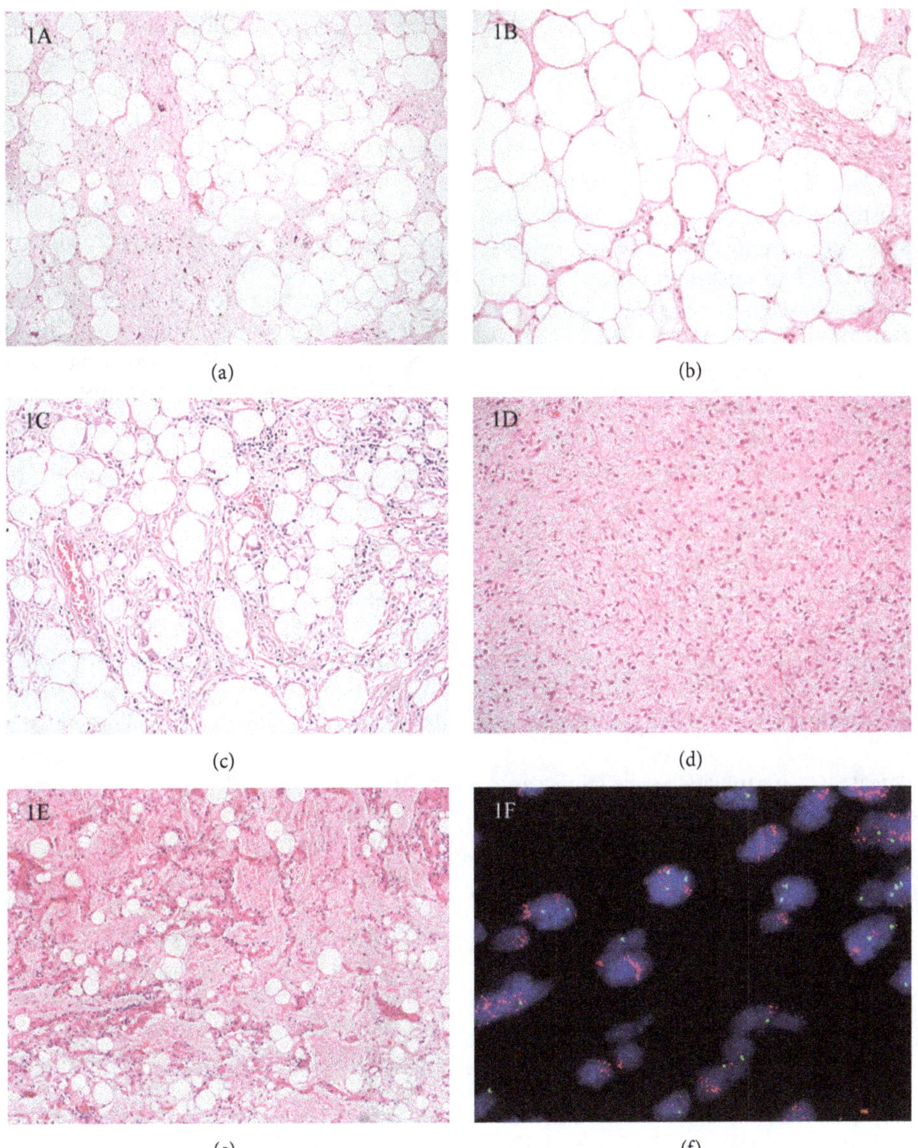

(a) (b) (c) (d) (e) (f)

FIGURE 1: (a) Well-differentiated liposarcoma (WDL). This typical example shows differentiated adipose tissue intersected by thick fibrous septa containing spindle cells with enlarged, hyperchromatic nuclei. (b) This WDL shows lobules of mature adipose tissue, with fibrous septa containing minimal atypia, and can be difficult to distinguish from fibrolipoma or lipoma with fat necrosis. (c) Fat necrosis. This can be extensive, with prominent histiocytes containing plump nuclei, making it difficult to distinguish from WDL. (d) Dedifferentiated liposarcoma (DDL) showing a "low grade" pattern of dedifferentiation can be mistaken for a variety of lesions, including benign neoplasms such as neurofibromas, those of intermediate biologic potential such as fibromatosis, or with other sarcomas such as low grade fibromyxoid sarcoma. FISH for assessment of *MDM2* amplification status is useful in supporting the diagnosis of DDL. (e) This myxoid variant of DDL bears a striking resemblance to myxoid liposarcoma (MLPS). Evidence of *MDM2* amplification with FISH is strongly supportive of DDL, as *MDM2* amplification is not described in MLPS. (f) Fluorescence in situ hybridization for *MDM2* amplification status. The green CEP 12 signals are located on the centromere of chromosome 12 and the red *MDM2* signals are located on the long arm of the same chromosome (12).

lesions and different pathologists' morphologic thresholds for making the diagnosis. Most recent studies have utilized FISH, using commercial probes for *MDM2* [21, 29]. While immunohistochemistry for MDM2 has high levels of accuracy, especially when coupled with that for CDK4 and p16 [29–35], the MDM2 antibody can be technically inconsistent [34] and p16 is nonspecific as it is expressed in a variety of nonadipocytic neoplasms. To this end, as FISH is shown to be a robust ancillary molecular cytogenetic technique [36] and its use becomes more widespread routinely; it seems reasonable to use it to assess for *MDM2* amplification in the first instance. Most reported series have used FISH as the diagnostic "gold standard," with review or reconsideration of the final diagnosis based on its results [37, 38]. However, other studies have based final diagnosis on histologic criteria [29, 39, 40] or a combination of techniques [29].

In this study, we found that where there was a firm histologic diagnosis of benign lipomatous tumor or of WDL/DDL, the concordance rates of histology with *MDM2* amplification results were high (92.6% and 96.5%, resp.). These results are broadly similar to the concordance rates of 85–100% in other published data [37–39, 41, 42], although those studies used cases in which firm histologic diagnoses had been made and did not consider "equivocal" diagnoses. Our series includes a large number of equivocal and uncertain histologic diagnoses, and it should be emphasized that the large majority of specimens analyzed by FISH in this study were those in which there was a level of diagnostic uncertainty; hence unequivocal cases of lipomas or DDL with adjacent WDL component were not tested. The concordance rate of histology and FISH seen here would almost certainly be higher if more diagnostically certain cases had been included. In dividing cases into two "levels" of histological uncertainty, we found that 31.6% of "possible" WDL were *MDM2* amplified, while 28.6% of "probable" WDL were *MDM2* amplified. All cases falling into this equivocal category therefore have a similar rate of positive FISH, and it would therefore seem prudent to perform FISH on any case of possible WDL with an element of uncertainty (irrespective of the degree of perceived histologic atypia).

In the 64 soft tissue neoplasms in which pure DDL was in the differential diagnosis, *MDM2* was amplified in only 21.9%. Most of these cases comprised spindle or pleomorphic sarcomas (not otherwise specified) without specific morphologic or immunohistochemical differentiation, other than scanty single marker expression (e.g., SMA only, or desmin only, or scanty CD34 only), which were not possible to further characterize. Small numbers of these cases were assigned provisional diagnoses, for example, rhabdomyosarcoma, if there was focal expression of appropriate markers (e.g., clear cut desmin with myogenin or MyoD1) (Table 2). The significance of this finding of *MDM2* amplification in 21.9% is uncertain, since up to 40% of other soft tissue sarcomas can harbor amplified *MDM2* [21, 22, 39, 40]. This and the fact that DDL can have a variety of appearances ranging from bland fibromatosis-like to UPS-like and exhibit several different types of heterologous differentiation [6, 7, 43–46] mean that unless there is an antecedent history of WDL or adjacent WDL component, a diagnosis of DDL cannot always be proven, even at sites where it is likely. Coindre et al. have previously shown that most retroperitoneal UPS represent DDL [43], although of our 30/64 sarcomas that were retroperitoneal, only 9 showed *MDM2* amplification, a lower figure than expected. It could be said that, for retroperitoneal sarcomas, FISH for *MDM2* is helpful in supporting a diagnosis of DDL rather than another sarcoma type. For example, of 201 spindle cell tumors studied by Kashima et al., 7 had *MDM2* amplification (3 spindle cell sarcomas NOS, 2 osteosarcomas, and 2 myxofibrosarcomas), of which all were retroperitoneal or intra-abdominal, with some on subsequent review showing WDL components, and these were all reclassified as DDL [41].

MDM2 amplification status by FISH could be of therapeutic importance, as amplified neoplasms, irrespective of precise histologic subtype, might be amenable in the future to targeted treatment with MDM2 antagonists. True retroperitoneal lipomas are rare but increasingly recognized [47] and show clinicopathologic and genetic features (including lack of *MDM2* amplification) more akin to lipomas than WDL [47] such that their identification by FISH is prognostically useful. Positive FISH for *MDM2* would also be useful in excluding pleomorphic and myxoid LPS (both of which can be mimicked by DDL but are virtually unknown intra-abdominally) [8, 9].

An interesting facet of this study is that despite the high histology:FISH concordance rates for clear-cut histologic lipomas and WDL/DDL (as also shown in previous studies), there is a dramatically lower histology:FISH concordance rate for equivocal cases of differentiated adipocytic neoplasms, despite histologic diagnoses by specialist soft tissue pathologists. This highlights that there exists a subgroup of microscopically equivocal well-differentiated lipomatous neoplasms that elude definitive histological diagnosis. If FISH was taken as gold standard, this questions whether, in specific contexts, prior detailed evaluation of differentiated adipocytic lesions by surgical pathologists might essentially be rendered less crucial than *MDM2* FISH. As with all ancillary tests that accompany histology and taking note of the small rate of both technical failures and what appear to be false negative results, we still recommend that FISH should be interpreted strictly in the context of the histological and clinical findings.

Since FISH is both labor and cost intensive and morphologically clear-cut cases of WDL/DDL do not require ancillary diagnostic confirmation, it is important to determine when it would be most useful and cost efficient for diagnosis. From their studies of trunk and extremity neoplasms, Zhang et al. recommended that lipomatous tumors that are recurrent and large (>15 cm) or show possible cytologic atypia are indications for FISH [37]. Neuville et al. also recommended that all poorly differentiated abdominal or retroperitoneal sarcomas be tested [42]. Le Guellec et al. recently showed similarities in histology, genomic profile, and clinical behavior of patients with peripheral UPS with *MDM2* amplification and peripheral conventional DDL which strongly suggested that peripheral UPS with *MDM2* amplification in fact represents DDL [48].

In this series, we found that, for histologically benign-appearing adipocytic neoplasms, *MDM2* amplification was more frequently found in those that were larger or in "classical" (intra-abdominal or inguinal) sites for WDL and in core biopsy specimens. Likewise, in cases of probable WDL/DDL a negative FISH result was more common in core biopsies, smaller lesions, and those not sited intra-abdominally or inguinally. External review cases that had FISH performed interestingly showed fewer discrepancies between histology (reviewed at our tertiary center) and FISH, but this highlights the robustness of FISH technique on referral material [4].

5. Conclusions

Our experience of FISH for testing *MDM2* amplification shows high concordance in established histological diagnoses of lipoma and WDL/DDL. The lower concordance for cases with equivocal histological diagnoses is an issue for debate, highlighting both the merit of using FISH as a diagnostic adjunct for all equivocal well-differentiated adipocytic neoplasms and the fact that there might exist a group of histologically differentiated adipocytic tumors needing more detailed morphologic and molecular characterization. There is particular value in performing FISH in core biopsies, larger adipocytic neoplasms with bland histology, and those occurring in "classical" inguinal or intra-abdominal sites. However, FISH results should not be relied on exclusively, and, as for any other ancillary diagnostic tests, should be interpreted in light of the histological and clinical findings.

Authors' Contribution

Khin Thway and Jayson Wang contributed equally to this work.

Acknowledgments

The authors acknowledge support from the NIHR Royal Marsden Hospital/ICR Biomedical Research Center. They are also very grateful to Melissa Dainton, Carol Brooker, and Frances Aldridge (Clinical Scientists and Cytogeneticists, Clinical Cytogenetics, Royal Marsden Hospital, Sutton, Surrey, UK) for their help in analyzing the cases.

References

[1] J. R. Goldblum, A. L. Folpe, and S. W. Weiss, "Benign lipomatous tumors," in *Enzinger and Weiss's Soft Tissue Tumors*, pp. 443–483, Elsevier, New York, NY, USA, 6th edition, 2014.

[2] A. G. Nascimento, "Dedifferentiated liposarcoma," *Seminars in Diagnostic Pathology*, vol. 18, no. 4, pp. 263–266, 2001.

[3] L. Laurino, A. Furlanetto, E. Orvieto, and A. P. D. Tos, "Well-differentiated liposarcoma (atypical lipomatous tumors)," *Seminars in Diagnostic Pathology*, vol. 18, no. 4, pp. 258–262, 2001.

[4] K. Thway and C. Fisher, "Histopathological diagnostic discrepancies in soft tissue tumours referred to a specialist centre," *Sarcoma*, vol. 2009, Article ID 741975, 7 pages, 2009.

[5] Z. K. Arbiser, A. L. Folpe, and S. W. Weiss, "Consultative (expert) second opinions in soft tissue pathology. Analysis of problem-prone diagnostic situations," *The American Journal of Clinical Pathology*, vol. 116, no. 4, pp. 473–476, 2001.

[6] W. H. Henricks, Y. C. Chu, J. R. Goldblum, and S. W. Weiss, "Dedifferentiated liposarcoma: a clinicopathological analysis of 155 cases with a proposal for an expanded definition of dedifferentiation," *The American Journal of Surgical Pathology*, vol. 21, no. 3, pp. 271–281, 1997.

[7] M. D. Kraus, L. Guillou, and C. D. M. Fletcher, "Well-differentiated inflammatory liposarcoma: an uncommon and easily overlooked variant of a common sarcoma," *The American Journal of Surgical Pathology*, vol. 21, no. 5, pp. 518–527, 1997.

[8] A. Mariño-Enríquez, C. D. M. Fletcher, P. D. Cin, and J. L. Hornick, "Dedifferentiated liposarcoma with 'homologous' lipoblastic (Pleomorphic Liposarcoma-like) differentiation: clinicopathologic and molecular analysis of a series suggesting revised diagnostic criteria," *American Journal of Surgical Pathology*, vol. 34, no. 8, pp. 1122–1131, 2010.

[9] R. S. A. de Vreeze, D. de Jong, I. H. G. Tielen et al., "Primary retroperitoneal myxoid/round cell liposarcoma is a nonexisting disease: an immunohistochemical and molecular biological analysis," *Modern Pathology*, vol. 22, no. 2, pp. 223–231, 2009.

[10] V. Billing, F. Mertens, H. A. Domanski, and A. Rydholm, "Deep-seated ordinary and atypical lipomas: histopathology, cytogenetics, clinical features, and outcome in 215 tumours of the extremity and trunk wall," *The Journal of Bone and Joint Surgery: British Volume*, vol. 90, no. 7, pp. 929–933, 2008.

[11] J. W. Serpell and R. Y. Y. Chen, "Review of large deep lipomatous tumours," *ANZ Journal of Surgery*, vol. 77, no. 7, pp. 524–529, 2007.

[12] D. McCormick, T. Mentzel, A. Beham, and C. D. M. Fletcher, "Dedifferentiated liposarcoma: clinicopathologic analysis of 32 cases suggesting a better prognostic subgroup among pleomorphic sarcomas," *The American Journal of Surgical Pathology*, vol. 18, no. 12, pp. 1213–1223, 1994.

[13] C. R. Antonescu, "The role of genetic testing in soft tissue sarcoma," *Histopathology*, vol. 48, no. 1, pp. 13–21, 2006.

[14] F. S. Leach, T. Tokino, P. Meltzer et al., "p53 mutation and MDM2 amplification in human soft tissue sarcomas," *Cancer Research*, vol. 53, no. 10, supplement, pp. 2231–2234, 1993.

[15] P. Dal Cin, P. Kools, R. Sciot et al., "Cytogenetic and fluorescence in situ hybridization investigation of ring chromosomes characterizing a specific pathologic subgroup of adipose tissue tumors," *Cancer Genetics and Cytogenetics*, vol. 68, no. 2, pp. 85–90, 1993.

[16] S. Pilotti, G. della Torre, C. Lavarino et al., "Distinct mdm2/p53 expression patterns in liposarcoma subgroups: implications for different pathogenetic mechanisms," *The Journal of Pathology*, vol. 181, no. 1, pp. 14–24, 1997.

[17] M. Nilbert, A. Rydholm, F. Mitelman, P. S. Meltzer, and N. Mandahl, "Characterization of the 12q13-15 amplicon in soft tissue tumors," *Cancer Genetics and Cytogenetics*, vol. 83, no. 1, pp. 32–36, 1995.

[18] F. Pedeutour, R. F. Suijkerbuijk, A. Forus et al., "Complex composition and co-amplification of SAS and MDM2 in ring and giant rod marker chromosomes in well-differentiated liposarcoma," *Genes Chromosomes and Cancer*, vol. 10, no. 2, pp. 85–94, 1994.

[19] J. S. Wunder, K. Eppert, S. R. Burrow, N. Gogkoz, R. S. Bell, and I. L. Andrulis, "Co-amplification and overexpression of CDK4, SAS and MDM2 occurs frequently in human parosteal osteosarcomas," *Oncogene*, vol. 18, no. 3, pp. 783–788, 1999.

[20] A. Neuville, F. Collin, P. Bruneval et al., "Intimal sarcoma is the most frequent primary cardiac sarcoma: clinicopathologic and molecular retrospective analysis of 100 primary cardiac sarcomas," *The American Journal of Surgical Pathology*, vol. 38, no. 4, pp. 461–469, 2014.

[21] J. Weaver, E. Downs-Kelly, J. R. Goldblum et al., "Fluorescence in situ hybridization for MDM2 gene amplification as a diagnostic tool in lipomatous neoplasms," *Modern Pathology*, vol. 21, no. 8, pp. 943–949, 2008.

[22] T. Nakayama, J. Toguchida, B.-I. Wadayama, H. Kanoe, Y. Kotoura, and M. S. Sasaki, "MDM2 gene amplification in bone and soft-tissue tumors: association with tumor progression in differentiated adipose-tissue tumors," *International Journal of Cancer*, vol. 64, no. 5, pp. 342–346, 1995.

[23] J. Rosai, M. Akerman, P. Dal Cin et al., "Combined morphologic and karyotypic study of 59 atypical lipomatous tumors: evalu-

ation of their relationship and differential diagnosis with other adipose tissue tumors (A report of the CHAMP study group)," *The American Journal of Surgical Pathology*, vol. 20, no. 10, pp. 1182–1189, 1996.

[24] J.-M. Coindre, F. Pédeutour, and A. Aurias, "Well-differentiated and dedifferentiated liposarcomas," *Virchows Archiv*, vol. 456, no. 2, pp. 167–179, 2010.

[25] A. E. Horvai, S. Devries, R. Roy, R. J. O'Donnell, and F. Waldman, "Similarity in genetic alterations between paired well-differentiated and dedifferentiated components of dedifferentiated liposarcoma," *Modern Pathology*, vol. 22, no. 11, pp. 1477–1488, 2009.

[26] A. P. dei Tos, C. Doglioni, S. Piccinin et al., "Coordinated expression and amplification of the MDM2, CDK4, and HMGI-C genes in atypical lipomatous tumours," *The Journal of Pathology*, vol. 190, no. 5, pp. 531–536, 2000.

[27] I. Hostein, M. Pelmus, A. Aurias, F. Pedeatour, S. Mathoulin-Pélissier, and J. M. Coindre, "Evaluation of MDM2 and CDK4 amplification by real-time PCR on paraffin wax-embedded metarial: a potential tool for the diagnosis of atypical lipomatous tomours/well-defferentiated liposarcomas," *Journal of Pathology*, vol. 202, no. 1, pp. 95–102, 2004.

[28] S. Shimada, T. Ishizawa, K. Ishizawa, T. Matsumura, T. Hasegawa, and T. Hirose, "The value of *MDM2* and *CDK4* amplification levels using real-time polymerase chain reaction for the differential diagnosis of liposarcomas and their histologic mimickers," *Human Pathology*, vol. 37, no. 9, pp. 1123–1129, 2006.

[29] N. Sirvent, J.-M. Coindre, G. Maire et al., "Detection of MDM2-CDK4 amplification by fluorescence in situ hybridization in 200 paraffin-embedded tumor samples: utility in diagnosing adipocytic lesions and comparison with immunohistochemistry and real-time PCR," *The American Journal of Surgical Pathology*, vol. 31, no. 10, pp. 1476–1489, 2007.

[30] P. B. Aleixo, A. A. Hartmann, I. C. Menezes, R. T. Meurer, and A. M. Oliveira, "Can MDM2 and CDK4 make the diagnosis of well differentiated/dedifferentiated liposarcoma? An immunohistochemical study on 129 soft tissue tumours," *Journal of Clinical Pathology*, vol. 62, no. 12, pp. 1127–1135, 2009.

[31] M. B. N. Binh, X. Sastre-Garau, L. Guillou et al., "MDM2 and CDK4 immunostainings are useful adjuncts in diagnosing well-differentiated and dedifferentiated liposarcoma subtypes: a comparative analysis of 559 soft tissue neoplasms with genetic data," *The American Journal of Surgical Pathology*, vol. 29, no. 10, pp. 1340–1347, 2005.

[32] M. He, S. Aisner, J. Benevenia, F. Patterson, H. Aviv, and M. Hameed, "p16 immunohistochemistry as an alternative marker to distinguish atypical lipomatous tumor from deep-seated lipoma," *Applied Immunohistochemistry and Molecular Morphology*, vol. 17, no. 1, pp. 51–56, 2009.

[33] S. Pilotti, G. D. Torre, A. Mezzelani et al., "The expression of *MDM2/CDK4* gene product in the differential diagnosis of well differentiated liposarcoma and large deep-seated lipoma," *British Journal of Cancer*, vol. 82, no. 7, pp. 1271–1275, 2000.

[34] K. Thway, R. Flora, C. Shah, D. Olmos, and C. Fisher, "Diagnostic utility of p16, CDK4, and MDM2 as an immunohistochemical panel in distinguishing well-differentiated and dedifferentiated liposarcomas from other adipocytic tumors," *The American Journal of Surgical Pathology*, vol. 36, no. 3, pp. 462–469, 2012.

[35] M. B. N. Binh, X. S. Garau, L. Guillo, A. Aurias, and J.-M. Coindre, "Reproducibility of MDM2 and CDK4 staining in soft tissue tumors," *The American Journal of Clinical Pathology*, vol. 125, no. 5, pp. 693–697, 2006.

[36] K. Thway, S. Rockcliffe, D. Gonzalez et al., "Utility of sarcoma-specific fusion gene analysis in paraffin-embedded material for routine diagnosis at a specialist centre," *Journal of Clinical Pathology*, vol. 63, no. 6, pp. 508–512, 2010.

[37] H. Zhang, M. Erickson-Johnson, X. Wang et al., "Molecular testing for lipomatous tumors: critical analysis and test recommendations based on the analysis of 405 extremity-based tumors," *The American Journal of Surgical Pathology*, vol. 34, no. 9, pp. 1304–1311, 2010.

[38] J. Cho, S. E. Lee, and Y.-L. Choi, "Diagnostic value of *MDM2* and *DDIT3* fluorescence *In Situ* hybridization in liposarcoma classification: a single-institution experience," *Korean Journal of Pathology*, vol. 46, no. 2, pp. 115–122, 2012.

[39] Y. Miura, Y. Keira, J. Ogino et al., "Detection of specific genetic abnormalities by fluorescence in situ hybridization in soft tissue tumors," *Pathology International*, vol. 62, no. 1, pp. 16–27, 2012.

[40] H. Kimura, Y. Dobashi, T. Nojima et al., "Utility of fluorescence in situ hybridization to detect MDM2 amplification in liposarcomas and their morphological mimics," *International Journal of Clinical and Experimental Pathology*, vol. 6, no. 7, pp. 1306–1316, 2013.

[41] T. Kashima, D. Halai, H. Ye et al., "Sensitivity of MDM2 amplification and unexpected multiple faint alphoid 12 (alpha 12 satellite sequences) signals in atypical lipomatous tumor," *Modern Pathology*, vol. 25, no. 10, pp. 1384–1396, 2012.

[42] A. Neuville, D. Ranchère-Vince, A. P. Dei Tos et al., "Impact of molecular analysis on the final sarcoma diagnosis: a study on 763 cases collected during a European epidemiological study," *The American Journal of Surgical Pathology*, vol. 37, no. 8, pp. 1259–1268, 2013.

[43] J.-M. Coindre, O. Mariani, F. Chibon et al., "Most malignant fibrous histiocytomas developed in the retroperitoneum are dedifferentiated liposarcomas: a review of 25 cases initially diagnosed as malignant fibrous histiocytoma," *Modern Pathology*, vol. 16, no. 3, pp. 256–262, 2003.

[44] J. C. Fanburg-Smith and M. Miettinen, "Liposarcoma with meningothelial-like whorls: a study of 17 cases of a distinctive histological pattern associated with dedifferentiated liposarcoma," *Histopathology*, vol. 33, no. 5, pp. 414–424, 1998.

[45] A. G. Nascimento, P. J. Kurtin, L. Guillou, and C. D. M. Fletcher, "Dedifferentiated liposarcoma: a report of nine cases with a peculiar neurallike whorling pattern associated with metaplastic bone formation," *The American Journal of Surgical Pathology*, vol. 22, no. 8, pp. 945–955, 1998.

[46] M. Hisaoka, S. Tsuji, H. Hashimoto, T. Aoki, and K. Uriu, "Dedifferentiated liposarcoma with an inflammatory malignant fibrous histiocytoma-like component presenting a leukemoid reaction," *Pathology International*, vol. 47, no. 9, pp. 642–646, 1997.

[47] R. S. MacArenco, M. Erickson-Johnson, X. Wang et al., "Retroperitoneal lipomatous tumors without cytologic atypia: are they lipomas?: a clinicopathologic and molecular study of 19 cases," *The American Journal of Surgical Pathology*, vol. 33, no. 10, pp. 1470–1476, 2009.

16

Analysis of the Intratumoral Adaptive Immune Response in Well Differentiated and Dedifferentiated Retroperitoneal Liposarcoma

William W. Tseng,[1,2] Shruti Malu,[3] Minying Zhang,[3] Jieqing Chen,[3] Geok Choo Sim,[3] Wei Wei,[4] Davis Ingram,[5] Neeta Somaiah,[6] Dina C. Lev,[5] Raphael E. Pollock,[7] Gregory Lizée,[3] Laszlo Radvanyi,[8,9] and Patrick Hwu[3,6]

[1]*Department of Surgery, Section of Surgical Oncology, University of Southern California, Los Angeles, CA 90033, USA*
[2]*Hoag Memorial Hospital Presbyterian, Newport Beach, CA 92663, USA*
[3]*Department of Melanoma Medical Oncology, The University of Texas MD Anderson Cancer Center, Houston, TX 77030, USA*
[4]*Department of Biostatistics, The University of Texas MD Anderson Cancer Center, Houston, TX 77030, USA*
[5]*Department of Cancer Biology, The University of Texas MD Anderson Cancer Center, Houston, TX 77030, USA*
[6]*Department of Sarcoma Medical Oncology, The University of Texas MD Anderson Cancer Center, Houston, TX 77030, USA*
[7]*Division of Surgical Oncology, The James Comprehensive Cancer Center, Ohio State University Medical Center, Columbus, OH 43210, USA*
[8]*Lion Biotechnologies, Woodland Hills, CA 91637, USA*
[9]*Department of Immunology, H. Lee Moffitt Cancer Center, Tampa, FL 33612, USA*

Correspondence should be addressed to William W. Tseng; william.tseng@med.usc.edu

Academic Editor: Peter C. Ferguson

Treatment options are limited in well differentiated (WD) and dedifferentiated (DD) retroperitoneal liposarcoma. We sought to study the intratumoral adaptive immune response and explore the potential feasibility of immunotherapy in this disease. Tumor-infiltrating lymphocytes (TILs) were isolated from fresh surgical specimens and analyzed by flow cytometry for surface marker expression. Previously reported immune cell aggregates known as tertiary lymphoid structures (TLS) were further characterized by immunohistochemistry. In all fresh tumors, TILs were found. The majority of TILs were CD4 T cells; however cytotoxic CD8 T cells were also seen (average: 20% of CD3 T cells). Among CD8 T cells, 65% expressed the immune checkpoint molecule PD-1. Intratumoral TLS may be sites of antigen presentation as DC-LAMP positive, mature dendritic cells were found juxtaposed next to CD4 T cells. Clinicopathologic correlation, however, demonstrated that presence of TLS was associated with worse recurrence-free survival in WD disease and worse overall survival in DD disease. Our data suggest that an adaptive immune response is present in WD/DD retroperitoneal liposarcoma but may be hindered by TLS, among other possible microenvironmental factors; further investigation is needed. Immunotherapy, including immune checkpoint blockade, should be evaluated as a treatment option in this disease.

1. Introduction

Although the majority of soft tissue sarcomas occur in the upper and lower extremities, approximately 20% are found in the retroperitoneum, where tumors can often cause significant morbidity and mortality [1]. Well differentiated (WD) and dedifferentiated (DD) liposarcoma are malignancies of adipocytic origin and the most common histologic subtype encountered in the retroperitoneum. WD tumors consist of mostly atypical adipocytes, whereas DD tumors have an additional, high grade, cellular portion [2, 3]. DD liposarcoma may arise from WD liposarcoma; however the precise relationship is still unproven.

In WD/DD retroperitoneal liposarcoma, surgery is the mainstay of treatment; however as tumors are typically massive in size (mean = 30 cm) and can invade adjacent visceral organs and critical structures, resection is often quite challenging [4, 5]. Locoregional recurrence occurs frequently and patients are subjected to multiple surgeries with the potential for increased complication rates [4]. Apart from surgery, few other effective treatment options exist. The role of radiation therapy is not well established [5]. Doxorubicin-based, cytotoxic chemotherapy is frequently given, especially for DD disease; however a recent, large retrospective analysis reported an objective response rate of only 12% [6].

In the past decade, significant advances have been made in the understanding of the molecular biology of WD/DD liposarcoma. The hallmark genetic change in this disease appears to be chromosomal amplification at 12q13–15 [2, 3, 5]. This region includes several hundred to thousands of genes, including MDM2 and CDK4. Amplification of MDM2 occurs in almost all tumors and detection by fluorescence in situ hybridization is often used in the diagnosis of WD/DD liposarcoma [2, 3]. Several novel therapies, driven by disease biology, have recently emerged and are currently being evaluated in early phase clinical trials [7]. Preliminary published data with small series of patients suggests that disease stabilization can be achieved; however, objective response rates are still dismally low: 5% for the MDM2 inhibitor, RG7112, and 3% for the CDK4/6 inhibitor, PD-0332991 [8, 9].

In melanoma, immune checkpoint blockade is an immunotherapeutic strategy that has recently been shown to have impressive objective response rates and even prolongation of survival, despite advanced stage of disease and heavy tumor burden [10–13]. These therapies inhibit the molecular checkpoints (CTLA4, PD-1) or "brakes" that arise naturally in an activated T cell. Unlike vaccines, immune checkpoint blockade does not induce targeting of a specific tumor antigen but instead maintains activation and cytotoxic function in tumor-infiltrating T cells that are already naturally sensitized to a variety of tumor antigens. By blocking both CTLA4 and PD-1 in patients with metastatic melanoma, Wolchok et al. an objective response rate of 53% with tumor shrinkage of up to 80% in many responders [12]. The clinical efficacy of immune checkpoint blockade is also being increasingly reported for other advanced solid tumors [14, 15].

Given the limited and ineffective treatment options currently available to patients with WD and DD retroperitoneal liposarcoma, we sought to study the natural tumor microenvironment from an immunologic standpoint as the first step to explore the potential feasibility of immunotherapy in this disease. In contrast to myxoid liposarcoma which have high expression of the cancer testis-antigen NY-ESO-1 [16], to our knowledge, no consistent and reliable tumor antigen has ever been identified in WD/DD liposarcoma, making vaccine strategies less appealing. Our aim was to study the adaptive immune response and specifically the tumor-infiltrating T cells and their expression of PD-1. This data can then be used to guide further evaluation of immune checkpoint blockade strategies in WD/DD liposarcoma.

2. Material and Methods

Approval for all portions of this study was obtained by the Institutional Review Board at The University of Texas, MD Anderson Cancer Center.

2.1. Fresh Tumor Processing and Analysis by Flow Cytometry. Fresh tumor resected at surgery was closely examined in pathology and nonnecrotic, more fibrous/less fatty portions of tumor were excised and brought to the laboratory for study. In a sterile tissue culture hood, tumor tissue was further dissected to remove visible blood vessels and areas of hypervascularity. Tissue processing techniques used for isolation of tumor-infiltrating lymphocytes (TILs) in melanoma [17, 18] were applied and optimized for liposarcoma. In brief, tumor tissues were placed in serum-free RPMI medium containing supplemental antibiotics and kept at 4°C until ready for use. Tumor chunks were processed by first sharply dicing tissue into smaller, 3-4 mm pieces followed by 2-3 h of enzymatic digestion at 37°C in a rocker, using a cocktail containing collagenase (3%), hyaluronidase (75 μg/mL), and DNAse (250 U/mL). The resulting cell suspension was then washed in PBS and pipetted across a 70 micron filter to remove debris. Ficoll density centrifugation (75%/100%) was then used to remove tumor cells and erythrocytes, enriching for immune cells. Fluorescently labeled antibodies against the cell surface markers CD3, CD56, CD19, CD4, CD8, PD-1, and 4-1BB (all from BD Biosciences, San Jose, CA) were incubated with immune cells, along with a viability marker (Live/Dead Fixable Aqua stain, Invitrogen, Life Technologies, Grand Island, NY). Surface marker expression on stained cells was determined using a multicolor FACS Canto II flow cytometer and the data was analyzed using FlowJo software.

2.2. Immunohistochemistry of FFPE Tissue. Formalin fixed paraformaldehyde embedded (FFPE) tumor tissue was obtained from our institutional pathology archives and 4-micrometer sections were cut. Tissue sections were deparaffinized in xylene and rehydrated through graded alcohols (100%, 95% to 80%). Antigen retrieval was carried out for 30 minutes in citric acid buffer (pH 6.0). After cooling down, the slides were thoroughly washed in distilled water and washed 3 times in 1xPBS, 2 minutes each. Endogenous peroxidase activity was quenched by immersion in 3% hydrogen peroxide (Sigma) in methanol for 10 minutes at room temperature followed by rinsing for 2 minutes in 1xPBS 3 times. Sections were then incubated with primary anti-DC-LAMP mouse antibody (clone 104G4, 1 : 100, Imgenex, San Diego, CA) for 30 minutes according to the manufacturers' instructions (Polink TS-MMR-Hu A Kit, GBI Labs, Bothell, WA). Visualization was performed with the DAB substrate supplied in the kit. Then mixed primary anti-CD4 mouse antibody (clone 4B12, 1 : 40, Leica Microsystems, Buffalo Grove, IL) and anti-CD8 rabbit antibody (clone EP1150Y, 1 : 200, Abcam, Boston, MA) were incubated and visualization was performed with AP-red for CD4 and emerald chromogen (green) for CD8 supplied in the kit. The slides were counterstained with hematoxylin and cover slipped with PerMount. For positive controls, sections of human tonsil tissues were used. Omission of the primary antibodies for tonsil tissue was used as negative controls for staining. Positive cells showed a brown, red, or green intense staining, while negative controls and unstained cells were blue.

2.3. Clinicopathologic Correlation and Statistical Methods. Clinical outcome data was obtained from a retrospective institutional sarcoma database for patients with and without TLS identified in available FFPE tumor sections. Kaplan-Meier curves were used to estimate recurrence-free and overall survival (RFS, OS) between patient groups. Comparisons of RFS and OS between patient groups were carried out using log-rank tests. All tests were two-sided and P values <0.05 were considered statistically significant. Statistical analysis was carried out using SAS version 9.3 (SAS Institute, Cary, NC). Statistical plotting was performed using Spotfire S+ 8.2 (TIBCO Inc., Palo Alto, CA).

3. Results

3.1. Tumor-Infiltrating Lymphocytes in Fresh Tissue. Tumor-infiltrating lymphocytes (TILs) were isolated from all resected retroperitoneal liposarcoma specimens ($n = 8$) included in the study (Table 1). TILs were identified independent of histology (WD versus DD), disease status (primary versus recurrent), or receipt of chemotherapy or radiation therapy prior to resection.

TILs consisted of a substantial population of CD3 T cells (Figure 1) and by flow cytometric analysis, the majority of these cells were CD4 "helper" T cells with a CD4 to CD8 ratio of 4.2 (range 2.0–8.6) (Table 1). CD8 "cytotoxic" T cells, however, were found in all tumors and represented an average of 20% (8–31) of the total CD3 T cell population. CD19 B cells and CD56 NK cells were seen in some tumors, generally with a low frequency (data not shown). Presence of select immune populations, including CD8 T cells, was verified by immunohistochemistry (Figure 1(b)).

Further analysis of surface marker expression on the cytotoxic CD8 T cell population demonstrated a high frequency of expression of the immune checkpoint molecule, PD-1, which was seen in 65% (57–73) of cells (Table 2, Figure 2). In contrast, there was a low frequency of CD8 T cells with expression of the costimulatory molecule, 4-1BB, seen in 10% (3–19) of cells (Table 2, Figure 2).

3.2. Tertiary Lymphoid Structures in FFPE and Clinical Correlation. Tissue sections from archived, FFPE tumor ($n = 35$) were analyzed by H&E and/or immunohistochemistry for presence of intratumoral tertiary lymphoid structures or TLS as described in WD liposarcoma, previously [19]. TLS were generally found in perivascular locations; however TLS could also be found in adipocytic areas of tumor. Varying levels of "architectural maturity" of TLS were observed, ranging from simple aggregates of immune cells to more complex structures resembling germinal centers, typically found within lymph nodes (Figure 3(a)). Occasionally, even macroscopic intratumoral TLS were seen (data not shown). No consistent differences in TLS characteristics (intratumoral location, maturity/size) were noted between WD and DD tumors. By immunohistochemistry, mature dendritic cells expressing DC-LAMP were identified within TLS (Figure 3(b)). Costaining for CD4 and CD8 demonstrated apparent juxtaposition of these mature dendritic cells next to CD4 T cells, suggestive of classic antigen presentation.

In total, TLS were identified in available tissue sections in 12 out of 25 (48%) of WD and 5 out of 10 (50%) of DD retroperitoneal liposarcoma tumors. Presence of TLS was associated with worse recurrence-free survival in patients with WD liposarcoma and worse overall survival in those with DD liposarcoma (Figure 3(c)). No differences in disease status (primary versus recurrent) or prior treatment (chemotherapy, radiation therapy) were noted between patients with and without intratumoral TLS for either histology.

4. Discussion and Conclusions

The first suggestion of an active immune component to WD/DD liposarcoma, at least in some tumors, was made in the late 1990s by two independent descriptions of an "inflammatory" variant of WD liposarcoma [20, 21]. Our own group reported a more contemporary characterization based on immunohistochemistry, which revealed the potential for a naturally occurring adaptive immune response [19]. In the current study, we expanded on our previous work to include all "noninflammatory" WD and DD retroperitoneal liposarcoma and also used flow cytometry to provide deeper analysis of the immune cells. We focused on T cells, a critical component of the adaptive immune response, found in the tumor microenvironment.

Tumor tissue obtained from surgery was used for study as this has direct relevance to patients and importantly, in WD/DD liposarcoma, there are no validated immunocompetent animal models available. The vast majority of preclinical models are xenografts established in immunodeficient mice [22]. Even in these xenograft models, in vivo growth is not consistent and in fact, tumor uptake is largely limited to the higher grade, DD tumors (personal communication, D. Lev). One exception is a report of a genetically engineered mouse model, in which spontaneous WD liposarcoma serendipitously developed in IL-22 overexpressing mice subjected to a high fat diet [23]. Tumors were shown to have MDM2 amplification confirming the diagnosis; however no further independent validation of this model has been done, to our knowledge. Interestingly, a prominent immune infiltrate was seen in tumors found in these mice, although further characterization was not reported.

The data from the current study confirms the presence of a naturally occurring, adaptive immune response within liposarcoma tumors, including presence of cytotoxic CD8 T cells (Figure 1). The high frequency of PD-1 expression and low 4-1BB expression (Figure 2) imply that these tumor-infiltrating CD8 T cells have been sensitized to tumor antigen but are no longer activated [24]. Interestingly, no clear differences in the frequency of CD8 T cells or the expression

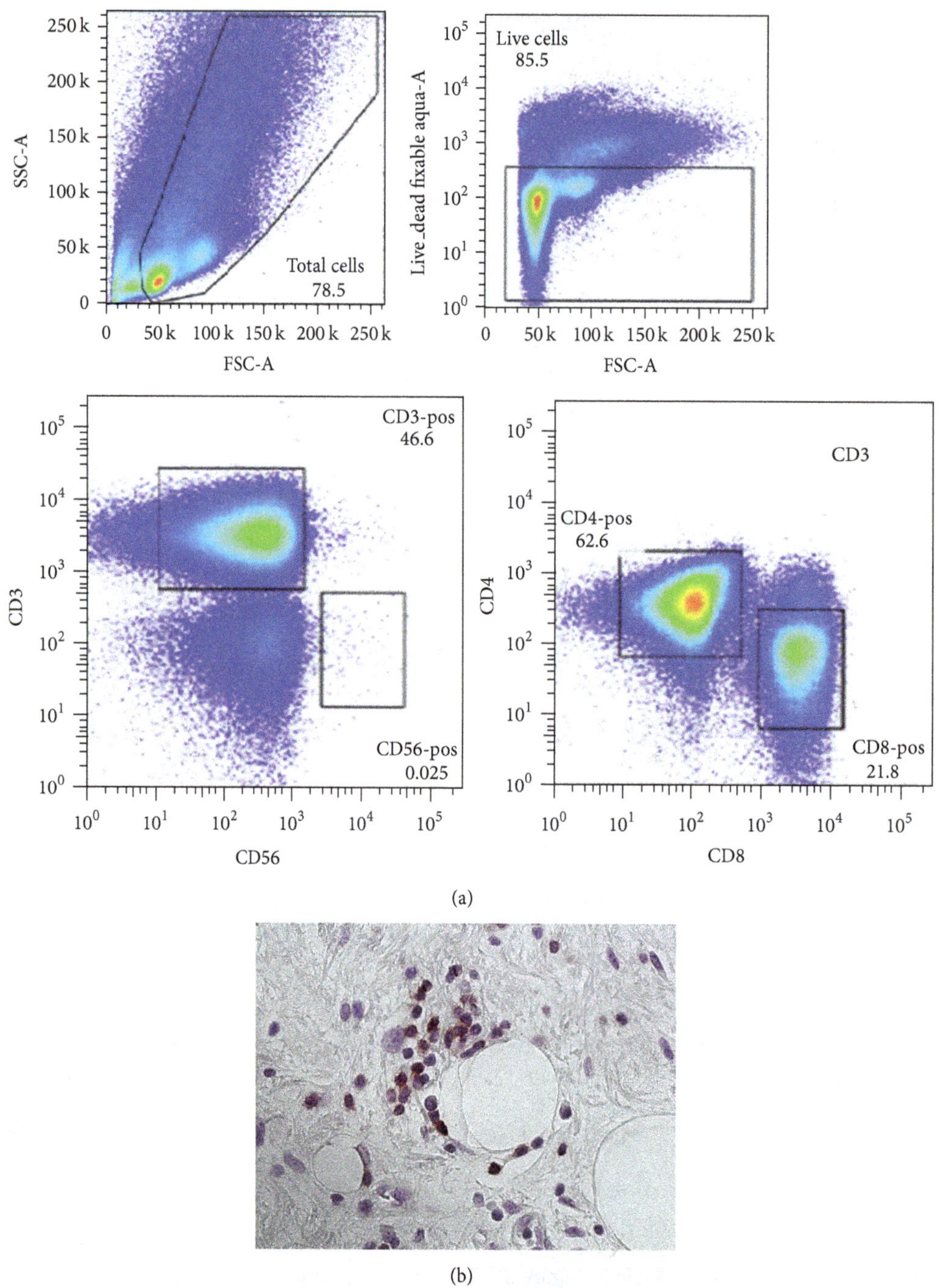

FIGURE 1: Tumor-infiltrating lymphocytes or TILs in WD/DD retroperitoneal liposarcoma. (a) Representative analysis by flow cytometry with gating schema for identification of CD3, CD4, and CD8 T cells. (b) Immunohistochemistry demonstrating intratumoral presence of CD8 T cells (brown), 400x magnification.

of PD-1/4-1BB were seen when comparing histology (WD versus DD, higher grade) or disease status (primary versus recurrent) (Tables 1 and 2). In separate experiments, we were able to expand these tumor-infiltrating lymphocytes or TILs in vitro, from 300 to almost 2000-fold using IL-2 and standard methods established for melanoma (data not shown). Taken together, our data suggests that in WD/DD retroperitoneal liposarcoma, the T cells can traffic to the tumor microenvironment and have the capacity to proliferate but lack effective antitumor function, likely from deactivation.

Although we did not directly analyze PD-1 expression by immunohistochemistry, the presence of this marker on immune cells within WD/DD liposarcoma tumors has been confirmed in a published report [25] and recently in an abstract presentation [Pollack et al., CTOS 2014]. Both studies looked at immunohistochemical expression of PD-1 in a variety of soft tissue sarcomas, which included a small cohort

TABLE 1: Tumor-infiltrating lymphocytes or TILs in WD/DD retroperitoneal liposarcoma.

Case	Histology	Disease status	Preop chemo	Preop Rad. Tx	Tumor size (g)	%CD4/%CD8
1	WD	R	N	N	12	61/31
2	WD	P	N	N	13	64/26
3	WD	R	N	N	2	71/28
4	WD	R	N	N	11	69/8
5	WD	R	N	N	2	57/12
6	DD	R	Y	N	6	63/22
7	DD	R	N	N	6	72/11
8	DD	P	Y	N	6	69/19

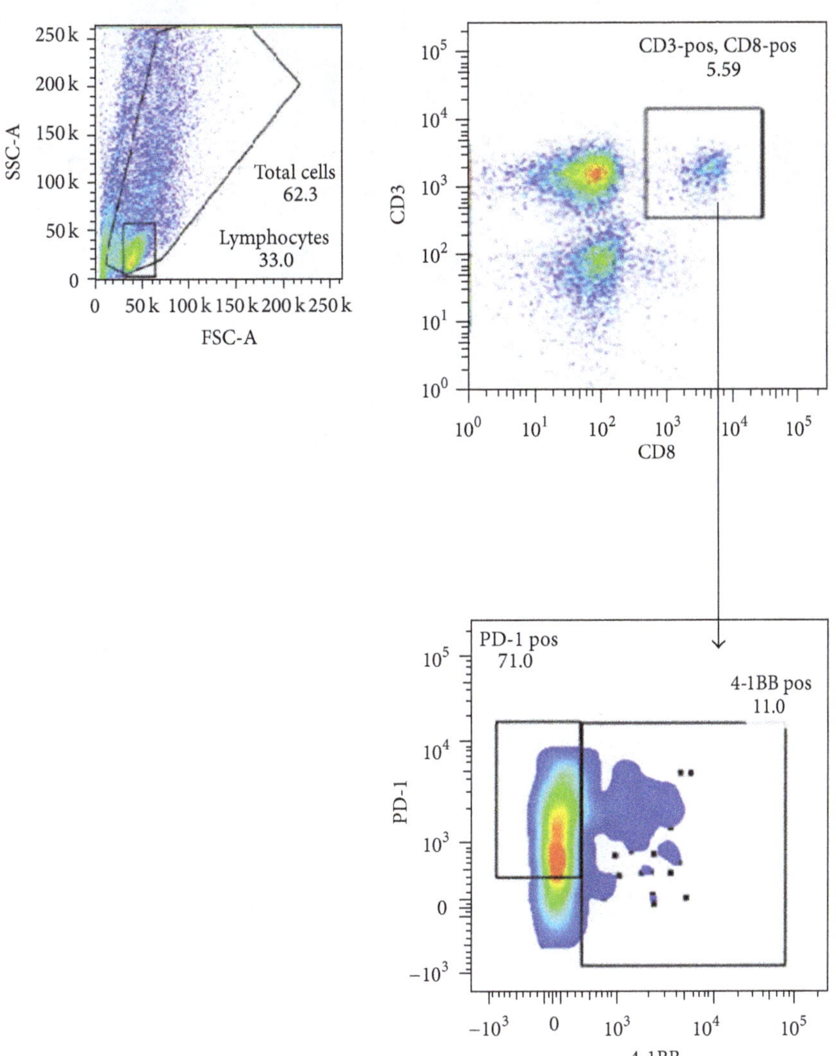

FIGURE 2: Expression of PD-1 and 4-1BB among the TIL CD8 population.

of liposarcoma cases. Our study is the first, to our knowledge, to demonstrate expression of this marker by flow cytometric analysis.

The etiology for cytotoxic CD8 T cell deactivation is unknown and likely multifactorial. The majority of the T cell population found in liposarcoma tumors are actually CD4 "helper" T cells. Intracellular staining with FoxP3 was positive in only a few, isolated cells (data not shown) suggesting that immunosuppressive, regulatory T cells are actually rare in the tumor microenvironment for WD/DD retroperitoneal liposarcoma. Other immunosuppressive cell types including myeloid derived suppressor cells or MDSCs and tumor-associated macrophages, however, likely also exist in the tumor microenvironment and are currently being

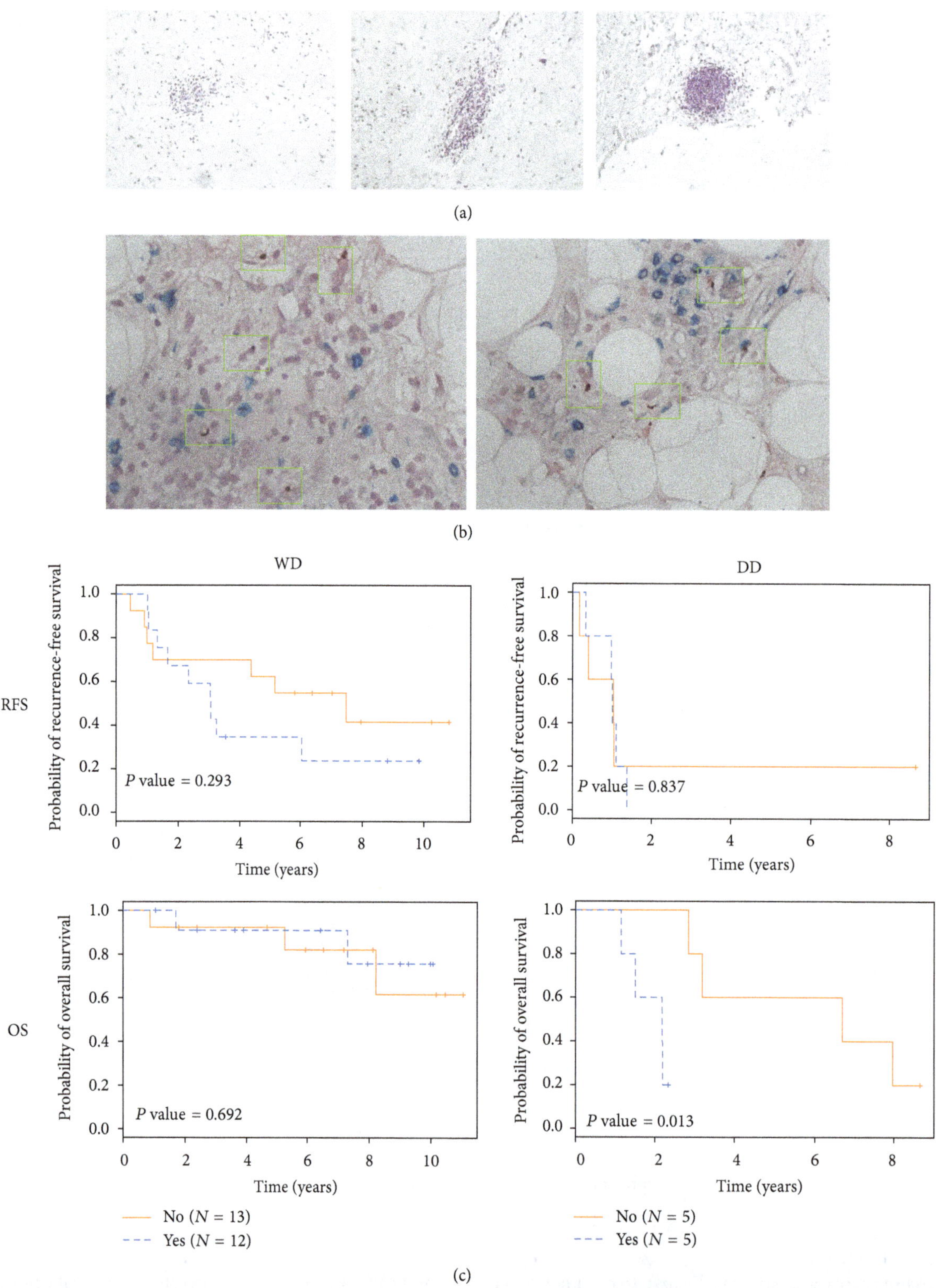

FIGURE 3: Intratumoral tertiary lymphoid structures (TLS) in WD/DD retroperitoneal liposarcoma. (a) General histologic appearance of TLS with varying levels of complexity and size, 100x magnification. (b) Immunohistochemistry for DC-LAMP (brown dots), a marker for mature dendritic cells, CD4 (red) and CD8 (green). Green boxes denote areas with DC-LAMP positive cells. 400x magnification. (c) Clinical outcome for patients with and without intratumoral TLS with recurrence-free survival (RFS) and overall survival (OS) shown.

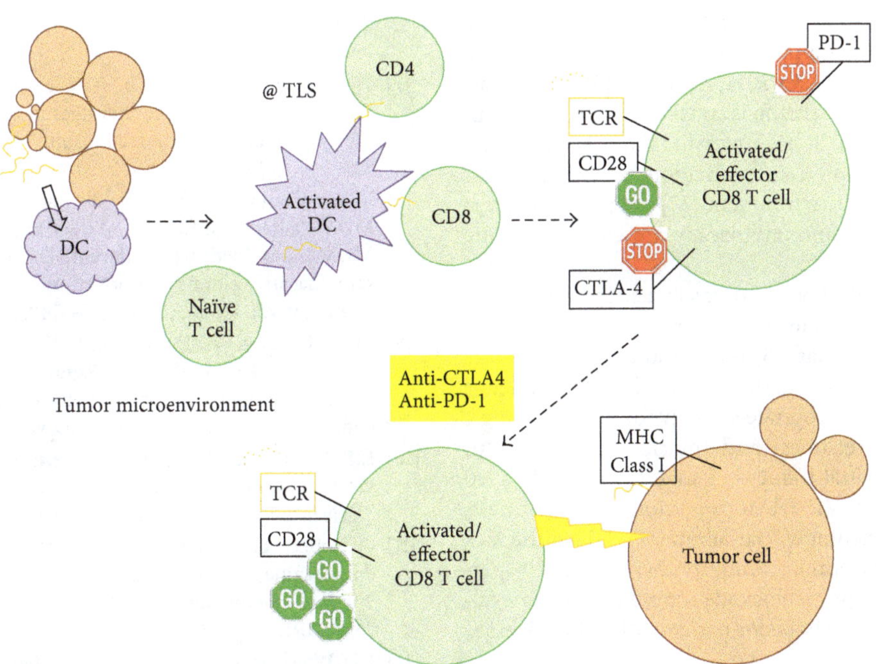

FIGURE 4: Summary of the intratumoral adaptive immune response in WD/DD retroperitoneal liposarcoma and the potential clinical utility of immune checkpoint blockade. Brown circles = tumor cell, yellow squiggle = tumor antigen, purple shapes = dendritic cell (DC), and green circles = T cell; TLS = tertiary lymphoid structure; TCR = T cell receptor; MHC = major histocompatibility complex.

TABLE 2: Expression of PD-1 and 4-1BB among the TIL CD8 population.

Histology	Disease status	% PD-1 (of CD8)	% 4-1BB (of CD8)
WD	P	73	3
DD	R	71	11
WD	R	61	11
WD	R	61	19
WD	P	57	5

investigated. A variety of tumor-derived factors both soluble (e.g., cytokines - IL-10, TGF-beta) and on the cell surface (e.g., PD-L1) may also lead to deactivation of CD8 T cells and remain to be defined.

Tertiary lymphoid structures or TLS may further hinder the antitumor response in WD/DD retroperitoneal liposarcoma. TLS have been described in non-small cell lung cancer, colorectal cancer, and melanoma and are likely intratumoral sites of antigen presentation or "ectopic" lymph nodes [26–28]. In liposarcoma, this concept is also supported by our observation of DC-LAMP positive, mature dendritic cells juxtaposed next to CD4 T cells (Figure 3(b)). In contrast to published reports in other solid tumors, our preliminary data suggest that, in liposarcoma, TLS may possibly be associated with worse clinical outcome. This data is limited by the relatively small number of cases studied and may be affected by sampling error with the sections of tumor that were available to us for TLS analysis. Nonetheless, our findings lead to the hypothesis that antigen presentation may be different on a cellular or cytokine level in liposarcoma versus other solid tumors. We observed varying levels of "architectural maturity" with TLS in liposarcoma (Figure 3(a)); given the typically large size of these tumors, perhaps TLS have evolved from antitumor to more protumor during the course of tumor growth. Alternatively, as liposarcomas have very few and inconsistent mutations in contrast to melanoma or lung cancer [29, 30], TLS in liposarcoma may be sites of antigen presentation against nonmutated antigens for which tolerance mechanisms are likely to exist. Finally, WD/DD liposarcoma does not disseminate to regional lymph nodes and having intratumoral TLS as potentially the only site antigen presentation may somehow negatively affect the antitumor immune response. Further studies with larger sample sizes are needed to validate our findings and explore these hypotheses.

From a treatment standpoint, our findings provide strong rationale to further evaluate the therapeutic potential of immunotherapy in WD/DD retroperitoneal liposarcoma. Immune checkpoint blockade (e.g., anti-CTLA4 or anti-PD-1) is particularly attractive as this can reactivate cytotoxic CD8 T cells, already sensitized to tumor antigen. The existence of an infiltrate of these immune cells within tumors puts WD/DD liposarcoma at an advantage in terms of potential for response to immune checkpoint blockade [31]. One potential biomarker to predict treatment response is PD-L1, the ligand for PD-1, found on tumor cells and antigen presenting cells [15]. In the current study, we did not analyze PD-L1 expression; however this data has been recently reported in soft tissue sarcoma [25]. Among the liposarcoma cases, 2 out of 4 (50%) WD and 2 out of 3 (67%) DD tumors expressed PD-L1 by immunohistochemistry. Other investigators have presented data in liposarcoma, thus far only in abstract form, showing the full spectrum of tumor PD-L1 expression from zero [D'Angelo et al., ASCO 2014] to 100% [Movva et al., ASCO 2014]. This wide variation is consistent with a previous report in melanoma which has suggested that PD-L1 expression fluctuates in relation to inflammation and other factors within the tumor microenvironment [32]. Other biomarkers for tumor response to immunotherapy are currently being explored.

We have summarized our findings in a schematic shown in Figure 4. Adaptive immune responses have been identified in other soft tissue sarcomas [33, 34]. Immunotherapy has the potential for efficacy in soft tissue sarcoma but the challenge will be to identify an appropriate strategy for each histologic subtype based on preclinical and translational data. Our results provide the initial framework to guide more detailed immunologic study in WD/DD retroperitoneal liposarcoma, which is currently ongoing in our laboratory. Given the lack of effective treatment options, immunotherapy and, in particular, immune checkpoint blockade should be further evaluated as it may offer new hope for patients with this disease.

Disclosure

This work was presented by William W. Tseng at the Connective Tissue Oncology Society 18th Annual Meeting, October 30 to November 2, 2013, in New York, NY. William W. Tseng and Raphael E. Pollock were previously affiliated with the Department of Surgical Oncology, The University of Texas MD Anderson Cancer Center, Houston, TX, USA. Laszlo Radvanyi was previously affiliated with the Department of Melanoma Medical Oncology, The University of Texas MD Anderson Cancer Center, Houston, TX, USA.

References

[1] M. A. Clark, C. Fisher, I. Judson, and J. M. Thomas, "Soft-tissue sarcomas in adults," *The New England Journal of Medicine*, vol. 353, no. 7, pp. 701–711, 2005.

[2] J.-M. Coindre, F. Pédeutour, and A. Aurias, "Well-differentiated and dedifferentiated liposarcomas," *Virchows Archiv*, vol. 456, no. 2, pp. 167–179, 2010.

[3] L. G. Dodd, "Update on liposarcoma: a review for cytopathologists," *Diagnostic Cytopathology*, vol. 40, no. 12, pp. 1122–1131, 2012.

[4] W. W. Tseng, B. W. Feig, D. C. Lev, and R. E. Pollock, "Surgery: chronic, primary treatment for well differentiated liposarcoma and a critical component of aggressive, multimodality treatment for dedifferentiated liposarcoma," in *Treatment Strategies—Oncology*, Cambridge Research Centre, London, UK, 2012.

[5] A. Hoffman, A. J. Lazar, R. E. Pollock, and D. Lev, "New frontiers in the treatment of liposarcoma, a therapeutically resistant malignant cohort," *Drug Resistance Updates*, vol. 14, no. 1, pp. 52–66, 2011.

[6] A. Italiano, M. Toulmonde, A. Cioffi et al., "Advanced well-differentiated/dedifferentiated liposarcomas: role of chemotherapy and survival," *Annals of Oncology*, vol. 23, no. 6, pp. 1601-1607, 2012.

[7] W. W. Tseng, N. Somaiah, A. J. Lazar, D. C. Lev, and R. E. Pollock, "Novel systemic therapies in advanced liposarcoma: a review of recent clinical trial results," *Cancers*, vol. 5, no. 2, pp. 529–549, 2013.

[8] I. Ray-Coquard, J.-Y. Blay, A. Italiano et al., "Effect of the MDM2 antagonist RG7112 on the P53 pathway in patients with MDM2-amplified, well-differentiated or dedifferentiated liposarcoma: an exploratory proof-of-mechanism study," *The Lancet Oncology*, vol. 13, no. 11, pp. 1133–1140, 2012.

[9] M. A. Dickson, W. D. Tap, M. L. Keohan et al., "Phase II trial of the CDK4 inhibitor PD0332991 in patients with advanced CDK4-amplified well-differentiated or dedifferentiated liposarcoma," *Journal of Clinical Oncology*, vol. 31, pp. 2024–2028, 2013.

[10] F. S. Hodi, S. J. O'Day, D. F. McDermott et al., "Improved survival with ipilimumab in patients with metastatic melanoma," *The New England Journal of Medicine*, vol. 363, pp. 711–723, 2010.

[11] C. Robert, L. Thomas, I. Bondarenko et al., "Ipilimumab plus dacarbazine for previously untreated metastatic melanoma," *The New England Journal of Medicine*, vol. 364, no. 26, pp. 2517–2526, 2011.

[12] J. D. Wolchok, H. Kluger, M. K. Callahan et al., "Nivolumab plus Ipilimumab in advanced melanoma," *The New England Journal of Medicine*, vol. 369, no. 2, pp. 122–133, 2013.

[13] O. Hamid, C. Robert, A. Daud et al., "Safety and tumor responses with lambrolizumab (anti-PD-1) in melanoma," *The New England Journal of Medicine*, vol. 369, no. 2, pp. 134–144, 2013.

[14] L. Calabrò, A. Morra, E. Fonsatti et al., "Tremelimumab for patients with chemotherapy-resistant advanced malignant mesothelioma: an open-label, single-arm, phase 2 trial," *The Lancet Oncology*, vol. 14, no. 11, pp. 1104–1111, 2013.

[15] S. L. Topalian, F. S. Hodi, J. R. Brahmer et al., "Safety, activity, and immune correlates of anti-PD-1 antibody in cancer," *The New England Journal of Medicine*, vol. 366, no. 26, pp. 2443–2454, 2012.

[16] S. M. Pollack, A. A. Jungbluth, B. L. Hoch et al., "NY-ESO-1 is a ubiquitous immunotherapeutic target antigen for patients with myxoid/round cell liposarcoma," *Cancer*, vol. 118, no. 18, pp. 4564–4570, 2012.

[17] M. E. Dudley, J. R. Wunderlich, T. E. Shelton, J. Even, and S. A. Rosenberg, "Generation of tumor-infiltrating lymphocyte cultures for use in adoptive transfer therapy for melanoma patients," *Journal of Immunotherapy*, vol. 26, no. 4, pp. 332–342, 2003.

[18] L. G. Radvanyi, C. Bernatchez, M. Zhang et al., "Specific lymphocyte subsets predict response to adoptive cell therapy using expanded autologous tumor-infiltrating lymphocytes in metastatic melanoma patients," *Clinical Cancer Research*, vol. 18, no. 24, pp. 6758–6770, 2012.

[19] W. W. Tseng, E. G. Demicco, A. J. Lazar, D. C. Lev, and R. E. Pollock, "Lymphocyte composition and distribution in inflammatory, well-differentiated retroperitoneal liposarcoma: clues to a potential adaptive immune response and therapeutic implications," *The American Journal of Surgical Pathology*, vol. 36, no. 6, pp. 941–944, 2012.

[20] P. Argani, F. Facchetti, G. Inghirami, and J. Rosai, "Lymphocyte-rich well-differentiated liposarcoma: report of nine cases," *The American Journal of Surgical Pathology*, vol. 21, no. 8, pp. 884–895, 1997.

[21] M. D. Kraus, L. Guillou, and C. D. M. Fletcher, "Well-differentiated inflammatory liposarcoma: an uncommon and easily

overlooked variant of a common sarcoma," *The American Journal of Surgical Pathology*, vol. 21, no. 5, pp. 518–527, 1997.

[22] T. Peng, P. Zhang, J. Liu et al., "An experimental model for the study of well-differentiated and dedifferentiated liposarcoma; deregulation of targetable tyrosine kinase receptors," *Laboratory Investigation*, vol. 91, no. 3, pp. 392–403, 2011.

[23] Z. Wang, L. Yang, Y. Jiang et al., "High fat diet induces formation of spontaneous liposarcoma in mouse adipose tissue with overexpression of interleukin 22," *PLoS ONE*, vol. 6, no. 8, Article ID e23737, 2011.

[24] A. Gros, P. F. Robbins, X. Yao et al., "PD-1 identifies the patient-specific $CD8^+$ tumor-reactive repertoire infiltrating human tumors," *The Journal of Clinical Investigation*, vol. 124, no. 5, pp. 2246–2259, 2014.

[25] J. R. Kim, Y. J. Moon, K. S. Kwon et al., "Tumor infiltrating PD1-positive lymphocytes and the expression of PD-L1 predict poor prognosis of soft tissue sarcomas," *PLoS ONE*, vol. 8, no. 12, Article ID e82870, 2013.

[26] M.-C. Dieu-Nosjean, M. Antoine, C. Danel et al., "Long-term survival for patients with non-small-cell lung cancer with intratumoral lymphoid structures," *Journal of Clinical Oncology*, vol. 26, no. 27, pp. 4410–4417, 2008.

[27] D. Coppola, M. Nebozhyn, F. Khalil et al., "Unique ectopic lymph node-like structures present in human primary colorectal carcinoma are identified by immune gene array profiling," *The American Journal of Pathology*, vol. 179, no. 1, pp. 37–45, 2011.

[28] J. L. Messina, D. A. Fenstermacher, S. Eschrich et al., "12-chemokine gene signature identifies lymph node-like structures in melanoma: potential for patient selection for immunotherapy?" *Scientific Reports*, vol. 2, article 765, 2012.

[29] J. Barretina, B. S. Taylor, S. Banerji et al., "Subtype-specific genomic alterations define new targets for soft-tissue sarcoma therapy," *Nature Genetics*, vol. 42, no. 8, pp. 715–721, 2010.

[30] B. S. Taylor, P. L. DeCarolis, C. V. Angeles et al., "Frequent alterations and epigenetic silencing of differentiation pathway genes in structurally rearranged liposarcomas," *Cancer Discovery*, vol. 1, no. 7, pp. 587–597, 2011.

[31] R.-R. Ji, S. D. Chasalow, L. Wang et al., "An immune-active tumor microenvironment favors clinical response to ipilimumab," *Cancer Immunology, Immunotherapy*, vol. 61, no. 7, pp. 1019–1031, 2012.

[32] J. M. Taube, R. A. Anders, G. D. Young et al., "Colocalization of inflammatory response with B7-H1 expression in human melanocytic lesions supports an adaptive resistance mechanism of immune escape," *Science Translational Medicine*, vol. 4, no. 127, Article ID 127ra37, 2012.

[33] S. P. D'Angelo, W. D. Tap, G. K. Schwartz, and R. D. Carvajal, "Sarcoma immunotherapy: past approaches and future directions," *Sarcoma*, vol. 2014, Article ID 391967, 13 pages, 2014.

[34] W. W. Tseng, N. Somaiah, and E. G. Engleman, "Potential for immunotherapy in soft tissue sarcoma," *Human Vaccines & Immunotherapeutics*. In press.

17

Evaluation of Quality of Life at Progression in Patients with Soft Tissue Sarcoma

Stacie Hudgens,[1] Anna Forsythe,[2] Ilias Kontoudis,[3] David D'Adamo,[2] Ashley Bird,[4] and Hans Gelderblom[5]

[1]*Clinical Outcomes Solutions, Tucson, AZ, USA*
[2]*Purple Squirrel Economics, New York, NY, USA*
[3]*Eisai Ltd., Hertfordshire, UK*
[4]*UT Southwestern Medical Center, Dallas, TX, USA*
[5]*Department of Medical Oncology, Leiden University Medical Center, Leiden, Netherlands*

Correspondence should be addressed to Stacie Hudgens; stacie.hudgens@clinoutsolutions.com

Academic Editor: Peter C. Ferguson

Introduction. Soft Tissue Sarcoma (STS) is a rare malignancy of mesodermal tissue, with international incidence estimates between 1.8 and 5 per 100,000 per year. Understanding quality of life (QoL) and the detrimental impact of disease progression is critical for long-term care and survival. *Objectives.* The primary objective was to explore the relationship between disease progression and health-related quality of life (HRQoL) using data from Eisai's study (E7389-G000-309). *Methods.* This was a 1:1 randomized, open-label, multicenter, Phase 3 study comparing the efficacy and safety of eribulin versus dacarbazine in patients with advanced STS. The QoL analysis was conducted for the baseline and progression populations using the European Organization for Research and Treatment of Cancer 30-item core QoL questionnaire (EORTC QLQ-C30). *Results.* There were no statistical differences between the two treatment arms at baseline for any domain ($p > 0.05$; $n = 452$). Of the 399 patients who experienced disease progression (unadjusted and adjusting for histology), dacarbazine patients had significantly lower Global Health Status, Physical Functioning scores, and significantly worse Nausea and Vomiting, Insomnia, and Appetite Loss ($p < 0.05$). *Conclusions.* These results indicate differences in HRQoL overall and at progression between dacarbazine and eribulin patients, with increases in symptom severity observed among dacarbazine patients.

1. Introduction

Soft Tissue Sarcoma (STS) is a rare malignancy of mesodermal tissue, with international incidence estimates between 1.8 and 5 per 100,000 per year [1]. Data from the Surveillance Epidemiology and End Results (SEER) database suggest that, despite low overall incidence, incidence is positively correlated with increases in age and is estimated to be as high as 18.2 cases per 100,00 among adults over the age of 70.2 years. Patients with STS account for approximately 0.7% of all new cancer cases and roughly 0.8% of all cancer deaths [2]. The rate of new STS diagnoses has increased steadily over time, with an average yearly increase of 1.8% between 2002 and 2012 [2]. The American Cancer Society estimates that 12,310 new cases of STS will be diagnosed in the United States (US) in 2016.

The 5-year overall survival estimate for STS is 64.9%, though this varies considerably between various staging levels. Exactly 81.4% of patients diagnosed with localized STS survive to year 5 compared to 17.3% among those diagnosed with metastatic STS. A 20-year longitudinal study discovered that 5-year survival rates increased by 28% in the period from 1992 to 2012, with improved detection and efficacy of radiotherapy listed as potential sources of the improvement [3].

Surgery is usually the initial management strategy for localized STS. Postoperative radiotherapy is encouraged in the National Comprehensive Cancer Network treatment guidelines for patients with STS to limit the rate of local recurrence and improve the progression-free survival (PFS). Even in cases in which optimal localized treatment was achieved, distant metastases occurred in many patients with STS, especially those with high-grade tumors. Studies examining the effect of adjuvant chemotherapy have produced equivocal results, and despite its wide use in the treatment of unresectable locally advanced or metastatic disease, a majority of patients ultimately relapsed such that overall survival was not affected [4].

For advanced STS, anthracyclines are considered the first-line therapy, with doxorubicin being prescribed most often for the systemic treatment of STS. Response rates exceeding 20% have been reported with doxorubicin alone or in combination with ifosfamide. However, the median survival of patients with metastatic STS has not improved beyond 12 months [5].

The standard second-line therapy in STS patients following failure of doxorubicin and ifosfamide is not defined. Some agents including pazopanib, gemcitabine, taxanes, trabectedin, and dacarbazine have shown promising activity. In addition, increasing evidence for "histology-tailored chemotherapy" has been observed in the last few years. However, recent evidence suggests that the combination of epirubicin and ifosfamide, regardless of the underlying histology, is superior to the selected histology-driven chemotherapy regimens [6–8]. Therefore, an understanding of the chemosensitivity of STS may result in more individualized treatment options. Recently, eribulin has been included also in an European Organization for Research and Treatment Cancer (EORTC) Phase 2 study of patients with STS and has been approved by the FDA for the treatment of liposarcomas [4, 9]. Accordingly, the quality of life (QoL) of STS patients has become an increasingly important endpoint of clinical trials for drug development and evaluation.

Several studies have been published indicating that STS and its treatment negatively impact patient health-related quality of life (HRQoL). Studies evaluating the impact of pre- and post-radiative surgery outcomes among patients with STS suggest that the magnitude of surgery-related impairment explained 54% of the decline in HRQoL, while participation restrictions (the ability to participate in activities with friends and families) explained 61% of the variation in HRQoL [10]. Other studies using the European Organization for Research and Treatment of Cancer 30-item core QoL questionnaire (EORTC QLQ-C30) indicate that disease progression is associated with a 30.26-point decline in Global Health Status [11]. When taken as a whole, these data suggest that differences between treatments on HRQoL impact are of potential utility when selecting a treatment regime for patients.

Understanding QoL/HRQoL and the detrimental impact of disease progression is critical for long-term care and survival and has become an increasingly important endpoint of clinical trials for drug development and evaluation. Therefore, QoL/HRQoL are our priority in the palliative care of all tumor patients, where curative treatment is no longer possible.

2. Objectives

The primary objective of this analysis was to explore the relationship between disease progression and HRQoL using patient-reported outcome data from Eisai's study E7389-G000-309 "A Randomized, Open-label, Multicenter, Phase 3 Study to Compare the Efficacy and Safety of Eribulin with Dacarbazine in Patients with Soft Tissue Sarcoma." Specifically, the purpose was twofold: (1) to identify differences in functional outcomes and symptom severity between eribulin and dacarbazine with respect to histology and (2) to determine the extent to which disease progression is associated with changes in HRQoL among patients with advanced or metastatic STS.

3. Methods

3.1. Study Design. This was a 1:1 randomized, open-label, multicenter, Phase 3 study comparing the efficacy and safety of eribulin (Treatment Arm A) versus dacarbazine (Treatment Arm B) in approximately 450 patients with advanced STS (either liposarcoma or leiomyosarcoma) at approximately 110 study sites globally. The entire study consisted of three consecutive phases: Prerandomization, Randomization, and an Optional Extension. All protocol deviations were reviewed and determined prior to database lock by the study director, the study statistician, the study data manager, and the study clinical operations manager. The review was conducted in a blinded manner without looking into subject treatment code or efficacy data.

The Prerandomization phase was no longer than 21 days and included two periods: screening (Day −21 to Day −2) and baseline (Day −1). During the Prerandomization phase, patients' eligibility and baseline data including demographics (age, gender, and race/ethnicity), New York Heart Association (NYHA) functional classification, Eastern Cooperative Oncology Group (ECOG) performance status, STS-specific screening assessments (diagnosis length, STS history and tumor grade, and pathological tumor node metastasis stage at diagnosis), and past treatment history data (surgical, medical, and radiation therapy) were examined or collected.

At Randomization (Day 0), the allocation of randomization numbers was performed using an interactive voice/web response system vendor based upon the following stratification factors: (a) histology (either liposarcoma or leiomyosarcoma), (b) region [Region 1: US and Canada; Region 2: Western Europe, Australia, and Israel; or Region 3: Eastern Europe, Latin America, and Asia], and (c) number of prior treatment regimens for advanced STS (≥ 2).

The randomization and extension phases each consisted of two periods: a treatment cycle and a follow-up period. A summary of each phase is provided in Figure 1.

3.2. Inclusion/Exclusion Criteria. The enrolled patients with STS were not responsive to surgery and/or radiotherapy and had disease progression within 6 months of randomization. The patients had measurable disease according to the Response Evaluation Criteria in Solid Tumors version 1.1

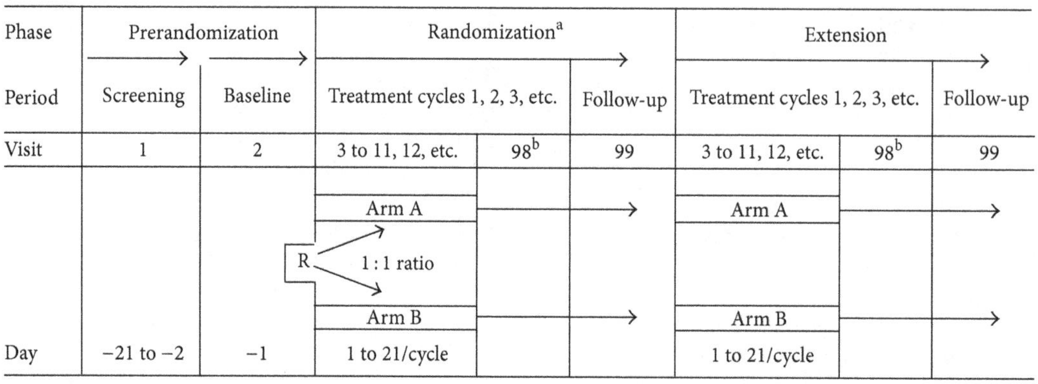

Phase	Prerandomization		Randomization[a]			Extension		
Period	Screening	Baseline	Treatment cycles 1, 2, 3, etc.		Follow-up	Treatment cycles 1, 2, 3, etc.		Follow-up
Visit	1	2	3 to 11, 12, etc.	98[b]	99	3 to 11, 12, etc.	98[b]	99
			Arm A		→	Arm A		→
			R: 1 : 1 ratio					
			Arm B		→	Arm B		→
Day	−21 to −2	−1	1 to 21/cycle			1 to 21/cycle		

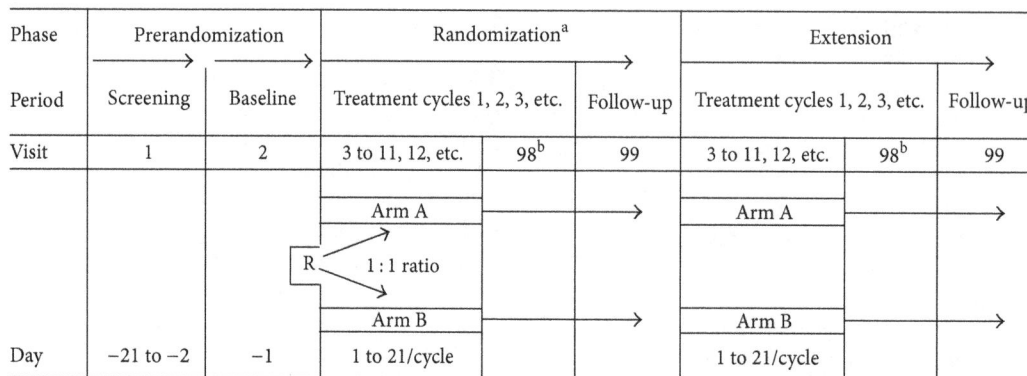

FIGURE 1: R: randomization. Arm A: eribulin mesylate 1.4 mg/m^2 IV on Days 1 and 8, every 21 days. Arm B: dacarbazine IV on Day 1, every 21 days. The starting dose must be selected from one of the following doses: 850 mg/m^2, 1,000 mg/m^2, or 1,200 mg/m^2. [a]The randomization phase will end at the time of data cut-off for the primary analysis when the target number of events has been observed. All subjects still on treatment with study treatment or in survival follow-up will then enter the extension phase. [b]Off-treatment visit.

(RECIST 1.1), with the modification that a chest X-ray could not be used for the assessment of chest lesions.

3.3. Analysis Populations. The analysis baseline population included all patients with available baseline data. Patients that did not meet all of the inclusion criteria or that met any of the exclusion criteria of the E7389-G000-309 clinical study were not eligible to receive study treatment. The analysis progression population included patients who met the criteria for disease progression. This schedule for tumor assessments was maintained irrespective of treatment delays.

3.4. Clinical Outcome Assessments. The QLQ-C30 consists of 30 questions that address five functional domains (Physical, Role, Cognitive, Emotional, and Social domains), nine symptom scales (Fatigue, Pain, Nausea and Vomiting, Dyspnea, Appetite Loss, Sleep Disturbance, Constipation, Diarrhea, and Financial Difficulties), and one global QoL scale. Items 29 (overall health) and 30 (overall QoL) are scaled from 1 "very poor" to 7 "excellent." All scale scores are transformed to a range of 0 to 100, with higher scale scores representing a higher response level.

3.5. Schedule of Assessments. The QLQ-C30 was administered at baseline, on Day 1 of each treatment cycle, and at the last visit of the randomization phase. Baseline questionnaires were completed in the clinic prior to randomization. Subsequent questionnaires were completed in the clinic before any study-related procedures for that visit and before tumor assessment results were communicated to the patient. Study patients were asked to complete questionnaires at each clinic visit, even if they had declined previously. Compliance was assessed by counting completed questionnaires.

The disease progression was determined during scheduled tumor assessments and was evaluated using the RECIST 1.1 progression criteria every 6 weeks from the date of randomization during the first 12 weeks and every 9 weeks thereafter or sooner, if clinically indicated, until disease progression was confirmed by investigator histology.

The schedule for tumor assessments was maintained irrespective of treatment delays.

4. Statistical Methods

Quality of life analysis was conducted for both the baseline and progression populations. Two different analyses were conducted: one adjusted for histology and treatment while the other adjusted for treatment only.

For the primary analysis, results were stratified by planned treatment and histology type (leiomyosarcoma versus liposarcoma). Statistically significant differences between treatment arms were evaluated by performing a multifactor analysis of variance (ANOVA) for the progression population. The two-way ANOVA was specified using planned treatment, histology type, and their interaction term as factors. Adjusted means and standard deviation (SD) of each respective domain score were reported for the baseline population at baseline and progression population at the time of progression.

For the secondary analysis, results were stratified by planned treatment and histology type. Statistically significant differences between treatment arms were evaluated by performing an ANOVA for each population. Adjusted means and SD of each respective domain score were reported for the baseline population at baseline and for the progression population at the time of progression. For both analyses, a p value of less than 0.05 was considered statistically significant.

Though change from baseline to time of progression was not conducted in this analysis due to the difference in sample size, it is important to note that a change greater than 10 points is considered meaningful for all EORTC functional domains and symptom scales [12].

5. Results

5.1. Descriptive Analysis. A total of 452 patients were randomized and included in the full analysis set (228 patients in the eribulin arm and 224 patients in the dacarbazine arm). All patients were between 24 and 83 years of age (n = 442

TABLE 1: Patients' baseline characteristics of cross-sectional population for QoL analysis.

Demographic items	Eribulin (n = 223)	DAC (n = 219)	Total (n = 442)	p value[1]
Age (years)				
n	223	219	442	
Mean (SD)	55.5 (11.09)	55.7 (10.46)	55.6 (10.77)	0.263
Median	56.0	56.0	56.0	
Min, Max	28.0, 83.0	24.0, 83.0	24.0, 83.0	
Gender				
Male	65 (29.1%)	79 (36.1%)	144 (32.6%)	0.120
Female	158 (70.9%)	140 (63.9%)	298 (67.4%)	
Race				
White	158 (70.9%)	164 (74.9%)	322 (72.9%)	
Black or African American	6 (2.7%)	6 (2.7%)	12 (2.7%)	
Japanese	1 (0.4%)	0 (0.0%)	1 (0.2%)	
Chinese	2 (0.9%)	1 (0.5%)	3 (0.7%)	0.865
Other Asian	15 (6.7%)	15 (6.8%)	30 (6.8%)	
Native Hawaiian or other Pacific Islander	1 (0.4%)	0 (0.0%)	1 (0.2%)	
Other	6 (2.7%)	4 (1.8%)	10 (2.3%)	
Missing	33 (15.2%)	29 (13.2%)	63 (14.3%)	
Region				
USA and Canada	85 (38.1%)	84 (38.4%)	169 (38.2%)	
Western Europe, Australasia, and Israel	104 (46.6%)	102 (46.6%)	206 (46.6%)	0.998
Eastern Europe, Latin America, and Asia	34 (15.2%)	33 (15.1%)	67 (15.2%)	
ECOG PS				
n	223	219	442	
Mean (SD)	0.5 (0.53)	0.7 (0.58)	0.6 (0.56)	0.661
Median	1.0	1.0	1.0	
Min, Max	0.0, 2.0	0.0, 2.0	0.0, 2.0	
NYHA				
Class I	144 (64.6%)	130 (59.4%)	274 (62.0%)	0.353
Class II	15 (6.7%)	19 (8.7%)	34 (7.7%)	
Prior regimens				
Number of prior regimens for advanced STS: 2	120 (53.8%)	120 (54.8%)	240 (54.3%)	0.836
Number of prior regimens for advanced STS: >2	103 (46.2%)	99 (45.2%)	202 (45.7%)	
Histology/cytology				
Liposarcoma	70 (31.4%)	71 (32.4%)	140 (31.9%)	0.816
Leiomyosarcoma	153 (68.6%)	148 (67.6%)	301 (68.1%)	

CSP, cross-sectional population; DAC, dacarbazine; ECOG PS, Eastern Cooperative Oncology Group Performance Status; NYHA, New York Heart Association; SD, standard deviation; STS, soft tissue sarcoma.
Of note, of the 452 patients randomized, only 442 patients (223 patients in the eribulin treatment arm and 219 patients in the DAC treatment arm) were included in the cross-sectional population (defined as any full analysis set patient with at least one item of QLQ-C30 or EQ-5D questionnaire at the time of randomization).
[1]From t-test on continuous variable or Chi-square test on categorical variables.

patients; mean [SD] age: 55.6 [10.77] years), male (n = 144 [32.6%] patients), white (n = 322 [72.9%] patients), from the US and Canada (169 [38.2%] patients), and of NYHA class I (n = 274 [62.0%] patients). There were higher percentages of patients with leiomyosarcoma than those with liposarcoma in the study (68.1% leiomyosarcoma versus 31.9% liposarcoma) overall and by treatment arm (see Table 1 for further details).

5.2. Baseline Results. At baseline, there were no statistical differences between the two treatment arms for any of the EORTC QLQ-C30 global health score and functioning domains ($p > 0.05$). Overall, patients had better Cognitive Functioning compared to the other domains (overall mean [SD] score of 84.2 [20.43]), but worse Global Health Status (mean [SD]: 65.1 [22.20]). The other functional domains

Table 2: Adjusted mean values at baseline and progression stratified by treatment.

Domain	Time point	Eribulin Mean (SD) BL $N = 228$ PD $N = 208$	DAC Mean (SD) BL $N = 224$ PD $N = 191$	Overall Mean (SD) BL $N = 452$ PD $N = 399$	p value
Global health score and functioning					
Global Health Status	Baseline	65.2 (23.49)	64.9 (20.63)	65.1 (22.10)	0.900
	Progression	62.1 (23.32)	56.1 (21.85)	59.3 (22.81)	0.008*
Physical Functioning	Baseline	76.6 (22.74)	76.5 (20.37)	76.6 (21.57)	0.970
	Progression	73.3 (22.69)	65.8 (26.35)	69.7 (24.77)	0.002*
Role Functioning	Baseline	74.0 (28.70)	74.2 (25.96)	74.1 (27.35)	0.925
	Progression	65.0 (32.95)	58.7 (31.61)	62.0 (32.43)	0.054
Emotional Functioning	Baseline	75.5 (21.73)	74.0 (22.72)	74.7 (22.21)	0.482
	Progression	71.7 (26.39)	69.4 (24.08)	70.6 (25.30)	0.365
Cognitive Functioning	Baseline	84.6 (19.49)	83.9 (21.39)	84.2 (20.43)	0.731
	Progression	81.0 (23.02)	78.7 (24.79)	79.1 (23.88)	0.337
Social Functioning	Baseline	71.7 (29.97)	73.3 (26.65)	72.5 (28.36)	0.554
	Progression	68.5 (29.59)	65.4 (28.94)	67.0 (29.29)	0.283
Symptoms Domains					
Fatigue	Baseline	31.4 (25.48)	32.0 (23.42)	31.7 (24.46)	0.788
	Progression	39.8 (26.29)	44.9 (28.38)	42.3 (27.39)	0.066
Nausea and Vomiting	Baseline	7.5 (15.02)	8.2 (18.05)	7.9 (16.58)	0.687
	Progression	7.8 (14.64)	13.7 (20.40)	10.7 (17.85)	0.001*
Pain	Baseline	26.6 (28.14)	30.5 (28.30)	28.5 (28.25)	0.149
	Progression	34.6 (29.89)	38.7 (30.87)	36.6 (30.39)	0.175
Dyspnea	Baseline	18.4 (24.89)	18.8 (25.16)	18.6 (24.99)	0.865
	Progression	22.2 (26.07)	27.4 (29.61)	24.7 (27.91)	0.064
Insomnia	Baseline	26.0 (28.02)	27.5 (29.10)	26.7 (28.54)	0.570
	Progression	26.7 (31.41)	33.2 (29.12)	29.8 (30.46)	0.035*
Appetite Loss	Baseline	16.8 (25.71)	18.3 (28.62)	17.6 (27.17)	0.555
	Progression	19.6 (27.26)	29.5 (32.58)	24.3 (30.30)	0.001*
Constipation	Baseline	17.6 (25.70)	15.0 (23.94)	16.3 (24.85)	0.276
	Progression	20.4 (27.36)	22.9 (28.11)	21.6 (27.72)	0.367
Diarrhea	Baseline	9.3 (19.89)	10.3 (21.79)	9.8 (20.83)	0.622
	Progression	13.4 (22.96)	10.3 (21.19)	11.9 (22.15)	0.168
Financial Difficulties	Baseline	24.3 (32.78)	25.7 (32.27)	25.0 (32.50)	0.669
	Progression	29.8 (35.87)	29.1 (32.35)	29.5 (34.19)	0.847

* indicates p values that are less than 0.05 and are considered statistically significant. DAC: dacarbazine.

(Physical, Role, Emotional, and Social) were comparable and had overall scores that ranged from 72.5 (28.36) to 76.6 (21.57) (Table 2).

In addition, overall patients had worse Fatigue (mean [SD]: 31.7 [24.46]), Pain (mean [SD]: 28.5 [28.25]), Insomnia (mean [SD]: 26.7 [28.54]), and Financial Difficulties (mean [SD]: 25.0 [32.50]) but better Nausea and Vomiting (mean [SD]: 7.9 [16.58]) and Diarrhea (mean [SD]: 9.8 [20.83]) compared to the other domains. All other mean symptom domains (Dyspnea, Appetite Loss, and Constipation) had scores that ranged from 16.3 (24.85) to 18.6 (24.99). When stratified by treatment arm, these results were not considered statistically different ($p > 0.05$) (Table 2).

When stratified by treatment and histology, no differences were observed between liposarcoma and leiomyosarcoma groups in either eribulin or dacarbazine patients for any of the EORTC QLQ-C30 domains (Table 3).

5.3. Quality of Life at Disease Progression. Of the 399 patients who experienced disease progression (both with and without adjusting for histology), dacarbazine patients had significantly lower Global Health Status ($p = 0.008$) and Physical Functioning scores ($p = 0.002$) compared to patients treated with eribulin at the time of progression. In addition, patients treated with dacarbazine also had significantly worse Nausea and Vomiting ($p = 0.001$), Insomnia ($p = 0.035$), and

TABLE 3: Adjusted mean values at baseline and progression stratified by treatment and histology.

Domain/time point	Eribulin		DAC		p value
	Liposarcoma Mean (SD) BL $N = 71$ PD $N = 53$	Leiomyosarcoma Mean (SD) BL $N = 157$ PD $N = 156$	Liposarcoma Mean (SD) BL $N = 72$ PD $N = 49$	Leiomyosarcoma Mean (SD) BL $N = 152$ PD $N = 142$	
Global health score and functioning					
Global Health Status					
Baseline	64.6 (24.40)	65.5 (23.15)	64.6 (20.93)	65.1 (20.55)	—
Progression	61.3 (23.52)	62.4 (23.33)	57.5 (20.29)	55.6 (22.42)	0.008*
Physical Functioning					
Baseline	73.2 (25.76)	78.2 (21.12)	76.8 (21.53)	76.4 (19.87)	—
Progression	71.4 (24.33)	74.0 (22.15)	63.9 (28.93)	66.4 (25.48)	0.002*
Role Functioning					
Baseline	69.8 (31.61)	75.9 (27.18)	75.0 (26.28)	73.9 (25.89)	—
Progression	57.9 (36.63)	67.4 (31.34)	60.2 (29.82)	58.2 (32.30)	0.054
Emotional Functioning					
Baseline	73.1 (23.10)	76.6 (21.05)	73.0 (24.51)	74.4 (21.88)	—
Progression	73.1 (27.33)	71.2 (26.13)	69.9 (23.50)	69.2 (24.40)	0.366
Cognitive Functioning					
Baseline	84.8 (19.26)	84.4 (19.66)	83.1 (21.83)	84.2 (21.24)	—
Progression	82.4 (20.26)	80.5 (23.94)	77.6 (24.90)	79.1 (24.82)	0.338
Social Functioning					
Baseline	64.7 (33.52)	74.8 (27.78)	71.8 (27.69)	74.0 (26.20)	—
Progression	62.3 (35.98)	70.6 (26.87)	63.2 (29.06)	66.1 (28.96)	0.282
Symptom scales					
Fatigue					
Baseline	34.1 (27.44)	30.1 (24.53)	32.6 (25.98)	31.7 (22.14)	—
Progression	39.2 (28.46)	40.1 (25.61)	43.5 (28.03)	45.4 (28.58)	0.067
Nausea and Vomiting					
Baseline	8.2 (17.30)	7.2 (13.92)	8.9 (18.00)	7.8 (18.12)	—
Progression	7.2 (11.09)	8.1 (15.70)	12.9 (22.12)	14.1 (19.85)	0.001*
Pain					
Baseline	28.3 (31.09)	25.9 (26.77)	31.9 (26.88)	29.9 (29.03)	—
Progression	35.8 (30.03)	34.2 (29.92)	34.4 (24.86)	40.3 (32.63)	0.175
Dyspnea					
Baseline	16.9 (22.60)	19.1 (25.91)	19.2 (27.98)	18.6 (23.77)	—
Progression	22.0 (25.27)	22.3 (26.42)	35.4 (33.62)	24.6 (27.70)	0.063
Insomnia					
Baseline	24.2 (29.64)	26.8 (27.32)	24.4 (28.71)	29.0 (29.27)	—
Progression	30.8 (33.56)	25.4 (30.65)	28.6 (27.22)	34.7 (29.67)	0.035*
Appetite Loss					
Baseline	16.9 (25.96)	16.8 (25.68)	18.3 (29.70)	18.4 (28.18)	—
Progression	18.2 (24.95)	20.0 (28.07)	29.9 (32.09)	29.3 (32.85)	0.001*
Constipation					
Baseline	19.8 (30.42)	16.6 (23.30)	17.4 (26.94)	13.8 (22.36)	—
Progression	20.7 (25.51)	20.2 (28.04)	23.8 (27.22)	22.5 (28.50)	0.368
Diarrhea					
Baseline	10.6 (21.76)	8.7 (19.03)	12.2 (23.39)	9.4 (20.99)	—
Progression	13.8 (18.98)	13.2 (24.23)	11.6 (25.05)	9.9 (19.77)	0.169

Table 3: Continued.

Domain/time point	Eribulin Liposarcoma Mean (SD) BL $N = 71$ PD $N = 53$	Eribulin Leiomyosarcoma Mean (SD) BL $N = 157$ PD $N = 156$	DAC Liposarcoma Mean (SD) BL $N = 72$ PD $N = 49$	DAC Leiomyosarcoma Mean (SD) BL $N = 152$ PD $N = 142$	p value
Financial Difficulties					
Baseline	26.1 (34.24)	23.5 (32.19)	25.4 (33.08)	25.8 (31.99)	—
Progression	37.1 (42.70)	27.3 (33.00)	34.7 (33.99)	27.2 (31.67)	0.846

∗ indicates p values that are less than 0.05 and are considered statistically significant. DAC: dacarbazine.

Appetite Loss ($p = 0.001$) compared to patients treated with eribulin at the time of progression (see Table 2).

Though no analysis of change in Physical Functioning from baseline was conducted for the progression population due to the difference in sample size at baseline, it is important to note that there was a greater than 10-point decrease in Physical Functioning scores for both liposarcoma and leiomyosarcoma histology groups in the dacarbazine arm. Role Functioning scores also decreased for eribulin patients with liposarcoma histology and both liposarcoma and leiomyosarcoma histology groups in dacarbazine-treated patients. In addition, both liposarcoma and leiomyosarcoma histology groups of dacarbazine patients had differences greater than the published threshold of 10 points in Fatigue and Appetite Loss, while eribulin patients had greater than 10-point differences in Fatigue for those with leiomyosarcoma histology and Financial Difficulties for those with liposarcoma histology. Dacarbazine patients also had changes in Pain for those with leiomyosarcoma and Dyspnea for those with liposarcoma histology.

Regardless of histology, the patients had a greater than 10-point change in dacarbazine and overall scores (total population) in Role Functioning from baseline to progression. In addition, dacarbazine patients had a greater than 10-point increase in Fatigue and Appetite Loss, while in the total population (overall), there was a greater than 10-point increase in Fatigue (see Table 3).

These differences in the mean values for the given health state are greater than the published interpretation threshold of 10 points. This indicates that it is possible to observe clinically meaningful differences between health states and the observed statistical significance.

6. Conclusions

Disease progression appears to be a key health state for evaluating QoL in patients with sarcoma and potentially lending additional supportive information for understanding progression-free survival. Overall, this article brings statistically relevant HRQoL results during the time of disease progression between the dacarbazine and eribulin treatment arms in the Phase 3 study of advanced/metastatic sarcoma patients. Notably higher increases in symptom severity were observed among dacarbazine patients relative to patients in the eribulin treatment arm in the areas of Fatigue, Nausea and Vomiting, and Appetite Loss. Significant differences between treatment arms were also observed in the EORTC functional scales, with the patients in the eribulin treatment arm reporting significantly higher levels of Global Health Status and Physical Functioning.

Dacarbazine patients and overall (total population) scores had a greater than 10-point change in mean value in Role Functioning at progression. Dacarbazine patients also had a greater than 10-point increase in Fatigue and Appetite Loss, while, overall, there was a greater than 10-point increase in Fatigue.

When taken as a whole, the differences in the mean value for a given health state are greater than the published interpretation threshold of 10 points and indicate that it is possible to observe clinically meaningful differences between health states and the observed statistical significance as well as illustrate worsening health states observed in the dacarbazine treatment arm.

Understanding QoL in a palliative patient population is critical for appropriately addressing a patient's needs and treatment options. The shift from extending survival to delaying deterioration in patient-reported symptom, function, and HRQoL is critical and an important goal of palliative treatment. As such, evaluation and interpretation of results of studies similar to this study bring the possibility for better treatment decisions in the future for patients with (advanced) STS. The results presented in this study suggest that HRQoL is a relevant consideration when determining therapeutic pathways for patients with advanced STS and provides support for the evaluation of patient-reported outcomes at various health states such as early treatment, ongoing treatment (e.g., progression-free survival), and postprogression.

Disclosure

Anna Forsythe was formerly affiliated with Eisai Inc., Woodcliff Lake, NJ, USA; Ilias Kontoudis was formerly affiliated with Eisai Ltd., Hertfordshire, United Kingdom; Ashley Bird was formerly affiliated with Clinical Outcomes Solutions, Tucson, AZ, USA.

Acknowledgments

The authors are grateful to Jamie Carroll, Senior Medical Writer, Clinical Outcomes Solutions. The preliminary study results were presented previously at the American Society of Clinical Oncology (ASCO) in 2016 [13]. This study was funded by Eisai, Inc.

References

[1] C. Wibmer, A. Leithner, N. Zielonke, M. Sperl, and R. Windhager, "Increasing incidence rates of soft tissue sarcomas? A population-based epidemiologic study and literature review," *Annals of Oncology*, vol. 21, no. 5, pp. 1106–1111, 2009.

[2] N. Howlader, A. M. Noone, M. Krapcho et al., *SEER Cancer Statistics Review, 1975–2012*, National Cancer Institute, Bethesda, Md, USA, 2015.

[3] *Cancer Facts & Figures 2016*, American Cancer Society, 2016.

[4] A. J. Jacobs, R. Michels, J. Stein, and A. S. Levin, "Improvement in overall survival from extremity soft tissue sarcoma over twenty years," *Sarcoma*, vol. 2015, Article ID 279601, 9 pages, 2015.

[5] National Comprehensive Cancer Network, *Practice Guidelines in Oncology*, 2016.

[6] M. Eriksson, "Histology-driven chemotherapy of soft-tissue sarcoma," *Annals of Oncology*, vol. 21, supplement 7, pp. vii270–vii276, 2010.

[7] A. Gronchi, S. Ferrari, V. Quagliuolo et al., "Full-dose neoadjuvant anthracycline+ ifosfamide chemotherapy is associated with a relapse free survival (RFS) and overall survival (OS) benefit in localized high-risk adult soft tissue sarcomas (STS) of the extremities and trunk wall: interim analysis of a prospective randomized trial," *Annals of Oncology*, vol. 27, supplement 6, article LBA6, 2016.

[8] R. Petrioli, A. Coratti, P. Correale et al., "Adjuvant epirubicin with or without ifosfamide for adult soft-tissue sarcoma," *American Journal of Clinical Oncology*, vol. 25, no. 5, pp. 468–473, 2002.

[9] P. Schoffski, I. L. Ray-Coquard, A. Cioffi et al., "Activity of eribulin mesylate (E7389) in patients with soft tissue sarcoma (STS): Phase II studies of the European Organisation for Research and Treatment of Cancer Soft Tissue and Bone Sarcoma Group (EORTC 62052)," *Journal of Clinical Oncology*, vol. 28, no. 15, pp. 10031–10031, 2010.

[10] D. Schreiber, R. S. Bell, J. S. Wunder et al., "Evaluating function and health related quality of life in patients treated for extremity soft tissue sarcoma," *Quality of Life Research*, vol. 15, no. 9, pp. 1439–1446, 2006.

[11] P. Reichardt, M. Leahy, X. Garcia del Muro et al., "Quality of life and utility in patients with metastatic soft tissue and bone sarcoma: the sarcoma treatment and burden of illness in North America and Europe (SABINE) study," *Sarcoma*, vol. 2012, Article ID 740279, 11 pages, 2012.

[12] M. T. King, "The interpretation of scores from the EORTC quality of life questionnaire QLQ-C30," *Quality of Life Research*, vol. 5, no. 6, pp. 555–567, 1996.

[13] S. Hudgens, A. Forsythe, I. Kontoudis, D. D'Adamo, A. Bird, and H. Gelderblom, "Evaluation of quality of life at progression in patients with soft tissue sarcoma," *Journal of Clinical Oncology*, vol. 34, abstract 11015, 2016.

18

Malignant Peripheral Nerve Sheath Tumors State of the Science: Leveraging Clinical and Biological Insights into Effective Therapies

AeRang Kim,[1] Douglas R. Stewart,[2] Karlyne M. Reilly,[3] David Viskochil,[4] Markku M. Miettinen,[5] and Brigitte C. Widemann[6]

[1]*Center for Cancer and Blood Disorders, Children's National Health System, 111 Michigan Ave NW, Washington, DC 20010, USA*
[2]*Clinical Genetics Branch, Division of Cancer Epidemiology and Genetics, National Cancer Institute, 9609 Medical Center Drive, Room 6E450, Bethesda, MD 20892, USA*
[3]*Rare Tumors Initiative, OD, CCR, National Cancer Institute, 37 Convent Drive, Bethesda, MD 20814, USA*
[4]*University of Utah, 295 Chipeta Way, Salt Lake City, UT 84108, USA*
[5]*Center for Cancer Research, National Cancer Institute, 10 Center Drive, Room 2S235C, Building 10, Bethesda, MD 20892, USA*
[6]*National Cancer Institute, Pediatric Oncology Branch, 10 Center Drive, Room 1-3742, Building 10, Bethesda, MD 20892, USA*

Correspondence should be addressed to AeRang Kim; aekim@childrensnational.org

Academic Editor: Alexander Lazar

Malignant peripheral nerve sheath tumor (MPNST) is the leading cause of mortality in patients with neurofibromatosis type 1. In 2002, an MPNST consensus statement reviewed the current knowledge and provided guidance for the diagnosis and management of MPNST. Although the improvement in clinical outcome has not changed, substantial progress has been made in understanding the natural history and biology of MPNST through imaging and genomic advances since 2002. Genetically engineered mouse models that develop MPNST spontaneously have greatly facilitated preclinical evaluation of novel drugs for translation into clinical trials led by consortia efforts. Continued work in identifying alterations that contribute to the transformation, progression, and metastasis of MPNST coupled with longitudinal follow-up, biobanking, and data sharing is needed to develop prognostic biomarkers and effective prevention and therapeutic strategies for MPNST.

1. Introduction

Neurofibromatosis type 1 (NF1) is an autosomal dominant, pan-ethnic disorder with an incidence of 1:3000 [1]. NF1 is characterized by diverse, progressive cutaneous, neurologic, skeletal, and neoplastic manifestations with limited therapeutic options. The leading cause of death in NF1 patients is the malignant peripheral nerve sheath tumor (MPNST), a highly aggressive soft tissue sarcoma [2]. Half of all MPNST develop in individuals with NF1, with a 5-year survival of about 20% to 50%, and the outcome is especially dismal in those with unresectable or metastatic disease [2, 3]. Most (65–88%) NF1 MPNST arise from plexiform neurofibromas (PN) [4], benign peripheral nerve sheath tumors that are a hallmark of NF1. The only known definitive therapy for MPNST is surgical resection with wide negative margins [4, 5], which is often not feasible or indicated due to location, size, and metastases [6, 7].

A 2002 MPNST consensus statement reviewed current knowledge, provided guidance for the diagnosis and management of MPNST, and identified research priorities [8]. While little progress has been made in the development of more effective therapies since then, there have been substantial advances in understanding MPNST natural history, biology, and preclinical modeling, and preclinical and clinical trial consortia have been established (Table 1). In this review, we update progress since 2002 in the (1) natural history of peripheral nerve sheath tumors, (2) pathogenesis of MPNST, (3) development of preclinical models, and (4) management and clinical trials for MPNST.

TABLE 1: Summary of progress in preclinical, clinical, and therapeutic MPNST research and clinical management since the 2002 international consensus conference.

Characteristic	2002	2016
Natural history of PN growth	(i) Unknown (ii) May be erratic	(i) Well characterized (ii) Identification of distinct nodular lesions (DNL) with different growth pattern
Imaging	(i) Role of FDG-PET unclear (ii) FLT PET should be considered	(i) FDG-PET has clear role (ii) FLT-PET under evaluation
Pathology	(i) ANF do not fit in category (ii) Locally aggressive (iii) Do not metastasize	(i) Identification of ANF as MPNST precursor
Risk for transformation ↑	(i) Nodular PN, large central PN, NF neuropathy	(i) Distinct nodular, FDG-avid lesions
Pathogenesis	(i) *NF1* microdeletion (ii) *p27, p53, p16*	(i) *CDKN2A/B* (ii) *SUZ12, EED*
Mouse models	(i) Briefly mentioned	(i) Preclinical trials consortium using GEMM
Chemotherapy targeted therapy	(i) Very few, if any, MPNST-specific data	(i) Prospective trial of chemotherapy completed (ii) MPNST-specific targeted trials ongoing (iii) SARC and NF clinical trials consortium
Access to tissue	(i) Importance of tissue banking	(i) CTF NF biobank
Data collection	(i) International database recommended	(i) No international database established

ANF: atypical neurofibroma; DNL: distinct nodular lesion; FDG-PET: fluorodeoxyglucose positron emission tomography; FLT-PET: fluorothymidine positron emission tomography; GEMM: genetically engineered mouse model; PN: plexiform neurofibroma; SARC: Sarcoma Alliance for Research through Collaboration (research and advocacy group); CTF: Children's Tumor Foundation.

2. Natural History of Peripheral Nerve Sheath Tumors

PN, a cardinal feature of NF1, are identified in up to 50% of individuals with NF1 [9]. They are a major source of morbidity [10], causing disfigurement, impairment of nerve function, pain, and in some cases transform to MPNST (Figure 1) [2, 3]. Magnetic resonance imaging (MRI) and fluorodeoxyglucose-(FDG-) positron emission tomography (PET) are utilized in the diagnosis of malignant transformation with features to aid in distinguishing MPNST from PN [11–14]. Since 2002, the use of whole-body and targeted longitudinal MRI with volumetric analysis has permitted the sensitive and reproducible characterization of PN growth [15–19]. Most PN growth occurs in children, and substantial PN volume increase is infrequent in adults. This is in contrast to distinct nodular lesions (DNL) which have been identified using longitudinal whole-body MRI and display different imaging and growth characteristics [20, 21]. On Short T1 Inversion Recovery (STIR) MRI, these lesions are nodular, ≥3 cm in longest diameter, and well demarcated and lack the "central dot" sign characteristic of PN. MRI imaging for MPNST demonstrate irregularly shaped, ill-defined margins, intratumoral lobulation, and inhomogeneous contrast enhancement [12]. DNL emerge after early childhood, their growth rate is not age-related, and they are frequently higher than that of surrounding or adjacent PN. In contrast to typical PN, most DNL are FDG-avid on FDG-PET [21, 22] more like MPNST [13]. Biopsy and excision of some radiographically detected DNL reveal histologically atypical neurofibromas (ANF). ANF share some features of low-grade MPNST and recognition of transformation of ANF to MPNST suggests that ANF are premalignant lesions of MPNST rather than variants of PN [23]. ANF have increased variable cellularity and have cells with enlarged, hyperchromatic nuclei and more pronounced fascicular growth [23, 24]. Taken together, these findings suggest that DNL have a distinct underlying biology compared to PN [20]. Genomic findings of *CDKN2A/B* loss in ANF and MPNST (but not PN) further support the hypothesis that ANF are precursor lesions for MPNST [22, 23, 25]. In a retrospective analysis of 76 ANF diagnosed in 63 patients with NF1, the majority ($n = 57$) were resected and have not recurred [22]. However, four ANF transformed into high grade MPNST. Sixteen patients had a history or developed MPNST in a different location, and patients with ANF may be at greater risk of developing MPNST [22]. Limited correlation of clinical outcome in surgical excision of ANF suggests that these lesions may not require aggressive surgery as MPNST. In a retrospective review of 23 patients who underwent surgical resection of a plexiform neurofibroma pathologically diagnosed as either low-grade MPNST or ANF had disease-specific survival of 100% with a median follow-up of 47 months despite 78% (18/23) of patients having microscopically positive margins [26]. No patients developed pulmonary metastasis. Further study is warranted, but focal surgical resection of premalignant ANF may play an important role in the prevention of MPNST.

3. Pathology of MPNST

Sarcoma arising from the peripheral nerve sheath is readily diagnosed as MPNST if the tumor clearly has nerve elements or arises in the context of NF1. Otherwise, the diagnosis of MPNST is more difficult, with a broad differential diagnosis of other sarcomas, and requires an extensive clinicopathologic assessment of immunohistochemical (IHC) markers,

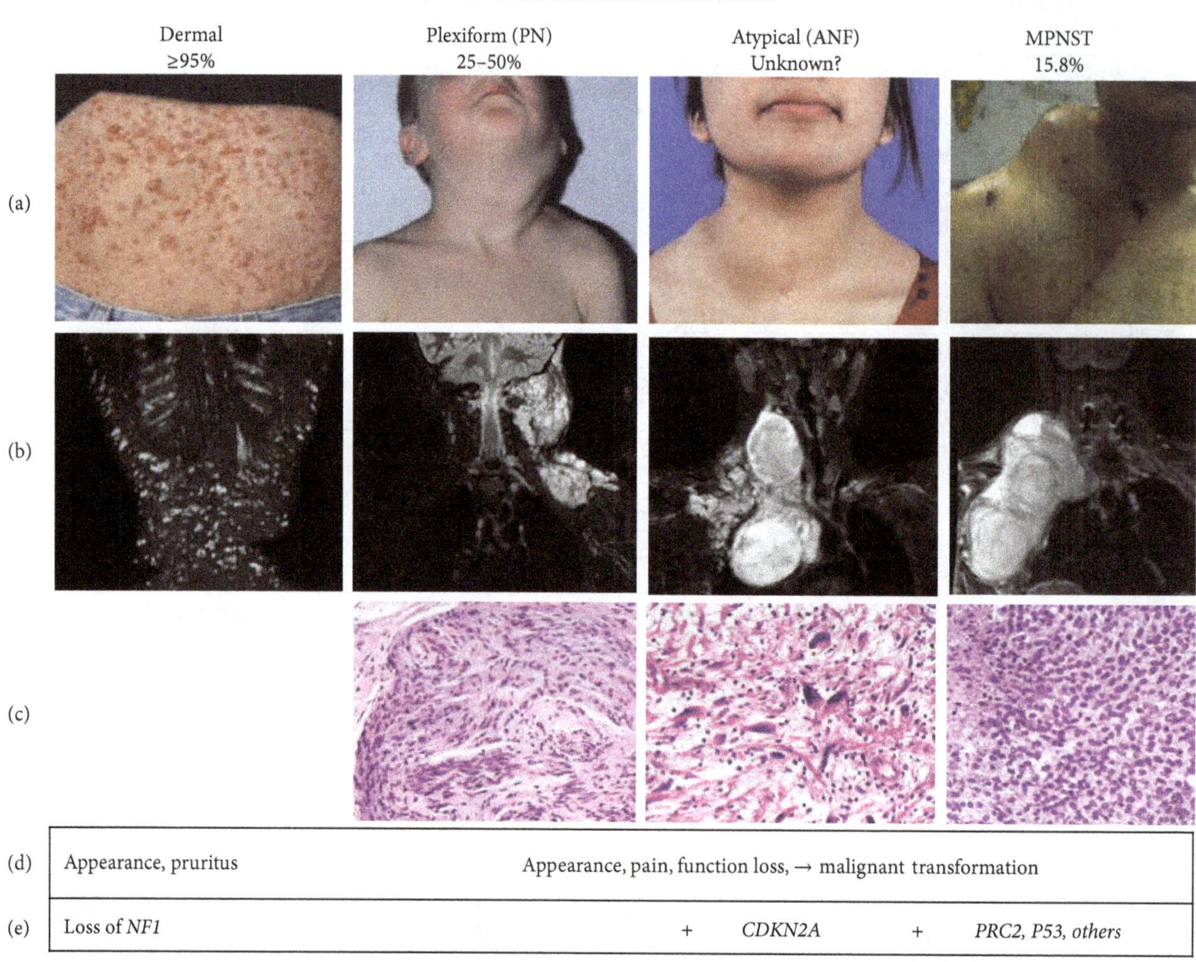

FIGURE 1: Pathogenesis of peripheral nerve sheath tumors in NF1. Percentages below each tumor type is the range of lifetime prevalence in individuals with NF1. Representative clinical photograph (a), MRI imaging (b), histology (c), clinical symptomology (d), and genetic features (e) of each tumor type are given. Histologically, plexiform neurofibroma shows mixture of areas of hypercellularity in the absence of other atypical features. Atypical neurofibroma shows atypical nuclei and higher cellularity. In contrast, MPNST are highly cellular with high mitotic activity and areas of necrosis.

tissue ultrastructure, and histologic findings [24, 27] to firmly establish a tumor diagnosis. High-grade MPNST are highly cellular with many mitotic figures and areas of necrosis. Low-grade MPNST are less cellular, have few mitotic figures and no areas of necrosis, and are difficult to distinguish from benign cellular neurofibromas and ANF. Various histologic patterns can coexist within a single specimen, making it imperative to examine as much of the tumor as possible to arrive at an appropriate diagnosis and grade [28]. Small biopsies are usually inadequate for clinical decision-making due to this intra-tumor heterogeneity.

IHC studies are helpful in distinguishing high-grade MPNST from other sarcomas but are less helpful in distinguishing ANF from low-grade MPNST. Typical staining includes in situ antibody studies on multiple formalin-fixed sections for S100 (calcium-binding motif as Schwann cell marker), Ki-67 (nuclear nonhistone protein marker of cell proliferation), TP53 (tumor suppressor marker for transformation), CD34 (sialomucin glycoprotein as nonspecific marker of endothelium and hematopoietic stem cells), and p16INK4a (cell-cycle inhibitory protein marker that is inactivated in MPNST). A standardized set of IHC markers has not been routinely applied to peripheral nerve sheath tumors across clinical pathology laboratories. Although they may be useful in characterizing MPNST [29], the pattern of IHC staining has not led to stratification of patients for personalized management of their tumor. Use of genetic markers in these tumors is emerging as another modality to more fully characterize peripheral nerve sheath tumors for clinical intervention.

4. Genetics and Genomics of MPNST

MPNST cells harbor complex rearranged genomes. Accumulated evidence suggests that *NF1* loss is necessary but not sufficient for MPNST development. As NF1-associated MPNST progress from *NF1*-nullizygous PN, they acquire mutations in other driver genes (e.g. *TP53* and *CDKN2A*). *NF1* loss is seen in a majority of sporadic MPNST, suggesting that *NF1* is an important tumor suppressor in all MPNST. Genetic alterations of *CDKN2A* and *TP53* are also observed in sporadic and radiation-associated MPNST [30]. Deletion of *CDKN2A* disrupts two encoded proteins (p16INK4A and p19ARF) and their associated regulatory cascades. *CDKN2A* deletions are also observed in ANF [23]. The first study of NF1-associated tumor progression in a single patient from PN to primary MPNST and MPNST metastasis using whole exome sequencing (WES) of biopsies [31] found biallelic *NF1* mutations in all tumor stages, chromosome 17p *(TP53)* loss in primary MPNST and metastasis, and no *CDKN2A* deletions or *EGFR* amplifications. Subsequent cytogenetic and array comparative genomic hybridization (aCGH) studies on MPNST have identified frequent losses on chromosomes 1p, 9p, 11, 12p, 14q, 18, 22q, X, and Y, with focal gains on chromosomes 7, 8q, and 15q [32]. There are no pathognomonic chromosomal translocations in MPNST. Amplification of genes encoding the epidermal growth factor (EGF) receptor, neuregulin-1 (NRG1) coreceptor erbB2, c-Kit, platelet-derived growth factor-α, and c-Met has been reported in MPNST [33].

In 2014, somatic mutations in *SUZ12* and *EED* encoding components of the polycomb repressive complex 2 (PRC2) were reported in NF1-associated and sporadic MPNST [30, 34, 35]. PRC2 is a histone methyltransferase and plays a critical role in marking chromatin for silencing. This finding suggests that transformation to MPNST involves a previously unsuspected epigenetic switch and points to potential epigenetic-based therapeutic strategies. Comprehensive genomic characterization of sporadic, NF1-, and radiation-associated MPNST shows recurrent inactivation of PRC2 from somatic mutation of *EED* and *SUZ12* [30, 35]. The *SUZ12* gene encodes a chromatin modifying protein, and its loss enhances colony growth of *NF1*-deficient (but not *NF1* wild-type) glioblastoma cells, suggesting that reduced PRC2 levels might promote tumorigenesis. Furthermore, *SUZ12* ablation causes loss of trimethylation at lysine 27 of histone H3 (H3K27me3) and increased H3K27 acetylation, establishing transcriptional activation marks to recruit bromodomain proteins that are potential drug targets for MPNST [34].

Frequent somatic alterations of *CDKN2A* and *NF1* significantly co-occur with PRC2 alteration. *SUZ12* is located near *NF1* in 17q11.2 and is involved in both type 1 and type 2 microdeletions at the *NF1* locus. Such microdeletions are associated with an increased risk of MPNST [36], leading to a model in which a "third hit" in *SUZ12* (the first two hits being the loss of *NF1* and one copy of *SUZ12* from a 17q11.2 microdeletion) drives transformation to MPNST [30]. PRC2 catalyzes trimethylation of H3K27 and multiple studies have found that significant loss of H3K27me3 in MPNST is associated with poor survival; furthermore, such loss is not observed in PN or ANF [37–39]. H3K27me3 loss or PRC2 mutation may be a useful biomarker to diagnose MPNST [35].

5. Preclinical Models

The primary model systems used to study MPNST have been (1) cell lines derived from MPNST patients, (2) xenograft models of patient-derived MPNST cells injected subcutaneously or into the sciatic nerve of immune compromised mice, (3) patient-derived xenografts (PDX) that have not been cultured, and (4) genetically engineered mouse models of sporadic MPNST.

5.1. Cell Culture Models. MPNST tumor lines from human and mouse have been used to elucidate the mechanism of action of neurofibromin [40]; study the role of tyrosine kinase receptors [41–47], growth factors [48–50], p53 [51, 52], microRNAs [30, 53], and sex hormones [54–56] in MPNST biology; and examine the effects of chemotherapy [57–67] and viral therapy [68–71] as potential treatments for MPNST. The most commonly used strains for grafting have been S462, ST88-14, and STS26T. STS26T was isolated from a metastatic lesion and has been shown to form metastases when injected into the tail vein of the mouse [62].

At least 33 NF1 or sporadic MPNST lines from primary or metastatic human tumors and mice tumors have been described in the literature to varying degrees (Supplemental Table 1, in Supplementary Material available online at https://doi.org/10.1155/2017/7429697). Mouse tumor lines have been made by isolating tumors with MPNST histology from $Nf1^{-/+}$:$Trp53^{-/+}$ *cis* mice (see below).

5.2. Xenograft/Orthograft Models. Over half of the described MPNST tumor lines have been used in grafting experiments to recapitulate the biology of MPNST in mice. The majority of these experiments studied human MPNST cells in immune-deficient mice. Although some cancer cell types are known to grow only on certain immune-deficient backgrounds (e.g., NSG), MPNST cells can engraft in hosts with residual immune function. MPNST cell lines that have been reported to engraft in mice and the type of mouse background used are listed in Supplemental Table 1. Xenograft models have been primarily used to test candidate therapeutics for MPNST.

5.3. Patient-Derived Xenograft (PDX) Models. Culture and xenograft models have been the mainstay of testing novel therapeutics for MPNST over the past 20 years. There is controversy regarding how well these models predict response in patients. This has led to the development of additional models that seek to better emulate the tumor microenvironment. Tumor cells passaged in culture adapt to the lack of extracellular matrix and culture-specific exogenous growth factors. PDX models are created by implanting patient tumor tissue directly into immune-deficient mice, so that the tumor cells grow directly within an in vivo environment. Very few of these models have been published. It is not clear how many have been maintained by passaging for use by other investigators. Bhola et al. [55] isolated tumor tissue from a male young adult NF1 patient and implanted small pieces subcutaneously into male NOD/SCID mice. The explants retained the histological and IHC characteristics of the parental tumor over more than 15 passages [72, 73].

5.4. Genetically Engineered Mouse Models (GEMMs). GEMMs develop MPNST spontaneously, permitting the coevolution

TABLE 2: Genetically engineered mouse models (GEMMs).

Tumor suppressors mutated	Method of mutation	Oncogenes overexpressed	Promoter overexpressed	Grade	Latency (months)	Penetrance (%)	REF
$Nf1^{-/+}$; $Ink4a^{-/-}$; $Arf^{-/-}$	Germline[1]			High	6.5	26	[79]
$Nf1^{flox/flox}$; $Pten^{flox/flox}$	Cre (Dhh^+ cells)			High	0.5	92	[80]
$Nf1^{flox/flox}$; $Pten^{flox/+}$	Cre (Dhh^+ cells)			Low	5.7	42	[80]
$Nf1^{flox/+}$; $Pten^{flox/flox}$	Cre (Dhh^+ cells)			Low	5.8	82	[80]
$Nf1^{flox/flox}$ + Nf1; p53shRNA	Cre (Periostin$^+$ cells)[4]			Low	6.1	56	[87]
$Nf1^{flox/-}$ + Nf1; p53shRNA	Cre ($GFAP^+$ cells)[4]			Low	3.0	73	[87]
$Nf1^{flox/flox}$; $Ink4a^{flox/flox}$; $Arf^{flox/flox}$	Cre (injection)			High	4.1	100	[86]
$Nf1^{-/+}$:$Trp53^{-/+}$	Germline[2]			High	5	81	[77, 78]
$Nf1^{flox/flox}$	Cre (Dhh^+ cells)	EGFR	CNP	High	~6	33	[81]
$Trp53^{-/+}$	Germline[3]	EGFR	CNP	Low-high	9.5	19	[84]
$Pten^{flox/+}$	Cre ($GFAP^+$ cells)	Kras-G12D	lox-STOP-lox[5]	High	~6	100	[82]
$Pten^{flox/flox}$	Cre (Dhh^+ cells)	EGFR	CNP	High	<1	100	[83]
$Trp53^{-/+}$	Germline[3]	GGFβ3	P0	Low-high	7.5	95	[57]
NA	NA	GGFβ3	P0	ND	8.7	71	[85]

[1]Spontaneous loss of NF1; [2]spontaneous loss of NF1 and p53; [3]spontaneous loss of p53; [4]injection of shRNA into sciatic nerve; [5]activation by Cre ($GFAP^+$ cells).
NA: not applicable; ND: not determined.

of microenvironment and tumor. One GEMM (*$Nf1^{-/+}$:$Trp53^{-/+}$ cis* mice) is being used for preclinical screening of drugs through the NF Therapeutic Consortium (NFTC) [34, 74–76]. The available GEMMs for MPNST use several approaches to initiate tumorigenesis: (1) spontaneous loss of heterozygosity of tumor suppressor genes, (2) expression of oncogenes by nervous system promoters, (3) Cre-lox system for mutation or conditional activation of genes during nerve development, or (4) adenoviral or lentiviral expression of shRNAs (Table 2). Heterozygous mutation of *Nf1* alone is not sufficient to drive MPNST tumorigenesis in mice; however, combining *Nf1* mutation with other mutations (*Trp53*, *Pten*, and *Cdkn2a*) gives rise to MPNST. In addition, MPNST GEMMs have been developed without mutation of *Nf1*, possibly recapitulating sporadic MPNST. The first MPNST GEMM was the *$Nf1^{-/+}$:$Trp53^{-/+}$cis* mouse [77, 78] with mutated copies of *Nf1* and *Trp53* in *cis* on mouse chromosome 11. Spontaneous loss of the wild-type alleles of these genes initiates tumorigenesis. Combining *Nf1* heterozygosity with loss of *Cdkn2a*, encoding $p16^{INK4A}$ and $p19^{ARF}$, gives rise to MPNST with low penetrance [79]. The Cre-lox system has been used in several GEMMs to mutate *Nf1*, *Trp53*, *Pten*, and/or *Cdkn2a* in cells of the developing nervous system [80–83], as well as to activate mutant Kras [82]. Some GEMMs have combined overexpression of the oncogenes *Egfr* or *Ggfb3* with tumor suppressor mutation by driving oncogene expression in nervous system cells using *CNP* or P_0 promoters, respectively [57, 80, 81, 84, 85]. More recently, MPNSTs have been modeled using injections into adult mouse sciatic nerve. Injection of adenovirus expressing Cre into mice carrying floxed alleles of *Nf1* and *Cdkn2a* drives high-grade MPNST through localized loss of neurofibromin, $p16^{Ink4a}$, and $p19^{Arf}$ in the nerve [86]. Low-grade MPNSTs form with the injection of shRNA for both *Nf1* and *Trp53* into mice that are either mutant for *Nf1* in all Periostin$^+$ cells or mutant for *Nf1* in $GFAP^+$ cells on a heterozygous mutant *Nf1* background [87]. Injection GEMMs have the advantage that tumorigenesis occurs in a more synchronized and spatially controlled manner; however, they require surgery for every mouse to expose the sciatic nerve for injection. GEMMs show different latencies for MPNST depending on the genes involved (*Cdkn2a, Pten, Trp53,* and *Egfr*) and the method used to mutate genes (shRNA knockdown versus genomic mutation through the Cre-lox system) (Table 2).

6. Clinical Trials Advances

Current treatment of MPNST is similar to treatment of soft tissue sarcomas as a whole and relies primarily on local control measures [5]. The only known definitive therapy for MPNST is surgical resection with wide negative margins, which may not be feasible due to variables such as tumor size, location, and/or metastases [7]. The role of adjuvant radiation is not defined; however, it is often recommended for high-grade lesions > 5 cm in size or with marginal excision [8, 88, 89]. For these patients, preoperative radiation should be considered [90]. Although radiation has shown improved local control, no effect on survival has been demonstrated [91, 92]. The role of chemotherapy is not defined. In a prospective study of chemotherapy (ifosfamide, doxorubicin, and etoposide) in NF1 associated and sporadic MPNST, a lower objective response rate was seen in NF1 patients (18%) compared with patients with sporadic MPNST patients (44%), similar to prior studies [93, 94]; however, disease stabilization was achieved in most patients at 4 cycles [95]. The best approach to treatment is by a multidisciplinary team of surgical, medical, and radiation oncologists, radiologists, and pathologists, all with sarcoma expertise. Patients with recurrent, unresectable, or metastatic disease have no known

TABLE 3: Targeted agents for treatment of MPNST: previous and ongoing clinical trials.

Drug	Target	Phase	n	Population	Outcome	Results	Ref.
Erlotinib	EGFR	II	24	≥18 y Refractory	Response WHO [101]	19/20 pts. PD at 2 months 1 SD	[96]
Sorafenib	C-Raf B-Raf VEGFR2 C-Kit PDGFR	II	12	≥18 y Refractory	Response RECIST [102]	No responses; median PFS 1.7 months	[97]
Imatinib	C-Kit PDGFR VEGFR	II	7	>10 y Refractory	Response RECIST [102]	No responses; 1 SD	[98]
Dasatinib	C-Kit SRC	II	14	≥13 y Refractory	Response CHOI [103]	No response or SD	[99]
Alisertib	AURKA	II	10	≥18 y Refractory	Response RECIST [102]	No response PFS 13 weeks	[100]
Bevacizumab/RAD001	Angiogenesis/mTOR	II	—	≥18 y Refractory	Response WHO [101]	Currently ongoing	—
Ganetespib/Sirolimus	Hsp90 mTOR	I/II	—	≥16 y Refractory	Response WHO [101]	Currently ongoing	—

curative options and enrollment in clinical trials should be considered.

The EGFR inhibitor erlotinib was the first targeted agent used in a histology-specific phase II trial for MPNST [96], based on the compelling preclinical observation that EGFR amplification was observed in MPNSTs and that Nf1/p53 murine MPNST were stimulated by EGF and inhibited by EGFR inhibitors [33]. Within 22 months, 24 patients were enrolled, but no activity was demonstrated. Subsequent trials of investigational agents (Table 3) have failed to demonstrate efficacy but show that the outcome for unresectable MPNST is poor with a median progression-free survival of less than 2 months and overall survival of less than 5 months [97–100]. These trials demonstrate that single histology trials in this rare disease are feasible and that MPNST progresses rapidly.

Selection, prioritization, and trial design are key challenges in the clinical development of effective therapies for MPNST. While preclinical drug discovery outpaces clinical development, the time and cost to evaluate promising therapies for MPNST are significant and patient numbers are limited. The Children's Tumor Foundation (CTF) and Neurofibromatosis Therapeutic Acceleration Program (NTAP) sponsor the preclinical NF Therapeutic Consortium (NFTC), which supports the conduct of preclinical trials of targeted therapies in GEMM targeting NF1 manifestations (e.g., MPNST and PN) to prioritize the selection of agents for clinical trials. There are no data yet demonstrating MPNST GEMM as valid surrogates for drug activity in humans. Through clinical consortia initiatives such as the Department of Defense (DoD) NF Clinical Trials Consortium and the SARC (Sarcoma Alliance for Research through Collaboration), therapies identified through these models are being translated into clinical trials specific for MPNST. Cooperative group participation allows for rapid accrual for early phase trials in MPNST. Approaches to accelerating testing of agents guided by preclinical rationale, with efficient endpoints, protocol design, and access to drugs, are needed. In turn, these trials can serve as a means to not only validate the best preclinical models, and information gained in the clinic can be used to help develop new therapeutic approaches at the bench.

7. Future Directions

Although the outcome for MPNST has not changed significantly since 2002, the more complete understanding of the natural history of peripheral nerve sheath tumors and of the genomic changes during malignant transformation of PN to ANF and MPNST offers hope for the development of more effective diagnostic, therapeutic, and prevention strategies for MPNST. Whole-body MRI and PET imaging may have utility for risk stratification and for implementation of surveillance and medical/surgical interventions as potential preventative therapies and for monitoring treatment response in large, irregular-shaped tumors. Research priorities should focus on the role of whole-body MRI to screen for PN-related tumor load and on longitudinal imaging to detect lesions concerning malignant transformation, such as DNL. The natural history of ANF needs to be better understood, including its clinical presentation, incidence of malignant transformation of DNL to ANF, and the role for timing and extent (wide versus limited) of surgical excision of these transitional tumors, while resource-intensive, prospective, longitudinal studies of individuals with NF1 and PN with whole-body MRI and other imaging modalities coupled with genomic and immunohistological data and collection of blood samples for potential
vention of MPNST.
biomarker development are predicted to have great value in advancing approaches to the diagnosis, treatment, and pre-

Great strides have been made in the development of preclinical models for understanding disease pathogenesis and drug testing in MPNST. Translating and validating preclinical models will require developing validated biomarkers of disease and outcome measures using new technologies that can be incorporated into clinical trials. The search for MPNST biomarkers must have new urgency. Circulating tumor DNA is essentially unstudied in MPNST and may offer great promise to screen and detect early cancers, score treatment response, and identify tumor recurrence. The importance of epigenetic mechanisms in MPNST pathogenesis has been underappreciated until the advent of comprehensive genomic studies which have offered clues to future therapies. An international MPNST database with phenotypic, genotypic, and treatment data is needed to share findings and inform next steps for research efforts and treatment strategies [104]. The tumor phenotype data should be comprehensive and include complete characterization of the tumors from clinical pathologists with expertise in sarcoma. To that end, standard and broadly accepted definitions of what constitutes benign cellular neurofibroma, DNL, ANF, low-grade MPNST, and high-grade MPNST need to be established. Molecular data needed for the MPNST database include constitutional DNA, tumor DNA, tumor expression patterns, circulating cell-free DNA, and possibly metabolic activity of the tumor. Treatment and outcome data need to be collated with the genotype-phenotype information in the database. Innovative clinical trial designs with efficient endpoints to accelerate testing of new drugs and access to novel agents for testing in combination are also needed.

Acknowledgments

This work has been supported in part by the NCI Center for Cancer Research and Division of Cancer Epidemiology and Genetics intramural research programs.

References

[1] R. E. Ferner, "Neurofibromatosis 1 and neurofibromatosis 2: a twenty first century perspective," *The Lancet Neurology*, vol. 6, no. 4, pp. 340–351, 2007.

[2] D. G. R. Evans, M. E. Baser, J. McGaughran, S. Sharif, E. Howard, and A. Moran, "Malignant peripheral nerve sheath tumours in neurofibromatosis," *Journal of Medical Genetics*, vol. 39, no. 5, pp. 311–314, 2002.

[3] E. Uusitalo, M. Rantanen, R. A. Kallionpää et al., "Distinctive cancer associations in patients with neurofibromatosis type 1," *Journal of Clinical Oncology*, vol. 34, no. 17, pp. 1978–1986, 2016.

[4] H. Meany, B. C. Widemann, and N. Ratner, "Malignant peripheral nerve sheath tumors: prognostic and diagnostic markers and therapeutic targets," in *Neurofibromatosis Type 1*, pp. 445–467, Springer, Berlin, Germany, 2012.

[5] C. L. Scaife and P. W. T. Pisters, "Combined-modality treatment of localized soft tissue sarcomas of the extremities," *Surgical Oncology Clinics of North America*, vol. 12, no. 2, pp. 355–368, 2003.

[6] P. W. Pisters, D. H. Leung, J. Woodruff, W. Shi, and M. F. Brennan, "Analysis of prognostic factors in 1,041 patients with localized soft tissue sarcomas of the extremities," *Journal of Clinical Oncology*, vol. 14, no. 5, pp. 1679–1689, 1996.

[7] G. Gupta, A. Mammis, and A. Maniker, "Malignant peripheral nerve sheath tumors," *Neurosurgery Clinics of North America*, vol. 19, no. 4, pp. 533–543, 2008.

[8] R. E. Ferner and D. H. Gutmann, "International consensus statement on malignant peripheral nerve sheath tumors in neurofibromatosis," *Cancer Research*, vol. 62, no. 5, pp. 1573–1577, 2002.

[9] V.-F. Mautner, F. A. Asuagbor, E. Dombi et al., "Assessment of benign tumor burden by whole-body MRI in patients with neurofibromatosis 1," *Neuro-Oncology*, vol. 10, no. 4, pp. 593–598, 2008.

[10] A. Kim, A. Gillespie, E. Dombi et al., "Characteristics of children enrolled in treatment trials for NF1-related plexiform neurofibromas," *Neurology*, vol. 73, no. 16, pp. 1273–1279, 2009.

[11] J. Wasa, Y. Nishida, S. Tsukushi et al., "MRI features in the differentiation of malignant peripheral nerve sheath tumors and neurofibromas," *American Journal of Roentgenology*, vol. 194, no. 6, pp. 1568–1574, 2010.

[12] A. Matsumine, K. Kusuzaki, T. Nakamura et al., "Differentiation between neurofibromas and malignant peripheral nerve sheath tumors in neurofibromatosis 1 evaluated by MRI," *Journal of Cancer Research and Clinical Oncology*, vol. 135, no. 7, pp. 891–900, 2009.

[13] R. E. Ferner, J. F. Golding, M. Smith et al., "[^{18}F]2-fluoro-2-deoxy-D-glucose positron emission tomography (FDG PET) as a diagnostic tool for neurofibromatosis 1 (NF1) associated malignant peripheral nerve sheath tumours (MPNSTs): a long-term clinical study," *Annals of Oncology*, vol. 19, no. 2, pp. 390–394, 2008.

[14] S. M. Broski, G. B. Johnson, B. M. Howe et al., "Evaluation of ^{18}F-FDG PET and MRI in differentiating benign and malignant peripheral nerve sheath tumors," *Skeletal Radiology*, vol. 45, no. 8, pp. 1097–1105, 2016.

[15] E. Dombi, S. L. Ardern-Holmes, D. Babovic-Vuksanovic et al., "Recommendations for imaging tumor response in neurofibromatosis clinical trials," *Neurology*, vol. 81, no. 21, supplement 1, pp. S33–S40, 2013.

[16] E. Dombi, J. Solomon, A. J. Gillespie et al., "NF1 plexiform neurofibroma growth rate by volumetric MRI: relationship to age and body weight," *Neurology*, vol. 68, no. 9, pp. 643–647, 2007.

[17] D. H. Gutmann, J. O. Blakeley, B. R. Korf, and R. J. Packer, "Optimizing biologically targeted clinical trials for neurofibromatosis," *Expert Opinion on Investigational Drugs*, vol. 22, no. 4, pp. 443–462, 2013.

[18] J. Solomon, K. Warren, E. Dombi, N. Patronas, and B. Widemann, "Automated detection and volume measurement of plexiform neurofibromas in neurofibromatosis 1 using magnetic resonance imaging," *Computerized Medical Imaging and Graphics*, vol. 28, no. 5, pp. 257–265, 2004.

[19] R. Nguyen, E. Dombi, B. C. Widemann et al., "Growth dynamics of plexiform neurofibromas: a retrospective cohort study of 201 patients with neurofibromatosis 1," *Orphanet Journal of Rare Diseases*, vol. 7, article 75, 2012.

[20] S. Akshintala, S. Bhaumik, A. Venkatesan et al., "Identification of lesions concerning for transformation to malignant peripheral nerve sheath tumors (MPNST) in Neurofibromatosis 1 (NF1)," in *Radiological Society of North America*, 2014.

[21] H. Meany, E. Dombi, J. Reynolds et al., "18-fluorodeoxyglucose-positron emission tomography (FDG-PET) evaluation of nodular lesions in patients with neurofibromatosis type 1 and plexiform neurofibromas (PN) or malignant peripheral nerve sheath

tumors (MPNST)," *Pediatric Blood and Cancer*, vol. 60, no. 1, pp. 59–64, 2013.

[22] C. Higham, E. Legius, N. Ullrich et al., *Atypical Neurofibromas in NF1: Clinical, Imaging and Pathology Characteristics*, Children's Tumor Foundation, Austin, Tex, USA, 2016.

[23] E. Beert, H. Brems, B. Daniëls et al., "Atypical neurofibromas in neurofibromatosis type 1 are premalignant tumors," *Genes Chromosomes and Cancer*, vol. 50, no. 12, pp. 1021–1032, 2011.

[24] F. J. Rodriguez, A. L. Folpe, C. Giannini, and A. Perry, "Pathology of peripheral nerve sheath tumors: diagnostic overview and update on selected diagnostic problems," *Acta Neuropathologica*, vol. 123, no. 3, pp. 295–319, 2012.

[25] B. Widemann, S. Bhaumik, S. Akshintala et al., "Identification of lesions concenring for malignant peripheral nerve sheath tumors in NF1," in *Proceedings of the CTOS Members Business Meeting*, Salt Lake City, Utah, USA, 2015.

[26] N. M. Bernthal, A. Putnam, K. B. Jones, D. Viskochil, and R. L. Randall, "The effect of surgical margins on outcomes for low grade MPNSTs and atypical neurofibroma," *Journal of Surgical Oncology*, vol. 110, no. 7, pp. 813–816, 2014.

[27] C. D. M. Fletcher, K. K. Unni, and F. Mertens, *WHO Classification of Tumours of Soft Tissue and Bone*, IARC, Lyons, France, 4th edition, 2013.

[28] B. W. Scheithauer, J. M. Woodruff, and R. A. Erlandson, *Tumors of the Peripheral Nervous System*, Atlas of Tumor Pathology Third Series, Armed Forces Institute of Pathology, Washington, DC, USA, 1999.

[29] M. Pekmezci, D. E. Reuss, A. C. Hirbe et al., "Morphologic and immunohistochemical features of malignant peripheral nerve sheath tumors and cellular schwannomas," *Modern Pathology*, vol. 28, no. 2, pp. 187–200, 2015.

[30] M. Zhang, Y. Wang, S. Jones et al., "Somatic mutations of SUZ12 in malignant peripheral nerve sheath tumors," *Nature Genetics*, vol. 46, no. 11, pp. 1170–1172, 2014.

[31] A. C. Hirbe, S. Dahiya, C. A. Miller et al., "Whole exome sequencing reveals the order of genetic changes during malignant transformation and metastasis in a single patient with NF1-plexiform neurofibroma," *Clinical Cancer Research*, vol. 21, no. 18, pp. 4201–4211, 2015.

[32] S. L. Carroll, "The challenge of cancer genomics in rare nervous system neoplasms: malignant peripheral nerve sheath tumors as a paradigm for cross-species comparative oncogenomics," *American Journal of Pathology*, vol. 186, no. 3, pp. 464–477, 2016.

[33] H. Li, S. Velasco-Miguel, W. C. Vass, L. F. Parada, and J. E. DeClue, "Epidermal growth factor receptor signaling pathways are associated with tumorigenesis in the Nf1:p53 mouse tumor model," *Cancer Research*, vol. 62, no. 15, pp. 4507–4513, 2002.

[34] T. De Raedt, E. Beert, E. Pasmant et al., "PRC2 loss amplifies Ras-driven transcription and confers sensitivity to BRD4-based therapies," *Nature*, vol. 514, no. 7521, pp. 247–251, 2014.

[35] W. Lee, S. Teckie, T. Wiesner et al., "PRC2 is recurrently inactivated through EED or SUZ12 loss in malignant peripheral nerve sheath tumors," *Nature Genetics*, vol. 46, no. 11, pp. 1227–1232, 2014.

[36] T. De Raedt, H. Brems, P. Wolkenstein et al., "Elevated risk for MPNST in NF1 microdeletion patients," *American Journal of Human Genetics*, vol. 72, no. 5, pp. 1288–1292, 2003.

[37] A. H. G. Cleven, G. A. Al Sannaa, I. Briaire-de Bruijn et al., "Loss of H3K27 tri-methylation is a diagnostic marker for malignant peripheral nerve sheath tumors and an indicator for an inferior survival," *Modern Pathology*, vol. 29, no. 6, pp. 582–590, 2016.

[38] C. N. Prieto-Granada, T. Wiesner, J. L. Messina, A. A. Jungbluth, P. Chi, and C. R. Antonescu, "Loss of H3K27me3 expression is a highly sensitive marker for sporadic and radiation-induced MPNST," *The American Journal of Surgical Pathology*, vol. 40, no. 4, pp. 479–489, 2016.

[39] M. Röhrich, C. Koelsche, D. Schrimpf et al., "Methylation-based classification of benign and malignant peripheral nerve sheath tumors," *Acta Neuropathologica*, vol. 131, no. 6, pp. 877–887, 2016.

[40] J. E. DeClue, A. G. Papageorge, J. A. Fletcher et al., "Abnormal regulation of mammalian p21ras contributes to malignant tumor growth in von Recklinghausen (type 1) neurofibromatosis," *Cell*, vol. 69, no. 2, pp. 265–273, 1992.

[41] J. J. Ryan, K. A. Klein, T. J. Neuberger et al., "Role for the stem cell factor/KIT complex in schwann cell neoplasia and mast cell proliferation associated with neurofibromatosis," *Journal of Neuroscience Research*, vol. 37, no. 3, pp. 415–432, 1994.

[42] A. Badache, N. Muja, and G. H. De Vries, "Expression of Kit in neurofibromin-deficient human Schwann cells: role in Schwann cell hyperplasia associated with type 1 neurofibromatosis," *Oncogene*, vol. 17, no. 6, pp. 795–800, 1998.

[43] J. E. DeClue, S. Heffelfinger, G. Benvenuto et al., "Epidermal growth factor receptor expression in neurofibromatosis type 1-related tumors and NF1 animal models," *The Journal of Clinical Investigation*, vol. 105, no. 9, pp. 1233–1241, 2000.

[44] I. Dang and G. H. DeVries, "Schwann cell lines derived from malignant peripheral nerve sheath tumors respond abnormally to platelet-derived growth factor-BB," *Journal of Neuroscience Research*, vol. 79, no. 3, pp. 318–328, 2005.

[45] N. Holtkamp, A. F. Okuducu, J. Mucha et al., "Mutation and expression of PDGFRA and KIT in malignant peripheral nerve sheath tumors, and its implications for imatinib sensitivity," *Carcinogenesis*, vol. 27, no. 3, pp. 664–671, 2006.

[46] M. Hakozaki, H. Hojo, M. Sato et al., "Establishment and characterization of a novel human malignant peripheral nerve sheath tumor cell line, FMS-1, that overexpresses epidermal growth factor receptor and cyclooxygenase-2," *Virchows Archiv*, vol. 455, no. 6, pp. 517–526, 2009.

[47] K. E. Torres, Q.-S. Zhu, K. Bill et al., "Activated MET is a molecular prognosticator and potential therapeutic target for malignant peripheral nerve sheath tumors," *Clinical Cancer Research*, vol. 17, no. 12, pp. 3943–3955, 2011.

[48] J. M. Eckert, S. J. Byer, B. J. Clodfelder-Miller, and S. L. Carroll, "Neuregulin-1β and neuregulin-1α differentially affect the migration and invasion of malignant peripheral nerve sheath tumor cells," *GLIA*, vol. 57, no. 14, pp. 1501–1520, 2009.

[49] C. Friedrich, N. Holtkamp, J. Cinatl Jr. et al., "Overexpression of Midkine in malignant peripheral nerve sheath tumor cells inhibits apoptosis and increases angiogenic potency," *International Journal of Oncology*, vol. 27, no. 5, pp. 1433–1440, 2005.

[50] M. Demestre, M. Y. Terzi, V. Mautner, P. Vajkoczy, A. Kurtz, and A. L. Piña, "Effects of pigment epithelium derived factor (PEDF) on malignant peripheral nerve sheath tumours (MPNSTs)," *Journal of Neuro-Oncology*, vol. 115, no. 3, pp. 391–399, 2013.

[51] H. Sonobe, T. Takeuchi, M. Furihata et al., "A new human malignant peripheral nerve sheath tumour-cell line, HS-sch-2, harbouring p53 point mutation," *International Journal of Oncology*, vol. 17, no. 2, pp. 347–352, 2000.

[52] N. Holtkamp, I. Atallah, A.-F. Okuducu et al., "MMP-13 and p53 in the progression of malignant peripheral nerve sheath tumors," *Neoplasia*, vol. 9, no. 8, pp. 671–677, 2007.

[53] M. Gong, J. Ma, M. Li, M. Zhou, J. M. Hock, and X. Yu, "MicroRNA-204 critically regulates carcinogenesis in malignant peripheral nerve sheath tumors," *Neuro-Oncology*, vol. 14, no. 8, pp. 1007–1017, 2012.

[54] G. Q. Perrin, H. Li, L. Fishbein et al., "An orthotopic xenograft model of intraneural NF1 MPNST suggests a potential association between steroid hormones and tumor cell proliferation," *Laboratory Investigation*, vol. 87, no. 11, pp. 1092–1102, 2007.

[55] P. Bhola, S. Banerjee, J. Mukherjee et al., "Preclinical in vivo evaluation of rapamycin in human malignant peripheral nerve sheath explant xenograft," *International Journal of Cancer*, vol. 126, no. 2, pp. 563–571, 2010.

[56] S. J. Byer, J. M. Eckert, N. M. Brossier et al., "Tamoxifen inhibits malignant peripheral nerve sheath tumor growth in an estrogen receptor-independent manner," *Neuro-Oncology*, vol. 13, no. 1, pp. 28–41, 2011.

[57] S. N. Brosius, A. N. Turk, S. J. Byer et al., "Neuregulin-1 overexpression and Trp53 haploinsufficiency cooperatively promote de novo malignant peripheral nerve sheath tumor pathogenesis," *Acta Neuropathologica*, vol. 127, no. 4, pp. 573–591, 2014.

[58] S. Imaizumi, T. Motoyama, A. Ogose, T. Hotta, and H. E. Takahashi, "Characterization and chemosensitivity of two human malignant peripheral nerve sheath tumour cell lines derived from a patient with neurofibromatosis type 1," *Virchows Archiv*, vol. 433, no. 5, pp. 435–441, 1998.

[59] Y. Hirokawa, H. Nakajima, C. O. Hanemann et al., "Signal therapy of NF1-deficient tumor xenograft in mice by the anti-PAK1 drug FK228," *Cancer Biology and Therapy*, vol. 4, no. 4, pp. 379–381, 2005.

[60] B. Barkan, S. Starinsky, E. Friedman, R. Stein, and Y. Kloog, "The Ras inhibitor farnesylthiosalicylic acid as a potential therapy for neurofibromatosis type 1," *Clinical Cancer Research*, vol. 12, no. 18, pp. 5533–5542, 2006.

[61] G. Johansson, Y. Y. Mahller, M. H. Collins et al., "Effective in vivo targeting of the mammalian target of rapamycin pathway in malignant peripheral nerve sheath tumors," *Molecular Cancer Therapeutics*, vol. 7, no. 5, pp. 1237–1245, 2008.

[62] M. P. Ghadimi, E. D. Young, R. Belousov et al., "Survivin is a viable target for the treatment of malignant peripheral nerve sheath tumors," *Clinical Cancer Research*, vol. 18, no. 9, pp. 2545–2557, 2012.

[63] W. Wang, W. Lin, B. Hong et al., "Effect of triptolide on malignant peripheral nerve sheath tumours in vitro and in vivo," *Journal of International Medical Research*, vol. 40, no. 6, pp. 2284–2294, 2012.

[64] J. Ohishi, M. Aoki, K. Nabeshima et al., "Imatinib mesylate inhibits cell growth of malignant peripheral nerve sheath tumors in vitro and in vivo through suppression of PDGFR-β," *BMC Cancer*, vol. 13, article 224, 2013.

[65] P. P. Patwardhan, O. Surriga, M. J. Beckman et al., "Sustained inhibition of receptor tyrosine kinases and macrophage depletion by PLX3397 and rapamycin as a potential new approach for the treatment of MPNSTs," *Clinical Cancer Research*, vol. 20, no. 12, pp. 3146–3158, 2014.

[66] G. Lopez, K. L. J. Bill, H. K. Bid et al., "HDAC8, A potential therapeutic target for the treatment of malignant peripheral nerve sheath tumors (MPNST)," *PLoS ONE*, vol. 10, no. 7, Article ID e0133302, 2015.

[67] P. Zhang, X. Yang, X. Ma et al., "Antitumor effects of pharmacological EZH2 inhibition on malignant peripheral nerve sheath tumor through the miR-30a and KPNB1 pathway," *Molecular Cancer*, vol. 14, no. 1, article 55, 2015.

[68] D. R. Deyle, D. Z. Escobar, K.-W. Peng, and D. Babovic-Vuksanovic, "Oncolytic measles virus as a novel therapy for malignant peripheral nerve sheath tumors," *Gene*, vol. 565, no. 1, pp. 140–145, 2015.

[69] A. R. Maldonado, C. Klanke, A. G. Jeßgga et al., "Molecular engineering and validation of an oncolytic herpes simplex virus type 1 transcriptionally targeted to midkine-positive tumors," *Journal of Gene Medicine*, vol. 12, no. 7, pp. 613–623, 2010.

[70] Y. Y. Mahller, S. S. Vaikunth, M. C. Ripberger et al., "Tissue inhibitor of metalloproteinase-3 via oncolytic herpesvirus inhibits tumor growth and vascular progenitors," *Cancer Research*, vol. 68, no. 4, pp. 1170–1179, 2008.

[71] T.-C. Liu, T. Zhang, H. Fukuhara et al., "Dominant-negative fibroblast growth factor receptor expression enhances antitumoral potency of oncolytic herpes simplex virus in neural tumors," *Clinical Cancer Research*, vol. 12, no. 22, pp. 6791–6799, 2006.

[72] Y. Takamiya, R. M. Friedlander, H. Brem, A. Malick, and R. L. Martuza, "Inhibition of angiogenesis and growth of human nerve-sheath tumors by AGM- 1470," *Journal of Neurosurgery*, vol. 78, no. 3, pp. 470–476, 1993.

[73] J. Castellsagué, B. Gel, J. Fernández-Rodríguez et al., "Comprehensive establishment and characterization of orthoxenograft mouse models of malignant peripheral nerve sheath tumors for personalized medicine," *EMBO Molecular Medicine*, vol. 7, no. 5, pp. 608–627, 2015.

[74] T. De Raedt, Z. Walton, J. L. Yecies et al., "Exploiting cancer cell vulnerabilities to develop a combination therapy for ras-driven tumors," *Cancer Cell*, vol. 20, no. 3, pp. 400–413, 2011.

[75] R. Lock, R. Ingraham, O. Maertens et al., "Cotargeting MNK and MEK kinases induces the regression of NF1-mutant cancers," *Journal of Clinical Investigation*, vol. 126, no. 6, pp. 2181–2190, 2016.

[76] C. F. Malone, J. A. Fromm, O. Maertens, T. DeRaedt, R. Ingraham, and K. Cichowski, "Defining key signaling nodes and therapeutic biomarkers in NF1-mutant cancers," *Cancer Discovery*, vol. 4, no. 9, pp. 1062–1073, 2014.

[77] K. Cichowski, T. S. Shih, E. Schmitt et al., "Mouse models of tumor development in neurofibromatosis type 1," *Science*, vol. 286, no. 5447, pp. 2172–2176, 1999.

[78] K. S. Vogel, L. J. Klesse, S. Velasco-Miguel, K. Meyers, E. J. Rushing, and L. F. Parada, "Mouse tumor model for neurofibromatosis type 1," *Science*, vol. 286, no. 5447, pp. 2176–2179, 1999.

[79] N. M. Joseph, J. T. Mosher, J. Buchstaller et al., "The loss of Nf1 transiently promotes self-renewal but not tumorigenesis by neural crest stem cells," *Cancer Cell*, vol. 13, no. 2, pp. 129–140, 2008.

[80] V. W. Keng, E. P. Rahrmann, A. L. Watson et al., "PTEN and NF1 inactivation in Schwann cells produces a severe phenotype in the peripheral nervous system that promotes the development and malignant progression of peripheral nerve sheath tumors," *Cancer Research*, vol. 72, no. 13, pp. 3405–3413, 2012.

[81] J. Wu, D. M. Patmore, E. Jousma et al., "EGFR-STAT3 signaling promotes formation of malignant peripheral nerve sheath tumors," *Oncogene*, vol. 33, no. 2, pp. 173–180, 2014.

[82] C. Gregorian, J. Nakashima, S. M. Dry et al., "PTEN dosage is essential for neurofibroma development and malignant transformation," *Proceedings of the National Academy of Sciences of the United States of America*, vol. 106, no. 46, pp. 19479–19484, 2009.

[83] V. W. Keng, A. L. Watson, E. P. Rahrmann et al., "Conditional inactivation of Pten with EGFR overexpression in Schwann

cells models sporadic MPNST," *Sarcoma*, vol. 2012, Article ID 620834, 12 pages, 2012.

[84] E. P. Rahrmann, B. S. Moriarity, G. M. Otto et al., "Trp53 haploinsufficiency modifies EGFR-driven peripheral nerve sheath tumorigenesis," *American Journal of Pathology*, vol. 184, no. 7, pp. 2082–2098, 2014.

[85] S. J. Kazmi, S. J. Byer, J. M. Eckert et al., "Transgenic mice overexpressing neuregulin-1 model neurofibroma-malignant peripheral nerve sheath tumor progression and implicate specific chromosomal copy number variations in tumorigenesis," *American Journal of Pathology*, vol. 182, no. 3, pp. 646–667, 2013.

[86] R. D. Dodd, J. K. Mito, W. C. Eward et al., "NF1 deletion generates multiple subtypes of soft-tissue sarcoma that respond to mek inhibition," *Molecular Cancer Therapeutics*, vol. 12, no. 9, pp. 1906–1917, 2013.

[87] A. C. Hirbe, S. Dahiya, D. Friedmann-Morvinski, I. M. Verma, D. Wade Clapp, and D. H. Gutmann, "Spatially- and temporally-controlled postnatal p53 knockdown cooperates with embryonic Schwann cell precursor Nf1 gene loss to promote malignant peripheral nerve sheath tumor formation," *Oncotarget*, vol. 7, no. 7, pp. 7403–7414, 2016.

[88] C.-C. H. Stucky, K. N. Johnson, R. J. Gray et al., "Malignant Peripheral Nerve Sheath Tumors (MPNST): The Mayo Clinic experience," *Annals of Surgical Oncology*, vol. 19, no. 3, pp. 878–885, 2012.

[89] W. W. Wong, T. Hirose, B. W. Scheithauer, S. E. Schild, and L. L. Gunderson, "Malignant peripheral nerve sheath tumor: analysis of treatment outcome," *International Journal of Radiation Oncology Biology Physics*, vol. 42, no. 2, pp. 351–360, 1998.

[90] A. Kaushal and D. Citrin, "The role of radiation therapy in the management of sarcomas," *Surgical Clinics of North America*, vol. 88, no. 3, pp. 629–646, 2008.

[91] J. C. Yang, A. E. Chang, A. R. Baker et al., "Randomized prospective study of the benefit of adjuvant radiation therapy in the treatment of soft tissue sarcomas of the extremity," *Journal of Clinical Oncology*, vol. 16, no. 1, pp. 197–203, 1998.

[92] J. Kahn, A. Gillespie, M. Tsokos et al., "Radiation therapy in management of sporadic and neurofibromatosis type 1-associated malignant peripheral nerve sheath tumors," *Frontiers in Oncology*, vol. 4, article 324, 2014.

[93] A. Ferrari, R. Miceli, A. Rey et al., "Non-metastatic unresected paediatric non-rhabdomyosarcoma soft tissue sarcomas: results of a pooled analysis from United States and European groups," *European Journal of Cancer*, vol. 47, no. 5, pp. 724–731, 2011.

[94] M. Carli, A. Ferrari, A. Mattke et al., "Pediatric malignant peripheral nerve sheath tumor: the Italian and German soft tissue sarcoma cooperative group," *Journal of Clinical Oncology*, vol. 23, no. 33, pp. 8422–8430, 2005.

[95] B. C. Widemann, D. K. Reinke, L. J. Helman et al., "SARC006: Phase II trial of chemotherapy in sporadic and neurofibromatosis type 1 (NF1)-associated high-grade malignant peripheral nerve sheath tumors (MPNSTs)," *Journal of Clinical Oncology*, vol. 31, Article ID 10522, 2013.

[96] K. Albritton, C. Rankin, C. M. Coffin et al., "Phase II trial of erlotinib in metastatic or unresectable malignant peripheral nerve sheath tumor (MPNST)," *Journal of Clinical Oncology*, vol. 24, Article ID 9518, 2006.

[97] R. G. Maki, D. R. D'Adamo, M. L. Keohan et al., "Phase II study of sorafenib in patients with metastatic or recurrent sarcomas," *Journal of Clinical Oncology*, vol. 27, no. 19, pp. 3133–3140, 2009.

[98] R. Chugh, J. K. Wathen, R. G. Maki et al., "Phase II multicenter trial of imatinib in 10 histologic subtypes of sarcoma using a bayesian hierarchical statistical model," *Journal of Clinical Oncology*, vol. 27, no. 19, pp. 3148–3153, 2009.

[99] S. Schuetze, K. Wathen, E. Choy et al., "Results of a Sarcoma Alliance for Research through Collaboration (SARC) phase II trial of dasatinib in previously treated, high-grade, advanced sarcoma," *Journal of Clinical Oncology*, vol. 28, Article ID 10009, 2010.

[100] M. A. Dickson, M. R. Mahoney, W. D. Tap et al., "Phase II study of MLN8237 (Alisertib) in advanced/metastatic sarcoma," *Annals of Oncology*, vol. 27, no. 10, pp. 1855–1860, 2016.

[101] A. B. Miller, B. Hoogstraten, M. Staquet, and A. Winkler, "Reporting results of cancer treatment," *Cancer*, vol. 47, no. 1, pp. 207–214, 1981.

[102] E. A. Eisenhauer, P. Therasse, J. Bogaerts et al., "New response evaluation criteria in solid tumours: revised RECIST guideline (version 1.1)," *European Journal of Cancer*, vol. 45, no. 2, pp. 228–247, 2009.

[103] H. Choi, C. Charnsangavej, S. C. Faria et al., "Correlation of computed tomography and positron emission tomography in patients with metastatic gastrointestinal stromal tumor treated at a single institution with imatinib mesylate: proposal of new computed tomography response criteria," *Journal of Clinical Oncology*, vol. 25, no. 13, pp. 1753–1759, 2007.

[104] D. Katz, A. Lazar, and D. Lev, "Malignant peripheral nerve sheath tumour (MPNST): the clinical implications of cellular signalling pathways," *Expert Reviews in Molecular Medicine*, vol. 11, article e30, 2009.

19

Multimodality Treatment in Ewing's Sarcoma Family Tumors of the Maxilla and Maxillary Sinus

David Thorn,[1] Christoph Mamot,[1] Fatime Krasniqi,[2] Frank Metternich,[3] and Sven Prestin[3]

[1]*Division of Medical Oncology, Cantonal Hospital Aarau, 5001 Aarau, Switzerland*
[2]*Division of Medical Oncology, University Hospital Basel, 4031 Basel, Switzerland*
[3]*Division of Ear, Nose and Throat, Head & Neck Surgery, Cantonal Hospital Aarau, 5001 Aarau, Switzerland*

Correspondence should be addressed to Sven Prestin; svenprestin@hotmail.com

Academic Editor: Uta Dirksen

The Ewing sarcoma family of tumors (ESFT) encompasses a group of highly aggressive, morphologically similar, malignant neoplasms sharing a common spontaneous genetic translocation that affect mostly children and young adults. These predominantly characteristic, small round-cell tumors include Ewing's sarcoma of the bone and soft tissue, as well as primitive neuroectodermal tumors (PNETs) involving the bone, soft tissue, and thoracopulmonary region (Askin's tumor). Extraosseous ESFTs are extremely rare, especially in the head and neck region, where literature to date consists of sporadic case reports and very small series. We hereby present a review of the literature published on ESFTs reported in the maxilla and maxillary sinus region from 1968 to 2016.

1. Introduction

Since the latest WHO classification of 2013 [1], Ewing sarcoma family of tumors (ESFT) encompasses a group of highly aggressive, morphologically similar, malignant neoplasms sharing a common spontaneous genetic translocation. These predominantly characteristic, small round-blue-cell tumors include classical Ewing's sarcoma of the bone, extraosseous and soft tissue Ewing's sarcoma, as well as primitive neuroectodermal tumors (PNETs) involving the bone, soft tissue, and the chest wall, and the latter also is referred to as Askin's tumor [2]. PNETs, a group of tumors classified by their common neuroectodermal origin were formerly subdivided into three major groups: (1) central PNETs (cPNET), including tumors arising from the central nervous system, such as medulloblastoma; (2) neuroblastoma, including tumors arising from the autonomic nervous system; and (3) peripheral PNETs (pPNET) referring to PNETs arising outside the central nervous system [3]. The classification and terminology of tumors belonging to the PNET-group were however not uniform and proved awkward from early on. Although the initial description of peripheral PNETs was made in 1918 by Stout [4], who described a malignant tumor of the forearm that grew axons in tissue culture, confirming its neural origin and association with neuroblastoma, Hart and Earle [5] introduced the term PNET in 1973 to characterize medulloblastoma-like lesions found in the cerebral hemispheres. In 1979, Askin et al. published a retrospective analysis of young patients with a diagnosis of small cell tumors of the thoracopulmonary region, encompassing the years from 1964 to 1976 [2]. Those small cell tumors, that did not fit the criteria of Ewing's sarcoma, lymphoma, rhabdomyosarcoma, or neuroblastoma, were designated as malignant, small cell tumors of the thoracopulmonary region, later on known as Askin's tumors. In the 1980s, the term peripheral PNET was reestablished to describe a group of soft tissue tumors of presumed neural-crest origin that presented outside the CNS and in the sympathetic nervous system.

Ewing's sarcoma, the second most common primary bone tumor in children and adolescents, was initially described by Ewing in 1921 [6] as an undifferentiated tumor involving the diaphysis of long bones that, in contrast to osteosarcomas, was radiation sensitive. PNETs have been notoriously difficult to differentiate from Ewing's sarcoma and other ESFTs considering their close molecular biological relationship. There have actually been many cases of PNETs confused with rhabdomyosarcoma, neuroblastoma, and even lymphoma. Light microscopically, PNETs are described as small, round cells that often form characteristic lobular or pseudorosette patterns, known as the Homer-Wright rosette. Their neuroectodermal differentiation is suggested by the presence of ganglion cells and neurofibrillary structures, which reveal electron-dense neurosecretory-like granules, filaments, and microtubules under the electron microscope [7–9]. Immunohistochemical evaluation shows positive staining for neuron-specific enolase, synaptophysin, S100 protein, and MB2 monoclonal antibodies [10, 11]. Diagnosis is therefore based on ultrastructural, immunohistochemical, and molecular biological investigations. When identifying tumor cells as PNETs and differentiating between Ewing's sarcoma and other small round-cell tumors, positive staining using polyclonal or monoclonal antibodies against at least two neuroendocrine or neural markers in combination with the histological detection of Homer-Wright rosettes is regarded confirmatory. As the possibilities in distinguishing between these entities constantly improved in the 80s and 90s, it was reported that the true incidence of PNETs might be indefinitely higher than assumed in older series [12–17].

Ewing's sarcoma cells, unlike PNETs, have been generally described to fail immunohistochemical staining with antibodies against neuron-specific enolase and S-100 protein [18–21], supporting the debate against their neural-crest origin. Alongside studies that report of positive immunohistochemical staining with antibodies against intermediate filaments [22], ultrastructural examination, and failure of staining with endothelial lysozyme, alpha-1 antitrypsin, alpha-1 antichymotrypsin, and immunoglobulin markers [23, 24], this forms a strong body of evidence suggesting Ewing's sarcoma cells originate from uncommitted, primitive mesenchymal cells. Both Ewing's sarcoma and PNETs show strong expression of the cell surface glycoprotein MIC2 (CD99) [25]; although not exclusively specific for these tumors, this marker is definitely regarded characteristic of them and very useful in the differential diagnosis from other small round-cell neoplasms.

Meanwhile, cytogenetic studies have led to the identification of the nonrandom t(11;22)(q24;q12) chromosome rearrangement [26, 27] in Ewing's sarcoma, PNET, Askin's tumor, and neuroepithelioma, thereby supplying strong proof of their common histogenesis. It is upon the basis of this mutual genetic aberration, which provides a valuable characteristic for their differential diagnosis from other small round-cell tumors that these entities are now collectively recognised as Ewing's sarcoma family of tumors (ESFT).

Different fusions of the EWS gene (EWSR1) on chromosome 22q12 with various members of the ETS gene family (FLI1, ERG, ETV1, ETV4, and FEV) have been described [28, 29]. The chimaeric fusion transcript EWS–FLI1 is the result of fusion of the EWS gene on 22q12 with the FLI1 gene on 11q24. Substitution of the EWS domain with a portion of the FLI1 transcriptional domain results in an EWS–FLI1 fusion transcript with increased transcriptional activity. The EWS-FLI1 fusion transcript is found in approximately 85% of cases and considered pathognomonic [28, 30]. In the remaining 15% of tumors, other EWS-ETS gene family rearrangements have been identified, the second most common being the t(21;22)(q22;q12) translocation resulting in fusion of EWS with the ERG gene on 21q22 [31].

The EWS-ETS fusion proteins have been shown to activate human telomerase activity in Ewing's sarcoma through upregulation of TERT (telomerase reverse transcriptase) gene expression, probably by functioning as a transcriptional coactivator [32]. The oncogenic effect of EWS-ETS fusion transcripts, may be partly mediated by upregulation of LAMB3 expression, a gene encoding the $\beta 3$ chain of laminin-5. Laminin-5 is frequently found to be strongly expressed in the cytoplasm of invading cancer cells, suggesting its role at the invasive front of colorectal, gastric, pancreatic, and breast tumors, alongside various others [33]. Many malignancies, experience loss of cell cycle control during multistage progression. In ESFTs, studies have demonstrated changes in G1/S regulatory genes after downregulation and forced expression of the EWS–FLI1 fusion gene [34], supporting the hypothesis that abrogation of the G1 checkpoint appears to be important in the progression and development of the clinical phenotype [35–37].

Although rare in adults, classical osseous Ewing's sarcoma constitutes the second most frequent primary bone cancer in children after osteosarcoma. Nevertheless, with an annual incidence of approximately 0.6/million total population, affecting 13/million 0–24 year olds each year in the UK [38], this is still a rare disease even among the adolescent population. Most commonly, patients are diagnosed with Ewing's sarcoma in the second decade of life, although 20–30% of cases are reported to occur in the first decade. The male to female ratio is approximately 1.3 : 1, so young boys are at a slightly higher risk than girls [39]. Caucasians are generally far more frequently affected than Asians, African-Americans, or Africans [40, 41]. Ewing's sarcoma usually involves the central and peripheral skeleton, namely, the pelvis and long bones, whereas involvement of nonosseous tissue is rare. ESFTs in the head and neck region are extremely rare, accounting for a mere 1%–7% of cases [39, 42, 43]. Generally, literature addressing Ewing's sarcoma family tumors in the head and neck region consists of sporadic case reports or very small series. Many of these series however fail to differentiate between the exact primary tumor locations by classifying "head and neck" as a collective potpourri [42, 44–48]. Although reported 5-year overall survival rates for Ewing's sarcoma family tumors in all sites have increased markedly thanks to modern multimodality treatment, reaching almost 70% in localized disease, only minimal data is available on the outcome of ESFTs located specifically in the head and neck region. Reports of pPNETs involving the maxilla and/or maxillary sinus are exceedingly rare; they predominantly lack immunohistochemical confirmation as well as long-term follow-up data after treatment. The following systematic review of the literature on ESFTs reported in the maxilla and maxillary sinus region aims to elucidate the background of these seldom neoplasms, detect analogies in their management, and give an overview of the modern multimodality treatment options available. We hope to offer guidance and support to clinicians facing the challenges of treating ESFTs in this confined region.

2. Methods

We performed a concise electronic research for reported cases of Ewing sarcoma family of tumors published in English medical literature, involving the maxilla and maxillary sinus only. The PubMed database was systematically searched for the terms Ewing's sarcoma, Ewing sarcoma family of tumors, Ewing, and PNET, in combination with the anatomical location sites:maxilla, maxillary sinus, upper jaw, and face, as well as head and neck. Single cases and case series describing ESFTs in this region were studied meticulously and the data extracted. Those cases of PNETs and Ewing's sarcomas not strictly limited to the maxilla or maxillary sinus, for instance, involving the mandible, the orbit, the palate, or the lower jaw, were then excluded, as were those cases that did not specify the exact location of the primary tumor.

3. Results

From 1968 to 2016, we found a total of 93 cases of ESFTs involving the maxilla or maxillary sinus published in the English medical literature (Table 1). Of these, 14 were further classified by the authors as being PNETS, mainly on account of their positivity for neuroendocrine markers. Of the 54 cases, in which patient's sex and age were specified, 32 were male (59.3%), 22 were female (just over 40%), and 36 patients were aged 25 or younger (66.6%). The slightly higher odds ratio for the male sex of 1.45, as well as the fact that the majority of cases describe patients in their first and second decade of life, seems congruent with the literature reported so far. All together 38 cases (40% of all the cases) reported positive immunohistochemical staining for MIC2/CD99. As from the year 1999, those cases including MIC2/CD99-status constitute 72% of total published cases and series. The transcription products EWS-FLI1, EWSR1, and EWS-ERG, on the other hand, were merely reported in 12 cases (only 13% of all cases), and 10 of these 12 cases were published since 2008. The vast majority of cases were identified as Ewing's sarcoma or PNETs on account of typical histological features, like Homer-Wright rosettes. 51 cases described patients' symptoms, probably leading to early diagnosis. Painless swelling was by far the most frequently reported symptom (31 cases, 60%), followed by congestion/obstruction (16 cases, 31%) and epistaxis (10 cases, 19.6%), while pain (5 cases) alongside proptosis with or without vision disorder (5 cases) seemed to occur seldom in less than 10% of patients. Mostly the onset of these symptoms occurred within the order of 3–6 months, thus leading to early diagnosis and therapeutic intervention accordingly. While only 4 cases failed to report therapy completely, 85 cases (91.4% of all cases) were treated with multimodality treatment, that is, the combination of at least local treatment (surgery and/or radiotherapy) plus systemic treatment. 11 cases reported the general term "chemoradiation" as the therapy implemented, without further specifying the exact cytostatic substances used, the radiation dose administered, or the sequence of these treatment modalities. The majority of 88 patients (95% of all cases) received some sort of local treatment via either radiotherapy, "chemoradiation," or surgical excision (usually maxillectomy or lateral rhinotomy), and the latter was often combined with further adjuvant radiotherapy. All together 81 patients (87%) received systemic treatment in the form of chemotherapy (either neoadjuvant chemotherapy, adjuvant chemotherapy, or as "chemoradiation" not further specified), just over a third of them received this chemotherapy neoadjuvantly (29 patients, 35.8%). Follow-up was reported in the majority of 79 cases (only 14 were not reported). Of these, in total 68 patients (86%) remained disease free during the period of observation, only 9 deaths and 2 recurrences were reported all together. Table 2 summarizes the follow-up and outcome data of the ESFT cases studied as a function of the implemented treatment modalities, respectively (only those cases including these specific data are represented; therefore, the case series by Biswas et al. [49] and Grevener et al. [50] were excluded). Maximum disease free periods were reported for radiochemotherapy with surgery (upon 16 years of follow-up [51]) and for radiotherapy without surgery (upon 23 years of follow-up [52]).

4. Discussion

4.1. Diagnosis and Differential Diagnosis of ESFTs. In the head and neck region, the differential diagnosis of small round-cell tumors includes lymphoma, malignant melanoma, rhabdomyosarcoma, olfactory neuroblastoma, undifferentiated carcinoma, and Ewing's sarcoma/pPNET. Melanoma, lymphoma and rhabdomyosarcoma can be identified with immunohistochemistry for S100, CD45, and desmin, respectively. In those cases of ESFTs which display focal positivity for S100 or desmin, additional immunohistochemical stains for melanoma markers (HMB45, Melan-A) and specific skeletal muscle markers (myogenin, myoD1) can be utilized to exclude melanoma and rhabdomyosarcoma. Carcinomas are generally diffusely positive for multiple keratins, whereas ESFTs typically stain focally for only one keratin marker [92]. Sometimes ESFTs can be positive for synaptophysin and other neuroendocrine markers (especially PNETs) but usually only stain focally. Almost 100% of ESFTs stain positively with CD99, while olfactory neuroblastomas do not [95]. The EWS-FLI1 fusion transcript, pathognomonic for ESFTs, does also not occur in neuroblastoma [96]. As outlined above, PNETs normally develop mainly in the central nervous system and soft tissue of children and young adults. When these tumors seldom occur outside the central nervous system, they are by definition termed peripheral primitive neuroectodermal tumor (pPNET). Peripheral primitive neuroectodermal tumors involving the maxilla are extremely rare disease entities [77]. In 1989, Coffin and Dehner described fewer than 10 reported cases of pPNETS involving the maxilla to have been published in English literature [97], while Mohindra et al. even spoke of less than 8 reported cases [83].

4.2. Prognostic Factors. Two-thirds of patients initially present with localized disease, which, when using multimodality treatment, is nowadays amenable to curation in approximately 70% of cases. However, patients presenting with primary metastatic disease (common sites being 10% in the lung, 10% in the bone/bone marrow, and 5% in combinations of lung and bone or other locations) generally

Table 1: Literature review 1968–2016.

Study	Year	Tumor/patient	Localisation	Symptoms	Therapy	Follow-up	IHC/Mol
Hunsuck [53]	1968	ES/m 33 y	Maxilla	Swelling	(1) RTX 3000 rads (2) Subtotal maxillectomy	18 mts: DF	n.s.
Roca et al. [54] REV.	1968	ES m/3 y	Maxilla	Proptosis	RTX 4000 r + resection	11 y: DF	n.s.
		ES m/7 y	Maxilla	Swelling	Curettage, RTX 5000 r + C	5 y: DF	n.s.
Brownson and Cook [55]	1969	ES f/6 y	Maxilla	Facial swelling	(1) RTX (n.f.s.) (2) VC	n.s.	n.s. n.s.
Fernandez et al. [56] REV.	1974	ES/2 Pat.	Maxilla	n.s.	Chemoradiation (n.f.s.)	n.s.	n.s.
Ferlito [57] REV.	1978	ES/m, 29 y	Maxilla	Congestion	RTX + Adr, V, Bl	10 mts: died	n.s.
		ES/m, 44 y	Maxilla	Swelling	Resection, RTX, Adr, V, CCNU	8 mts: DF	n.s.
		ES/m, 43 y	Maxilla	Epistaxis	RTX + Adr, V, CCNU	1 y: died	n.s.
		ES/m, 44 y	Maxilla	Epistaxis	RTX + Adr, V, CCNU	3 mts: DF	n.s.
Komray [58]	1979	ES/m, 15 y	Max sin	Epistaxis, exopht.	(1) RTX 6000 rads (2) VAdC	1 y: DF	n.s.
Strong et al. [52] REV.	1979	ES/m, 3 y	Maxilla	n.s.	AMC + RTX 4000 rads	23 y: DF	n.s.
		ES/m, 7 y	Maxilla	n.s.	C + RTX 6500 rads	14 y: died	n.s.
		ES/m, 9 y	Maxilla	n.s.	CVAD + RTX 6000 rads	4 y: DF	n.s.
Pontius and Sebek [59]	1981	ES/m, 39 y	Max. sin.	Obstruct., lacrimat.	(1) Resection (2) RTX 7500 rads	2 y: DF	n.s.
Hossfeld et al. [60]	1982	ES/n.s.	Maxilla	n.s.	Chemoradiation (n.f.s.)	n.s.	n.s.
Slootweg et al. [61]	1983	PNET/m, 10 y	Maxilla	Swelling	(1) Subtotal maxillectomy (2) RTX 50 Gy	3 y: DF	n.s.
Bacchini et al. [62]	1986	ES/f, 7 y	Maxilla	n.s.	(1) Curettage, RTX 6000 rads (2) Adj. CVAD	5 y 6 mts: DF	n.s.
Siegal et al. [42] REV.	1987	ES/m, 14 y	Maxilla	Swelling	VCD/VACD + RTX 4300 rads	10 y: DF	n.s.
		ES/m, 9 y	Maxilla	Swelling	VCD/VACD + RTX 6000 rads	8 y: DF	n.s.
		ES/f, 8 y	Maxilla	Swelling	VCD/VACD + RTX 6550 rads	7 y 5 mts: DF	n.s.
		ES/f, 15 y	Maxilla	Swelling	VCD/VACD + RTX 5500 rads	11 mts: DF	n.s.

Table 1: Continued.

Study	Year	Tumor/patient	Localisation	Symptoms	Therapy	Follow-up	IHC/Mol
Amin et al. [63]	1990	ES/f, 10 y	Maxilla	Obstruct., swelling	(1) Lateral rhinotomy (2) RTX, not performed	n.s.	n.s.
Yeo et al. [64]	1991	PNET/f, 7 y	Maxilla	Swelling, pain	(1) Neoadj. VAC (2) Partial maxillectomy (3) Adj. C + RTX 50 Gy	9 y: DF	n.s.
Filiatrault et al. [65]	1993	PNET/f, 11 y	Max sin	Obstruct.	Chemoradiation (n.f.s.)	10 mts: SD	n.s.
Jones and McGill [66] REV.	1995	PNET/f, 13 y	Max sin	n.s.	Chemoradiation (n.f.s.)	2 y: DF	n.s.
Shah et al. [67]	1995	PNET/m, 42 y	Max sin	Swelling	(1) CAVCisPt, I, VP-16, E (2) RTX (n.f.s.)	9 mts: died	n.s.
Ibarburen et al. [68]	1996	PNET/f, 20 mts	Maxilla	Swelling	n.s.	3 y: DF	n.s.
Fiorillo et al. [69]	1996	ES/m, 7 y ES/f, 22 y	Maxilla Maxilla	Swelling Swelling	CVAIE + RTX 6000 cGy CVAIE + RTX 6000 cGy	52 mts: DF 41 mts: DF	n.s. n.s.
Zheng et al. [70]	1998	ES/m, 16 y	Maxilla	Swelling	n.s.	n.s.	n.s.
Allam et al. [71] REV.	1999	ES/9 Pat.	Maxilla	n.s.	(1) RTX + VAdC + IEP/VAIA (2) Surgery, n.s.	3.4 y (mean)	n.s.
Toda et al. [72]	1999	PNET/f, 57 y	Max. sin.	Obstruct.	(1) VAdC (2) RTX 40 Gy	3 mts: died	MIC2–
Daw et al. [51]	2000	ES	Maxilla	n.s.	(1) Resection, RTX 3500 cGy (2) Adj. CVAD, Carm	16 y 9 mts: DF	n.s.
Wexler et al. [73]	2003	ES	Max sin	Congestion, swelling	(1) Neoadj. VAdC + IE (2) Subtotal maxillectomy (3) Adjuv. chemotherapy (n.f.s.)	3 y: DF	MIC2+, EWS-FLI1
Kao et al. [74]	2002	PNET/m, 74 y	Maxilla	Swelling	CisPtEI	4 mts: died	$CD99^{+}$
Alobid et al. [75]	2003	PNET/f, 23 y	Max. sin.	Obstruct.	(1) Lateral rhinotomy (2) Adj. CVAD + RTX 60 Gy	59 mts: DF	$CD99^{+}$
Harman et al. [76]	2003	ES/f, 40 y	Max sin	Obstruct.	(1) VAC (2) RTX 2000 cGy	n.s.	$CD99^{+}$
Windfuhr [44] REV.	2004	PNET/m, 7 y	Max. sin.	Exopht., vision loss	(1) Lateral rhinotomy (2) Adj. VIDE/VACD (3) RTX 45 Gy	17 mts: DF	n.s.
Howarth et al. [43]	2004	ES/m, 9 y	Maxilla	Swelling	(1) VIDE (inoperable) (2) RTX (n.f.s.)	n.s.	$CD99^{+}$

Table 1: Continued.

Study	Year	Tumor/patient	Localisation	Symptoms	Therapy	Follow-up	IHC/Mol
Sun et al. [77]	2007	PNET/f, 49 y	Maxilla	Swelling	(1) Total right maxillectomy (2) Radiotherapy 60 Gy	3 mts: DF	$CD99^+$, EWS-FLI1
Infante-Cossio et al. [78]	2005	ES/m, 17 y	Max. sin.	Swelling	(1) Neoadj. VCAIE (2) Complete resection (3) Adj. chemotherapy (n.f.s.)	8 y: DF	$CD99^+$
Coskun et al. [79]	2005	ES/f, 16 y	Max sin	Swelling	(1) Surgery declined (2) RTX + CVAD/IE	1 y: DF	$CD99^+$
Varshney et al. [80]	2007	ES	Maxilla	Swelling	(1) Resection (2) Adj. VAC + RTX 2000 cGy	n.s.	$CD99^+$
Thariat et al. [81]	2008	ES/m, 26 y	Max. sin.	Swelling	(1) Neoadj. CD (2) Surgery (3) Adj. AV	11 y: local recurrence	t(11;22) EWSR1
Prasad et al. [82]	2008	ES/m, 18 y	Maxilla	Swelling	(1) Extended maxillectomy (2) Adj. chemotherapy (n.f.s.)	1 y: DF	n.s.
Mohindra et al. [83]	2008	PNET/m, 5 y	Max. sin.	Swelling, exopht.	(1) VIDECAdr (2) RTX 55.8 Gy	n.s.	$CD99^+$, EWS-FLI1
Bornstein et al. [84]	2008	ES/f, 19 y	Max. sin.	Pain in teeth	(1) neoadj. VIDE (EU-Ew99) (2) Hemimaxillectomy (3) Adj. VAC + RTX 46 Gy	n.s.	$CD99^+$, EWS-FLI1
Kawabata et al. [85] REV.	2008	ES, PNET/m, 12 y	Max sin	Swelling	(1) VDCIE (2) RTX 45 Gy	20 mts: DF	$CD99^+$, EWS-ERG
Ataergin et al. [86]	2009	ES/n.s.	Maxilla	n.s.	(1) Neoadj. IEAM (2) Resection (3) Adj. RTX (n.f.s.), VD IE AC	died	n.s.
Piloni et al. [87]	2009	ES/2 Pat.	n.s.	n.s.	n.s.	n.s.	n.s.
Gupta et al. [88]	2009	ES/m, 30 y	Maxilla	Swelling, congestion	(1) Excision (2) Adj. chemoradiation (n.f.s.)	n.s.	$CD99^+$

Table 1: Continued.

Study	Year	Tumor/patient	Localisation	Symptoms	Therapy	Follow-up	IHC/Mol
Hormozi et al. [89]	2010	PNET/f, 28 y	Maxilla Metastasis Parasellar	Diplopia	(1) Maxillectomy (2) γ-knife (optic chiasma) (3) Adj. VAI + RTX 80 Gy	6 mts: DF	$CD99^{+}$
Dadhe et al. [90]	2010	ES/m, 12 y	Max. sin.	Swelling, pain	(1) Extended maxillectomy (2) Adj. chemotherapy (n.f.s.)	1 y: DF	n.s.
Davido et al. [91]	2011	ES/m, 25 y	Max. sin.	Swelling, pain	(1) Neoadj. IDCisPt (2) Part maxillectomy (3) Adj. IDCisPt	5 y: DF	$CD99^{+}$
Hafezi et al. [92] REV.	2011	ES/f, 69 y ES/f, 45 y ES/m, 54 y ES/m, 25 y ES/f, 13 y ES/f, 15 y	Max. sin. Max. sin. Maxilla Max. sin. Max. sin. Max. sin.	Obstruct., epistaxis Obstruct., epistaxis Obstruct., epistaxis Obstruct., epistaxis Obstruct., epistaxis Obstruct., epistaxis	Chemoradiation (n.f.s.) Chemoradiation (n.f.s.) Chemoradiation (n.f.s.) Surgery (n.f.s.) Surgery (n.f.s.) Chemoradiation (n.f.s.)	6 mts: DF 14 mts: died 17 mts: died 26 mts: DF 4 mts: DF 14 y: DF	$CD99^{+}$, EWS-FLI1 $CD99^{+}$, EWS-FLI1 $CD99^{+}$ EWSR1 $CD99^{+}$ EWSR1 $CD99^{+}$ EWSR1 $CD99^{+}$ EWSR1
Yeshvanth et al. [93]	2012	ES/f, 29 y	Maxilla	Obstruct., epistaxis	(1) Neoadj. VACDex (2) Resection	1 y: DF	$CD99^{+}$
Kaler and Sheriff [94]	2013	ES/m, 22 y	Maxilla & orbit	Swelling, pain	(1) Craniofacial resection (2) Chemoradiation (n.f.s.)	2 y: local recurrence	$CD99^{+}$
Biswas et al. [49]	2014	ES/14 Pat.	Maxilla (sin.)	n.s.	(1) VDCIE (2) RTX or surgery ± RTX 50–60 Gy (3) Adj. chemotherapy (n.f.s.)	58 mts (median)	$CD99^{+}$
Grevener et al. [50]	2016	ES/7 Pat.	Maxilla	n.s.	(1) VIDE (2) RTX or surgery ± RTX 44–54 Gy	3.3 y (median)	n.s.

TABLE 2: ESFT, outcome as a function of treatment modality.

	Chemo TX, alone	Surgery, alone	Radio(chemo)TX (VAC, VCAD, VIDE) no surgery	Radio(chemo)TX (VAC, VCAD, VIDE) plus surgery	Treatment not specified
PNET	1 case [74]	—	6 cases	6 cases	1 case
Ewing	—	3 cases	23 cases	29 cases	3 cases
Disease free upon follow-up ≥ 1 year	—	1 case [92]	12 cases	15 cases	1 case [68]
Max. follow-up	4 months [74]	26 months [92]	23 years [52]	>16 years [51]	3 years [68]
Status upon max. follow-up	Dead	Disease free	Disease free	Disease free	Disease free

have a poor chance of long-term survival, as this is the most important adverse prognostic factor. Therefore, complete staging, including at least CT of the chest and MRI with or without CT of the primary site, as well as PET scan and/or bone scan is regarded obligatory. In the staging of ESFTs, the combination of PET or PET/CT with conventional imaging has demonstrated sensitivity and specificity > 90% [98]. Other established adverse prognostic factors are increased tumor size, as unfavourable outcome has been shown for tumor volumes > 200 mL [39, 50], poor or no response to preoperative chemotherapy, as defined by >10% viability of residual tumor after neoadjuvant therapy [99, 100], elevated serum LDH level, axial localization, and older age (>15 years). The individual risk of relapse or disease progression however remains difficult to predict. While the EWS-ETS fusion type was shown to be prognostic within the retrospective de Alava et al. study [101], prospective evaluation of different EWS-FLI1 fusion architecture failed to reach statistical significance as independent prognostic markers [100]. When modern effective therapies are implemented, as reported from the EURO-EWING 99 study and the Children's Oncology Group study, patients with Ewing's sarcomas have similar outcomes, regardless of fusion subtype [100, 102].

4.3. Imaging and Staging. Classical Ewing's sarcoma, typically involving the long bones, radiologically presents as "onion skinning" periosteal reaction; although also described as a characteristic feature of neuroectodermal tumor lesions, this feature is definitely less frequently observed in the facial skeleton [78, 103]. Osteolytic lesions are not a pathognomonic radiologic feature of ESFTs, because other diseases like osteosarcoma, neuroblastoma, lymphosarcoma, osteomyelitis, and metastatic carcinoma can exhibit a similar image pattern [62]. In the skull, these tumors present as permeative, destructive lesions with large associated soft tissue components without calcifications, reflecting their aggressive nature. Radiologic features include "moth-eaten" permeative bony destruction, exuberant periosteal reaction (onion skin, sunburst, spiculated, hair on end), cortical erosion, and presence of an associated soft tissue mass. CT of Ewing's sarcoma of the PNS shows a diffusely enhancing soft tissue mass with bone destruction [57, 104–107]. Usually, no calcification is noted. Similar changes, however, might be seen in the other PNS tumors (squamous cell carcinoma, esthesioneuroblastoma, lymphoma, etc.). MRI findings of Ewing's sarcoma of the skull show an unusual pattern of reactive sclerosis [108]. MRI of Ewing's sarcoma typically shows the lesion as hypointense to isointense on T1W1 and hypointense to hyperintense on T2W1.

4.4. Local Therapy. Although there are no randomized studies comparing surgery and radiotherapy, data from retrospective analyses suggest better local control of early ESFTs achieved by surgery (with or without postoperative radiotherapy) than by radiotherapy alone [109]. Combined analysis from the CESS 81, CESS 86, and EICESS 92 trials even showed the rate of local failure after surgery to be significantly lower than after definitive radiotherapy without prior excision [109]. Therefore, if technically possible, complete surgical excision should be regarded the mainstay of local control. Only in those cases where complete surgical excision is not feasible (see below), should radiotherapy be applied alone at a dose of 45–60 Gy and then, however, preferably combined with systemic treatment. Mere surgical debulking procedures, aimed at tumor-downsizing without achieving complete resection, do not improve local control compared to definitive radiotherapy and should not be advocated as they are associated with additional morbidity. Data from the CESS and EICESS trials, showed that patients who had an intralesional resection followed by radiotherapy had the same local control rates as patients who received radiotherapy alone [109], thereby clearly negating the benefit of intralesional surgery. When local treatment modalities like surgery or radiotherapy are used without systemic chemotherapy, 5-year survival often remains <10%. Modern treatment protocols including systemic polychemotherapy regimens in multimodality trials render survival rates of up to 70% in localized and 20%–30% in metastatic disease, depending upon metastatic sites and burden [110, 111]. Grevener et al. have recently studied the outcome of Ewing sarcomas of the head and neck by analyzing the German Society for Pediatric Hematology and Oncology database between 1999 and 2009. This publication also included 7 cases of ESFTs involving the maxilla but found no difference in event free survival or overall survival when comparing the local treatment modalities: surgery, radiotherapy or combined surgery followed by adjuvant radiotherapy [50]. In our review of ESFTs confined to the maxilla and maxillary sinus, we found that a total of 88 patients (95% of all cases) received some sort of local treatment via either radiotherapy, "chemoradiation," or surgical excision. Maxillectomy and lateral rhinotomy were the most frequently performed surgical techniques. Some of these patients then received further local control postoperatively by adjuvant radiotherapy. Several case series failed to discriminate between the exact modality of local therapy utilized, that is, merely reporting "radiotherapy or surgical resection" (with or without adjuvant radiotherapy). For this reason, it will not be possible to make a general recommendation concerning the optimal local treatment strategy based on this review data. The best treatment option for local tumor control in the maxilla or maxillary sinus will always need to be assessed individually, as each and every clinical case will present its unique challenges to the team of specialists involved.

Morbidity of local therapy is one of these key issues, which, when facing ESFTs in the maxilla and maxillary sinus region, will tremendously impact the choice of local treatment modality. Surgery of the middle face and skull is technically demanding. Radical tumor excision is often limited by the proximity of adjacent critical structures and complicated by the wish to preserve function and cosmesis. Extensive, mutilating facial surgery, leading to loss of physiognomy, functional defects, and cosmetic problems, will often provoke a multitude of further complications and severely compromise patients' quality of life, without therapeutic benefit in the long run. Major concerns related to surgical management, especially in children and adolescents, include deleterious effects on respiratory function, nutrition and deglutition, speech, and vision as well as overall facial appearance and cosmesis. On the other hand, the use of modern surgical techniques, implementing microvascular flaps, immediate reconstruction using PEEK (Polyetheretherketone) implants, titanium grid-plates, titanium-enforced Medpore-foils, obturator prosthesis, dental prosthesis, and other reconstructive surgical materials, often enable the surgeon to perform excellent functional and esthetical results nowadays [112]. Taking this into account, whenever complete surgical excision is threatening to provoke morbidity at a high cost for the patient, or even deemed to be technically impossible, then alternatively, considering ESFTs' pronounced radiosensitivity, radiotherapy may constitute a valid option for effective local tumor control. While radiation may seem less burdensome, it is certainly not without both early and late sequelae. Organ preservation does not automatically mean functional preservation. Radiotherapy in this region may also lead to serious adverse effects, such as mucositis and stomatitis, with consecutive loss of taste and appetite, as well as severe pain. Radiotherapy may harm the function of salivary and nasal glands, be detrimental to dental health status, and compromise nasal inspiration by injuring mucous membranes as well as causing a multitude of ocular disorders, like irritations and dryness, conjunctivitis, lens opacification, or even total blindness. Other late effects of radiotherapy in the facial region include auditory and vestibular defects. In the child and adolescent, long-term adverse effects on growth, behavioral problems, and cognitive deficits have also been reported. Modern intensity modulated radiotherapy (IMRT) protocols applied by radiooncology departments in specialized sarcoma centers can of course substantially reduce the risk of morbidity, by calculating and programming defined radiation tangents in order to minimize scattered radiation, otherwise harming surrounding structures. When IMRT is implemented accordingly, it can, for instance, avoid orbital sequelae as has been previously shown in the treatment of sinonasal tumors [113]. Radiation induced secondary tumors are another well-known late effect, especially an increased risk for osteosarcomas has frequently been described; these however tend to occur more often after treatment of ESFTs involving the extremities. The phenomenon of radiation induced secondary malignancy is clearly dose related; a significant increased risk for secondary tumors arises with administered radiation doses above 40 Gy [114, 115]. When radiotherapy has been administered as the primary local treatment modality (e.g., neoadjuvantly), subsequent surgery can lead to common complications, including wound infections, fistula formation, and the need for surgical revision, whereas flap survival does not seem to be negatively impacted by prior radiation [116]. Needless to say, it is imperative that local treatment modalities for ESFTs in the maxillary region be discussed multidisciplinary early on. Highly experienced maxillofacial surgeons, radiooncologists, and radiation-physicists, as well as medical oncologists and specialized nursing staff should be involved, thereby outweighing the advantages and risks of implementing a given therapeutic local strategy. As always in ESFT-management, but especially for ESFTs involving the confined maxillary region, the possibility of tumor downstaging by neoadjuvant systemic chemotherapy, alongside combating early micrometastatic disease, needs to be carefully evaluated and preferably utilized whenever possible.

4.5. Systemic Therapy. While high-dose chemotherapy followed by hematopoietic stem cell transplantation, although employed in some trial protocols in high-risk localized and metastatic ES [117], is still clearly considered investigational, the most active substances so far are regarded to be doxorubicin, cyclophosphamide, ifosfamide, vincristine, dactinomycin, and etoposide [39, 109, 118–120]. Combinations of these agents are initially employed neoadjuvantly during 3–6 cycles at 2-3-week intervals after histological diagnosis is confirmed by biopsy to downstage the tumor and increase the probability of achieving microscopically negative resection margins. Following surgical resection, further 6 to 10 cycles of adjuvant polychemotherapy have been shown to improve relapse free survival and overall survival [118, 119, 121–123]. Thereby, overall treatment duration usually reaches approximately 10–12 months. In the attempt of perfecting efficacy, a variety of regimens have been analyzed prospectively and retrospectively.

Data from the IESS-I and IESS-II trials could show that adjuvant chemotherapy with VACD (vincristine, dactinomycin, cyclophosphamide, and doxorubicin) leads to a significantly better 5-year relapse free survival (60% versus 24%) and overall survival (65% versus 28%) compared to VAC (vincristine, dactinomycin, and cyclophosphamide) when applied together with radiotherapy in localized non-metastatic disease [119].

When ifosfamide and etoposide were added to this regimen (VACD-IE) in the Pediatric Oncology Group-Children's Cancer Group (POG-CCG) study, the 5-year event free survival rate (69% versus 54%) and the 5-year overall survival rate (72% versus 61%) were superior to VACD [124]. VACD-IE also showed lower cumulative incidences of local failure (11%) compared to VACD (30%), irrespective of the type of local control therapy [124]. In the INT 0091 study, patients with metastatic disease, however, did not profit from adding IE as there were no significant differences in 5-year event free survival or OS between VACD and VACD-IE [118]. In line with this data, the addition of etoposide to VAIA (EVAIA) was seemingly associated with a survival benefit (although not statistically significant) in the subgroup of patients without metastases in the EICESS-92 study [120]. The Euro-EWING 99 protocol for the treatment of localized disease is largely based on the same drug combinations used in the previous Cooperative Ewing's Sarcoma Study (CESS) and the European Intergroup Cooperative Ewing's Sarcoma Study (EICESS). Multiagent induction chemotherapy with six courses of VIDE (vincristine, ifosfamide, doxorubicin, and etoposide) followed by local treatment (surgery and/or RT) and HDT/SCT (high-dose chemotherapy/stem cell transplantation) were designed to evaluate efficacy and safety in patients with primary disseminated Ewing's sarcoma [99]. Of the 93 cases of ESFTs found in the maxilla or maxillary sinus region described in our review, only 7 failed to receive chemotherapy of some sort. The overwhelming majority was treated with polychemotherapy regimens including doxorubicin, cyclophosphamide, ifosfamide, vincristine, dactinomycin, and etoposide.

Complications and toxicities caused by chemotherapy are numerous and agent dependent. Besides the most common and often expected adverse effects, like fatigue, mucositis, and hemotoxicity, many cytostatic substances can cause agent-specific toxicity. For example, anthracyclines, including doxorubicin, may induce a dose-related cardiomyopathy leading to congestive heart failure. Alkylating agents, like cyclophosphamide and ifosfamide, are associated with infertility, especially male infertility, so that sperm cryopreservation should be offered to postpubertal boys and men wishing to father children, prior to the initiation of chemotherapy. Chemotherapy has also been associated with inducing secondary malignancies. There have been reports of 1%-2% increased rates of secondary leukemia following a sequence of chemotherapy protocols utilized for treating Ewing's sarcoma, and usually these malignancies occurred within 3 years of initial ESFT-diagnosis and therapy [118].

4.6. Follow-Up and Outcome. Upon completion of multimodality treatment for ESFTs of the maxilla or maxillary sinus, patients should be controlled clinically and radiologically in regular fixed intervals. In our review of the literature of ESFTs involving the maxilla and maxillary sinus, follow-up was reported in the majority of 79 cases (see Tables 1 and 2; only 14 cases failed to report follow-up at all). Of these, an overwhelming 68 Patients (86%) remained disease free during the period of observation, and only 9 deaths and 2 recurrences were reported all together. This can be accounted for mainly by the fact that all but one of the cases reported documented early ESFTs confined to the maxilla or maxillary sinus, thereby ruling out (or failing to mention) metastatic disease. The greater amount of tumor recurrences has however previously been described to take place within the first 2 years of follow-up [44]. Therefore, as some of the follow-up periods mentioned in this review are less than one year, some case series included median follow-up periods and others even failed to precisely outline deaths with respect to the exact primary tumor-site, and the actual numbers of true relapses and tumor-associated deaths may be indefinitely higher and so underrepresented by these figures. Taking these caveats into account, the overall prognosis for early ESFTs confined to the maxilla and maxillary sinus, as represented (see Table 2), seems nonetheless very optimistic. So bearing in mind, of course, that the collected data presented in this review are of selected cases only, these findings do stand in line with previous reports that tend to show a more favourable prognosis for ESFTs occurring in the head and neck region [50].

4.7. Recommendations for Daily Practice. In daily clinical practice, when facing a patient, especially pediatric patient or adolescent, presenting symptoms of acute or chronic unexplained facial swelling, a painless (or painful) mass of the upper jaw and nasal congestion or obstruction, as well as unexplained nose bleeding, we recommend further timely diagnostic procedures. These should at least include meticulous clinical examination of the jaw and oral cavity, endoscopy, biopsy for histology, and local imaging by X-ray or if necessary computed tomography. Once histologically confirmed, ESFTs should then be transferred to, or treated under close supervision of, a sarcoma center from an early stage. The necessity for further imaging (i.e., MRI of the head and neck, CT, and PET/CT), neoadjuvant treatment strategies, and precise preoperative surgical and/or radiotherapeutical planning is vital and needs to be evaluated by the involved MDT-specialists as soon as possible. This interdisciplinary decision-making process is just as important as the definitive skills and expertise of the sarcoma surgeon or radiooncologist involved in the next steps of treatment. In localized ESFTs of the maxilla and/or maxillary sinus, we recommend always preoperatively consulting a team of experienced maxillofacial surgeons alongside surgeons with profound experience in the field of plastic reconstructive surgery of the upper jaw and surgical dentistry. Radiooncologist and medical oncologists should be included in preoperative decision-making as well. Whenever feasible, neoadjuvant chemotherapy ideally within a clinical trial, containing a well-known and efficacious regimen like VIDE, should be administered and closely monitored by an experienced team of medical and/or pediatric oncologists. Therapeutic success (tumor-shrinkage) should be checked in regular 8–12-week intervals, radiologically as well as clinically if possible. The aim hereby should always be to boost the probability of complete R0-tumor-resection leading to microscopically free margins by maximum tumor-shrinkage, as well as destroying occult micrometastasis. If the risk of debilitating surgery causing serious personal morbidity to the patient, or the risk of incomplete tumor excision itself, is deemed high, then alternatively IMRT to the radiologically predefined tumor-bed should be evaluated by experienced radiooncologists. Decisions concerning the modality of adjuvant treatment following local tumor control should, when applicable, be made upon the defined histological regression grade, that is, pathologically reported vitality of the remaining tumor tissue (see above) excised after neoadjuvant systemic treatment. This treatment, once again, should ideally be performed under the umbrella of a randomized clinical trial; if not available, however, then at least it should be performed in close analogy to renown therapeutic protocols as, for instance, the EWING 99 study. Upon completion of multimodality treatment for ESFTs of the maxilla or maxillary sinus, patients should be controlled clinically and radiologically in regular fixed intervals. As most relapses have been reported to occur within the first two years after treatment [44], we would advocate close follow-up during the first 5 years by experienced clinicians at a sarcoma center. Endoscopic controls, when possible also performed behind a surgically placed prosthesis (ideally provisional and not definitely fixed during the first 3 years), as well as MRIs of the head and face and X-ray of the chest, should follow a strict 3–6 monthly schedule. After the first 5 years, it may be sufficient to perform follow-ups in greater intervals of 6–12 months, always, however, considering the patient's individual relapse-risk depending upon that mentioned above (resection margin status, radiotherapy dose, remission status following chemotherapy, etc.).

5. Conclusions

Although rare and potentially highly aggressive, ESFTs limited to the maxilla and maxillary sinus seem well manageable when utilizing modern multimodality treatment strategies. As described in the literature to date, outcome and prognosis of this specific entity seem more favourable compared to ESFTs occurring in the common primary sites located in the long bones or pelvis. This may in part be due to the fact, that patients presenting with ESFTs in the maxilla or maxillary sinus frequently experience symptoms like facial swelling, nasal congestion or even epistaxis at an early stage of tumor growth, ultimately leading to earlier diagnosis and successful treatment. Contrary to expectations, ESFTs occurring in the confined spatial proportions of the maxilla and maxillary sinus, often less amenable to complete surgical resection with clear tumor margins, may be equally successfully treated with a combination of radiotherapy and chemotherapy without surgery. Especially in those cases, in which the risk for morbidity by mutilating surgery seems high or complete surgical excision technically impossible, radiotherapy (combined with neoadjuvant and/or adjuvant chemotherapy) may prove to be similarly efficacious for achieving good local control without compromising long-term survival. In general we recommend consulting a sarcoma reference center early on in treatment planning, thereby ensuring for multidisciplinary expertise in favour of best clinical practice. As always, when available, patients with such rare tumor entities should definitely be enrolled in clinical trials or at least treated in accordance with modern trial protocols. So using well-established chemotherapy regimens neoadjuvantly and adjuvantly, in combination with surgery and/or radiotherapy for local control, will aim to achieve maximum possible treatment outcome.

Abbreviations

IHC: Immunohistochemistry
Mol: Molecular analysis
DF: Disease free
n.s.: Not specified
n.f.s.: Not further specified
RTX: Radiotherapy
VC: Vincristine and cyclophosphamide
Adr: Adriamycin
V: Vincristine
Bl: Bleomycin
CCNU: Chloroethylcyclohexylnitrosourea
VAdC: Vincristine, Adriamycin, and cyclophosphamide
AMC: Amethopterin and Cyclophosphamide
C: Cyclophosphamide
CVAD: Cyclophosphamide, vincristine, actinomycin, and doxorubicin
VCD: Vincristine, cyclophosphamide, and dactinomycin
VAC: Vincristine, actinomycin, and Cyclophosphamide
VACD: Vincristine, Adriamycin, cyclophosphamide, and dactinomycin
CAVCisPt: Cyclophosphamide, Adriamycin, vincristine, and cisplatin
I: Ifosfamide
E: Etoposide
VAIA: Vincristine, Adriamycin, ifosfamide, and actinomycin
CVAIE: Cyclophosphamide, Vincristine, actinomycin, ifosfamide, and etoposide
IEP: Ifosfamide, etoposide, and cisplatin
Carm: Carmustine
IE: Ifosfamide and etoposide
CisPtEI: Cisplatin, etoposide, and ifosfamide
VIDE: Vincristine, ifosfamide, doxorubicin, and etoposide
VCAIE: Vincristine, cyclophosphamide, actinomycin, ifosfamide, and etoposide
VIDECAdr: Vincristine, ifosfamide, dactinomycin, etoposide, cyclophosphamide, and Adriamycin
VDCIE: Vincristine, doxorubicin, cyclophosphamide, ifosfamide, and etoposide
IEAM: Ifosfamide, etoposide, actinomycin, and melphalan
VD IE AC: Vincristine, dactinomycin, ifosfamide, etoposide, doxorubicine, and cyclophosphamide
VAI: Vincristin, actinomycin, and ifosfamide
IDCisPt: Ifosfamide, doxorubicin, and cisplatin
CD: Cyclophosphamide and doxorubicine
AV: Actinomycin and vincristine
VACDex: Vincristine, Adriamycin, cyclophosphamide, and dexamethasone.

Competing Interests

The authors declare that they have no competing interests.

References

[1] C. D. M. Fletcher, J. A. Bridge, P. Hogendoorn, and F. Martens, *World Health Organization (WHO) Classification of Tumours of Soft tissue and Bone. Pathology and Genetics*, IARC Press, Lyon, France, 2013.

[2] F. B. Askin, J. Rosal, and R. K. Sibley, "Malignant small cell tumor of the thoracopulmonary region in childhood: a distinctive clinicopathologic entity of uncertain histogenesis," *Cancer*, vol. 43, no. 6, pp. 2438–2451, 1979.

[3] N. G. Nikitakis, A. R. Salama, B. W. O'Malley Jr., R. A. Ord, and J. C. Papadimitriou, "Malignant peripheral primitive neuroectodermal tumor-peripheral neuroepithelioma of the head and neck: a clinicopathologic study of five cases and review of the literature," *Head and Neck*, vol. 25, no. 6, pp. 488–498, 2003.

[4] A. P. Stout, "A tumor of the ulnar nerve," *Proceedings of the New York Pathological Society*, vol. 18, pp. 2–12, 1918.

[5] N. M. Hart and K. M. Earle, "Primitive neuroectodermal tumors in children," *Cancer*, vol. 32, pp. 172–188, 1973.

[6] J. Ewing, "Diffuse endothelioma of bone," *CA: A Cancer Journal for Clinicians*, vol. 22, no. 2, pp. 95–98, 1972.

[7] P. Moerman, P. Goddeeris, J.-P. Fryns, and J. M. Lauweryns, "Primitive neuroectodermal tumor: a newly recognized cause of early fetal death," *Pediatric Pathology*, vol. 4, no. 1-2, pp. 137–142, 1985.

[8] L. Dehner, "Peripheral and central primitive neuroectodermal tumors: a nosologic concept seeking a consensus," *Archives of Pathology and Laboratory Medicine*, vol. 110, no. 11, pp. 997–1005, 1986.

[9] K. Chowdhury, J. J. Manoukian, L. Rochon, and L. R. Begin, "Extracranial primitive neuroectodermal tumor of the head and neck," *Archives of Otolaryngology—Head and Neck Surgery*, vol. 116, no. 4, pp. 475–478, 1990.

[10] H. J. Kahn and P. S. Thorner, "Monoclonal antibody MB2: a potential marker for ewing's sarcoma and primitive neuroectodermal tumor," *Fetal and Pediatric Pathology*, vol. 9, no. 2, pp. 153–162, 1989.

[11] B. H. Kushner, S. I. Hajdu, S. C. Gulati, R. A. Erlandson, P. R. Exelby, and P. H. Lieberman, "Extracranial primitive neuroectodermal tumors. The Memorial Sloan-Kettering Cancer Center experience," *Cancer*, vol. 67, no. 7, pp. 1825–1829, 1991.

[12] C. Kimber, A. Michalski, L. Spitz, and A. Pierro, "Primitive neuroectodermal tumours: anatomic location, extent of surgery, and outcome," *Journal of Pediatric Surgery*, vol. 33, no. 1, pp. 39–41, 1998.

[13] A. Llombart-Bosch, M. J. Terrier-Lacombe, A. Peydro-Olaya, and G. Contesso, "Peripheral neuroectodermal sarcoma of soft tissue (peripheral neuroepithelioma): a pathologic study of ten cases with differential diagnosis regarding other small, round-cell sarcomas," *Human Pathology*, vol. 20, no. 3, pp. 273–280, 1989.

[14] H. Jurgens, V. Bier, D. Harms et al., "Malignant peripheral neuroectodermal tumors. A retrospective analysis of 42 patients," *Cancer*, vol. 61, no. 2, pp. 349–357, 1988.

[15] B. H. Kushner, S. I. Hajdu, S. C. Gulati, R. A. Erlandson, P. R. Exelby, and P. H. Lieberman, "Extracranial primitive neuroectodermal tumors. The Memorial Sloan-Kettering Cancer Center experience," *Cancer*, vol. 67, no. 7, pp. 1825–1829, 1991.

[16] H. Hashimoto, M. Enjoji, and H. Kiryu, "Malignant neuroepithelioma (peripheral neuroblastoma). A clinicopathologic study of 15 cases," *American Journal of Surgical Pathology*, vol. 7, no. 4, pp. 309–318, 1983.

[17] D. Schmidt, D. Harms, and S. Burdach, "Malignant peripheral neuroectodermal tumours of childhood and adolescence," *Virchows Archiv A, Pathological Anatomy and Histopathology*, vol. 406, no. 3, pp. 351–365, 1985.

[18] S. C. Loeffel, G. Y. Gillespie, S. A. Mirmiran et al., "Cellular immunolocalization of S100 protein within fixed tissue sections by monoclonal antibodies," *Archives of Pathology and Laboratory Medicine*, vol. 109, no. 2, pp. 117–122, 1985.

[19] M. J. Finegold, T. J. Triche, and F. B. Askin, "Neuroblastoma and the differential diagnosis of small-, round-, blue-cell tumors," *Human Pathology*, vol. 14, no. 7, pp. 569–595, 1983.

[20] Y. Nakamura, L. E. Becker, and A. Marks, "S-100 protein in tumors of cartilage and bone. An immunohistochemical study," *Cancer*, vol. 52, no. 10, pp. 1820–1824, 1983.

[21] S. W. Weiss, J. M. Langloss, and F. M. Enzinger, "Value of S-100 protein in the diagnosis of soft tissue tumors with particular reference to benign and malignant Schwann cell tumors," *Laboratory Investigation*, vol. 49, no. 3, pp. 299–308, 1983.

[22] M. Miettinen, V. P. Lehto, and I. Virtanen, "Histogenesis of Ewing's sarcoma: an evaluation of intermediate filaments and endothelial cell markers," *Virchows Archiv Abteilung B: Cell Pathology*, vol. 41, no. 3, pp. 277–284, 1982.

[23] P. S. Dickman, L. A. Liotta, and T. J. Triche, "Ewing's sarcoma: characterization in established cultures and evidence of its histogenesis," *Laboratory Investigation*, vol. 47, no. 4, pp. 375–382, 1982.

[24] J. J. Navas-Palacios, R. Aparicio-Duque, and M. D. Valdes, "On the histogenesis of Ewing's sarcoma: an ultrastructural, immunohistochemical, and cytochemical study," *Cancer*, vol. 53, no. 9, pp. 1882–1901, 1984.

[25] K. Scotlandi, M. Serra, M. C. Manara et al., "Immunostaining of the $p30/32^{MIC2}$ antigen and molecular detection of EWS rearrangements for the diagnosis of Ewing's sarcoma and peripheral neuroectodermal tumor," *Human Pathology*, vol. 27, no. 4, pp. 408–416, 1996.

[26] A. Aurias, C. Rimbaut, D. Buffe, J.-M. Zucker, and A. Mazabraud, "Translocation involving chromosome 22 in Ewing's Sarcoma. A cytogenetic study of four fresh tumors," *Cancer Genetics and Cytogenetics*, vol. 12, no. 1, pp. 21–25, 1984.

[27] C. Turc-Carel, I. Philip, M.-P. Berger, T. Philip, and G. M. Lenoir, "Chromosome study of Ewing's Sarcoma (ES) cell lines. Consistency of a reciprocal translocation t(11;22)(q24;q12)," *Cancer Genetics and Cytogenetics*, vol. 12, no. 1, pp. 1–19, 1984.

[28] O. Delattre, J. Zucman, T. Melot et al., "The Ewing family of tumors—a subgroup of small-round-cell tumors defined by specific chimeric transcripts," *The New England Journal of Medicine*, vol. 331, no. 5, pp. 294–299, 1994.

[29] C. T. Denny, "Gene rearrangements in Ewing's sarcoma," *Cancer Investigation*, vol. 14, no. 1, pp. 83–88, 1996.

[30] S. A. Burchill, "Ewing's sarcoma: diagnostic, prognostic, and therapeutic implications of molecular abnormalities," *Journal of Clinical Pathology*, vol. 56, no. 2, pp. 96–102, 2003.

[31] P. H. B. Sorensen and T. J. Triche, "Gene fusions encoding chimaeric transcription factors in solid tumours," *Seminars in Cancer Biology*, vol. 7, no. 1, pp. 3–14, 1996.

[32] A. Takahashi, F. Higashino, M. Aoyagi et al., "EWS/ETS fusions activate telomerase in Ewing's tumors," *Cancer Research*, vol. 63, no. 23, pp. 8338–8344, 2003.

[33] H. Irifune, H. Nishimori, G. Watanabe et al., "Aberrant laminin $\beta 3$ isoforms downstream of EWS-ETS fusion genes in ewing family tumors," *Cancer Biology and Therapy*, vol. 4, no. 4, pp. 449–455, 2005.

[34] Y. Matsumoto, K. Tanaka, F. Nakatani, T. Matsunobu, S. Matsuda, and Y. Iwamoto, "Downregulation and forced expression of EWS-Fli1 fusion gene results in changes in the expression of G_1 regulatory genes," *British Journal of Cancer*, vol. 84, no. 6, pp. 768–775, 2001.

[35] H. Kovar, G. Jug, D. N. T. Aryee et al., "Among genes involved in the RB dependent cell cycle regulatory cascade, the p16 tumor suppressor gene is frequently lost in the Ewing family of tumors," *Oncogene*, vol. 15, no. 18, pp. 2225–2232, 1997.

[36] J. A. López-Guerrero, A. Pellín, R. Noguera, C. Carda, and A. Llombart-Bosch, "Molecular analysis of the 9p21 locus and p53 genes in Ewing family tumors," *Laboratory Investigation*, vol. 81, no. 6, pp. 803–814, 2001.

[37] A. Maitra, H. Roberts, A. G. Weinberg, and J. Geradts, "Aberrant expression of tumor suppressor proteins in the Ewing family of tumors," *Archives of Pathology and Laboratory Medicine*, vol. 125, no. 9, pp. 1207–1212, 2001.

[38] S. J. Cotterill, L. Parker, A. J. Malcolm, M. Reid, L. More, and A. W. Craft, "Incidence and survival for cancer in children and young adults in the North of England, 1968–1995: a report from the Northern Region Young Persons' Malignant Disease Registry," *British Journal of Cancer*, vol. 83, no. 3, pp. 397–403, 2000.

[39] M. Bernstein, H. Kovar, M. Paulussen et al., "Ewing's sarcoma family of tumors: current management," *Oncologist*, vol. 11, no. 5, pp. 503–519, 2006.

[40] J. G. Gurney, A. R. Swensen, and M. Bulterys, "Malignant bone tumors," in *Cancer Incidence and Survival Among Children and Adolescents: United States SEER Program 1975–1995*, L. A. G. Ries, M. A. Smith, J. G. Gurney et al., Eds., pp. 99–110, NIH, Bethesda, MD, USA, 1999.

[41] H. W. Hense, S. Ahrens, M. Paulussen et al., "Descriptive epidemiology of Ewing's tumor—analysis of German patients from EICESS 1980–1997," *Clinical Pediatrics*, vol. 211, pp. 271–275, 1999.

[42] G. P. Siegal, W. R. Oliver, W. R. Reinus et al., "Primary Ewing's sarcoma involving the bones of the head and neck," *Cancer*, vol. 60, no. 11, pp. 2829–2840, 1987.

[43] K. L. Howarth, I. Khodaei, A. Karkanevatos, and R. W. Clarke, "A sinonasal primary Ewing's sarcoma," *International Journal of Pediatric Otorhinolaryngology*, vol. 68, no. 2, pp. 221–224, 2004.

[44] J. P. Windfuhr, "Primitive neuroectodermal tumor of the head and neck: incidence, diagnosis, and management," *Annals of Otology, Rhinology and Laryngology*, vol. 113, no. 7, pp. 533–543, 2004.

[45] J. P. Vaccani, V. Forte, A. L. de Jong, and G. Taylor, "Ewing's sarcoma of the head and neck in children," *International Journal of Pediatric Otorhinolaryngology*, vol. 48, no. 3, pp. 209–216, 1999.

[46] R. B. Raney, L. Asmar, J. Newton et al., "Ewing's sarcoma of soft tissues in childhood: a report from the Intergroup Rhabdomyosarcoma Study, 1972 to 1991," *Journal of Clinical Oncology*, vol. 15, no. 2, pp. 574–582, 1997.

[47] B. M. Wenig, P. Dulguerov, S. P. Kapadia, M. L. Prasad, J. C. Fanburgsmith, and L. D. Thompson, "Neuroectodermal tumors," in *World Health Organization Classification of Tumours. Pathology and Genetics of Head and Neck Tumours*, E. L. Barnes, J. W. Eveson, P. Reichart, and D. Sidransky, Eds., pp. 65–70, IARC Press, Lyon, France, 2005.

[48] T. H. La, P. A. Meyers, L. H. Wexler et al., "Radiation therapy for Ewing's sarcoma: results from Memorial Sloan-Kettering in the modern era," *International Journal of Radiation Oncology Biology Physics*, vol. 64, no. 2, pp. 544–550, 2006.

[49] B. Biswas, A. Thakar, B. K. Mohanti, S. Vishnubhatla, and S. Bakhshi, "Prognostic factors in head & neck Ewing sarcoma family of tumors," *Laryngoscope*, vol. 125, no. 3, pp. E112–E117, 2014.

[50] K. Grevener, L. M. Haveman, A. Ranft et al., "Management and outcome of ewing sarcoma of the head and neck," *Pediatric Blood & Cancer*, vol. 63, no. 4, pp. 604–610, 2016.

[51] N. C. Daw, H. H. Mahmoud, W. H. Meyer et al., "Bone sarcomas of the head and neck in children," *Cancer*, vol. 88, no. 9, pp. 2172–2180, 2000.

[52] L. C. Strong, J. Herson, B. M. Osborne, and W. W. Sutow, "Risk of radiation-related subsequent malignant tumors in survivors of Ewing's sarcoma," *Journal of the National Cancer Institute*, vol. 62, no. 6, pp. 1401–1406, 1979.

[53] E. E. Hunsuck, "Ewing's sarcoma of the maxilla. Report of a case," *Oral Surgery, Oral Medicine, Oral Pathology*, vol. 25, no. 6, pp. 923–928, 1968.

[54] A. N. Roca, J. L. Smith Jr., W. S. MacComb, and B.-S. Jing, "Ewing's sarcoma of the maxilla and mandible: study of six cases," *Oral Surgery, Oral Medicine, Oral Pathology*, vol. 25, no. 2, pp. 194–203, 1968.

[55] R. J. Brownson and R. P. Cook, "Ewing's sarcoma of the maxilla," *Annals of Otology, Rhinology & Laryngology*, vol. 78, pp. 1–6, 1969.

[56] C. H. Fernandez, R. D. Lindberg, W. W. Sutow, and M. L. Samuels, "Localized Ewing's sarcoma—treatment and results," *Cancer*, vol. 34, no. 1, pp. 143–148, 1974.

[57] A. Ferlito, "Primary Ewing's sarcoma of the maxilla: a clinicopathological study of four cases," *Journal of Laryngology and Otology*, vol. 92, no. 11, pp. 1007–1024, 1978.

[58] R. R. Komray, "Resident's page. Pathologic quiz case 2. Ewing's sarcoma of the right maxilla," *Archives of Otolaryngology*, vol. 105, no. 2, pp. 108–111, 1979.

[59] K. I. Pontius and B. A. Sebek, "Extraskeletal Ewing's sarcoma arising in the nasal fossa. Light- and electron-microscopic observations," *American Journal of Clinical Pathology*, vol. 75, no. 3, pp. 410–415, 1981.

[60] D. K. Hossfeld, S. Seeber, E. Siemers, C. G. Schmidt, and E. Scherer, "Early results of combined modality therapy of patients with Ewing's sarcoma," *Recent Results in Cancer Research*, vol. 80, pp. 124–127, 1982.

[61] P. J. Slootweg, W. Straks, and F. N. van der Dussen, "Primitive neuroectodermal tumour of the maxilla. Light microscopy and ultrastructural observations," *Journal of Oral and Maxillofacial Surgery*, vol. 11, no. 2, pp. 54–57, 1983.

[62] P. Bacchini, C. Marchetti, L. Mancini, D. Present, F. Bertoni, and G. Stea, "Ewing's sarcoma of the mandible and maxilla: a report of three cases from the Istituto Beretta," *Oral Surgery, Oral Medicine, Oral Pathology*, vol. 61, no. 3, pp. 278–283, 1986.

[63] M. N. Amin, K. M. Islam, A. N. Ahmed, P. G. Datta, A. S. Amin, and M. Abdullah, "Ewing's sarcoma of maxilla—a case report," *Bangladesh Medical Research Council Bulletin*, vol. 16, no. 1, pp. 42–45, 1990.

[64] J. F. Yeo, H. S. Loh, and I. Sng, "Primitive neuroectodermal tumour in the oral cavity. Case report," *Australian Dental Journal*, vol. 36, no. 5, pp. 337–341, 1991.

[65] D. Filiatrault, S. Jéquier, and P. Brochu, "Pediatric case of the day. Primitive neuroectodermal tumor (PNET) of the right maxillary sinus," *RadioGraphics*, vol. 13, no. 6, pp. 1397–1399, 1993.

[66] J. E. Jones and T. McGill, "Peripheral primitive neuroectodermal tumors of the head and neck," *Archives of Otolaryngology—Head and Neck Surgery*, vol. 121, no. 12, pp. 1392–1395, 1995.

[67] N. Shah, A. Roychoudhury, and Ch. Sarkar, "Primitive neuroectodermal tumor of maxilla in an adult," *Oral Surgery, Oral Medicine, Oral Pathology, Oral Radiology, and Endodontics*, vol. 80, no. 6, pp. 683–686, 1995.

[68] C. Ibarburen, J. J. Haberman, and E. A. Zerhouni, "Peripheral primitive neuroectodermal tumors. CT and MRI evaluation," *European Journal of Radiology*, vol. 21, no. 3, pp. 225–232, 1996.

[69] A. Fiorillo, F. Tranfa, G. Canale et al., "Primary Ewing's sarcoma of the maxilla, a rare and curable localization: report of two new cases, successfully treated by radiotherapy and systemic chemotherapy," *Cancer Letters*, vol. 103, no. 2, pp. 177–182, 1996.

[70] P. Zheng, X. Lu, and K. Zheng, "Ewing's sarcoma of the maxilla," *Chinese Medical Journal*, vol. 111, no. 4, pp. 377–378, 1998.

[71] A. Allam, G. El-Husseiny, Y. Khafaga et al., "Ewing's sarcoma of the head and neck: a retrospective analysis of 24 cases," *Sarcoma*, vol. 3, no. 1, pp. 11–15, 1999.

[72] T. Toda, E. Atari, A. M. Sadi, M. Kiyuna, and S. Kojya, "Primitive neuroectodermal tumor in sinonasal region," *Auris Nasus Larynx*, vol. 26, no. 1, pp. 83–90, 1999.

[73] L. H. Wexler, A. Kacker, J. D. Piro, J. Haddad Jr., and L. G. Close, "Combined modality treatment of Ewing's sarcoma of the maxilla," *Head & Neck*, vol. 25, no. 2, pp. 168–172, 2003.

[74] S. Y. Kao, J. Yang, A. H. Yang, K. W. Chang, and R. C. S. Chang, "Peripheral primitive neuroectodermal tumor of the maxillary gingivae with metastasis to cervical lymph nodes: report of a case," *Journal of Oral and Maxillofacial Surgery*, vol. 60, no. 7, pp. 821–825, 2002.

[75] I. Alobid, M. Bernal-Sprekelsen, L. Alós, P. Benítez, J. Traserra, and J. Mullol, "Peripheral primitive neuroectodermal tumour of the left maxillary sinus," *Acta Oto-Laryngologica*, vol. 123, no. 6, pp. 776–778, 2003.

[76] M. Harman, F. Kiroglu, M. Kösem, and Ö. Ünal, "Primary Ewing's sarcoma of the paranasal sinus with intracranial extension: imaging features," *Dentomaxillofacial Radiology*, vol. 32, no. 5, pp. 343–346, 2003.

[77] G. Sun, Z. Li, J. Li, and C. Wang, "Peripheral primitive neuroectodermal tumour of the maxilla," *British Journal of Oral and Maxillofacial Surgery*, vol. 45, no. 3, pp. 226–227, 2007.

[78] P. Infante-Cossio, J. L. Gutierrez-Perez, A. Garcia-Perla, M. Noguer-Mediavilla, and F. Gavilan-Carrasco, "Primary Ewing's sarcoma of the maxilla and zygoma: report of a case," *Journal of Oral and Maxillofacial Surgery*, vol. 63, no. 10, pp. 1539–1542, 2005.

[79] B. U. Coskun, U. Cinar, H. Savk, T. Basak, and B. Dadas, "Isolated maxillary sinus Ewing's sarcoma," *Rhinology*, vol. 43, no. 3, pp. 225–228, 2005.

[80] S. Varshney, S. S. Bist, N. Gupta, and R. Bhatia, "Primary extraskeletal Ewing's sarcoma of the maxilla with intraorbital extension," *Indian Journal of Otolaryngology and Head and Neck Surgery*, vol. 59, no. 3, pp. 273–276, 2007.

[81] J. Thariat, A. Italiano, F. Peyrade et al., "Very late local relapse of Ewing's sarcoma of the head and neck treated with aggressive multimodal therapy," *Sarcoma*, vol. 2008, Article ID 854141, 4 pages, 2008.

[82] B. V. Prasad, B. R. A. Mujib, T. S. Bastian, and P. D. Tauro, "Ewing's sarcoma of the maxilla," *Indian Journal of Dental Research*, vol. 19, no. 1, pp. 66–69, 2008.

[83] P. Mohindra, B. Zade, A. Basu et al., "Primary PNET of maxilla: an unusual presentation," *Journal of Pediatric Hematology/Oncology*, vol. 30, no. 6, pp. 474–477, 2008.

[84] M. M. Bornstein, T. von Arx, and H. J. Altermatt, "Loss of pulp sensitivity and pain as the first symptoms of a Ewing's sarcoma in the right maxillary sinus and alveolar process: report of a case," *Journal of Endodontics*, vol. 34, no. 12, pp. 1549–1553, 2008.

[85] M. Kawabata, K. Yoshifuku, Y. Sagara, and Y. Kurono, "Ewing's sarcoma/primitive neuroectodermal tumour occurring in the maxillary sinus," *Rhinology*, vol. 46, no. 1, pp. 75–78, 2008.

[86] S. Ataergin, A. Ozet, L. Solchaga et al., "Long-lasting multiagent chemotherapy in adult high-risk Ewing's sarcoma of bone," *Medical Oncology*, vol. 26, no. 3, pp. 276–286, 2009.

[87] M. J. Piloni, G. Molina, and A. Keszler, "Malignant oral-maxillary neoplasm in children and adolescents. A retrospective analysis from the biopsy service at a school of dentistry in Argentina," *Acta Odontológica Latinoamericana*, vol. 22, no. 3, pp. 233–238, 2009.

[88] S. Gupta, O. P. Gupta, S. Mehrotra, and D. Mehrotra, "Ewing sarcoma of the maxilla: a rare presentation," *Quintessence International*, vol. 40, no. 2, pp. 135–140, 2009.

[89] A. K. Hormozi, M. R. Ghazisaidi, and S. N. Hosseini, "Unusual presentation of peripheral primitive neuroectodermal tumor of the maxilla," *Journal of Craniofacial Surgery*, vol. 21, no. 6, pp. 1761–1763, 2010.

[90] D. P. Dadhe, B. G. Janardan, and M. B. Sambhus, "Ewing's sarcoma of maxilla in an adolescent boy," *Journal of the International Clinical Dental Research Organization*, vol. 2, no. 3, pp. 153–156, 2010.

[91] N. Davido, A. Rigolet, S. Kerner, F. Gruffaz, and Y. Boucher, "Case of Ewing's sarcoma misdiagnosed as a periapical lesion of maxillary incisor," *Journal of Endodontics*, vol. 37, no. 2, pp. 259–264, 2011.

[92] S. Hafezi, R. R. Seethala, E. B. Stelow et al., "Ewing's family of tumors of the sinonasal tract and maxillary bone," *Head and Neck Pathology*, vol. 5, no. 1, pp. 8–16, 2011.

[93] S. K. Yeshvanth, K. Ninan, S. K. Bhandary, K. P. H. Lakshinarayana, J. K. Shetty, and J. H. Makannavar, "Rare case of extraskeletal Ewings sarcoma of the sinonasal tract," *Journal of Cancer Research and Therapeutics*, vol. 8, no. 1, pp. 142–144, 2012.

[94] A. Kaler and S. Sheriff, "Primary ewing's sarcoma of the paranasal sinuses and orbit," *Innovative Journal of Medical and Health Science*, vol. 3, pp. 1–3, 2013.

[95] A. Llombart-Bosch, I. Machado, S. Navarro et al., "Histological heterogeneity of Ewing's sarcoma/PNET: an immunohistochemical analysis of 415 genetically confirmed cases with clinical support," *Virchows Archiv*, vol. 455, no. 5, pp. 397–411, 2009.

[96] P. Argani, B. Perez-Ordoñez, H. Xiao, S. M. Caruana, A. G. Huvos, and M. Ladanyi, "Olfactory neuroblastoma is not related to the Ewing family of tumors: absence of EWS/FLI1 gene fusion and MIC2 expression," *American Journal of Surgical Pathology*, vol. 22, no. 4, pp. 391–398, 1998.

[97] C. M. Coffin and L. P. Dehner, "Peripheral neurogenic tumors of the soft tissues in children and adolescents: a clinicopathologic study of 139 cases," *Pediatric Pathology*, vol. 9, no. 4, pp. 387–407, 1989.

[98] G. Treglia, M. Salsano, A. Stefanelli, M. V. Mattoli, A. Giordano, and L. Bonomo, "Diagnostic accuracy of 18F-FDG-PET and PET/CT in patients with Ewing sarcoma family tumours: a systematic review and a meta-analysis," *Skeletal Radiology*, vol. 41, no. 3, pp. 249–256, 2012.

[99] C. Juergens, C. Weston, I. Lewis et al., "Safety assessment of intensive induction with vincristine, ifosfamide, doxorubicin, and etoposide (VIDE) in the treatment of ewing tumors in the EURO-E.W.I.N.G. 99 Clinical Trial," *Pediatric Blood and Cancer*, vol. 47, no. 1, pp. 22–29, 2006.

[100] M.-C. Le Deley, O. Delattre, K.-L. Schaefer et al., "Impact of EWS-ETS fusion type on disease progression in Ewing's sarcoma/peripheral primitive neuroectodermal tumor: prospective results from the cooperative Euro-E.W.I.N.G. 99 trial," *Journal of Clinical Oncology*, vol. 28, no. 12, pp. 1982–1988, 2010.

[101] E. de Alava, A. Kawai, J. H. Healey et al., "EWS-FLI1 fusion transcript structure is an independent determinant of prognosis in Ewing's sarcoma," *Journal of Clinical Oncology*, vol. 16, no. 4, pp. 1248–1255, 1998.

[102] J. A. van Doorninck, L. Ji, B. Schaub et al., "Current treatment protocols have eliminated the prognostic advantage of type 1 fusions in Ewing sarcoma: a report from the Children's Oncology Group," *Journal of Clinical Oncology*, vol. 28, no. 12, pp. 1989–1994, 2010.

[103] S. L. P. C. Lopes, S. M. de Almeida, A. L. F. Costa, V. A. Zanardi, and F. Cendes, "Imaging findings of Ewing's sarcoma in the mandible," *Journal of Oral Science*, vol. 49, no. 2, pp. 167–171, 2007.

[104] B. Velche-Haag, F. Proust, A. Laquerrière, D. Dehesdin, and P. Fréger, "Ewing's sarcoma of the ethmoid bone. Case report," *Neurochirurgie*, vol. 48, no. 1, pp. 25–29, 2002.

[105] B. Velche-Haag, D. Dehesdin, F. Proust, J. P. Marie, J. Andrieu-Guitrancourt, and A. Laquerriere, "Ewing's sarcoma of the head and neck: a case report," *Annales d'Oto-Laryngologie et de Chirurgie Cervico Faciale*, vol. 119, no. 6, pp. 363–368, 2002.

[106] L. V. Csokonai, B. Liktor, G. Arató, and F. Helffrich, "Ewing's sarcoma in the nasal cavity," *Otolaryngology—Head and Neck Surgery*, vol. 125, no. 6, pp. 665–667, 2001.

[107] A. Böör, I. Jurkovic, I. Friedmann, L. Plank, and P. Kocan, "Extraskeletal Ewing's sarcoma of the nose," *Journal of Laryngology and Otology*, vol. 115, no. 1, pp. 74–76, 2001.

[108] M. P. Freeman, C. M. Currie, G. F. Gray Jr., and J. J. Kaya, "Ewing sarcoma of the skull with an unusual pattern of reactive sclerosis: MR characteristics," *Journal of Computer Assisted Tomography*, vol. 12, pp. 14–36, 1985.

[109] A. Schuck, S. Ahrens, M. Paulussen et al., "Local therapy in localized Ewing tumors: results of 1058 patients treated in the CESS 81, CESS 86, and EICESS 92 trials," *International Journal of Radiation Oncology, Biology, Physics*, vol. 55, no. 1, pp. 168–177, 2003.

[110] R. Ladenstein, U. Pötschger, M. C. Le Deley et al., "Primary disseminated multifocal Ewing sarcoma: results of the Euro-EWING 99 trial," *Journal of Clinical Oncology*, vol. 28, no. 20, pp. 3284–3291, 2010.

[111] S. J. Cotterill, S. Ahrens, M. Paulussen et al., "Prognostic factors in Ewing's tumor of bone: analysis of 975 patients from the European Intergroup Cooperative Ewing's Sarcoma Study Group," *Journal of Clinical Oncology*, vol. 18, no. 17, pp. 3108–3114, 2000.

[112] E. Garfein, M. Doscher, O. Tepper, J. Gill, R. Gorlick, and R. V. Smith, "Reconstruction of the pediatric midface following oncologic resection," *Journal of Reconstructive Microsurgery*, vol. 31, no. 5, pp. 336–342, 2015.

[113] I. Madani, K. Bonte, L. Vakaet, T. Boterberg, and W. De Neve, "Intensity-modulated radiotherapy for sinonasal tumors: Ghent University Hospital update," *International Journal of Radiation Oncology, Biology, Physics*, vol. 73, no. 2, pp. 424–432, 2009.

[114] J. Kuttesch, L. H. Wexler, R. B. Marcus et al., "Second malignancies after Ewing's sarcoma: radiation dose-dependency of secondary sarcomas," *Journal of Clinical Oncology*, vol. 14, no. 10, pp. 2818–2825, 1996.

[115] J. Dunst, S. Ahrens, M. Paulussen et al., "Second malignancies after treatment for Ewing's sarcoma: a report of the CESS-studies," *International Journal of Radiation Oncology, Biology, Physics*, vol. 42, no. 2, pp. 379–384, 1998.

[116] C. Klug, D. Berzaczy, H. Reinbacher et al., "Influence of previous radiotherapy on free tissue transfer in the head and neck region: evaluation of 455 cases," *Laryngoscope*, vol. 116, no. 7, pp. 1162–1167, 2006.

[117] S. Ferrari, K. Sundby Hall, R. Luksch et al., "Nonmetastatic Ewing family tumors: high-dose chemotherapy with stem cell rescue in poor responder patients. Results of the Italian Sarcoma Group/Scandinavian Sarcoma Group III protocol," *Annals of Oncology*, vol. 22, no. 5, pp. 1221–1227, 2011.

[118] H. E. Grier, M. D. Krailo, N. J. Tarbell et al., "Addition of ifosfamide and etoposide to standard chemotherapy for Ewing's sarcoma and primitive neuroectodermal tumor of bone," *The New England Journal of Medicine*, vol. 348, no. 8, pp. 694–701, 2003.

[119] M. E. Nesbit Jr., E. A. Gehan, E. O. Burgert Jr. et al., "Multimodal therapy for the management of primary, nonmetastatic Ewing's sarcoma of bone: a long-term follow-up of the First Intergroup study," *Journal of Clinical Oncology*, vol. 8, no. 10, pp. 1664–1674, 1990.

[120] M. Paulussen, A. W. Craft, I. Lewis et al., "Results of the EICESS-92 study: two randomized trials of Ewing's sarcoma treatment—cyclophosphamide compared with ifosfamide in standard-risk patients and assessment of benefit of etoposide added to standard treatment in high-risk patients," *Journal of Clinical Oncology*, vol. 26, no. 27, pp. 4385–4393, 2008.

[121] E. O. Burgert, M. E. Nesbit, L. A. Gamsey et al., "Multimodal therapy fort he management of nonpelvic, localized Ewing's sarcoma of bone: a long-term follow up of the First Intergroup study," *Journal of Clinical Oncology*, vol. 8, pp. 1664–1674, 1990.

[122] R. C. Shamberger, M. P. LaQuaglia, M. C. Gebhardt et al., "Ewing sarcoma/primitive neuroectodermal tumor of the chest wall: impact of initial versus delayed resection on tumor margins, survival, and use of radiation therapy," *Annals of Surgery*, vol. 238, no. 4, pp. 563–568, 2003.

[123] M. J. Krasin, A. M. Davidoff, C. Rodriguez-Galindo et al., "Definitive surgery and multiagent systemic therapy for patients with localized Ewing sarcoma family of tumors: local outcome and prognostic factors," *Cancer*, vol. 104, no. 2, pp. 367–373, 2005.

[124] T. I. Yock, M. Krailo, C. J. Freyer et al., "Local control in pelvic ewing sarcoma: analysis from INT-0091-a report from the children's oncology group," *Journal of Clinical Oncology*, vol. 24, no. 24, pp. 3838–3843, 2006.

20

Limb-Salvage Surgery of Soft Tissue Sarcoma with Sciatic Nerve Involvement

Hussein Sweiti,[1] **Noor Tamimi**,[2] **Fabian Bormann**,[1] **Markus Divo**,[3] **Daniela Schulz-Ertner**,[4] **Marit Ahrens**,[5] **Ulrich Ronellenfitsch**,[6] **and Matthias Schwarzbach**[1]

[1]*Department of Surgery, Clinical Center Frankfurt Höchst, Frankfurt, Germany*
[2]*Department of Trauma and Orthopedic Surgery, BG Trauma Center, Frankfurt, Germany*
[3]*Institute for Pathology, Clinical Center Frankfurt Höchst, Frankfurt, Germany*
[4]*Radiological Institute, Agaplesion Markus Hospital, Frankfurt, Germany*
[5]*Department of Hematology and Oncology, University Hospital Frankfurt, Frankfurt, Germany*
[6]*Department of Vascular and Endovascular Surgery, Heidelberg University Hospital, Heidelberg, Germany*

Correspondence should be addressed to Hussein Sweiti; hsweiti@gmail.com

Academic Editor: Valerae O. Lewis

Background. The surgical resection of soft tissue sarcomas (STS) with sciatic nerve involvement presents a significant surgical and oncological challenge. Current treatment strategies pursue a multimodal approach with the aim of limb preservation. We aim to evaluate the outcomes of limb-sparing surgery of STS in a patient cohort and to propose a classification for STS with sciatic nerve involvement. *Methods.* Patients receiving limb-preserving resections for STS with sciatic nerve involvement between 01/2010 and 01/2017 were included. Clinical and oncological data were prospectively collected in a computerized database and retrospectively analyzed. Sciatic nerve involvement in STS was classified preoperatively as follows: type A for nerve encasement; type B for nerve contact; and type C for no nerve involvement. *Results.* A total of 364 patients with STS were treated, of which 27 patients had STS with sciatic nerve involvement. Eight patients with type A tumors (29.6%) underwent sciatic nerve resection, and 19 patients with type B tumors (70.4%) received epineural dissections. Disease progression was observed in 8 patients (29.6%) with a local recurrence of 11.1% and distant metastasis in 29.6%. The type of nerve resection significantly influenced leg function but had no impact on disease recurrence or overall survival. *Conclusion.* In a cohort of carefully selected patients with STS and sciatic nerve involvement, the extent of sciatic nerve resection had no significant impact on disease recurrence or survival. Precise classification of neural involvement may therefore be useful in selecting the appropriate degree of nerve resection, without compromising oncological outcome or unnecessarily sacrificing leg function.

1. Introduction

Soft tissue sarcomas (STS) are a rare and heterogeneous group of mesenchymal tumors, representing only 1% of all adult malignancies [1, 2]. The incidence in Europe has been reported as 4 per 100,000 people per year [3]. These tumors vary in their tendency for aggressive behavior and can occur in all age groups and in a variety of anatomic sites [4]. The lower extremity, however, is the most commonly affected site with approximately 28% of all STS arising there [5]. At least 50 histologic subtypes have been identified, with undifferentiated pleomorphic sarcoma (UPS) and liposarcoma being the most common subtypes [6].

Local disease control is essential in the management of STS, with surgical resection being the only treatment modality capable of achieving complete tumor cell eradication [7]. Achieving negative microscopic margins upon resection of STS has been shown to significantly reduce the risk of local recurrence [8]. The ability to obtain wide margins may however be particularly challenging if the tumor is in close proximity to important neurovascular structures. For STS with vascular involvement, reasonable oncological outcomes have been reported with vessel reconstruction in limb-salvage surgery [9–11]. Nerve reconstruction, on the other hand, does not guarantee preservation of function [12]. Tumor infiltration of the sciatic nerve has previously been an

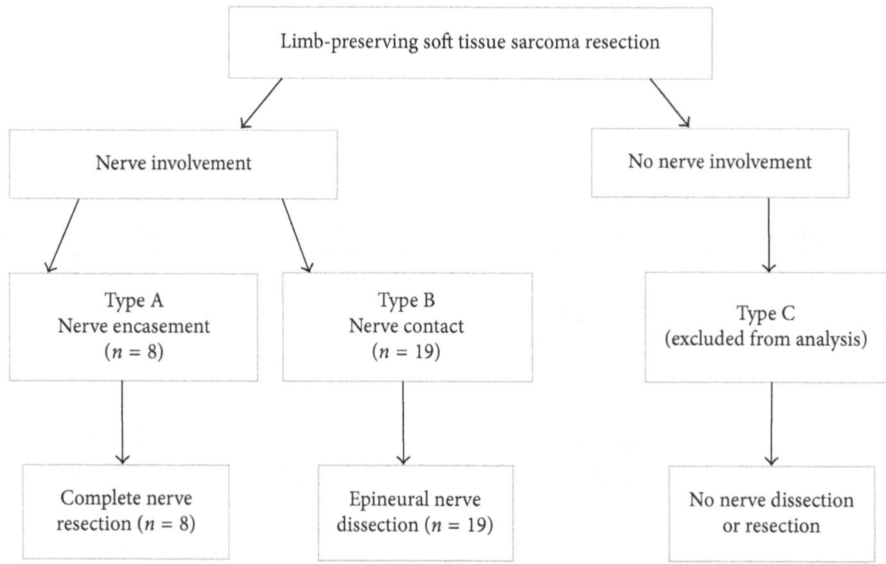

Figure 1: Classification of sciatic nerve involvement and surgical treatment algorithm for lower limb STS.

indication for limb amputation [13], but more recent studies have shown limb-sparing surgery with partial or complete sciatic nerve resection to be an excellent alternative [14–17].

The aim of this study is to analyze the oncological and functional outcomes of limb-sparing surgery in STS with sciatic nerve involvement. In addition, we aim to classify the degree of nerve involvement and suggest a suitable therapeutic approach for neural involvement.

2. Methods

2.1. Study Design, Setting, and Participants. The data of all adult patients with STS (extremities, trunk, and retroperitoneal) undergoing surgical treatment at the Clinical Center Frankfurt Hoechst from January 1st, 2010 until January 31st, 2017 were collected in a computerized database on an ongoing basis and was retrospectively analyzed. Patients with STS of the lower extremity with sciatic nerve involvement who underwent limb-preserving tumor resections were selected from the database and included in this study. All patients consented on the use of their clinical data for research purposes. The study was approved by the ethics committee of the Medical Council of the State of Hesse, Germany.

Involvement of the sciatic nerve was confirmed preoperatively when CT or MRI scans showed no layer of normal tissue between the tumor and the sciatic nerve. Lower limb sarcomas arising from the sciatic nerve or those extending towards the sciatic nerve were included.

2.2. Classification of Nerve Involvement. The extent of neural involvement was assessed using high-resolution CT and/or MRI scans. STS with encasement of the nerve were classified as type A. Encasement was defined as ≥180° of nerve contact with the tumor. These tumors were reassessed intraoperatively and underwent en bloc compartmental resection together with the nerve, if the classification was confirmed. STS which revealed direct contact with the nerve (<180°)

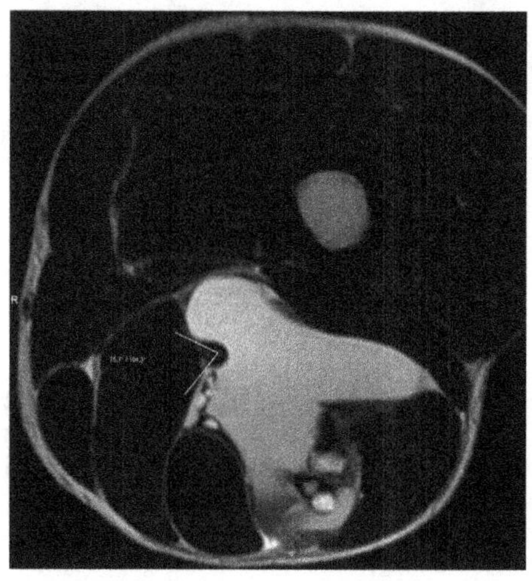

Figure 2: Preoperative MRI scan in a patient with type A sciatic nerve involvement and G3 pleomorphic sarcoma.

without encasement or disruption of its continuity were classified as type B and were treated with a compartmental resection of the tumor with epineural dissection. STS without nerve involvement were classified as type C and were resected without nerve dissection or resection (Figure 1). MRI scans from two of our patients illustrating type A and type B sciatic nerve involvement are displayed in Figures 2 and 3, respectively.

Intraoperative reassessment of sciatic nerve involvement was done by visually scrutinizing and palpating the relationship of the nerve to the tumor, if possible. In selected cases, intraoperative ultrasound was employed to visualize the extent of contact of the tumor to the nerve.

2.3. General and Perioperative Variables. In addition to basic patient demographic data (age, gender, and affected side), the status of each patient at the time of presentation (primary tumor, local recurrence, and presence of metastasis)

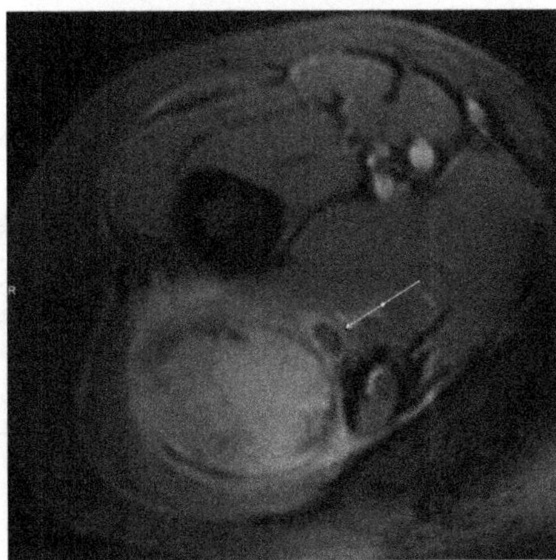

FIGURE 3: Preoperative MRI scan in a patient with type B sciatic nerve involvement and G2 liposarcoma.

was also noted. All therapeutic measures (external radiation therapy, chemotherapy, isolated limb perfusion, or surgical resection) were carried out upon recommendation by a multidisciplinary tumor board. En bloc compartmental resections were carried out in accordance with the surgical standards described by Enneking et al. [18, 19]. Assessment of tumor specimens was carried out by the in-house pathologists and confirmed by the reference pathological department of Heidelberg University Hospital. Specimens were assessed for histological entity, tumor size (maximal diameter), grade, microscopic margins, and nerve infiltration. Tumor grading was based on the criteria of the "Fédération Nationale des Centres de Lutte Contre le Cancer" (FNCLCC), which takes cell differentiation, mitotic activity, and necrosis into consideration. Finally, duration of surgery, surgical and medical complications, reoperations, and the duration of hospital stay were recorded.

2.4. Survival, Disease Progression, and Functional Outcome. Following discharge, patients were seen at regular intervals as part of their cancer follow-up care. Patients with intermediate- and high-grade tumors received quarterly clinical exams and MRI studies during the first two postoperative years, every six months during the third year, and on an annual basis afterwards for two more years. Chest CT scans were carried out every six months. Patients with low-grade tumors received clinical exams and MRI studies every six months during the first two postoperative years, and annually for three more years. Chest CT-scans or X-rays were offered on a yearly basis. Information on the functional outcome was recorded by examining the lower limb for function and range of motion (categories: normal, limited, and severely limited). Limited function was defined as a reduced knee flexion of 90°–110° and/or weakness of the intrinsic foot muscles; movement of the foot was possible but reduced. Patients with severely limited function of the leg had a severely reduced knee flexion (<90°), and minimal or no movements of the foot were possible. Patients were also asked about the presence of chronic swelling, paresthesia, or chronic pain as well as their walking range, the use of walking aids, and their satisfaction with limb preservation. Finally, the musculoskeletal tumor society (MSTS) rating score modified by Enneking was calculated in the 20 surviving patients [20]. This scoring system consists of six main categories: pain, limb function, walking aids, walking distance, gait, and emotional acceptance. A score of 0–5 is assigned to each category; higher scores are associated with a greater level of function. The scores out of a total of 30 were then converted to percentages.

2.5. Statistical Methods. Statistical analyses were performed with IBM SPSS Statistics 24. Continuous variables were expressed as median and range, and correlations between continuous variables were explored using the Pearson correlation test. The X^2 test and Fischer exact test were used when comparing categorical variables. When comparing categorical variables with continuous variables, the Kolmogorov–Smirnov–Lilliefors test was implemented in determining whether data followed a normal distribution. The independent *t*-Test was used with normally distributed data, and the Wilcoxon–Mann–Whitney *U* test was used with nonnormally distributed data.

The Kaplan–Meier method was used to calculate the survival and disease progression curves, and the log-rank test was used to calculate differences between groups. A p value of ≤0.05 was considered significant.

3. Results

3.1. Participants. A total of 364 patients with STS underwent surgical resection between January 1st, 2010 and January 31st, 2017. The lower extremity was affected in 179 patients (49.2%) and the upper extremity was affected in 19 patients (5.2%). Twenty-seven patients (15.1% of all patients with lower limb STS) had sciatic nerve involvement (type A or B) and were included for further analysis.

3.2. Preoperative Characteristics. Descriptive analysis of the 27 included patients revealed a median age of 57 years (interquartile range (IQR): 46–74 years). Six patients (22.2%) presented with a local recurrence while the remaining 21 patients (77.8%) presented with primary tumors. None of the patients presented with primarily metastasized disease. The tumor entity was confirmed in all cases via trucut or incisional biopsy. Based on the proposed neural involvement classification system, 19 patients (70.4%) had STS with direct contact with the sciatic nerve (type B) and 8 patients (29.6%) revealed encasement of the sciatic nerve (type A). Additional general and preoperative characteristics are summarized in Table 1.

3.3. Surgical Therapy and Histopathologic Results. All surgical resections of STS were carried out by one experienced surgeon (Matthias Schwarzbach). A macroscopically complete resection without amputation was achieved in all patients. The median operative duration was 5.17 hours (IQR: 3.92–6.54 hours). Eight patients (29.6%) with type A sciatic nerve involvement underwent complete resection of

Table 1: General and preoperative characteristics.

Characteristic	Number of patients ($N = 27$)	%
Gender		
Male	12	44.4
Female	15	55.6
Sides		
Right	16	59.3
Left	11	40.7
Presentation status		
Primary tumor	21	77.8
Local recurrence	6	22.2
Sciatic nerve involvement		
Type A	8	29.6
Type B	19	70.4
Neoadjuvant therapy		
External beam radiation therapy	10	37.0
Chemotherapy	6	22.2
Isolated limb perfusion	5	18.5

the sciatic nerve, and the remaining 19 patients with type B nerve involvement underwent epineural dissection. The preoperative radiological categorization of type A and type B nerve involvement was confirmed intraoperatively in all 27 cases. Liposarcoma was the most common histopathologic entity (48.1%), with 9 out of 13 liposarcomas diagnosed as low grade (G1). The median tumor size measured by the pathologist following resection was 15 cm (IQR: 8.5–26.5 cm). The negative margin rate in our series was 92.6% with a median margin of 5 mm (IQR: 3–10 mm). Two patients with positive margins (R1) were initially classified as type B. They both received adjuvant radiotherapy and were disease-free at the latest follow-up appointments (22 and 17 months postoperatively). Table 2 summarizes additional histopathologic findings.

3.4. Postoperative Course. Seven patients (25.9%) received adjuvant radiation therapy (60–66 Gy total dose), and one patient (3.7%) received adjuvant radiochemotherapy. Five other patients (18.5%) were subject to adjuvant chemotherapy. A total of 20 patients (74.1%) developed a surgical morbidity, and 6 patients (22.2%) developed a medical complication. Wound-related morbidity, such as necrosis, dehiscence, or infection, was the most common complication affecting 10 patients (37.0%), followed by hematomas or seromas which affected 6 patients (22.2%). In addition, two patients (7.4%) suffered a fracture of the operated extremity following discharge. No hospital mortalities took place, and the median hospital stay was 30 days (IQR: 22–48 days). Table 3 provides a list of all complications.

3.5. Oncological Outcome. Patients were followed up for a maximum duration of 5 years postoperatively. The median postoperative follow-up duration was 23 months (IQR: 15.5–50 months). Eight patients (29.6%) were found to have progression of disease (local recurrence or metastasis). All 8 patients had metastatic disease, 3 of which (11.1%) also developed a local recurrence. The most common site of metastasis was the lung, with 5 patients developing pulmonary metastases. A secondary limb amputation was carried out in one patient due to a local recurrence. The overall mortality rate in our series was 25.9% ($n = 7$), with a tumor-related mortality rate of 22.2% ($n = 6$). A significant association between the development of metastasis and mortality was demonstrated by the Kaplan–Meier survival analysis ($p < 0.001$), as shown in Figure 4.

Various general, perioperative, and histopathologic parameters were investigated for their association with disease progression or mortality. Patient age, initial presentation with recurrent disease, tumor size, tumor histology, type of nerve resection, duration of surgery, and duration of hospital stay were not found to have a statistically significant impact on the development of postoperative complications, disease progression, or survival. Resection margin in millimeters positively correlated with postoperative survival ($p = 0.014$).

Table 2: Histopathologic findings.

Characteristic	Number of patients ($N = 27$)	%
Histologic entity		
Liposarcoma (all subtypes)	13	48.1
Pleomorphic sarcoma (all subtypes)	11	40.7
Malignant giant cell tumor	1	3.7
Myxofibrosarcoma	1	3.7
Primitive neuroectodermal tumor	1	3.7
Grade		
Low grade (G1)	10	37.0
Intermediate grade (G2)	5	18.5
High grade (G3)	12	44.4
Maximum tumor diameter (cm)		
≥30	5	18.5
20–29	4	14.8
10–19	9	33.3
<10	9	33.3
Margin		
Microscopically negative margins (R0)	25	92.6
Microscopically positive margins (R1)	2	7.4

Table 3: Postoperative morbidity.

	Number of patients ($N = 27$)	%
Surgical complications		
Wound necrosis/dehiscence	10	37.0
Hematoma/seroma	6	22.2
Fracture (after discharge)	2	7.4
Bleeding	1	3.7
Reoperations (total)	13	48.1
Wound revisions	10	37.0
Hemorrhage control	1	3.7
Reduction and internal fixation	2	7.4
Medical complications		
Pneumonia	2	7.4
Urinary tract infection	2	7.4
Sepsis	1	3.7
Deep venous thrombosis	1	3.7
Hospital mortality	0	0

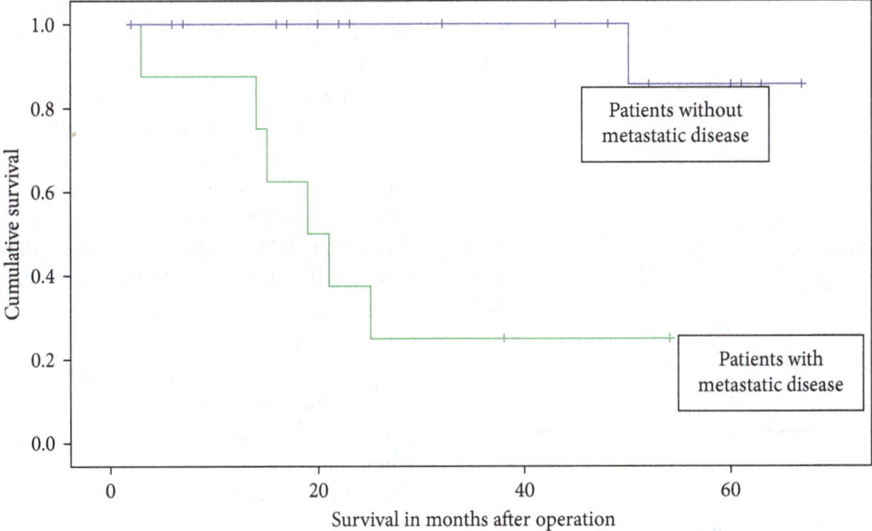

FIGURE 4: Development of metastatic disease and overall survival ($p < 0.001$).

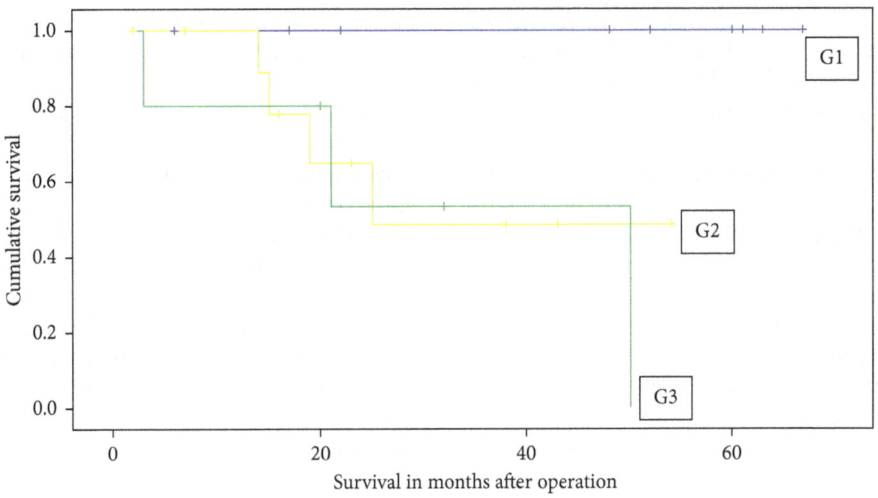

FIGURE 5: Tumor grade (G1/G2/G3) and overall survival ($p = 0.023$).

Higher tumor grades (G2 and G3) were significantly associated with the development of distant metastatic disease ($p = 0.010$) as well as mortality ($p = 0.020$), compared to low grade tumors (G1). Figure 5 shows the Kaplan–Meier survival curve for different tumor grades ($p = 0.023$).

3.6. Functional Outcome. The postoperative functional outcome assessment revealed that 50% of surviving patients had an MSTS score of 83% or higher. Five patients (25%) scored between 67% and 80%, and the remaining 5 patients had a score of less than 67%. The main functional outcomes are summarized in Table 4.

Complete sciatic nerve resection was found to be significantly associated with the development of leg edema ($p = 0.017$), chronic pain ($p = 0.003$), reduced leg function ($p < 0.001$), and lower MSTS scores ($p = 0.001$) when compared to epineural nerve dissection. All patients, including those with complications or recurrence of disease, expressed their satisfaction with their decision in opting for limb-sparing surgery as opposed to amputation of the leg.

4. Discussion

Our study has shown reasonable oncological and functional outcomes following limb-sparing surgery in a patient cohort with STS and sciatic nerve involvement treated in a specialized center. The frequency of local recurrence (11.1%) and distant metastasis (29.6%) compare well with a large prospective study of 1,041 patients with STS, which reported rates of 17% and 22%, respectively [21]. More recent studies, however, demonstrated local recurrence rates of 10% or less [6, 22–25]. Pisters et al. found that high-grade lesions were a significant prognostic factor in the development of metastatic disease, which was also confirmed in our patient cohort [21].

Liposarcoma and pleomorphic sarcoma were the two most common histopathological entities in our study population, which is analogous to the current literature [6].

Table 4: Functional outcome.

	Number of patients ($N = 27$)	%
Chronic leg edema	15	55.6
Paresthesia	18	66.7
Chronic pain	12	44.4
Walking aids/braces	17	63.0
Leg function/range of motion		
Severely limited/no function	9	33.3
Limited	12	44.4
Normal	6	22.2
Walking distance		
>500 m	15	55.6
100–500 m	9	33.3
<100 m	3	11.1

The histopathological subtype was not found to be of prognostic significance in our study, which may be due to our small population size. Other studies have shown the histological subtype to be an independent prognostic factor. Resection margins have also been shown to be an independent prognostic factor in local and distant disease control [26–28]. This was confirmed in our study, as the size of the margins was significantly correlated with survival after surgery.

The overall 5-year survival of patients with metastatic STS has been shown to be poor [6]. Our study confirmed the correlation between the development of metastatic disease and mortality, which has been shown in previous studies [21]. Williard et al. reported a tumor-related mortality rate of greater than 50% despite local tumor control, independent of whether patients were treated with limb amputation or limb-sparing surgery, further emphasizing the need to improve systemic disease control [29].

This is a series of large, deep, and in 7 cases recurrent STS with sciatic nerve involvement undergoing compartmental tumor resections as part of a multimodal therapeutic approach. Wound necrosis or dehiscence and the collection of hematomas or seromas were particularly common postoperative complications, occurring in 37.0% and 22.2% of cases, respectively. These factors contributed, in our opinion, to a high reoperation rate of 48.1% as well as a median hospital stay of 30 days.

In the past, some authors recommended hip disarticulation or hindquarter amputation when complete resection of the sciatic nerve was indicated, as a limb without tactile sensations was not considered worth saving from a functional perspective [13, 29–32]. Several authors have, however, reported acceptable functional outcomes after complete resection of the sciatic nerve [11, 15–17, 33], with some studies demonstrating superior function when comparing sciatic nerve resection with amputation of the leg [34, 35]. In our study, all patients expressed their satisfaction with the decision to undergo limb-sparing surgery, despite functional limitations which were particularly apparent in the sciatic nerve resection group. It is important that patients are properly instructed preoperatively regarding adequate foot care of their postoperative insensate feet to minimize skin complications, particularly the development of foot ulcers, which can ultimately lead to a secondary amputation of the limb [16].

The extent of nerve resection was not found to affect the local or distant recurrence probability or have an impact on survival in our study. Similar local recurrence rates were also reported by Clarkson et al. in their cohort of 94 patients when comparing sciatic nerve resection with epineural dissection [17]. Their study also demonstrated superior functional outcomes with patients receiving epineural nerve dissection compared to complete nerve resection. Our study further confirms these findings, as there was a significant association in the development of chronic leg edema, chronic pain, poor leg function, and lower MSTS scores in patients who had undergone a complete nerve resection when compared with nerve dissection. In addition, O'Donnell et al. found that sparing adjacent critical structures did not increase the risk of a local recurrence or reduce survival rates and led to superior functional outcomes in 169 patients with STS and positive margins after tumor resection [36]. We therefore propose that the sciatic nerve is resected only when there is tumor encasement of the nerve (>180°), which is similar to the recommendations made by Clarkson et al. [17].

Our proposed classification system provides a simple and clinically applicable algorithm to facilitate the choice between nerve resection or epineural dissection in patients undergoing limb-sparing surgery due to STS with sciatic nerve involvement. The significance of this classification lies in its potential to encourage a limited epineural dissection in eligible patients (type B) without compromising the oncological outcome or unnecessarily sacrificing the leg function. In addition, this classification may help establish limb-salvage surgery as the procedure of choice in patients requiring complete sciatic nerve resection (type A). The initial assessment of nerve involvement is radiological followed by an intraoperative confirmation. Hence, this classification may be used in the preoperative setting to inform and consent the patient on the expected procedure and its alternatives. It is essential to validate the proposed classification and to critically assess its applicability for different nerves separately, due to variations in their sensorimotor functions and in the degree of compensation following nerve resection.

The present study is one of the largest published series on STS with sciatic nerve involvement to date, as most prior studies were limited to a cohort of less than 20 patients [14–17, 26]. Nevertheless, the small number of patients with this rare constellation of soft tissue sarcoma with sciatic nerve involvement limits the statistical power of our analysis. In addition, the proposed classification does not take significant prognostic parameters, such as grading, into consideration. The tumor grade may influence the extent of surgical resection and could potentially be incorporated into the treatment algorithm. For example, a nerve-sparing surgical resection should be thoroughly considered in a young patient with a well-differentiated liposarcoma and type A sciatic nerve involvement to minimize the loss of function. This is because these tumors rarely metastasize, and the risk of local recurrence may be reduced by incorporating adjuvant or neoadjuvant radiotherapy. In addition, the established classification for vascular involvement in STS by Schwarzbach et al. could also be combined with our proposed classification for nerve involvement, enabling STS with neurovascular involvement to be more accurately classified [9, 37]. Furthermore, the effects of neoadjuvant and adjuvant therapy on both functional and oncological outcomes were not addressed in our study, and no patient-reported functional outcomes were reported in the current series. This data may be used in future studies to compare preoperative and postoperative functions, as it has been suggested that patients with worse function preoperatively have more room to improve postoperatively [15].

5. Conclusions

This is the first study to date to classify the extent of sciatic nerve involvement in STS and to suggest a surgical treatment algorithm. In our study, the extent of nerve resection had no significant impact on disease recurrence or overall survival. Hence, precise classification of nerve involvement is useful in selecting the appropriate degree of nerve resection, without compromising oncological outcome or unnecessarily sacrificing leg function. Additional studies are necessary to validate and optimize this classification.

References

[1] P. F. Choong and H. A. Rudiger, "Prognostic factors in soft-tissue sarcomas: what have we learnt?," *Expert Review of Anticancer Therapy*, vol. 8, no. 2, pp. 139–146, 2008.

[2] R. Siegel, J. Ma, Z. Zou, and A. Jemal, "Cancer statistics, 2014," *CA: A Cancer Journal for Clinicians*, vol. 64, no. 1, pp. 9–29, 2014.

[3] P. G. Casali, L. Jost, S. Sleijfer, J. Verweij, J. Y. Blay, and ESMO Guidelines Working Group, "Soft tissue sarcomas: ESMO clinical recommendations for diagnosis, treatment and follow-up," *Annals of Oncology*, vol. 20, no. 4, pp. 132–136, 2009.

[4] E. G. Elias, S. D. Brown, and W. J. Culpepper, "Experience in the management of 52 patients with soft tissue sarcoma. The results of a median follow-up of seven years," *Cancer Therapy*, vol. 6, pp. 47–54, 2008.

[5] M. F. Brennan, C. R. Antonescu, N. Moraco, and S. Singer, "Lessons learned from the study of 10,000 patients with soft tissue sarcoma," *Annals of Surgery*, vol. 260, no. 3, pp. 416–422, 2014.

[6] L. M. Nystrom, N. B. Reimer, J. D. Reith et al., "Multidisciplinary management of soft tissue sarcoma," *Scientific World Journal*, vol. 2013, Article ID 852462, 11 pages, 2013.

[7] D. L. Flugstad, C. P. Wilke, M. A. McNutt, R. A. Welk, M. J. Hart, and W. C. McQuinn, "Importance of surgical resection in the successful management of soft tissue sarcoma," *Archives of Surgery*, vol. 134, no. 8, pp. 856–861, 1999.

[8] C. H. Gerrand, J. S. Wunder, R. A. Kandel et al., "Classification of positive margins after resection of soft-tissue sarcoma of the limb predicts the risk of local recurrence," *The Journal of Bone and Joint Surgery*, vol. 83, no. 8, pp. 1149–1155, 2001.

[9] M. H. Schwarzbach, Y. Hormann, U. Hinz et al., "Results of limb-sparing surgery with vascular replacement for soft tissue sarcoma in the lower extremity," *Journal of Vascular Surgery*, vol. 42, no. 1, pp. 88–97, 2005.

[10] T. Koperna, B. Teleky, S. Vogi et al., "Vascular reconstruction for limb salvage in sarcoma of the lower extremity," *Archives of Surgery*, vol. 131, no. 10, pp. 1103–1107, 1996.

[11] R. N. Nambisan and C. P. Karakousis, "Vascular reconstruction for limb salvage in soft tissue sarcomas," *Surgery*, vol. 101, no. 6, pp. 668–677, 1987.

[12] D. X. Lun, Y. C. Hu, and H. C. Huang, "Management of great vessels and nerves in limb-salvage surgery for bone and soft tissue tumors," *Orthopaedic Surgery*, vol. 5, no. 4, pp. 233–238, 2013.

[13] J. E. Thomas, D. G. Piepgras, B. Scheithauer, B. M. Onofrio, and T. C. Shives, "Neurogenic tumors of the sciatic nerve: a clinicopathologic study of 35 cases," *Mayo Clinic Proceedings*, vol. 58, no. 10, pp. 640–647, 1983.

[14] J. Bickels, J. C. Wittig, Y. Kollender, K. Kellar-Graney, M. M. Malawer, and I. Meller, "Sciatic nerve resection: is that truly an indication for amputation?," *Clinical Orthopaedics and Related Research*, vol. 399, pp. 201–204, 2002.

[15] A. D. Brooks, J. S. Gold, D. Graham et al., "Resection of the sciatic, peroneal, or tibial nerves: assessment of functional status," *Annals of Surgical Oncology*, vol. 9, no. 1, pp. 41–47, 2002.

[16] B. Fuchs, A. M. Davis, J. S. Wunder et al., "Sciatic nerve resection in the thigh: a functional evaluation," *Clinical Orthopaedics and Related Research*, vol. 382, pp. 34–41, 2001.

[17] P. W. Clarkson, A. M. Griffin, C. N. Catton et al., "Epineural dissection is a safe technique that facilitates limb salvage surgery," *Clinical Orthopaedics and Related Research*, vol. 438, pp. 92–96, 2005.

[18] W. F. Enneking, *Musculoskeletal Tumor Surgery*, Churchill Livingstone, New York, NY, USA, 1983.

[19] W. F. Enneking, S. S. Spanier, and M. A. Goodman, "A system for surgical staging of musculoskeletal sarcoma," *Clinical Orthopaedics and Related Research*, vol. 415, pp. 4–18, 2003.

[20] W. F. Enneking, W. Dunham, M. C. Gebhardt, M. Malawar, and D. J. Pritchard, "A system for the functional evaluation of reconstructive procedures after surgical treatment of tumors of the musculoskeletal system," *Clinical Orthopaedics and Related Research*, vol. 286, pp. 241–246, 1993.

[21] P. W. Pisters, D. H. Leung, J. Woodruff, W. Shi, and M. F. Brennan, "Analysis of prognostic factors in 1,041 patients with localized soft tissue sarcomas of the extremities," *Journal of Clinical Oncology*, vol. 14, no. 5, pp. 1679–1689, 1996.

[22] B. O' Sullivan, A. M. Davis, R. Turcotte et al., "Preoperative versus postoperative radiotherapy in soft-tissue sarcoma of the limbs: a randomised trial," *The Lancet*, vol. 359, no. 9325, pp. 2235–2241, 2002.

[23] R. Dagan, D. J. Indelicato, L. McGee et al., "The significance of a marginal excision after preoperative radiation therapy for soft tissue sarcoma of the extremity," *Cancer*, vol. 118, no. 12, pp. 3199–3207, 2012.

[24] S. Abatzoglou, R. E. Turcotte, A. Adoubali, M. H. Isler, and D. Roberge, "Local recurrence after initial multidisciplinary management of soft tissue sarcoma: is there a way out?," *Clinical Orthopaedics and Related Research*, vol. 468, no. 11, pp. 3012–3018, 2010.

[25] E. N. Novais, B. Demiralp, J. Alderete, M. C. Larson, P. S. Rose, and F. H. Sim, "Do surgical margin and local

recurrence influence survival in soft tissue sarcomas?," *Clinical Orthopaedics and Related Research*, vol. 468, no. 11, pp. 3003–3011, 2010.

[26] S. H. Herbert, B. W. Corn, L. J. Solin et al., "Limb-preserving treatment for soft tissue sarcomas of the extremities. The significance of surgical margins," *Cancer*, vol. 72, no. 4, pp. 1230–1238, 1993.

[27] I. J. Spiro, A. E. Rosenberg, D. Springfield, and H. Suit, "Combined surgery and radiation therapy for limb preservation in soft tissue sarcoma of the extremity: the Massachusetts General Hospital experience," *Cancer Investigation*, vol. 13, no. 1, pp. 86–95, 1995.

[28] R. G. Bevilacqua, A. Rogatko, S. I. Hajdu, and M. F. Brennan, "Prognostic factors in primary retroperitoneal soft-tissue sarcomas," *Archives of Surgery*, vol. 126, no. 3, pp. 328–334, 1991.

[29] W. C. Williard, S. I. Hajdu, E. S. Casper, and M. F. Brennan, "Comparison of amputation with limb-sparing operations for adult soft tissue sarcoma of the extremity," *Annals of Surgery*, vol. 215, no. 3, pp. 269–275, 1992.

[30] E. U. Conrad, D. Springfield, and T. D. Peabody, "Pelvis," in *Surgery for Bone and Soft Tissue Tumors*, M. A. Simon and D. Springfield, Eds., pp. 323–341, Lippincott-Raven, Philadelphia, PA, USA, 1998.

[31] P. Hohenberger, J. R. Allenberg, P. M. Schlag, and P. Reichardt, "Results of surgery and multimodal therapy for patients with soft tissue sarcoma invading to vascular structures," *Cancer*, vol. 85, no. 2, pp. 396–408, 1999.

[32] T. W. Prewitt, H. R. Alexander, and W. F. Sindelar, "Hemipelvectomy for soft tissue sarcoma: clinical results in fifty-three patients," *Surgical Oncology*, vol. 4, no. 5, pp. 261–269, 1995.

[33] M. J. Dorsi, Z. S. Zwagil, W. Hsu, and A. J. Belzberg, "Epithelioid sarcoma of the tibial portion of the sciatic nerve," *Clinical Neurology and Neurosurgery*, vol. 113, no. 6, pp. 506–508, 2011.

[34] A. M. Davis, M. Devlin, A. M. Griffin, J. S. Wunder, and R. S. Bell, "Functional outcome in amputation versus limb sparing of patients with lower extremity sarcoma: a matched case-control study," *Archives of Physical Medicine and Rehabilitation*, vol. 80, no. 6, pp. 615–618, 1999.

[35] M. I. O'Connor, "Surgical management of malignant soft tissue tumors," in *Surgery for Bone and Soft Tissue Tumors*, M. A. Simon and D. Springfield, Eds., pp. 555–565, Lippincott-Raven, Philadelphia, PA, USA, 1998.

[36] P. W. O'Donnell, A. M. Griffin, W. C. Eward et al., "The effect of the setting of a positive surgical margin in soft tissue sarcoma," *Cancer*, vol. 120, no. 18, pp. 2866–2875, 2014.

[37] M. H. Schwarzbach, Y. Hormann, U. Hinz et al., "Clinical results of surgery for retroperitoneal sarcoma with major blood vessel involvement," *Journal of Vascular Surgery*, vol. 44, no. 1, pp. 46–55, 2006.

21

Confirmed Activity and Tolerability of Weekly Paclitaxel in the Treatment of Advanced Angiosarcoma

Gaetano Apice,[1] Antonio Pizzolorusso,[1] Massimo Di Maio,[1] Giovanni Grignani,[2] Vittorio Gebbia,[3] Angela Buonadonna,[4] Annarosaria De Chiara,[1] Flavio Fazioli,[1] Giampaolo De Palma,[1] Danilo Galizia,[2] Carlo Arcara,[3] Nicola Mozzillo,[1] and Francesco Perrone[1]

[1]*Istituto Nazionale Tumori IRCCS "Fondazione G. Pascale", Via Mariano Semmola, 80131 Napoli, Italy*
[2]*Institute for Cancer Research and Treatment, Strada Provinciale, km 3.95, Candiolo, 10060 Turin, Italy*
[3]*Medical Oncology Unit, La Maddalena Hospital, Via San Lorenzo Colli 312/d, 90146 Palermo, Italy*
[4]*Departments of Radiation Oncology and Medical Oncology, CRO, National Cancer Institute, Via Franco Gallini 2, 33081 Aviano, Italy*

Correspondence should be addressed to Gaetano Apice; gaetanoapice@virgilio.it

Academic Editor: C. Verhoef

Background. In several prospective and retrospective studies, weekly paclitaxel showed promising activity in patients with angiosarcoma. *Patients and Methods.* Our study was originally designed as a prospective, phase II multicenter trial for patients younger than 75, with ECOG performance status 0–2, affected by locally advanced or metastatic angiosarcoma. Patients received paclitaxel 80 mg/m^2 intravenously, at days 1, 8, and 15 every 4 weeks, until disease progression or unacceptable toxicity. Primary endpoint was objective response. *Results.* Eight patients were enrolled but, due to very slow accrual, the trial was prematurely stopped and further 10 patients were retrospectively included in the analysis. Out of 17 evaluable patients, 6 patients obtained an objective response (5 partial, 1 complete), with an objective response rate of 35% (95% confidence interval 17%–59%). Of note, five responses were obtained in pretreated patients. In the paper, details of overall survival, progression-free survival, and tolerability are reported. *Conclusions.* In this small series of patients with locally advanced or metastatic angiosarcoma, weekly paclitaxel was confirmed to be well tolerated and active even in pretreated patients.

1. Introduction

Angiosarcomas are very rare tumors (incidence < 1/100.000/year) of vascular or lymphatic origin characterized by a clinical heterogeneity in terms of presentation and behavior. This subgroup of sarcomas represent about 1-2% of all soft tissue tumors and can occur in any anatomic site of the body but most commonly originate in the skin of head and neck and in breast area [1].

Although etiology is unknown, several risk factors for angiosarcoma have been described: previous exposure to radiation therapy [2, 3], vinyl chloride [4], chronic lymphedema [5], and prolonged immunosuppression [6, 7].

Regardless of morphology, angiosarcoma is considered as a high-grade tumor [8] and constitutes one of the most aggressive subtypes of soft tissue sarcomas with overall median survival of <4 years. In our experience even angiosarcomas histologically classified as low grade can develop distant metastasis.

Wide surgical resection followed as much as possible by adjuvant radiation therapy is the mainstay of therapy in patients with localized disease [9, 10].

As for other soft tissue sarcomas chemotherapy is still not a standard treatment in adjuvant setting, despite the fact that angiosarcomas develop distant metastasis in up to 50% of cases [11, 12].

Doxorubicin-based chemotherapy remains the first-line standard treatment of metastatic or unresectable angiosarcoma providing a progression-free survival of 3.7–5.4 months and response rate between 40% and 65% [11].

Taxanes have been found effective in patients affected by vascular-derived tumors, such as Kaposi sarcoma [13]. Paclitaxel is potent antiangiogenic drug and, at least *in vitro*, exhibits its efficacy on human endothelial cells at low-dose concentration as well as cytotoxic effect at regular concentration [14–16].

In this paper we report a retrospective series of 17 patients with advanced angiosarcoma treated with weekly paclitaxel in 4 centers of Italian Sarcoma Group.

2. Patients and Methods

2.1. Patients. The study was originally designed as a prospective, phase II multicenter trial with the aim of assessing activity and toxicity of the weekly schedule of paclitaxel. Patients with histological diagnosis of angiosarcoma, with locally advanced or metastatic disease, and not eligible for surgery or recurrent after previous surgery were eligible for the inclusion in the study. Previous chemotherapy was allowed, but it had to be stopped at least 4 weeks before the inclusion in the protocol. Main exclusion criteria were age younger than 75, performance status worse than 2 according to Eastern Cooperative Oncology Group, other malignant diseases in the previous 5 years (with the exception of nonmelanomatous skin cancer or carcinoma *in situ* of the uterine cervix), and brain metastases or inadequate laboratory values (neutrophils < 2000/mm^3, platelets < 100000/mm^3, hemoglobin < 10 g/dL, serum creatinine level > 1.5 x upper normal limit (UNL), sAST or sALT > 1.25xUNL in the absence of liver metastases or >2.5xUNL in the presence of liver metastases, and serum bilirubin > 1.25xUNL in the absence of liver metastases or >1.5xUNL in the presence of liver metastases). The study protocol was approved by the ethical committees of all participating institutions, and all patients prospectively enrolled in the trial provided written informed consent.

2.2. Study Treatment. Patients received paclitaxel 80 mg/m^2 intravenously (IV), at days 1, 8, and 15 every 4 weeks until disease progression or unacceptable toxicity. Standard premedication with dexamethasone and H1 (promethazine) and H2 (ranitidine) receptor antagonists was prescribed by protocol, before each administration of paclitaxel. Chemotherapy could be postponed, at Investigator's discretion, for up to 14 days for persistent hematological toxicity (neutrophils < 1500/mm^3; platelets < 100000/mm^3; hemoglobin < 8 g/dL) or persistent nonhematological toxicities grade ≥2. A 25% dose reduction (60 mg/m^2) for paclitaxel was planned in case of previous grade 4 neutropenia lasting more than 3 days or in case of previous platelets < 50000/mm^3. After disease progression, there was no predetermined salvage treatment planned by study protocol; however further chemotherapy was allowed at Investigators' discretion.

2.3. Assessment Procedures. Patients were evaluated at baseline with a complete history and physical examination, routine hematology and biochemistry, chest X-ray, chest CT scan, abdominal ultrasound, and CT scan (or magnetic resonance or ultrasound) for specific sites of disease.

Tumor response was assessed by repeating instrumental exams every two cycles of chemotherapy, by using RECIST criteria version 1.0 [17].

Toxicity was codified according to National Cancer Institute Common Terminology Criteria (version 2.0). During treatment, routine hematology, biochemistry, and physical examination were performed every 3 administrations of paclitaxel, before the next cycle. Hematology was also repeated before each weekly administration of chemotherapy.

2.4. Sample Size and Statistical Analysis. Objective response was the primary endpoint of the trial, and the sample size of the study was determined according to Gehan's two-stage design, based on the requirement of stopping the study at an early stage if the response rate was below 20%, and of estimating the response rate with a standard error less than 0.10 [18]. If no objective tumor response was observed among the first 14 evaluable patients, recruitment of patients would stop, whilst additional (1, 6, 9, or 11) patients had to be included if there were responses (1, 2, 3, or more than 3, resp.) in the first 14 patients.

Median follow-up was calculated according to the reverse Kaplan-Meier technique [19]. Overall survival (OS) was calculated from the date of treatment start to the date of death, or the date of last follow-up for alive patients. Progression-free survival (PFS) was defined as the time from the date of treatment start to the date of disease progression, or the date of death for patients that died without progression, or the date of last follow-up for patients alive and without progression at the end of the study. OS and PFS curves were estimated according to the Kaplan-Meier product limit method.

Statistical analyses were performed with S-PLUS software (S-PLUS 6.0 Professional, release 1, Insightful Corporation, Seattle, WA, USA).

3. Results

Between October 2002 and March 2006, 8 patients were enrolled in the prospective trial by 5 Italian institutions. The trial was prematurely stopped, due to very slow accrual, although the planned number of 14 patients had not been reached. Further 10 patients, who started treatment with weekly paclitaxel between April 2003 and November 2011, were retrospectively included in the analysis.

One patient enrolled in the prospective trial has been excluded from the analysis due to lack of postregistration data. Baseline characteristics of the 17 evaluable patients, overall and scattered by prospective versus retrospective group, are summarized in Table 1. Median age was 64 years (range 20–80), and most patients had ECOG performance status 0 or 1. The majority of patients had metastatic disease (13, 76%) and had received previous surgery. All the 7 patients enrolled in the prospective trial were pretreated with chemotherapy for advanced disease, whilst 7 out of 10 patients retrospectively analyzed received paclitaxel as first-line of treatment for advanced disease. Individual characteristics of all the treated patients are listed in Table 2.

TABLE 1: Baseline characteristics.

	Prospective group (n = 7)	Retrospective group (n = 10)	Study population (n = 17)
Gender			
Males	3 (43%)	5 (50%)	8 (47%)
Females	4 (57%)	5 (50%)	9 (53%)
Age			
Median (range)	63 (20–74)	68 (46–80)	64 (20–80)
ECOG performance status (3 missing data items)			
0	3 (43%)	2 (29%)	5 (36%)
1	3 (43%)	5 (71%)	8 (57%)
2	1 (14%)	—	1 (7%)
Stage			
Locally advanced	1 (14%)	3 (30%)	4 (24%)
Metastatic	6 (86%)	7 (70%)	13 (76%)
Grading (1 missing data item)			
G1	—	—	—
G2	3 (43%)	4 (44%)	7 (44%)
G3	4 (57%)	5 (56%)	9 (56%)
Previous surgery			
Yes	5 (71%)	9 (90%)	14 (82%)
Previous chemotherapy			
None	—	5 (50%)	5 (29%)
Only adjuvant	—	2 (20%)	2 (12%)
Advanced disease	7 (100%)	3 (30%)	10 (59%)

TABLE 2: Individual characteristics of the 17 patients included in the analysis.

Patient code	Type of study	Gender	Age	PS	Stage	Grading	Previous surgery	Previous chemotherapy	Best response	PFS (months)	OS (months)
1	P	F	35	2	Metastatic	G3	Yes	Yes	PD	0.9	0.9^+
2	P	M	64	0	Metastatic	G3	No	Yes	PD	10.1^+	10.1^+
4	P	M	20	0	Metastatic	G3	Yes	Yes	PR	1.5^+	1.5^+
5	P	F	50	1	Metastatic	G2	Yes	Yes	PR	9.0	17.7
6	P	F	63	0	Metastatic	G2	Yes	Yes	PD	10.0	33.2
7	P	F	67	1	Loc. adv.	G3	No	Yes	SD	62.2^+	62.2^+
8	P	M	74	1	Metastatic	G2	Yes	Yes	SD	5.5	45.9^+
1001	R	M	73	1	Loc. adv.	G3	Yes	No	SD	2.7	9.6^+
1002	R	M	70	1	Metastatic	G3	Yes	Yes	PD	4.6	7.1
1003	R	F	66	0	Metastatic	G2	Yes	Yes	PR	6.6	8.6^+
1004	R	F	75	0	Metastatic	G3	Yes	Yes	PR	3.0	16.5
1005	R	M	46	1	Metastatic	n.a.	Yes	Yes	SD	3.5	7.6^+
1006	R	F	61	1	Metastatic	G2	Yes	Yes	CR	1.8	2.0
1007	R	F	62	n.a.	Metastatic	G3	Yes	No	PR	2.0	20.8^+
1008	R	M	71	n.a.	Loc. adv.	G2	Yes	No	PD	3.8	7.3
1009	R	M	80	1	Loc. adv.	G3	No	No	SD	6.0	9.9
1010	R	F	47	n.a.	Metastatic	G2	Yes	No	SD	1.8	18.6

P: prospective; R: retrospective; M: male; F: female; PS: performance status; n.a.: not available; loc. adv.: locally advanced; CR: complete response; PR: partial response; SD: stable disease; PD: progressive disease; PFS: progression-free survival; OS: overall survival; +: patient censored without event at the last observation.

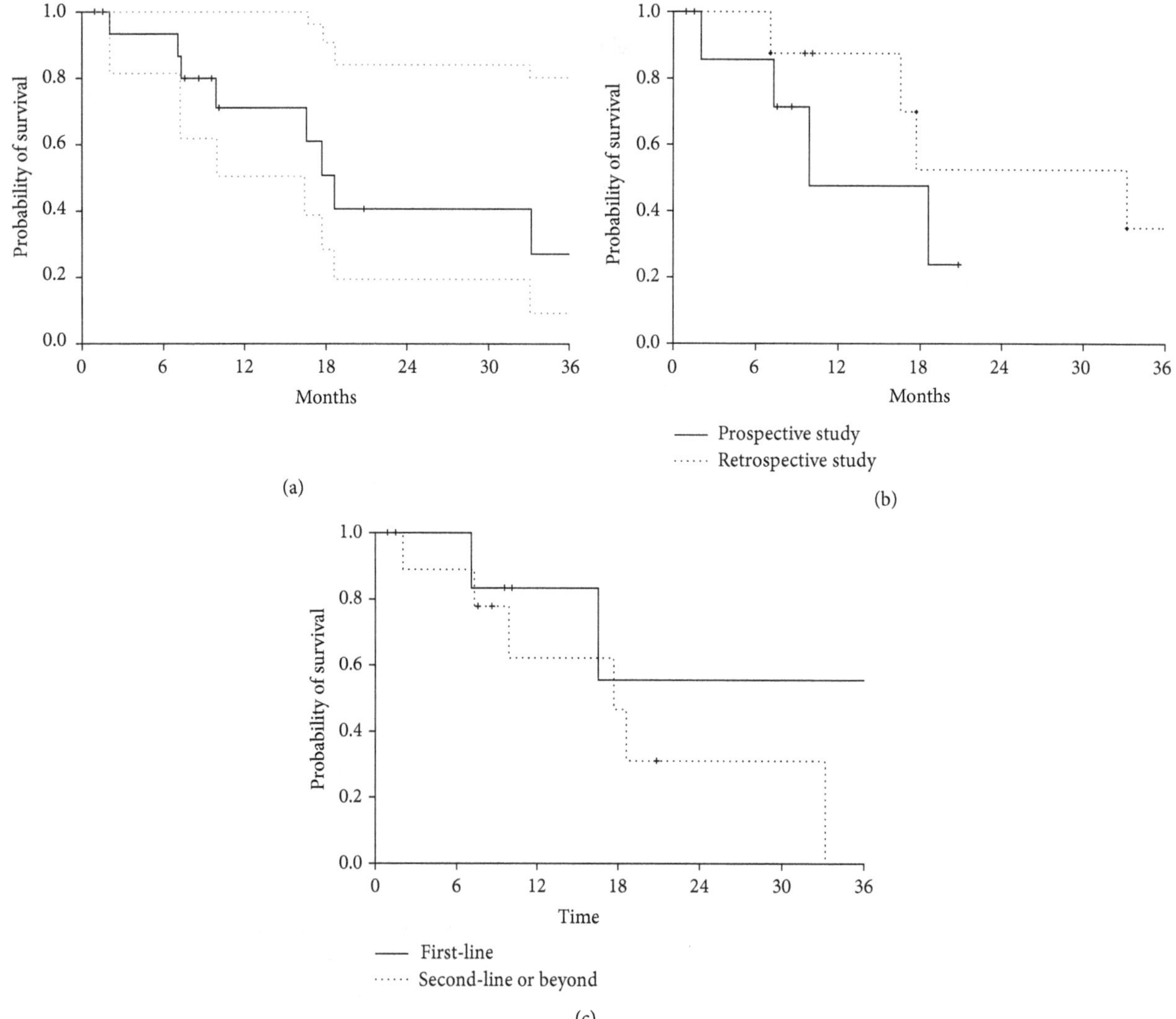

FIGURE 1: Kaplan-Meier curves of overall survival. (a) Overall survival in the whole series of patients (prospective + retrospective). Dotted lines represent 95% confidence intervals. (b) Overall survival according to type of study: continuous line refers to patients enrolled in the prospective study; dotted line refers to patients included in the retrospective study. (c) Overall survival according to line of treatment: continuous line refers to patients treated with paclitaxel as first-line; dotted line refers to patients receiving paclitaxel as second-line or further line.

Median number of paclitaxel administrations in the 17 evaluable patients was 12 (range, 4–30). Two patients received more than 6 cycles of treatment, stopping because of disease progression after 8 and 10 cycles, respectively. Median number of paclitaxel administrations in the 7 patients enrolled in the prospective study was 8 (range, 6–18). Median number of paclitaxel administrations in the 10 patients enrolled in the retrospective study was 13.5 (range, 4–30).

Median dose intensity of paclitaxel in the 17 evaluable patients was 60 mg/m^2/week (range, 43–80). Median dose intensity of paclitaxel in the 7 patients enrolled in the prospective study was 60 mg/m^2/week (range, 44–68). Median dose intensity of paclitaxel in the 10 patients enrolled in the retrospective study was 61 mg/m^2/week (range, 42–80).

Overall, 6 patients obtained an objective response (5 partial responses, 1 complete response). Objective response rate was 35% (95% confidence interval 17%–59%). Of note, five of the objective responses were obtained in patients already pretreated with chemotherapy. Considering only the 7 patients enrolled in the prospective trial, 2 partial responses were observed (objective response rate 29%, 95% confidence interval 8%–64%).

After a median follow-up of 20.8 months, 14 progressions (82%) and 8 deaths (47%) were recorded in the 17 evaluable patients. In the prospective group, after a median follow-up of 20.8 months, 7 progressions (100%) and 4 deaths (57%) were recorded. In the retrospective group, after a median follow-up of 45.9 months, 7 progressions (70%) and 4 deaths (40%) were recorded.

Median overall survival was 18.6 months (95% confidence interval (CI) 16.5–n.a.) (Figure 1(a)). In the prospective group, median overall survival was 9.9 months (95% CI

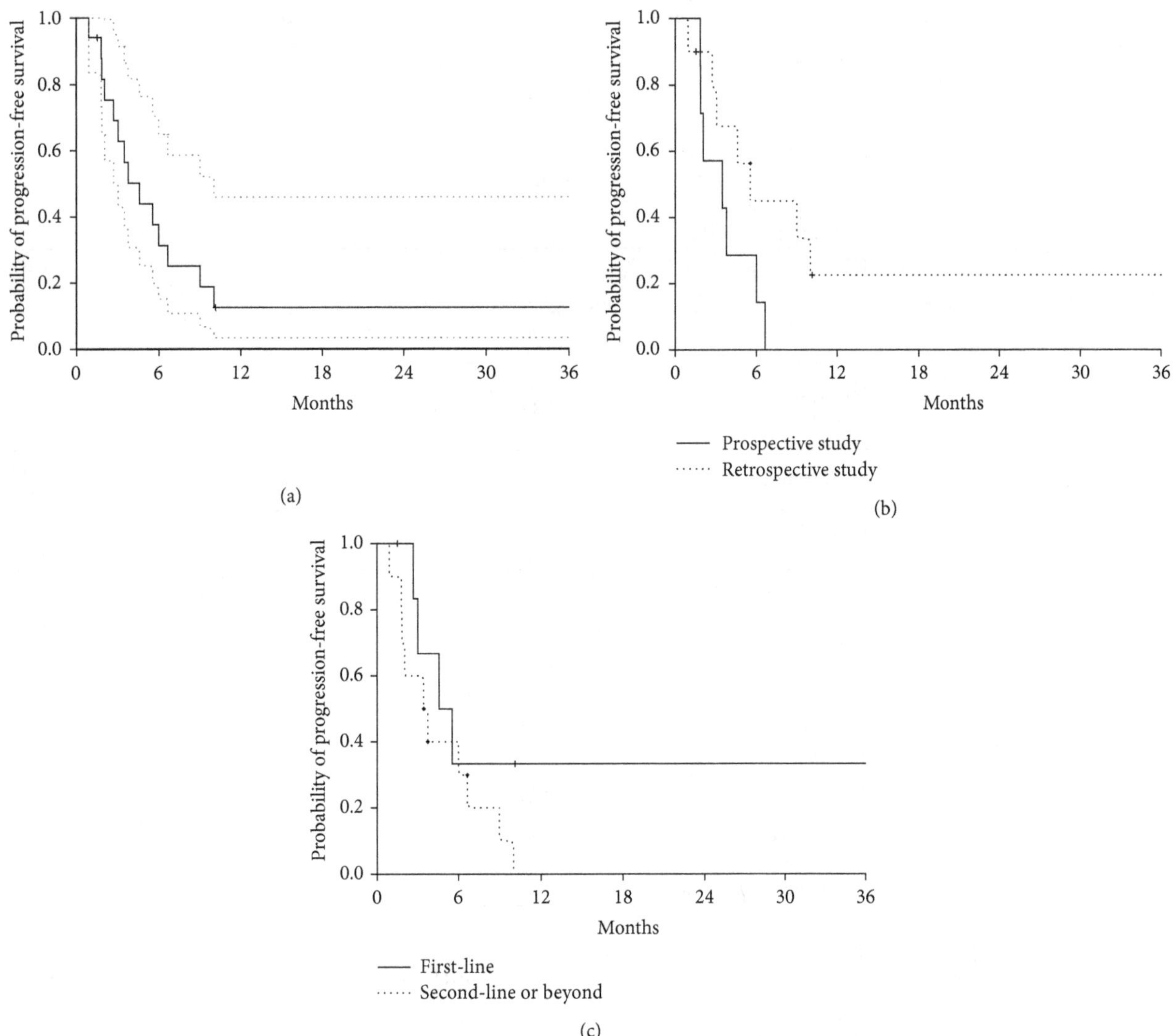

FIGURE 2: Kaplan-Meier curves of progression-free survival. (a) Progression-free survival in the whole series of patients (prospective + retrospective). Dotted lines represent 95% confidence intervals. (b) Progression-free survival according to type of study: continuous line refers to patients enrolled in the prospective study; dotted line refers to patients included in the retrospective study. (c) Progression-free survival according to line of treatment: continuous line refers to patients treated with paclitaxel as first-line; dotted line refers to patients receiving paclitaxel as second-line or further line.

7.3–n.a.), whilst, in the retrospective group, median overall survival was 33.2 months (95% CI 16.5–n.a.) (Figure 1(b)). In patients receiving experimental treatment as first-line, median overall survival was not reached (95% CI 16.5–n.a.), whilst, in patients receiving experimental treatment as second-line or further line, median overall survival was 17.7 months (95% CI 9.9–n.a.) (Figure 1(c)).

Median progression-free survival was 4.6 months (95% confidence interval (CI) 2.7–10.0) (Figure 2(a)). In the prospective group, median progression-free survival was 3.5 months (95% CI 1.8–n.a.), whilst, in the retrospective group, median progression-free survival was 5.5 months (95% CI 3.0–n.a.) (Figure 2(b)). In patients receiving experimental treatment as first-line, median progression-free survival was 5.1 months (95% CI 3.0–n.a.), whilst, in patients receiving experimental treatment as second-line or further line, median progression-free survival was 3.6 months (95% CI 1.8–n.a.) (Figure 2(c)).

Mild or moderate anemia was reported during treatment in ten patients (59%), grade 1 in 9 patients and grade 2 in 1 patient. Any grade neutropenia was reported in 4 patients (24%), grade 3-4 neutropenia was reported in 2 patients, and there was no case of febrile neutropenia. Any grade thrombocytopenia was reported in 5 patients (29%), grade 3-4 thrombocytopenia was reported in 2 patients, and there were no relevant bleeding episodes. Mild or moderate asthenia was reported in 6 patients (35%), mild or moderate skin toxicity in 3 patients (18%), grade 1-2 diarrhea in 3 patients (18%), grade 1 constipation in 3 patients (18%), and grade 1-2 nausea or vomiting in 2 patients (12%). Neuropathy was reported in 5 patients (grade 3 in 1, grade 2 in 1, and grade 1 in 3 patients). No severe organ toxicities were described.

Table 3: Main characteristics and results obtained in the studies with paclitaxel in patients with advanced angiosarcoma.

Author, year [ref]	Type of study	Paclitaxel dose and schedule	Period of treatment	Number of patients	Response rate (%)	PFS (median)	OS (median)
Fata et al., 1999 [20]	Retrospective	250 mg/m^2 continuous infusion for 24 h every 3 weeks or 175 mg/m^2 every 3 weeks or 90 mg/m^2 weekly	1992–1998	9	89	TTP 5 months	n.a.
Schlemmer et al., 2008 [21]	Retrospective	135–175 mg/m^2 every 3 weeks ($n = 21$) or 75–100 mg/m^2 weekly ($n = 11$)	1996–2005	32	62	TTP 7.6 months	n.a.
Penel et al., 2008 [22]	Prospective	80 mg/m^2 on days 1, 8, and 15, every 4 weeks	2005–2006	30 (assessable 27)	18-19	TTP 4 months	8 months
Penel et al., 2012 [9]	Retrospective	Weekly schedule	1996–2009	47	45	TTP 5.6 months	13.1 months
Italiano et al., 2012 [23]	Retrospective	80 mg/m^2 on days 1, 8, and 15, every 4 weeks	1990–2010	75	53	5.8 months	10.3 months
Ray-Coquard et al., 2015 [24]	Prospective	Control arm: paclitaxel 90 mg/m^2 on days 1, 8, and 15, every 4 weeks, for 6 cycles	2010–2013	26		PFS: 6.8 mo Progression-free rate at 6 months: 57%	Overall survival at 1 year: 55%
		Experimental arm: same as control arm + bevacizumab 10 mg/kg on days 1, 8, and 15 followed by maintenance therapy 15 mg/kg/3 wks until intolerance/progression	2010–2013	26		PFS: 6.9 mo Progression-free rate at 6 months: 57%	Overall survival at 1 year: 58%
Our study	Prospective + retrospective	80 mg/m^2 on days 1, 8, and 15, every 4 weeks	Prospective: 2002–2006 Retrospective: 2003–2011	18 (17 evaluable)	35	4.6 months	18.6 months

PFS: progression-free survival; OS: overall survival; TTP: time-to-progression; n.a.: not available.

4. Discussion

In recent years, after the start of our study, several experiences with paclitaxel in patients with advanced or metastatic angiosarcoma have been published [20–23]. Table 3 reports the main characteristics and results obtained in these studies and in our series. The EORTC soft tissue and bone sarcoma group published a retrospective study about the use of paclitaxel in 32 patients [21]. Only 11 patients of this series received a weekly schedule of paclitaxel; the others were treated with the classical, every-3-week schedule. In the whole series, response rate was 62% and median progression-free survival was 7.6 months; however many of the patients were not pretreated with chemotherapy. These results prompted the authors to define paclitaxel as active agent, warranting prospective trials in this setting. Similarly, weekly paclitaxel was associated with promising efficacy in a retrospective analysis of patients treated between 1996 and 2009 in the French Sarcoma Group [23].

In a prospective phase II trial, 30 patients were treated with weekly paclitaxel, at the same schedule tested in our study. In that series of patients (11 pretreated with chemotherapy and 19 not pretreated), weekly paclitaxel produced 18% response rate, a median time-to-progression of 4 months, and a median overall survival of 8 months. Similar to our series, results were considered encouraging also in the subgroup of patients who had already failed previous chemotherapy, with similar progression-free survival compared to those who were treatment naïve.

Recently, a randomized phase II trial testing the addition of bevacizumab to weekly paclitaxel in patients with advanced or metastatic angiosarcoma was presented [24]. In that trial, patients assigned to control arm received paclitaxel 90 mg/m^2 at days 1, 8, and 15 every 4 weeks, and patients assigned to experimental arm received the same schedule with the addition of bevacizumab. Unfortunately, the addition of the antiangiogenic monoclonal antibody was not associated with any benefit in PFS nor in overall survival.

The retrospective fraction of this study did not allow us to describe exhaustively the adverse events related to chemotherapy. However no important toxicities were reported. There were no cases of febrile neutropenia and no relevant bleeding episodes, whilst grade 3-4 neutropenia was reported in 2 cases and only 1 patient exhibited grade 3 neuropathy. In conclusion, our experience confirms that weekly paclitaxel is well tolerated and active in patients with advanced and metastatic angiosarcomas, even though, in our experience, duration of response was quite short. Further studies of this agent are warranted, also in combination with other drugs. An interesting schedule with taxanes and doxorubicin, an active combination in other tumors, may be a major issue, particularly in neoadjuvant setting, whereas the combination of anthracycline plus ifosfamide can be difficult to administer in many angiosarcoma patients due to the age and clinical conditions.

References

[1] V. T. Devita, S. A. Rosenberg, and T. S. Lawrence, *Cancer: Principles and Practice of Oncology*, Lippincott Williams & Wilkins, Philadelphia, Pa, USA, 8th edition, 2008.

[2] S. B. Williams and M. Reed, "Cutaneous angiosarcoma after breast conserving treatment for bilateral breast cancers in a BRCA-1 gene mutation carrier—a case report and review of the literature," *Surgeon*, vol. 7, no. 4, article 250, 2009.

[3] P. Karlsson, E. Holmberg, A. Samuelsson, K.-A. Johansson, and A. Wallgren, "Soft tissue sarcoma after treatment for breast cancer—a Swedish population-based study," *European Journal of Cancer*, vol. 34, no. 13, pp. 2068–2075, 1998.

[4] J. A. Abraham, F. J. Hornicek, A. M. Kaufman et al., "Treatment and outcome of 82 patients with angiosarcoma," *Annals of Surgical Oncology*, vol. 14, no. 6, pp. 1953–1967, 2007.

[5] J. Fayette, E. Martin, S. Piperno-Neumann et al., "Angiosarcomas, a heterogeneous group of sarcomas with specific behavior depending on primary site: a retrospective study of 161 cases," *Annals of Oncology*, vol. 18, no. 12, pp. 2030–2036, 2007.

[6] I. Ahmed and K. L. Hamacher, "Angiosarcoma in a chronically immunosuppressed renal transplant recipient: report of a case and review of the literature," *American Journal of Dermatopathology*, vol. 24, no. 4, pp. 330–335, 2002.

[7] J. J. Goedert, T. R. Coté, P. Virgo et al., "Spectrum of AIDS-associated malignant disorders," *The Lancet*, vol. 351, no. 9119, pp. 1833–1839, 1998.

[8] S. W. Weiss, J. Lasota, and M. M. Miettinem, "Angiosarcoma of soft tissue," in *WHO Classification Tumours of Soft Tissue and Bone*, C. D. M. Fletcher, K. K. Unni, and F. Mertens, Eds., pp. 175–177, IARC Press, Lyon, France, 2002.

[9] N. Penel, A. Italiano, I. Ray-coquard et al., "Metastatic angiosarcomas: doxorubicin-based regimens, weekly paclitaxel and metastasectomy significantly improve the outcome," *Annals of Oncology*, vol. 23, no. 2, pp. 517–523, 2012.

[10] N. Penel, A. Lansiaux, and A. Adenis, "Angiosarcomas and taxanes," *Current Treatment Options in Oncology*, vol. 8, no. 6, pp. 428–434, 2007.

[11] M. G. Fury, C. R. Antonescu, K. J. Van Zee, M. F. Brennan, and R. G. Maki, "A 14-year retrospective review of angiosarcoma: clinical characteristics, prognostic factors, and treatment outcomes with surgery and chemotherapy," *Cancer Journal*, vol. 11, no. 3, pp. 241–247, 2005.

[12] S. A. Vorburger, Y. Xing, K. K. Hunt et al., "Angiosarcoma of the breast," *Cancer*, vol. 104, no. 12, pp. 2682–2688, 2005.

[13] J. Stebbing, A. Wildfire, S. Portsmouth et al., "Paclitaxel for anthracyclin-resistant AIDS-related Kaposi's sarcoma: clinical and angiogenic correlations," *Annals of Oncology*, vol. 14, no. 11, pp. 1660–1660, 2003.

[14] E. Pasquier, S. Honore, B. Pourroy et al., "Antiangiogenic concentrations of paclitaxel induce an increase in microtubule dynamics in endothelial cells but not in cancer cells," *Cancer Research*, vol. 65, no. 6, pp. 2433–2440, 2005.

[15] J. R. Merchan, D. R. Jayaram, J. G. Supko, X. He, G. J. Bubley, and V. P. Sukhatme, "Increased endothelial uptake of paclitaxel as a potential mechanism for its antiangiogenic effects: potentiation by Cox-2 inhibition," *International Journal of Cancer*, vol. 113, no. 3, pp. 490–498, 2005.

[16] M. A. Jordan, R. J. Toso, D. Thrower, and L. Wilson, "Mechanism of mitotic block and inhibition of cell proliferation by taxol at low concentrations," *Proceedings of the National Academy of Sciences of the United States of America*, vol. 90, no. 20, pp. 9552–9556, 1993.

[17] P. Therasse, S. G. Arbuck, E. A. Eisenhauer et al., "New guidelines to evaluate the response to treatment in solid tumors," *Journal of the National Cancer Institute*, vol. 92, no. 3, pp. 205–216, 2000.

[18] E. A. Gehan, "The determination of the number of patients required in a preliminary and a follow-up trial of a new chemotherapeutic agent," *Journal of Chronic Diseases*, vol. 13, no. 4, pp. 346–353, 1961.

[19] M. Schemper and T. L. Smith, "A note on quantifying follow-up in studies of failure time," *Controlled Clinical Trials*, vol. 17, no. 4, pp. 343–346, 1996.

[20] F. Fata, E. O'Reilly, D. Ilson et al., "Paclitaxel in the treatment of patients with angiosarcoma of the scalp or face," *Cancer*, vol. 86, no. 10, pp. 2034–2037, 1999.

[21] M. Schlemmer, P. Reichardt, J. Verweij et al., "Paclitaxel in patients with advanced angiosarcomas of soft tissue: a retrospective study of the EORTC soft tissue and bone sarcoma group," *European Journal of Cancer*, vol. 44, no. 16, pp. 2433–2436, 2008.

[22] N. Penel, B. N. Bui, J.-O. Bay et al., "Phase II trial of weekly paclitaxel for unresectable angiosarcoma: the ANGIOTAX study," *Journal of Clinical Oncology*, vol. 26, no. 32, pp. 5269–5274, 2008.

[23] A. Italiano, A. Cioffi, N. Penel et al., "Comparison of doxorubicin and weekly paclitaxel efficacy in metastatic angiosarcomas," *Cancer*, vol. 118, no. 13, pp. 3330–3336, 2012.

[24] I. L. Ray-Coquard, J. Domont, E. Tresch-Bruneel et al., "Paclitaxel given once per week with or without bevacizumab in patients with advanced angiosarcoma: a randomized phase II trial," *Journal of Clinical Oncology*, vol. 33, no. 25, pp. 2797–2802, 2015.

22

Notch Signaling Mediates Skeletal Muscle Atrophy in Cancer Cachexia Caused by Osteosarcoma

Xiaodong Mu,[1,2] Rashmi Agarwal,[3] Daniel March,[3] Adam Rothenberg,[3] Clifford Voigt,[4] Jessica Tebbets,[3] Johnny Huard,[1,2] and Kurt Weiss[3]

[1]Department of Orthopaedic Surgery, University of Texas Health Science Center at Houston, Houston, TX 77030, USA
[2]Center for Regenerative Sports Medicine, Steadman Philippon Research Institute, Vail, CO 81657, USA
[3]Cancer Stem Cell Laboratory, Department of Orthopaedic Surgery, University of Pittsburgh, Pittsburgh, PA 15213, USA
[4]Department of Orthopaedic Surgery, Lenox Hill Hospital, New York, NY 10075, USA

Correspondence should be addressed to Kurt Weiss; weiskr@upmc.edu

Academic Editor: Michelle Ghert

Skeletal muscle atrophy in cancer cachexia is mediated by the interaction between muscle stem cells and various tumor factors. Although Notch signaling has been known as a key regulator of both cancer development and muscle stem cell activity, the potential involvement of Notch signaling in cancer cachexia and concomitant muscle atrophy has yet to be elucidated. The murine K7M2 osteosarcoma cell line was used to generate an orthotopic model of sarcoma-associated cachexia, and the role of Notch signaling was evaluated. Skeletal muscle atrophy was observed in the sarcoma-bearing mice, and Notch signaling was highly active in both tumor tissues and the atrophic skeletal muscles. Systemic inhibition of Notch signaling reduced muscle atrophy. *In vitro* coculture of osteosarcoma cells with muscle-derived stem cells (MDSCs) isolated from normal mice resulted in decreased myogenic potential of MDSCs, while the application of Notch inhibitor was able to rescue this repressed myogenic potential. We further observed that Notch-activating factors reside in the exosomes of osteosarcoma cells, which activate Notch signaling in MDSCs and subsequently repress myogenesis. Our results revealed that signaling between tumor and muscle via the Notch pathway may play an important role in mediating the skeletal muscle atrophy seen in cancer cachexia.

1. Introduction

Cachexia is a clinical condition characterized by weight loss, muscle atrophy, fatigue, and weakness in an individual who is not trying to lose weight. The metabolic milieu of cachexia is defined by the progressive decreases of skeletal muscle and adipose tissue and negative protein balance. While cachexia may accompany a number of diseases (e.g., renal failure, COPD, AIDS, and tuberculosis), it frequently occurs in patients with cancer, wherein it is referred to as cancer-associated cachexia (CAC). CAC is a prevalent and debilitating comorbidity of malignancy. CAC is present in over 50% of oncology patients at the time of death and is the immediate cause of death in around 30%. Although Hippocrates wrote about cachexia in antiquity, it remains a clinical problem in dire need of a solution: there are no management strategies or pharmacologic adjuvants that effectively treat or prevent cancer cachexia [1–4].

Cachexia is distinguished from conditions of decreased caloric intake such as anorexia or starvation, in which muscle mass is generally spared [5, 6]. Starvation-associated wasting can be ameliorated by caloric replacement or hyperalimentation, but cachexia is refractory to nutritional support. This may be due to the systemic inflammation of cachexia. There is overproduction of inflammatory cytokines such as tumor necrosis factor-α (TNF-α) and interleukin-1 (IL-1) in response to chronic systemic pathology, which results in the dysregulation of muscle homeostasis and a catabolic state [5–7]. Inflammatory cytokines have been shown to inhibit myogenic differentiation through the activation of NF-κB [8–10], a pathway known to play a role in muscular dystrophies and inflammatory myopathies [9–12]. Interestingly, close crosstalk between NF-κB and Notch signaling in the regulation of tumor development and metastasis has been reported [13–15].

Notch signaling is involved in the preservation of stem cell quiescence and the maintenance of a stem cell pool in skeletal muscle, helping to keep stem cells in an undifferentiated state [16–18]. Thus, Notch signaling functions as a repressor of myogenesis, and sustained activation of Notch in muscle stem cells has an adverse effect on muscle regeneration [19–23]. Constitutive activation of the Notch1 Intracellular Domain (NICD) in muscle cells results in impaired skeletal muscle regeneration, as well as an increased number of undifferentiated Pax7+ stem cells (satellite cells) [24]. A recent study of pancreatic cancer-associated muscle atrophy demonstrated enrichment of Pax7+ stem cells in skeletal muscle, which is associated with impaired myogenic potential and reduced myotube fusion [1]. Based on these observations, we hypothesized that Notch signaling might play a role in mediating the skeletal muscle atrophy present in CAC.

Sarcoma encompasses a diverse group of malignancies that arise from cells of mesenchymal origin. Although sarcoma represents only 1% of new cancer diagnoses, it accounts for 2% of cancer deaths. Fifty percent of patients with soft tissue sarcoma develop fatal pulmonary metastatic disease. The outlook for these patients is abysmal: they are considered to be incurable and have a median survival of approximately twelve months [25–35]. Because sarcomas arise in tissues such as muscle, bone, cartilage, and adipose, sarcoma patients not only face the morbidity imparted by the disease itself, but also often experience significant musculoskeletal impairment secondary to aggressive surgical treatment ranging from tumor removal to limb amputation. This musculoskeletal morbidity leaves sarcoma patients uniquely susceptible to the debilitating effects of CAC; however, virtually nothing is known regarding the mechanisms of sarcoma-associated cachexia (SAC).

In this study, a sarcoma-carrying mouse model was established, utilizing the murine osteosarcoma cell line K7M2. K7M2 has high metastatic potential and has previously been shown to feature increased Notch signaling when compared with nonmetastatic osteosarcoma cells [36]. The level of Notch signaling was studied in both the tumors and the atrophic skeletal muscles of the mice. *In vitro* coculture of K7M2 cells with muscle-derived stem cells (MDSCs) isolated from normal wild-type (WT) mice without cancer was performed to determine if activated Notch signaling can be transferred from tumor cells to muscle cells and if the myogenic potential of muscle cells could be altered. Additionally, because exosomes have been recognized as important to intercellular communication among tumor cells [37], the potential role of exosomes in remotely delivering Notch-activating factors from tumor cells to muscle cells was evaluated. Finally, because TNF-α is known as a key mediator of muscle atrophy in cancer cachexia [38–41] and crosstalk between the TNF-α and Notch pathways has been described in cancer development and metastasis [14, 15, 42], we also investigated the potential of TNF-α to mediate Notch activation in muscle cells.

2. Materials and Methods

2.1. Animals and Osteosarcoma Cell Lineages. Wild-type (WT) mice (C57BL/6J) were obtained from Jackson Laboratories (Bar Harbor, ME) and used for the isolation of muscle-derived stem cells (MDSCs). SCID/beige mice (CB17.Cg-$Prkdc^{scid}Lyst^{bg\text{-}J}$/Crl, female, 4-week-old) were obtained from Charles River and used for experiments on cancer cachexia. At least six mice were used in each experimental sample group. All procedures were approved by the Institutional Animal Care and Use Committee (IACUC) at the University of Pittsburgh. Murine osteosarcoma cell lineages K7M2 and K12 used in this study were the generous gift of Drs. Lee Helman and Chand Khanna at the National Cancer Institute. K7M2 and K12 are related murine osteosarcoma cell populations with differing metastatic potentials: K7M2 is highly metastatic to the lung but K12 is virtually non-metastatic [43]. K7M2 cells and K12 cells were cultured with proliferation medium [PM, DMEM with 10% FBS and 1% penicillin-streptomycin (P/S) antibiotics].

2.2. Transplantation of Osteosarcoma Cells. K7M2 cells were locally injected into the right hindlimbs of 4-week-old SCID/beige mice; the cortex of the proximal tibia was punctured with a 30 g needle, and cells were injected into the intramedullary canal (2.0×10^5 cells/per mouse). Osteosarcoma tumor development was then permitted, and muscle tissues were collected for study six weeks after cell transplantation.

2.3. Stem Cell Isolation from Skeletal Muscle. Muscle-derived stem cells (MDSCs) were isolated from the skeletal muscle of WT mice (4-week-old) using the modified preplate technique [44]. Mice were sacrificed in a carbon dioxide chamber followed by cervical dislocation according to the IACUC protocol. The cells were cultured in the growth medium [GM: DMEM supplemented with 20% Fetal Bovine Serum (FBS), 1% P/S antibiotics, and 0.5% chick embryo extract (CEE)] at 37°C in 5% CO_2.

2.4. Cell Coculture Experiment, Myogenesis Assay, and Notch Inhibition. Cell coculture was conducted with a transwell system (Corning Transwell) illustrated in Figure 5(a), with a cell nonpermeable filter (0.4 μm). MDSCs (20,000/well in 12-well plate) were cultured in the lower chamber, while the same number of K7M2 or K12 cells was cultured in the upper chamber to determine the influence of osteosarcoma cells on the expression of Notch genes and myogenesis of MDSCs. A control group was provided by MDSCs cocultured with MDSCs, themselves. The γ-secretase inhibitor DAPT (N-[N-(3,5-difluorophenacetyl-L-alanyl)]-S-phenylglycine t-butyl ester; Calbiochem) (10 μM in DMSO) was added to the MDSCs cocultured with K7M2 cells to observe the effect of Notch inhibition on myogenesis. Cell coculture was performed in growth medium for two days, with and without DAPT treatment. Then the upper chambers were removed and the medium was switched to myogenic differentiation medium (DM, DMEM supplemented with 2% Horse Serum and 1% P/S antibiotics) for an additional 2 days. Progression of myogenesis of MDSCs was then tracked by immunostaining of the fixed cells with antibody to fast-myosin heavy chain (f-MHC) (Sigma).

2.5. Exosome Isolation and Treatment of Muscle-Derived Stem Cells (MDSCs). K7M2 cells were plated at 60% confluence in plastic flasks and cultured for 2 days. Exosome isolation was performed with the "Total Exosome Isolation Reagent (from cell culture media)" kit (Life Technologies), as instructed. Briefly, 10 mL of cell culture media was harvested and centrifuged at 2000 ×g for 30 minutes to remove cells and debris. The reagent was added to the cell-free culture media (1 : 2), and the solution was incubated overnight at 4°C. The precipitated exosomes were recovered by standard centrifugation at 10,000 ×g for 60 min. The pellet was then added to 10 mL of fresh culture medium for the treatment of MDSCs.

2.6. In Vivo Notch Inhibition. MK-0752 (Merck) is a potent γ-secretase inhibitor that has been used in clinical trials to inhibit Notch activity in tumor development [45, 46]. In order to observe the effect of Notch inhibition on cancer cachexia in the mice, low doses of MK-0752 (50 mg/kg) [47] (5 mg/mL in 10% DMSO) were injected via an intraperitoneal (IP) route 3 times per week, starting two weeks after K7M2 cell injection. MK-0752 injections were continued for 4 weeks. Mice receiving the vehicle (10% DMSO) served as a control.

2.7. mRNA Analysis with Semiquantitative Reverse Transcriptase-PCR. Total RNA was obtained from cells or frozen tissues using the RNeasy Mini Kit (Qiagen, Inc., Valencia, CA) according to the manufacturer's instructions. Reverse transcription was performed using the iScript cDNA Synthesis Kit (Bio-Rad Laboratories, Inc., Hercules, CA). The primer sequences are as follows: GAPDH (Forward: TCCATGACAACTTTGGCATTG; Reverse: TCACGCCACAGCTTTCCA); Notchl (Forward: GCCGCAAGAGGCTTGAGAT; Reverse: GGAGTCCTGGCATCGTTGG); Hesl (Forward: CCAGCCAGTGTCAACACGA; Reverse: AATGCCGGGAGCTATCTTTCT); TNF-α (Forward: GATTATGGCTCAGGGTCCAA; Reverse: CTCCCTTTGCAGAACTCAGG); and Klotho (Forward: CCCAAACCATCTATGAAAC; Reverse: CTACCGTATTCTATGCCTTC). PCR reactions were performed using an iCycler Thermal Cycler (Bio-Rad Laboratories, Inc.). The cycling parameters used for all primers were as follows: incubation of the reaction mix at 95°C for 10 minutes, PCR, 40 cycles of 30 seconds at 95°C for denaturation, 1 minute at 54°C for annealing, and 30 seconds at 72°C for extension. Products were separated and visualized on a 1.5% agarose gel stained with ethidium bromide. All data were normalized to the expression of GAPDH (glyceraldehyde 3-phosphate dehydrogenase).

2.8. Histology. Tissue sections of skeletal muscles or tumors were fixed with 4% formalin (10 min) and rinsed with PBS. For Masson Trichrome staining, sections were incubated in Weigert's iron hematoxylin working solution for 10 min and then rinsed under running water for 10 min. Slides were transferred to Biebrich scarlet-acid fuchsin solution for 15 min, followed by incubation in aniline blue solution for another 5 min. Slides were then rinsed, dehydrated, and mounted. For hematoxylin and eosin (H&E) staining, sections were incubated for 5 min in hematoxylin solution prior to counterstaining with eosin. For immunofluorescent staining, the frozen tissue sections were fixed with 4% formalin and the primary antibodies to Pax7 (DHSB) and Notch3 (Santa Cruz) were applied at 1 : 100~1 : 200. All slides were analyzed using fluorescence microscopy (Leica Microsystemic Inc., IL) and were photographed at 40–400x magnification.

2.9. Measurement of Results and Statistical Analysis. The measurement of results from images was performed using commercially available software (Northern Eclipse, version 6.0, Empix Imaging, Inc., Mississauga, ON, Canada) and Image J software (version 1.32j, National Institutes of Health, Bethesda, MD). Data from at least three samples from each subject were pooled for statistical analysis. Results are given as the mean ± standard deviation (SD). Statistical significance of any difference was calculated using Student's t-test, with $P < 0.05$ being considered statistically significant.

3. Results

3.1. Skeletal Muscle Atrophy Occurs in Osteosarcoma-Bearing Mice. To establish an orthotopic model of sarcoma, K7M2 murine osteosarcoma cells were injected into the right tibias of SCID/beige mice. Six weeks after K7M2 cell injection, sarcoma tumors over 1 cm in diameter were observed in the right hindlimbs of the mice (Figure 1(a), green arrow). Compared to the control mice, both the size of skeletal muscle from the uninjected left hindlimb (Figures 1(b) and 1(c)) and the volume of abdominal adipose tissue (Figure 1(a), circles) were found to be diminished in mice with tumors. The dramatic loss of muscle and adipose tissue in these mice confirm the presence of CAC.

3.2. Sarcoma-Bearing Mice Demonstrated Skeletal Muscle Atrophy Characterized by Smaller Myofibers and Enhanced Fibrosis. H&E staining and trichrome staining were performed on histologic slides of skeletal muscle tissue from tumor-bearing mice. Compared with normal mice, there was an infiltration of mononuclear cells into the skeletal muscle of tumor-bearing mice (Figure 2(a), magnified area). Also, compared to the normal mice, the myofibers within the skeletal muscle of tumor-bearing mice were smaller (Figures 2(b) (magnified area) and 2(c)) and fibrosis, reflected by collagen deposition, was increased (Figures 2(b) and 2(d)). These histologic findings corroborated the gross observation of CAC and muscle atrophy in tumor-bearing mice.

3.3. Notch Signaling Is Increased in Both the Tumor Tissue and Skeletal Muscle of Sarcoma-Bearing Mice. Semiquantitative Reverse Transcriptase-PCR (RT-PCR) was performed to compare the differential gene expression patterns of tumor, normal muscle (from mice without tumor), and atrophic muscle (from sarcoma-bearing mice). The expression of

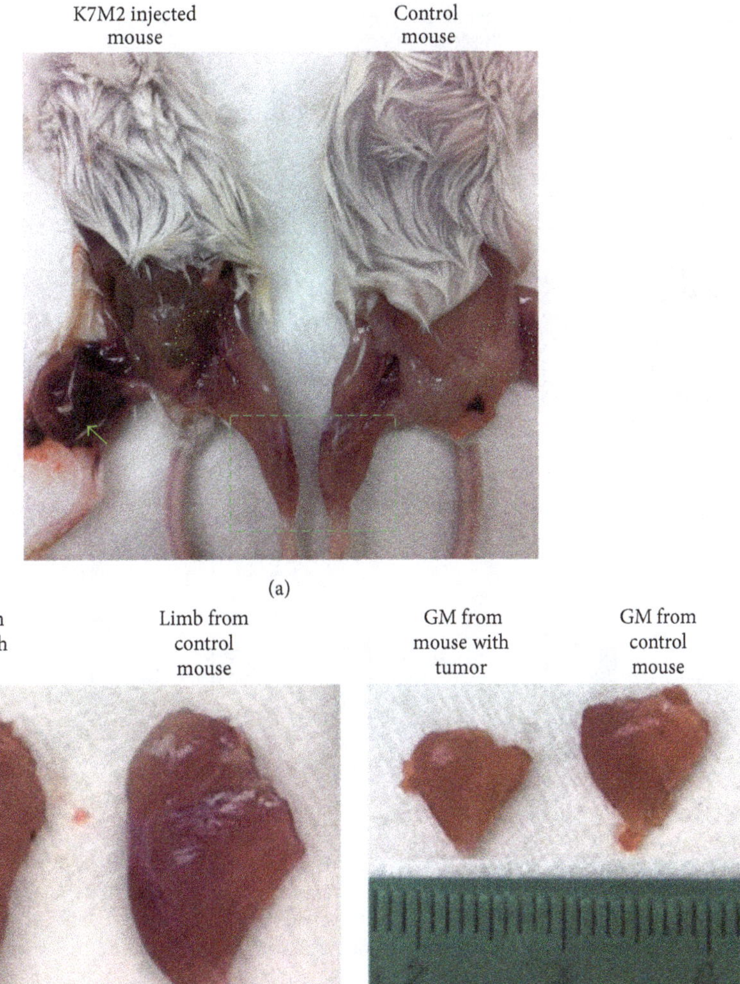

FIGURE 1: Cancer cachexia in osteosarcoma-bearing mice. (a) Six weeks after the injection of K7M2 cells into tibias of mice, tumor development can be observed in right hindlimb (green arrow). The tumor-bearing mice showed smaller muscle size (outlined with rectangle) and reduced adipose tissue (outlined with circles). (b) Left hindlimbs from mice with and without tumor. (c) Gastrocnemius (GM) muscles from mice with and without tumor.

TNF-α and Hes1 (a downstream effector of Notch signaling) in tumor tissue was higher than both normal muscle and atrophic muscle, while the expression of Klotho [an anti-inflammatory factor [48, 49]] was lower (Figures 3(a) and 3(b)). When normal muscle and atrophic muscle were compared, the expression of TNF-α and Hes1 was higher in atrophic muscle, while the expression of Klotho was lower (Figures 3(a) and 3(b)). These observations suggest that both proinflammatory signaling and Notch signaling are greater in atrophic muscle compared with normal muscle.

In agreement with the observation obtained at the mRNA level, immunostaining for the Notch3 protein further demonstrated an increased number of Notch3+ cells in the tumor tissue (Figure 3(c)). Additionally, there were more Notch3+ cells in atrophic muscle when compared with normal muscle (Figures 3(d) and 3(e)). Pax7 is a cell marker for muscle stem cells (satellite cells), and NF-κB-mediated enrichment of undifferentiated Pax7+ cells in muscles has been shown to promote CAC [1]. We also observed an increased number of Pax7+ cells in atrophic muscle compared with normal muscle. Some of these Pax7+ cells in atrophic muscle were also Notch3+ (Pax7+/Notch3+) (Figure 3(d)). This observation suggests that there are more undifferentiated muscle stem cells in atrophic muscle, possibly due to the activation of Notch signaling.

3.4. Systemic Inhibition of Notch Signaling in Tumor-Bearing Mice Reduces Muscle Atrophy and Fibrosis but Does Not Affect Tumor Size. While the effect of Notch inhibition on cancer development has been extensively studied [50–52], its effect in CAC has not been addressed. In this study, a low dose of the *in vivo* Notch inhibitor MK-0752 (50 mg/kg) [47] was injected intraperitoneally starting 2 weeks after cell injection, when tumors began to appear. Injection of MK-0752 was performed 3 times a week for 4 weeks. Results showed that the size of the primary osteosarcoma tumors was not significantly decreased by Notch inhibition (Figure 4(a)). However, trichrome staining of the muscle revealed reduced

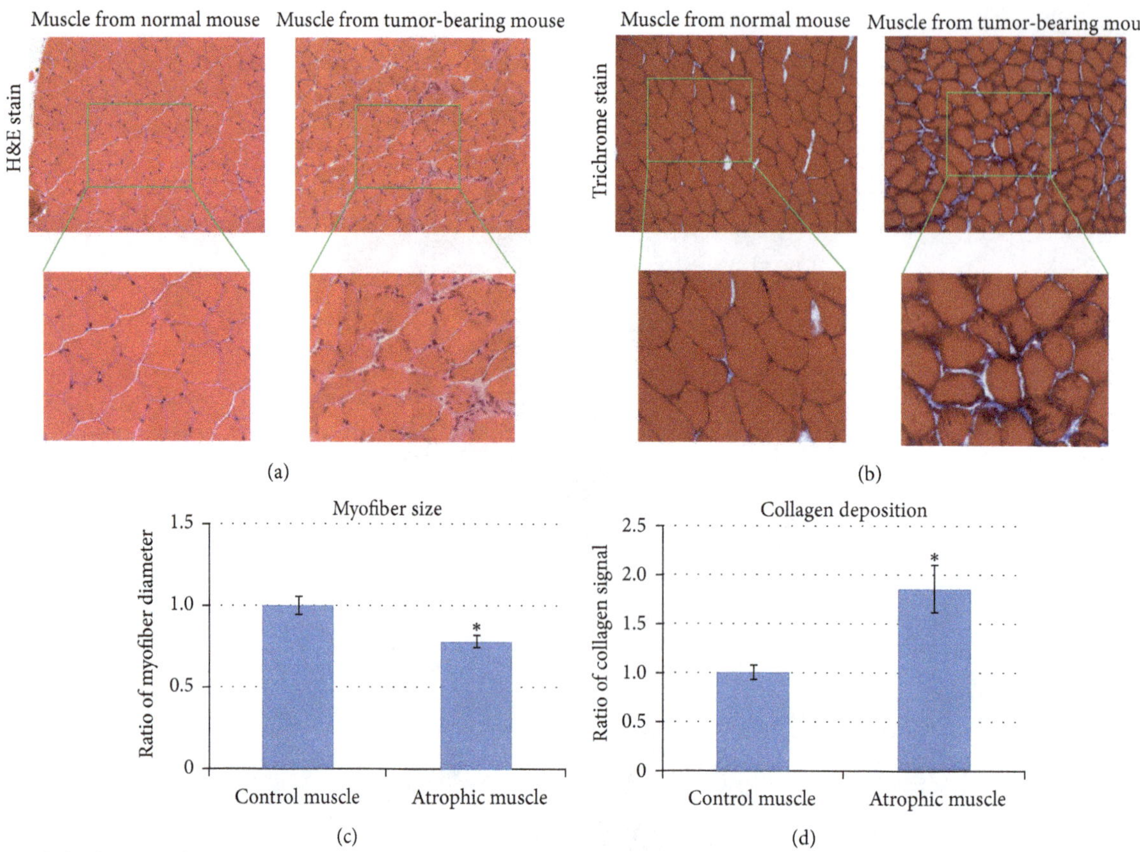

FIGURE 2: Skeletal muscle from tumor-carrying mice developed muscle atrophy. (a) H&E staining of GM muscles, revealing relative myofiber size and number of mononuclear cells (i.e., macrophages or undifferentiated muscle stem cells) in mice with and without tumor. $N = 4$ mice in each group. (b) Trichrome staining of GM muscles, demonstrating differential myofiber size and collagen deposition. $N = 4$ mice in each group. (c) Myofiber size in GM muscles. (d) Collagen deposition in GM muscles. "*" in the bar chart indicates $P < 0.05$.

fibrosis formation (Figure 4(b)) and increased myofiber size (Figures 4(b) and 4(c)). These observations indicate that although Notch inhibition may not efficiently repress *in situ* osteosarcoma tumor growth, the muscle atrophy associated with cancer cachexia could be ameliorated by Notch inhibition.

3.5. Coculture of K7M2 Cells with MDSCs from Normal Muscle Yields Repressed Myogenesis of MDSCs and the Upregulation of Notch Signaling Genes. To investigate the potential influence of osteosarcoma cells on muscle stem cells, MSDCs isolated from 4-week-old control mice were cocultured with K7M2 cells, K12 cells (nonmetastatic murine osteosarcoma cells), or MDSCs themselves in a transwell system with a 0.4 μm cell nonpermeable filter (Figure 5(a)). Compared with the control MDSCs (MDSC/MDSC or MDSC/K12), MDSCs cocultured with K7M2 (MDSC/K7M2) developed reduced myogenic potential, as demonstrated by the decreased immunostaining of myosin heavy chain (MHC)+ myotubes (Figures 5(b) and 5(c)). This observation indicates that tumor cells may release soluble factors that repress the myogenic differentiation of MDSCs.

To determine if Notch signaling could mediate the repressed myogenesis in MDSCs/K7M2, MDSCs cocultured with K7M2 cells were treated with the *in vitro* Notch inhibitor DAPT (γ-secretase inhibitor, 10 μM) for 2 days and then underwent 2 days of a myogenesis assay. The myogenic potential of MDSCs/K7M2 treated with DAPT was improved compared with the MDSCs/K7M2 without DAPT treatment (Figures 5(b) and 5(c)). This observation suggests that Notch inhibition could rescue the myogenic potential of MDSCs repressed by coculture with K7M2 cells.

Our previous studies demonstrated that Notch signaling was greatly increased in K7M2 cells compared with nonmetastatic K12 cells [36]. Here, we directly compared the expression levels of Notch pathway genes between K7M2 cells and MDSCs and found they were greater in K7M2 cells (Figures 5(d) and 5(e)). We also observed that the expression of Notch pathway genes in MDSCs was upregulated upon being cocultured with K7M2 cells when compared with control MDSCs cocultured with MDSCs (Figures 5(f) and 5(g)). This observation explains the effect of DAPT treatment in rescuing the repressed myogenic potential of MDSCs (Figures 5(b) and 5(c)) and indicates that tumor cells may release a Notch-activating factor that leads to increased Notch signaling in MDSCs.

3.6. Exosomes from K7M2 Cells Increase Notch Activation and Repress MDSC Myogenic Potential. We sought to identify the Notch-activating factors that were potentially generated and

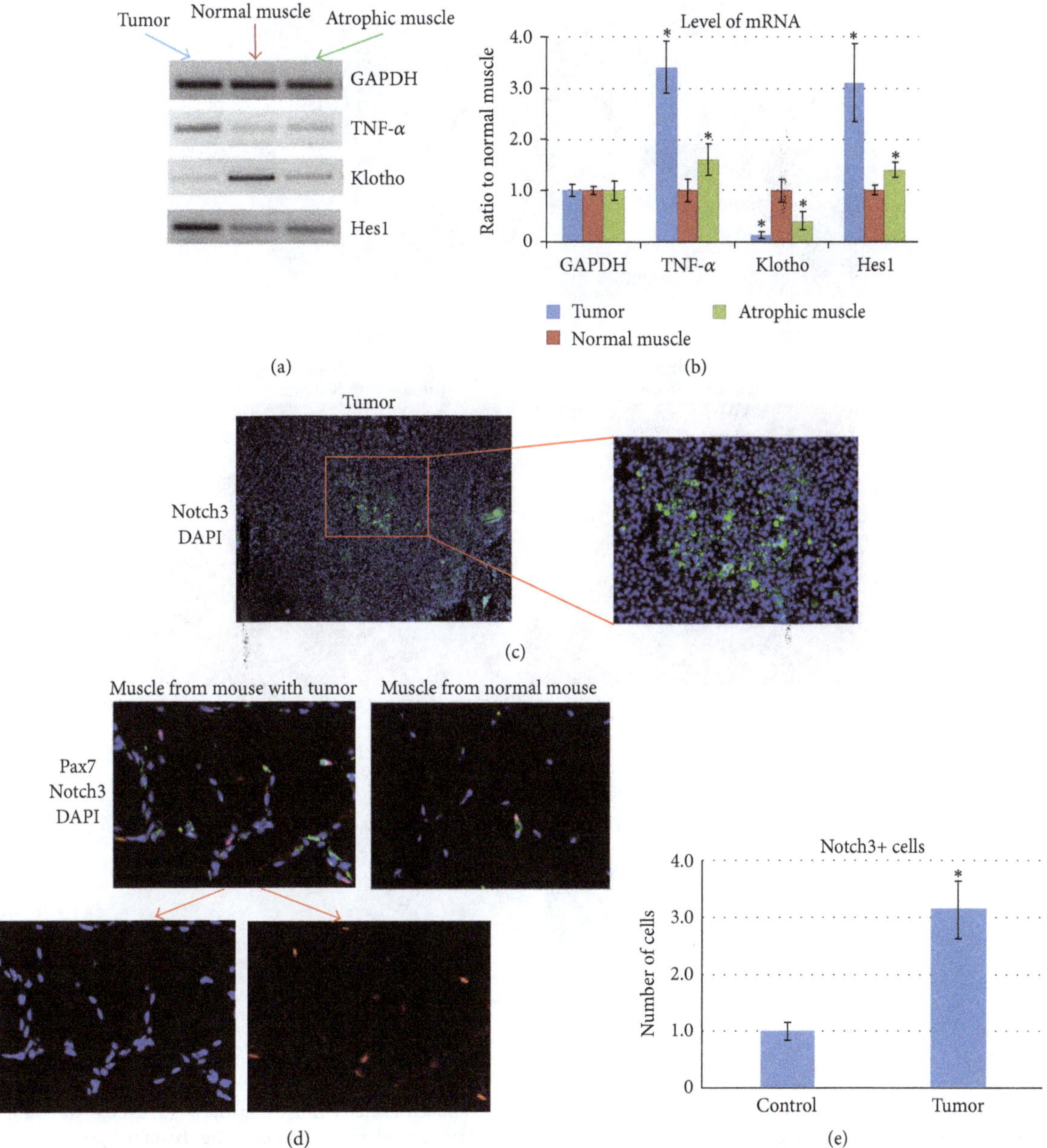

Figure 3: Increased Notch activation in both tumor tissues and skeletal muscle of tumor-bearing mice. (a) Semiquantitative PCR showed the gene expression of TNF-α, Hesl, and Klotho in tumor, normal muscle, and atrophic muscle. (b) mRNA levels of TNF-α, Hesl, and Klotho in 3 types of tissues. "$*$" in the bar chart indicates $P < 0.05$ compared to normal muscle. (c) Immunostaining of tumor tissue with antibody to Notch3, showing enrichment of Notch3+ cells in tumor. (d) Immunostaining of muscle tissue with antibody to Notch3 and Pax7, showing increased numbers of Pax7+ cells, Notch3+ cells, and Pax7+/Notch3+ cells in the muscle of tumor-bearing mice. The colocations of Pax7 and DAPI are indicated with arrows in the images. (e) The quantification of Notch3+ cells in muscle of normal mice (control) and mice bearing tumor (tumor). "$*$" in the bar chart indicates $P < 0.05$.

released by K7M2 cells. Exosomes released by cancer cells have been identified as important mediators of intercellular communication [37, 53]. The filter (0.4 μm) used in the cell coculture system described above was permissive for translocation of exosomes (<0.1 μm). To determine if exosomes might carry factors that could regulate MDSC myogenic potential, exosomes in the culture medium of K7M2 cells were isolated and added to the culture medium of MDSCs. K7M2 exosome treatment of MDSCs repressed myogenesis in a manner similar to their inhibition with K7M2 coculture (Figure 6(a)). Additionally, the expression of Notch signaling genes in MDSCs was found to be upregulated by K7M2 exosome treatment, in contrast to MSDCs treated with exosomes isolated from MDSCs (MDSC exosomes) (Figures 6(b) and 6(c)). These observations indicate that Notch-activating factors could have been delivered from K7M2 cells to MDSCs by exosomes. Further, coapplication of DAPT with K7M2 exosomes rescued the repressed myogenesis

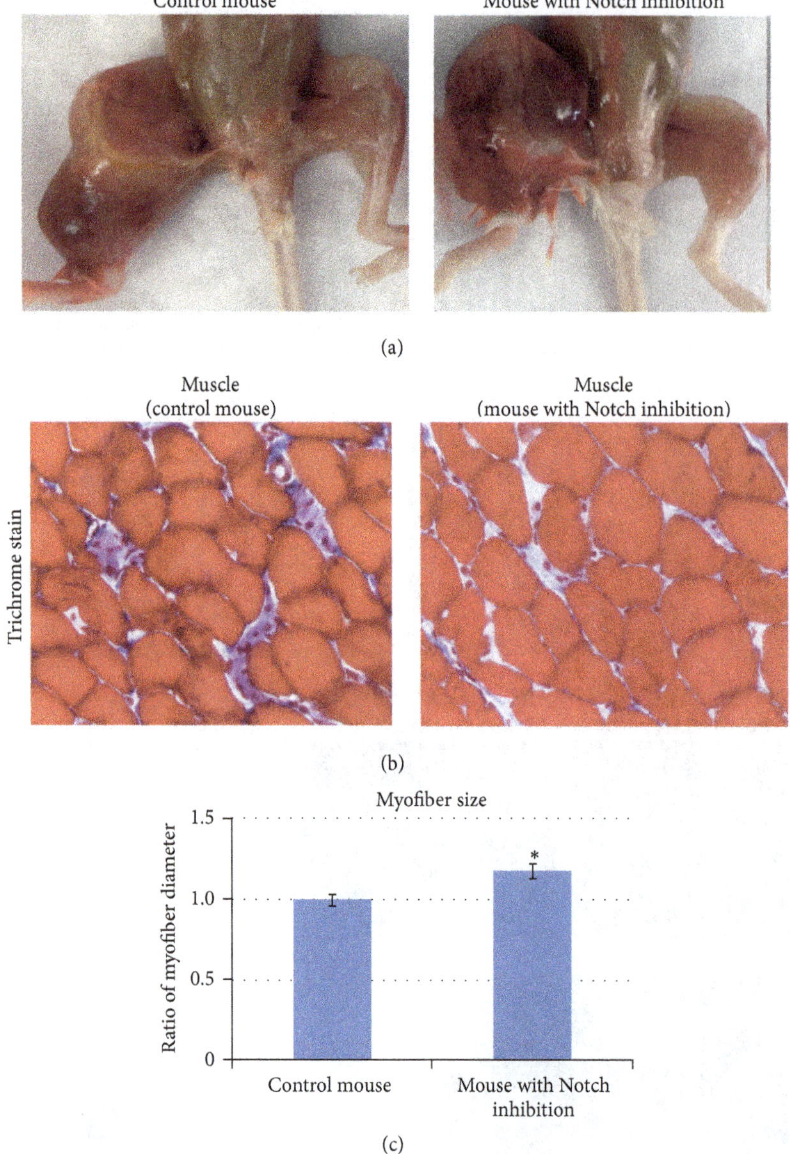

FIGURE 4: *In vivo* inhibition of Notch signaling in tumor-bearing mice reduced skeletal muscle atrophy. (a) Notch inhibitor MK-0752 (50 mg/kg) was injected starting two weeks after K7M2 cell injection, three times a week for four weeks. The size of the primary osteosarcoma tumor was unaffected by MK-0752 injection. $N = 4$ mice in each group. (b) Trichrome staining showing decreased fibrosis formation in muscles with Notch inhibition. (c) Differential myofiber size with and without MK-0752 injection. "$*$" in the bar chart indicates $P < 0.05$.

of MDSCs (Figure 6(a)). These observations indicate that exosomes from K7M2 cells may be the delivery vehicles for Notch-activating factors, which in turn upregulate Notch signaling in MDSCs and repress myogenesis.

3.7. TNF-α Treatment Increases Notch Activation and Represses the Myogenesis of MDSCs. Previous studies have revealed that proinflammatory factors, such as TNF-α, function as the key mediators of muscle atrophy in cancer cachexia [38–41]. Because elevated TNF-α expression was observed in sarcoma tumors (Figure 3), we hypothesized that another potential mechanism for Notch activation could be TNF-α released by the tumor into the systemic circulation exerting an effect on skeletal muscle. TNF-α has been found to closely interact with Notch signaling in regulating cancer development and metastasis [14, 15, 42]. Here we observed that the myogenesis of MDSCs was repressed with TNF-α treatment (Figure 6(d)), and TNF-α treatment (20 ng/mL) of MDSCs also caused the upregulation of Notch signaling genes (Notchl and Hesl) (Figures 6(e) and 6(f)).

4. Discussion

The key role of Notch signaling in the regulation of skeletal muscle regeneration and stem cell function has been previously established [16–18]. The importance of Notch signaling in mediating denervation-induced muscle atrophy is also well documented [54, 55]. However, although skeletal muscle

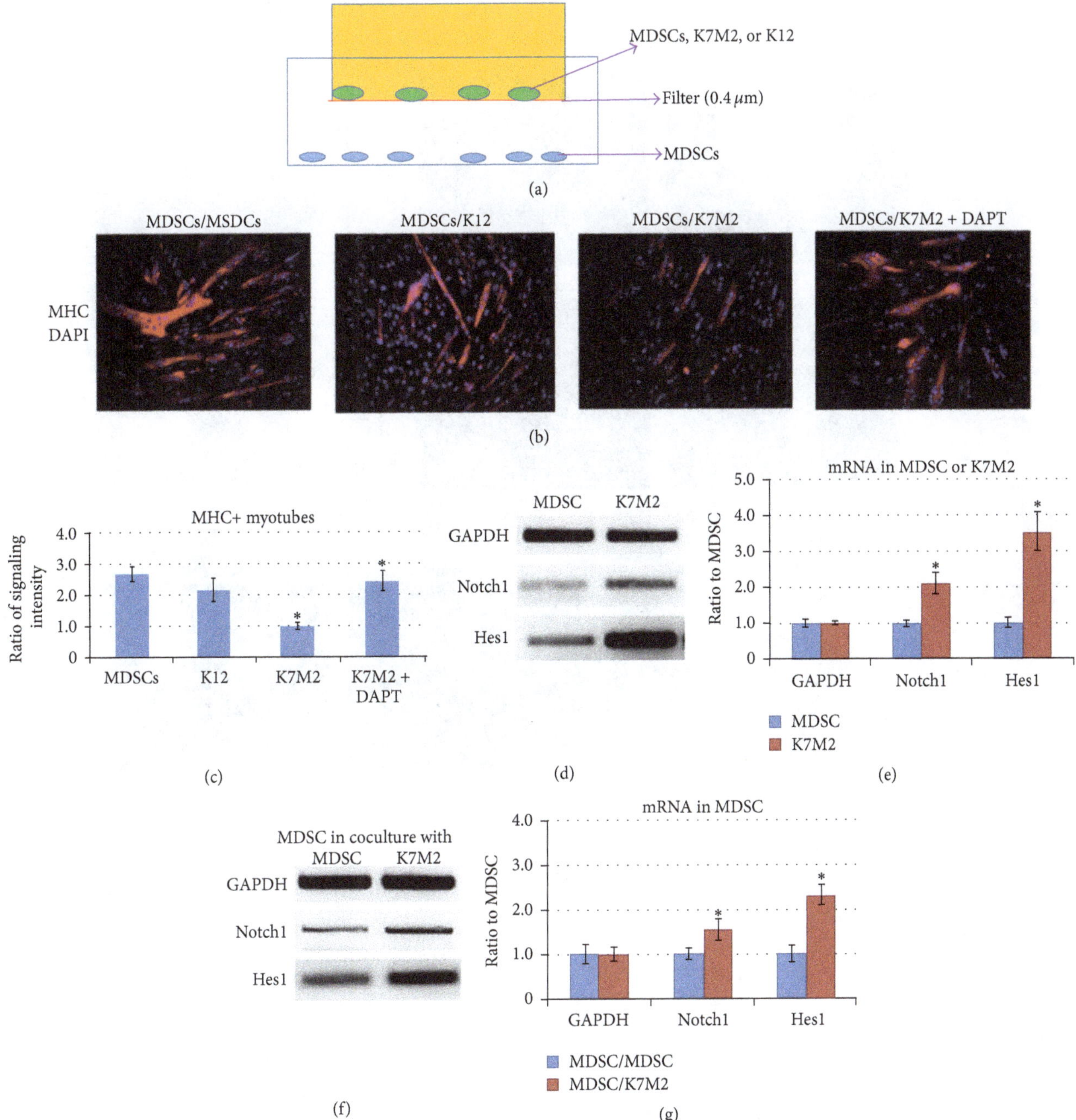

FIGURE 5: Coculture of K7M2 cells and MDSCs (from normal muscle) resulted in repressed myogenesis of MDSCs and upregulated expression of Notch genes. (a) The transwell system used in this study, including the upper chamber seeded with MDSCs, K7M2 cells, or K12 cells on the cell nonpermeable filter (0.4 μm) and the lower chamber seeded with MDSCs. (b) Myogenesis (myotube formation) of cocultured MDSCs was measured by immunostaining of myosin heavy chain (MHC). K7M2 cells repressed the myogenesis potential of MSDCs, while the coadministration of DAPT could rescue the repressed myogenesis. (c) Ratio of MHC+ myotubes formed by cocultured MDSCs. $N = 3$ replicates for each group. (d) Semiquantitative PCR revealed higher mRNA levels of Notchl and Hesl genes in K7M2 cells, compared to MDSCs. (e) Differential expression of Notch genes in K7M2 cells versus MDSCs. (f) Semiquantitative PCR revealed higher mRNA levels of Notchl and Hesl genes in MDSCs cocultured with K7M2 cells, compared to MDSCs cocultured with MDSCs. (g) Differential expression of Notch genes in MDSCs/K7M2 versus MDSCs/MDSCs. "$*$" in the bar chart indicates $P < 0.05$.

atrophy is the key feature of CAC, the potential role of Notch in skeletal muscle biology and stem cell function in CAC is still unknown. Notch activation in the stem cell niche is known to mediate the quiescence of muscle stem cells in skeletal muscle, which is important for maintaining the integrity and function of the stem cell pool. However, constant activation of Notch signaling adversely affects muscle regeneration and the downregulation of Notch signaling is preferred during certain stages of muscle regeneration [24, 56]. This study is the first attempt

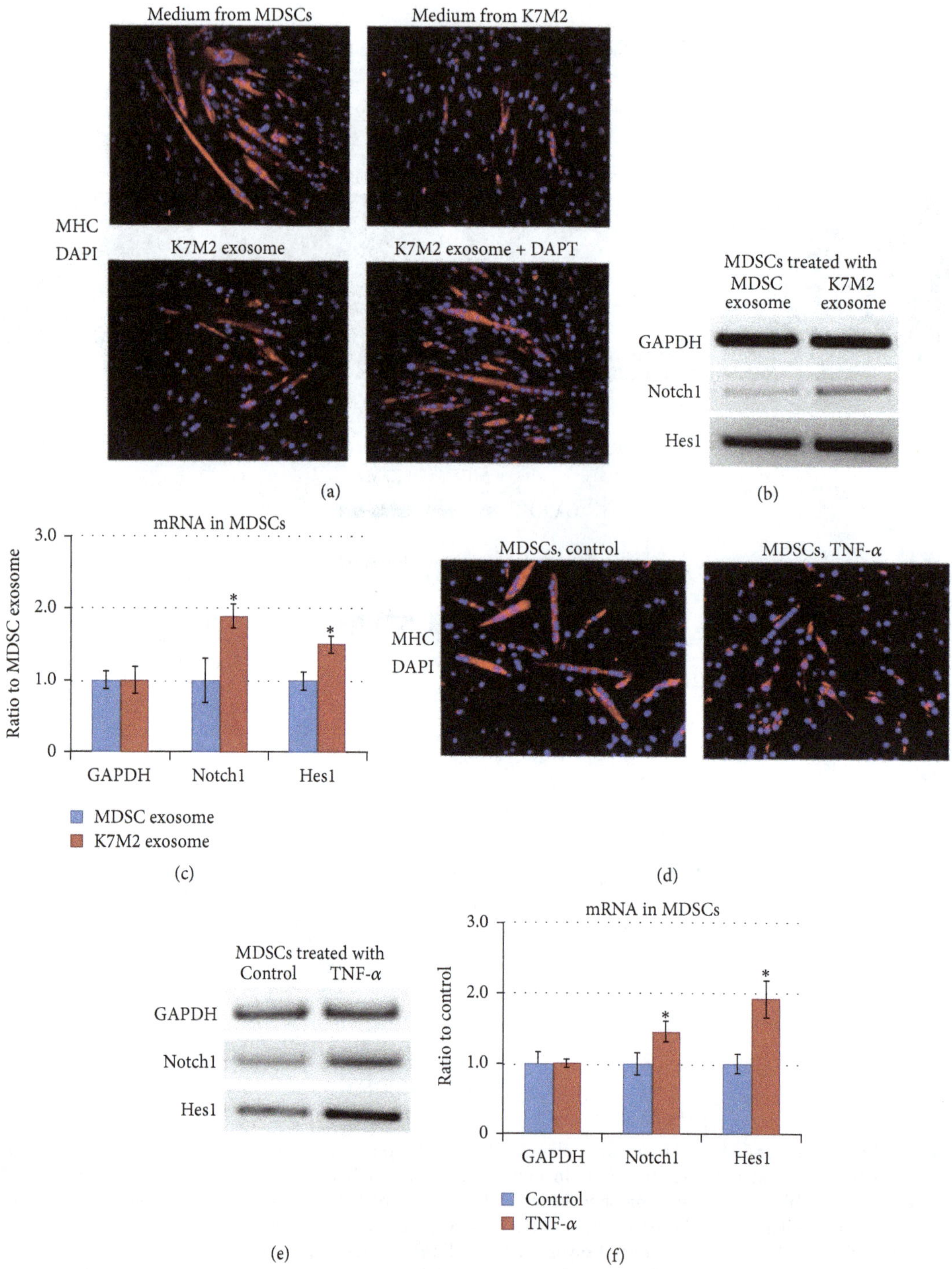

FIGURE 6: Exosomes from K7M2 cells increased Notch activation and repressed the myogenesis of MDSCs, and TNF-α treatment of MDSCs repressed myogenesis by activating Notch signaling. (a) MDSCs were treated with culture medium of MDSCs, culture medium of K7M2 cells, exosomes isolated from the culture medium of K7M2 cells (K7M2 exosomes), and K7M2 exosomes plus DAPT. Myotube formation was measured with immunostaining against MHC. (b) The expression of Notchl and Hesl in MDSCs treated with K7M2 exosomes or MDSC exosomes was compared with semiquantitative PCR. (c) Differential expression of Notchl and Hesl in MDSCs/K7M2 exosome versus MDSCs/MDSC exosome. (d) Myogenesis of MDSCs with and without TNF-α treatment was compared using immunostaining of MHC. (e) TNF-α treatment (20 ng/mL) of MDSCs upregulated the expression of Notchl and Hesl. (f) Differential expression of Notchl and Hesl in K7M2 with or without TNF-α treatment. "$*$" in the bar chart indicates $P < 0.05$.

to understand the role of Notch signaling in cancer-associated cachexia.

We have previously shown that the osteosarcoma cell line K7M2 actively expresses Notch genes (Notchl, Notch2, and Notch4; Hesl), but not Notch3 [36]. In the described coculture study of MDSCs and K7M2 cells, the increased expression of Notchl and Hesl in the MDSCs was found to correlate with the repressed myogenic potential of the cells (Figure 5(f)), while the expression of Notch3 was not obviously changed (data not shown). Although western blot was not performed to confirm the production of Notchl and Notch3 proteins, the increased expression of Hesl (a key downstream Notch effector) indicates that the overall Notch signaling in MDSCs was increased through coculture with K7M2 OS cells. Future studies will evaluate Notchl Intracellular Domain (NICD) expression and protein production, as well as Hesl expression, which could build an even stronger case for our hypothesis. This current result also reveals the coactivation of proinflammatory signaling and Notch signaling in both the K7M2-induced osteosarcoma tumor and the atrophic muscles of tumor-bearing mice (Figure 3). Proinflammatory factors, such as TNF-α, have been shown as key mediators of cancer cachexia [38–41]. Close correlation of TNF-α with Notch in the regulation of cancer development and metastasis has also been described [14, 15, 42]. TNF-α/NF-κB can activate Notch by inducing Jaggedl expression, and Notch activation in turn could sustain excessive proinflammatory signaling [13, 14, 57, 58]. However, the interaction of Notch signaling and TNF-α/NF-κB signaling in CAC has not been described. In this study, we have observed that the atrophic muscles in sarcoma-bearing mice feature the upregulated expression of both Notch genes and TNF-α, while the expression of anti-inflammation factor Klotho was downregulated (Figure 3). Therefore, we suggest that TNF-α may have circulated from the tumor to skeletal muscle and interfered with muscle stem cell activity and muscle regeneration via interaction with Notch signaling.

In addition to proinflammatory factors (e.g., TNF-α), our results indicate that exosomes from tumor cells may also serve to activate Notch signaling in the skeletal muscle. Previous studies have demonstrated that microRNAs (miRNAs) play an important role in exosome-mediated intercellular communication in cancer cells [59, 60]. MicroRNAs have been recently recognized to play critical roles in the Notch signaling pathway, and crosstalk between miRNA and Notch signaling pathways in tumor development has been demonstrated [61]. Candidate miRNAs that could mediate Notch-activating signaling may include miRNA199b-5p [62] or miRNA-21 [63]. The delivery of Notch ligand DLL4 via exosomes has also been demonstrated as a novel mechanism for Notch ligands to expand their signaling potential beyond cell-cell contact [64]. Therefore, we suggest that exosomes from K7M2 cells may contain miRNAs, Notch ligands (e.g., DLLs or Jagged), or both, allowing transfer of the Notch-activating signal from tumor to muscle.

Strategies to therapeutically modulate Notch signaling have been of great interest in the research and treatment of cancer. Notch inhibitors, including γ-secretase inhibitors, have been extensively studied in clinical trials in patients with solid tumors [51, 52, 65]; MK-0752, a potent inhibitor of γ-secretase, has been utilized in clinical trials to study its effect on Notch inhibition and cancer development [45, 46]. Our current study illustrated that although systemic MK-0752 treatment of tumor-carrying mice at a lower dosage may not efficiently repress the gross development of osteosarcoma, it could still improve the histology of atrophic muscle. The systemic effect of MK-0752 on osteosarcoma metastasis is currently under investigation.

5. Conclusion

Our current results demonstrate that Notch signaling is overactivated in the skeletal muscle of sarcoma-bearing mice and is involved in the development of muscle atrophy. *In vitro* studies further reveal that Notch-activating signals could be transferred from tumor cells (K7M2) to muscle stem cells (MDSCs) via exosomes or TNF-α released by the tumor cells. Our results reveal a novel role for Notch signaling in the mediation of skeletal muscle atrophy in CAC. Therefore, in addition to the role of Notch signaling in cancer development and metastasis, the role of Notch in cancer cachexia should also be further investigated.

Abbreviations

MDSCs: Muscle-derived stem cells
CAC: Cancer-associated cachexia
SAC: Sarcoma-associated cachexia
f-MHC: Fast-myosin heavy chain
NICD: Notchl Intracellular Domain.

Competing Interests

There are no competing interests to disclose.

Acknowledgments

The authors would acknowledge the funding support from NIH granted to Dr. Kurt Weiss (K08 CA177927) and the Sarcoma Foundation of America (SFA). They also acknowledge the support of the University of Pittsburgh Cancer Institute, Pittsburgh Cure Sarcoma, and the Houy family in loving memory of Jon Houy.

References

[1] W. A. He, E. Berardi, V. M. Cardillo et al., "NF-κB-mediated Pax7 dysregulation in the muscle microenvironment promotes cancer cachexia," *The Journal of Clinical Investigation*, vol. 123, no. 11, pp. 4821–4835, 2013.

[2] C. Elabd, W. Cousin, P. Upadhyayula et al., "Oxytocin is an age-specific circulating hormone that is necessary for muscle maintenance and regeneration," *Nature Communications*, vol. 5, article 4082, 2014.

[3] S.-J. Lee and D. J. Glass, "Treating cancer cachexia to treat cancer," *Skeletal Muscle*, vol. 1, no. 1, article 2, 2011.

[4] X. Zhou, J. L. Wang, J. Lu et al., "Reversal of cancer cachexia and muscle wasting by ActRIIB antagonism leads to prolonged survival," *Cell*, vol. 142, no. 4, pp. 531–543, 2010.

[5] S. Dodson, V. E. Baracos, A. Jatoi et al., "Muscle wasting in cancer cachexia: clinical implications, diagnosis, and emerging treatment strategies," *Annual Review of Medicine*, vol. 62, pp. 265–279, 2011.

[6] J. K. Onesti and D. C. Guttridge, "Inflammation based regulation of cancer cachexia," *BioMed Research International*, vol. 2014, Article ID 168407, 7 pages, 2014.

[7] J. E. Morley, D. R. Thomas, and M.-M. G. Wilson, "Cachexia: pathophysiology and clinical relevance," *The American Journal of Clinical Nutrition*, vol. 83, no. 4, pp. 735–743, 2006.

[8] R. C. J. Langen, A. M. W. J. Schols, M. C. J. M. Kelders, E. F. M. Wouters, and Y. M. W. Janssen-Heininger, "Inflammatory cytokines inhibit myogenic differentiation through activation of nuclear factor-κB," *The FASEB Journal*, vol. 15, no. 7, pp. 1169–1180, 2001.

[9] S. Baghdiguian, M. Martin, I. Richard et al., "Calpain 3 deficiency is associated with myonuclear apoptosis and profound perturbation of the IκB α/NF-κB pathway in limb-girdle muscular dystrophy type 2A," *Nature Medicine*, vol. 5, no. 5, pp. 503–511, 1999.

[10] A. Lu, J. D. Proto, L. Guo et al., "NF-κB negatively impacts the myogenic potential of muscle-derived stem cells," *Molecular Therapy*, vol. 20, no. 3, pp. 661–668, 2012.

[11] M. C. Monici, M. Aguennouz, A. Mazzeo, C. Messina, and G. Vita, "Activation of nuclear factor-κB in inflammatory myopathies and Duchenne muscular dystrophy," *Neurology*, vol. 60, no. 6, pp. 993–997, 2003.

[12] R. B. Hunter and S. C. Kandarian, "Disruption of either the Nfkb1 or the Bcl3 gene inhibits skeletal muscle atrophy," *Journal of Clinical Investigation*, vol. 114, no. 10, pp. 1504–1511, 2004.

[13] L. Espinosa, S. Cathelin, T. D'Altri et al., "The Notch/Hes1 pathway sustains NF-κB activation through CYLD repression in T cell leukemia," *Cancer Cell*, vol. 18, no. 3, pp. 268–281, 2010.

[14] E. Maniati, M. Bossard, N. Cook et al., "Crosstalk between the canonical NF-κB and Notch signaling pathways inhibits Pparγ expression and promotes pancreatic cancer progression in mice," *Journal of Clinical Investigation*, vol. 121, no. 12, pp. 4685–4699, 2011.

[15] L. Li, F. Zhao, J. Lu et al., "Notch-1 signaling promotes the malignant features of human breast cancer through NF-κB activation," *PLoS ONE*, vol. 9, no. 4, Article ID e95912, 2014.

[16] C. R. R. Bjornson, T. H. Cheung, L. Liu, P. V. Tripathi, K. M. Steeper, and T. A. Rando, "Notch signaling is necessary to maintain quiescence in adult muscle stem cells," *Stem Cells*, vol. 30, no. 2, pp. 232–242, 2012.

[17] P. Mourikis, R. Sambasivan, D. Castel, P. Rocheteau, V. Bizzarro, and S. Tajbakhsh, "A critical requirement for notch signaling in maintenance of the quiescent skeletal muscle stem cell state," *STEM CELLS*, vol. 30, no. 2, pp. 243–252, 2012.

[18] S.-I. Fukada, M. Yamaguchi, H. Kokubo et al., "Hesr1 and Hesr3 are essential to generate undifferentiated quiescent satellite cells and to maintain satellite cell numbers," *Development*, vol. 138, no. 21, pp. 4609–4619, 2011.

[19] R. Kopan, J. S. Nye, and H. Weintraub, "The intracellular domain of mouse Notch: a constitutively activated repressor of myogenesis directed at the basic helix-loop-helix region of MyoD," *Development*, vol. 120, no. 9, pp. 2385–2396, 1994.

[20] K. Kuroda, S. Tani, K. Tamura, S. Minoguchi, H. Kurooka, and T. Honjo, "Delta-induced Notch signaling mediated by RBP-J inhibits MyoD expression and myogenesis," *The Journal of Biological Chemistry*, vol. 274, no. 11, pp. 7238–7244, 1999.

[21] J. N. Waddell, P. Zhang, Y. Wen et al., "Dlk1 is necessary for proper skeletal muscle development and regeneration," *PLoS ONE*, vol. 5, no. 11, Article ID e15055, 2010.

[22] M. F. Buas, S. Kabak, and T. O. M. Kadesch, "Inhibition of myogenesis by notch: evidence for multiple pathways," *Journal of Cellular Physiology*, vol. 218, no. 1, pp. 84–93, 2009.

[23] T. Kitamoto and K. Hanaoka, "Notch3 null mutation in mice causes muscle hyperplasia by repetitive muscle regeneration," *STEM CELLS*, vol. 28, no. 12, pp. 2205–2216, 2010.

[24] Y. Wen, P. Bi, W. Liu, A. Asakura, C. Keller, and S. Kuang, "Constitutive Notch activation upregulates Pax7 and promotes the self-renewal of skeletal muscle satellite cells," *Molecular and Cellular Biology*, vol. 32, no. 12, pp. 2300–2311, 2012.

[25] "Adjuvant chemotherapy for localised resectable soft tissue sarcoma in adults," *Cochrane Database of Systematic Reviews*, no. 4, Article ID CD001419, 2000.

[26] D. J. Biau, P. C. Ferguson, P. Chung et al., "Local recurrence of localized soft tissue sarcoma: a new look at old predictors," *Cancer*, vol. 118, no. 23, pp. 5867–5877, 2012.

[27] J.-Y. Blay, M. van Glabbeke, J. Verweij et al., "Advanced soft-tissue sarcoma: a disease that is potentially curable for a subset of patients treated with chemotherapy," *European Journal of Cancer*, vol. 39, no. 1, pp. 64–69, 2003.

[28] R. Grimer, I. Judson, D. Peake, and B. Seddon, "Guidelines for the management of soft tissue sarcomas," *Sarcoma*, vol. 2010, Article ID 506182, 15 pages, 2010.

[29] S. R. Grobmyer and M. F. Brennan, "Predictive variables detailing the recurrence rate of soft tissue sarcomas," *Current Opinion in Oncology*, vol. 15, no. 4, pp. 319–326, 2003.

[30] A. Italiano, S. Mathoulin-Pelissier, A. Le Cesne et al., "Trends in survival for patients with metastatic soft-tissue sarcoma," *Cancer*, vol. 117, no. 5, pp. 1049–1054, 2011.

[31] L. Mariani, R. Miceli, M. W. Kattan et al., "Validation and adaptation of a nomogram for predicting the survival of patients with extremity soft tissue sarcoma using a three-grade system," *Cancer*, vol. 103, no. 2, pp. 402–408, 2005.

[32] N. Pervaiz, N. Colterjohn, F. Farrokhyar, R. Tozer, A. Figueredo, and M. Ghert, "A systematic meta-analysis of randomized controlled trials of adjuvant chemotherapy for localized resectable soft-tissue sarcoma," *Cancer*, vol. 113, no. 3, pp. 573–581, 2008.

[33] P. W. Pisters, D. H. Leung, J. Woodruff, W. Shi, and M. F. Brennan, "Analysis of prognostic factors in 1,041 patients with localized soft tissue sarcomas of the extremities," *Journal of Clinical Oncology*, vol. 14, no. 5, pp. 1679–1689, 1996.

[34] A. I. Spira and D. S. Ettinger, "The use of chemotherapy in soft-tissue sarcomas," *Oncologist*, vol. 7, no. 4, pp. 348–359, 2002.

[35] M. Van Glabbeke, A. T. van Oosterom, J. W. Oosterhuis et al., "Prognostic factors for the outcome of chemotherapy in advanced soft tissue sarcoma: an analysis of 2,185 patients treated with anthracycline-containing first-line regimens—a European organization for research and treatment of cancer soft tissue and bone sarcoma group study," *Journal of Clinical Oncology*, vol. 17, no. 1, pp. 150–157, 1999.

[36] X. Mu, C. Isaac, N. Greco, J. Huard, and K. Weiss, "Notch signaling is associated with ALDH activity and an aggressive metastatic phenotype in murine osteosarcoma cells," *Frontiers in Oncology*, vol. 3, article 143, 2013.

[37] W.-X. Chen, Y.-Q. Cai, M.-M. Lv et al., "Exosomes from docetaxel-resistant breast cancer cells alter chemosensitivity by delivering microRNAs," *Tumor Biology*, vol. 35, no. 10, pp. 9649–9659, 2014.

[38] D. Coletti, V. Moresi, S. Adamo, M. Molinaro, and D. Sassoon, "Tumor necrosis factor-α gene transfer induces cachexia and inhibits muscle regeneration," *Genesis*, vol. 43, no. 3, pp. 120–128, 2005.

[39] M. Figueras, S. Busquets, N. Carbó, V. Almendro, J. M. Argilés, and F. J. López-Soriano, "Cancer cachexia results in an increase in TNF-α receptor gene expression in both skeletal muscle and adipose tissue," *International Journal of Oncology*, vol. 27, no. 3, pp. 855–860, 2005.

[40] M. J. Tisdale, "Catabolic mediators of cancer cachexia," *Current Opinion in Supportive and Palliative Care*, vol. 2, no. 4, pp. 256–261, 2008.

[41] J. Gelin, L. L. Moldawer, C. Lönnroth, B. Sherry, R. Chizzonite, and K. Lundholm, "Role of endogenous tumor necrosis factor alpha and interleukin 1 for experimental tumor growth and the development of cancer cachexia," *Cancer Research*, vol. 51, no. 1, pp. 415–421, 1991.

[42] S. H. Lee, H. S. Hong, Z. X. Liu et al., "TNFα enhances cancer stem cell-like phenotype via Notch-Hes1 activation in oral squamous cell carcinoma cells," *Biochemical and Biophysical Research Communications*, vol. 424, no. 1, pp. 58–64, 2012.

[43] C. Khanna, J. Prehn, C. Yeung, J. Caylor, M. Tsokos, and L. Helman, "An orthotopic model of murine osteosarcoma with clonally related variants differing in pulmonary metastatic potential," *Clinical and Experimental Metastasis*, vol. 18, no. 3, pp. 261–271, 2000.

[44] B. Gharaibeh, A. Lu, J. Tebbets et al., "Isolation of a slowly adhering cell fraction containing stem cells from murine skeletal muscle by the preplate technique," *Nature Protocols*, vol. 3, no. 9, pp. 1501–1509, 2008.

[45] I. Krop, T. Demuth, T. Guthrie et al., "Phase I pharmacologic and pharmacodynamic study of the gamma secretase (Notch) inhibitor MK-0752 in adult patients with advanced solid tumors," *Journal of Clinical Oncology*, vol. 30, no. 19, pp. 2307–2313, 2012.

[46] M. Fouladi, C. F. Stewart, J. Olson et al., "Phase I trial of MK-0752 in children with refractory CNS malignancies: a pediatric brain tumor consortium study," *Journal of Clinical Oncology*, vol. 29, no. 26, pp. 3529–3534, 2011.

[47] J. J. Cook, K. R. Wildsmith, D. B. Gilberto et al., "Acute γ-secretase inhibition of nonhuman primate CNS shifts Amyloid Precursor Protein (APP) metabolism from amyloid-β production to alternative APP fragments without amyloid-β rebound," *The Journal of Neuroscience*, vol. 30, no. 19, pp. 6743–6750, 2010.

[48] D. E. Arking, A. Krebsova, M. Macek Sr. et al., "Association of human aging with a functional variant of klotho," *Proceedings of the National Academy of Sciences of the United States of America*, vol. 99, no. 2, pp. 856–861, 2002.

[49] F. Liu, S. Wu, H. Ren, and J. Gu, "Klotho suppresses RIG-I-mediated senescence-associated inflammation," *Nature Cell Biology*, vol. 13, no. 3, pp. 254–262, 2011.

[50] V. Bolós, J. Grego-Bessa, and J. L. de la Pompa, "Notch signaling in development and cancer," *Endocrine Reviews*, vol. 28, no. 3, pp. 339–363, 2007.

[51] B. Purow, "Notch inhibition as a promising new approach to cancer therapy," *Advances in Experimental Medicine and Biology*, vol. 727, pp. 305–319, 2012.

[52] N. Takebe, D. Nguyen, and S. X. Yang, "Targeting Notch signaling pathway in cancer: clinical development advances and challenges," *Pharmacology and Therapeutics*, vol. 141, no. 2, pp. 140–149, 2014.

[53] C. Roma-Rodrigues, A. R. Fernandes, and P. V. Baptista, "Exosome in tumour microenvironment: overview of the crosstalk between normal and cancer cells," *BioMed Research International*, vol. 2014, Article ID 179486, 10 pages, 2014.

[54] X.-H. Liu, S. Yao, R.-F. Qiao et al., "Nandrolone reduces activation of Notch signaling in denervated muscle associated with increased Numb expression," *Biochemical and Biophysical Research Communications*, vol. 414, no. 1, pp. 165–169, 2011.

[55] P. Nagpal, P. J. Plant, J. Correa et al., "The ubiquitin ligase Nedd4-1 participates in denervation-induced skeletal muscle atrophy in mice," *PLoS ONE*, vol. 7, no. 10, Article ID e46427, 2012.

[56] A. S. Brack, I. M. Conboy, M. J. Conboy, J. Shen, and T. A. Rando, "A temporal switch from notch to Wnt signaling in muscle stem cells is necessary for normal adult myogenesis," *Cell Stem Cell*, vol. 2, no. 1, pp. 50–59, 2008.

[57] T. Quillard and B. Charreau, "Impact of Notch signaling on inflammatory responses in cardiovascular disorders," *International Journal of Molecular Sciences*, vol. 14, no. 4, pp. 6863–6888, 2013.

[58] J. Bash, W.-X. Zong, S. Banga et al., "Rel/NF-κB can trigger the Notch signaling pathway by inducing the expression of Jagged1, a ligand for Notch receptors," *The EMBO Journal*, vol. 18, no. 10, pp. 2803–2811, 1999.

[59] B. N. Hannafon and W.-Q. Ding, "Intercellular communication by exosome-derived microRNAs in cancer," *International Journal of Molecular Sciences*, vol. 14, no. 7, pp. 14240–14269, 2013.

[60] S. A. Melo, H. Sugimoto, J. T. O'Connell et al., "Cancer exosomes perform cell-independent MicroRNA biogenesis and promote tumorigenesis," *Cancer Cell*, vol. 26, no. 5, pp. 707–721, 2014.

[61] Z. Wang, Y. Li, D. Kong, A. Ahmad, S. Banerjee, and F. H. Sarkar, "Cross-talk between miRNA and Notch signaling pathways in tumor development and progression," *Cancer Letters*, vol. 292, no. 2, pp. 141–148, 2010.

[62] K. Y. Won, Y. W. Kim, H.-S. Kim, S. K. Lee, W.-W. Jung, and Y.-K. Park, "MicroRNA-199b-5p is involved in the Notch signaling pathway in osteosarcoma," *Human Pathology*, vol. 44, no. 8, pp. 1648–1655, 2013.

[63] Y. Xiong, Y.-Y. Zhang, Y.-Y. Wu et al., "Correlation of over-expressions of miR-21 and Notch-1 in human colorectal cancer with clinical stages," *Life Sciences*, vol. 106, no. 1-2, pp. 19–24, 2014.

[64] H. Sheldon, E. Heikamp, H. Turley et al., "New mechanism for Notch signaling to endothelium at a distance by delta-like 4 incorporation into exosomes," *Blood*, vol. 116, no. 13, pp. 2385–2394, 2010.

[65] E. R. Andersson and U. Lendahl, "Therapeutic modulation of Notch signalling—are we there yet?" *Nature Reviews Drug Discovery*, vol. 13, no. 5, pp. 357–378, 2014.

23

Correlation of High-Risk Soft Tissue Sarcoma Biomarker Expression Patterns with Outcome following Neoadjuvant Chemoradiation

John M. Kane III,[1] Anthony Magliocco,[2] Qiang Zhang,[3] Dian Wang,[4] Alex Klimowicz,[5] Jonathan Harris,[3] Jeff Simko,[6] Thomas DeLaney,[7] William Kraybill,[8] and David G. Kirsch[9]

[1]*Roswell Park Cancer Institute, Buffalo, NY, USA*
[2]*H. Lee Moffitt Cancer Center, Tampa, FL, USA*
[3]*NRG Oncology Statistics and Data Management Center, Philadelphia, PA, USA*
[4]*Rush University Medical Center, Chicago, IL, USA*
[5]*Tom Baker Cancer Centre, Calgary, AB, Canada*
[6]*University of California, San Francisco, CA, USA*
[7]*Massachusetts General Hospital, Boston, MA, USA*
[8]*The Ohio State University, Columbus, OH, USA*
[9]*Duke University Medical Center, Durham, NC, USA*

Correspondence should be addressed to John M. Kane III; john.kane@roswellpark.org

Academic Editor: Akira Kawai

Background. Sarcoma mortality remains high despite adjuvant chemotherapy. Biomarker predictors of treatment response and outcome could improve treatment selection. *Methods.* Tissue microarrays (TMAs) were created using pre- and posttreatment tumor from two prospective trials (MGH pilot and RTOG 9514) of neoadjuvant/adjuvant MAID chemotherapy and preoperative radiation. Biomarkers were measured using automated computerized imaging (AQUA or ACIS). Expression was correlated with disease-free survival (DFS), distant disease-free survival (DDFS), and overall survival (OS). *Results.* Specimens from 60 patients included 23 pretreatment (PRE), 40 posttreatment (POST), and 12 matched pairs (MPs). In the MP set, CAIX, GLUT1, and PARP1 expression significantly decreased following neoadjuvant therapy, but p53 nuclear/cytoplasmic (N/C) ratio increased. In the PRE set, no biomarker expression was associated with DFS, DDFS, or OS. In the POST set, increased p53 N/C ratio was associated with a significantly decreased DFS and DDFS (HR 4.13, $p = 0.017$; HR 4.16, $p = 0.016$), while increased ERCC1 and XPF expression were associated with an improved DFS and DDFS. No POST biomarkers were associated with OS. *Conclusions.* PRE biomarker expression did not predict survival outcomes. Expression pattern changes after neoadjuvant chemoradiation supports the concepts of tumor reoxygenation, altered HIF-1α signaling, and a p53 nuclear accumulation DNA damage response. *Clinical Trial Registration.* NRG Oncology RTOG 9514 is registered with ClinicalTrials.gov.

1. Introduction

Despite major improvements in local control/limb salvage, survival for "high-risk" soft tissue sarcomas (STSs) has not significantly changed over time. Almost half of patients with a large, deep, high-grade sarcoma (stage III) will die within 5 years of their diagnosis. Consequently, the potential benefits of adjuvant chemotherapy have been explored. Several studies have reported improvements in overall survival of 4–19% [1–3]. However, toxicity has been significant, including both acute hematologic toxicity and late myelodysplasia/leukemia [2, 4, 5]. In addition, it has been impossible to identify which subset of "high-risk" patients truly benefit from adjuvant chemotherapy based upon standard prognostic variables (age, location, histologic subtype, size, and grade) [1].

Beginning in 1989, Massachusetts General Hospital (MGH) performed a pilot trial of neoadjuvant MAID chemotherapy (mesna, Adriamycin, ifosfamide, and dacarbazine), 44 Gy interdigitated preoperative radiation, and adjuvant systemic chemotherapy in 48 patients with high-risk extremity STSs (high grade, ≥8 cm) [4]. Actuarial 5-year overall survival (OS) was 87%, significantly higher than that of a corresponding historical control group. Long-term follow-up for these patients was also available as part of a larger study [6]. At a median follow-up of 46 months, 5-year OS was still 86%. Based upon the promising results of the MGH pilot trial, the Radiation Therapy Oncology Group (RTOG) opened trial 9514 in 1997, a phase II study of neoadjuvant chemotherapy and radiation for "high-risk" soft tissue sarcomas of the extremities and trunk [5]. Sixty-four patients were treated using a regimen almost identical to that in the MGH pilot trial. With long-term follow-up, the estimated 5-year OS was an impressive 71.2% [7].

As part of NRG Oncology RTOG 9514, the original biopsy and surgical resection specimens for many of the participating patients were stored in the RTOG Tissue Bank. In addition, one of the principal investigators for the MGH pilot trial was also involved in NRG Oncology RTOG 9514, providing access to many of the pathology specimens from the MGH pilot trial. Both studies had long-term follow-up information on a group of large, high-grade STS patients treated with the same neoadjuvant chemoradiation/adjuvant chemotherapy regimens. This afforded a unique opportunity to construct tissue microarrays (TMAs) of the tumor specimens, which could be used to potentially correlate candidate biomarker expression with outcome in a uniform cohort of "high-risk" STS patients.

2. Methods

2.1. Specimen Acquisition. After obtaining institutional review board approval from MGH, available diagnostic biopsy and surgical resection specimens from the pilot trial were pathologically reviewed to assure the presence of viable tumor. The representative paraffin blocks were then sent to the RTOG Tissue Bank at the University of San Francisco. Representative 0.6 mm punch biopsies were obtained in order to create a TMA, and the blocks were returned to the parent institution. Many of the specimens from NRG Oncology RTOG 9514 were already housed in the RTOG Tissue Bank as part of the original protocol. An attempt was made to obtain any missing specimens by contacting the treating institutions.

The original pretreatment diagnostic biopsy for patients in both trials was typically a core needle or limited incisional biopsy specimen. Therefore, it was only a representative portion of a larger tumor. In contrast, the final surgical specimen following neoadjuvant therapy often contained tissue blocks from several different areas. To minimize the sampling error from biomarker expression heterogeneity and to maximize the acquisition of adequate quality tumor for immunohistochemistry (IHC) analysis (e.g., nonnecrotic tissue), the parent institution was asked to provide two blocks representing different areas of assessable tumor (ideally, one central and one peripheral). H&E sections from these blocks were reviewed, and areas of highest tumor concentration circled to act as guides for punching the TMA cores. As the potential for tumor heterogeneity was considered, TMAs were constructed in triplicate.

2.2. Candidate Biomarkers. All of the patients in this study came from either the MGH pilot trial or RTOG 9514, which were large, deep, "high-risk" STSs. Therefore, some of the biomarkers chosen were previously associated with STS outcome in smaller, more heterogeneous studies. In addition, all of the patients had received neoadjuvant chemoradiation. Consequently, other biomarkers had potential relationships to the cellular responses to chemoradiation damage. Although many biomarkers were available for assessment, nine candidate biomarkers were chosen for this initial TMA analysis for the reasons outlined above.

Ki67 is a nuclear nonhistone protein that is expressed in proliferating cells [8]. Increased Ki67 expression in STSs has been associated with a decreased metastasis-free survival [9, 10].

p53 is a multifunctional "tumor suppressor" protein, which can be induced by DNA damage to cause cell cycle arrest to allow for DNA damage repair, activate DNA repair proteins, and initiate apoptosis [11]. p53 mutations and overexpression on IHC, especially as assessed by N-terminal binding antibodies, are associated with decreased STS survival [12, 13].

Ataxia-telangiectasia mutated (ATM) kinase is a serine-threonine kinase that mediates cell cycle checkpoint control following exposure to agents that produce double-stranded DNA breaks, such as ionizing radiation [14]. ATM-dependent arrest of the cell cycle in G1 following radiation is through activation of p53 [15].

Poly (ADP-ribose) polymerase-1 (PARP1) is activated by DNA damage, playing a role in DNA base excision repair, but can also regulate transcription [16]. Loss of PARP1 activity leads to enhanced cancer cell death. Doxorubicin has been anecdotally shown to decrease PARP1 expression/activity [17].

Excision repair cross-complementation group 1 (ERCC1) is a rate-limiting protein in the nucleotide excision repair and interstrand crosslink repair pathways, including removing platinum chemotherapy adducts [18]. In STS patients undergoing trabectedin therapy, high expression correlated with improved progression-free survival and OS [19].

Xeroderma pigmentosum group F-complementing protein (XPF) is the catalytic component of the ERCC1 structure-specific DNA repair endonuclease complex [18].

Carbonic anhydrase IX (CAIX) is a transmembrane protein that catalyzes the hydration of carbon dioxide to carbonic acid, modulating pH [20]. Significant upregulation can occur with tumor hypoxia [21]. Expression has been associated with a decreased disease-specific survival and OS in large, deep, high-grade STSs [22].

Glucose transporter 1 (GLUT1) facilitates the transport of glucose across the plasma membranes of mammalian cells. It can be upregulated by hypoxic conditions, facilitating tumor cell generation of ATP via anaerobic glycolysis [23]. Bone and

STS patients with glut-1 overexpression had a significantly worse OS as compared to those without overexpression [24].

Hypoxia-inducible factor 1-alpha (HIF-1α) is a subunit of the transcription factor that regulates the cellular responses to hypoxia and may increase expression of proteins necessary for the development of metastases [25–27]. Increased HIF-1α expression in STSs has been associated with a shorter OS [28]. HIF-1α can also mediate resistance to radiation therapy [29].

2.3. TMA Construction, Staining, and Scoring. TMAs were constructed, stained, and scored using commercially available reagents and previously described, well-validated techniques [30–33].

2.4. TMA Construction. Two consecutive representative sections were recut from each specimen block. One was banked for future reference, if necessary. The other recut slide was stained with hematoxylin and eosin and used to determine the optimal locations for the 0.6 mm core biopsies of the specimen block. For the smaller-sized pretreatment biopsy specimens, one block was processed in this manner. For the larger posttreatment surgical resection specimens, if available, two blocks from noncontiguous areas of the tumor were processed. This algorithm produced 2-3 cores/patient (1 pretreatment and 1-2 posttreatment) on the TMA block. The blocks were arrayed using consecutive patients in order. Representative tissues with known IHC positivity to each of the study biomarkers were chosen by the Tissue Bank and also placed on the master TMA block to serve as positive controls.

As previously noted, three copies of the TMA were made by taking punches from different parts of the available tumor and stained with each marker to allow for consideration of expression heterogeneity across different areas of the tumor.

Construction of the TMA block was performed using the automated instruments at the RTOG Tissue Bank (Beecher Instruments, Sun Prairie, WI). Recipient paraffin blocks were made using standard jumbo metal molds commonly used for tissue embedding with standard plastic histology cassettes on top (Sakura Finetek, Torrance, CA). Type 9 embedding paraffin (Richard-Allan Scientific, Kalamazoo, MI) was used to make the paraffin recipient TMA block. A supplied H&E slide marked to represent the area of interest and its corresponding paraffin tissue block was used to accurately punch out the donor cores for each case and placed into the TMA. Heat strips were glued to the recipient block holder on the TMA instrument. The recipient block was then heated to approx. 100°F.

After each array block was constructed, a glass slide heated up to 80°C was set on the warmed block and allowed to melt the surface. The heated glass slide set the punches, eliminating the oven step used in the original method for array construction. The glass slide and array block were then turned over and allowed to cool on a room temperature tabletop for 5 minutes before chilling on an ice tray (slide down) before separating. The microtome used was the Microm HM 355-S (Thermo Fischer Scientific, Waltham, MA). The microtome chuck was adjusted manually to the flat surface of the array block. Since the block warmer was used when punching the array blocks, the punch surface was already flat, eliminating the need to trim into the block. Sections were taken almost directly off the surface. TMA blocks were sectioned at 4 microns and gently placed on a water bath at 38°C. Individual sections were maneuvered onto plus-charged slides with a probe. For quality control, a section from each TMA was stained with H&E. Each TMA core was checked to verify the presence or absence of tumor by the biobank pathologist (JPS), followed by a subsequent recheck by the pathologist performing the immunohistochemical studies (TM).

2.5. Fluorescence Immunohistochemistry. TMA sections (4 microns) were deparaffinized in xylene, rinsed in ethanol, and rehydrated as previously described [32]. Heat-induced epitope retrieval (HIER) was performed using a Decloaking Chamber (Biocare Medical, Concord, CA) for all target biomarkers by heating slides to 121°C for either 3 or 6 minutes, in either a citrate-based (pH 6.0) target retrieval solution (S1699, DAKO, Mississauga, Canada), or a Tris/EDTA-based (pH 9.0) target retrieval solution (S2367, DAKO). Supplementary 2 summarizes all target antibody specifics and their HIER conditions.

Slides were then processed using a DAKO Autostainer. Endogenous peroxidase activity was quenched with a 10-minute incubation of peroxidase block (K4007, DAKO), followed by a 15-minute protein block (SignalStain®; 8112L, Cell Signaling, Danvers, MA) to prevent nonspecific antibody binding.

All primary antibodies were diluted in SignalStain and applied for 60 minutes at room temperature along with either rat anti-vimentin (MAB2105, clone 280618, 1:100, R&D Systems, Minneapolis, MN, USA) or rabbit anti-vimentin (2707-1, clone EPR3776, 1:250, Epitomics, Burlingame, CA) to identify tumor cells. Slides were washed in Tris-buffered saline and Tween® 20 (TBST) wash buffer (S3006, DAKO) and then treated for 60 minutes with either goat anti-rabbit EnVision + (K4011, DAKO) or goat anti-mouse EnVision + (K4007, DAKO) secondary antibody. Either Alexa-488-conjugated goat anti-rat antibody (A-11006, polyclonal, 1:200, Invitrogen, Burlington, ON, Canada) or Alexa-555-conjugated goat anti-rabbit antibody (A-21429, polyclonal, 1:200, Invitrogen) was applied along with the anti-rabbit and anti-mouse secondary antibodies, respectively, to detect vimentin. Slides were then treated for 5 minutes with a TSA-Plus Cy5 tyramide signal amplification reagent (NEL745B001KT, PerkinElmer, Waltham, MA), coverslipped using ProLong Gold antifade mounting medium with 4′,6-diamidino-2-phenylindole (DAPI) (P36935, Invitrogen), and stored at 4°C.

2.6. Automated Image Acquisition and Analysis. Compartment-specific expression of all biomarkers was quantified using the HistoRx AQUA® platform (Branford, CT). Automated image acquisition was performed using the HistoRx PM-2000™ slide scanner, and digital images were analyzed using AQUAnalysis® software version 2.3.4.1 as previously described [33]. Briefly, seamless high-resolution images were acquired using an 8-bit monochrome TDI line-image capture camera with filters specific for DAPI to define the nuclear compartment, either fluoroscein isothiocyanate (FITC) or Cyanine 3 (Cy3) to define the vimentin-positive tumor cytosolic compartment, and Cy5 to define all target markers. A tumor-specific mask was generated to distinguish cancer cells from surrounding stromal tissue by thresholding the vimentin images to create a binary mask that identified the presence or absence of tumor cells by the presence of a pixel that was "on" or "off," respectively.

Images were cropped to exclude unusable areas from final analysis and then processed using optimized threshold values. Images were validated according to the following: (1) >10% of the tissue area is vimentin positive and (2) >50% of the image was usable (i.e., not compromised due to overlapping or out of focus tissue).

Compartment-specific AQUA scores, representing protein expression for all markers, were calculated as the average concentration of Cy5 pixel intensity within the compartment area for each TMA core. For each patient sample, the average compartment-specific AQUA score over triplicate cores was used to define the tumor score (tAQUA). Representative staining for CAIX and GLUT1 is shown in Supplementary 1.

2.7. 3′-Diaminobenzidine Tetrahydrochloride (DAB) Immunohistochemistry (Ki67 Only). Deparaffinized and rehydrated TMA sections underwent HIER using the PT-Link (DAKO) by heating slides at 97°C for 20 minutes in DAKO EnVision™ FLEX, Low pH (Link) target retrieval solution. After cooling to 65°C, slides were then placed in 1x EnVision FLEX wash buffer for 5 minutes prior to running the slides on the DAKO Autostainer Link 48. The FLEX monoclonal mouse anti-human Ki67 antigen (clone MIB-1) ready-to-use antibody (DAKO, IR626) for the Link platform was used following the manufacturer's specifications using EnVision FLEX reagents (DAKO, K8002) with counterstaining performed on the autostainer using hematoxylin (Link) (DAKO, K8008).

All images were reviewed by one of the study pathologists (TM) as a quality control step in data acquisition. Immunohistochemical staining was quantitatively assessed using ACIS® III Automated Cellular Imaging System (DAKO). Briefly, the ACIS III digitizes and reports a region score using proprietary software to generate a specific algorithm for Ki67 that identifies color thresholds (blue (hematoxylin overlay) and light brown and dark brown (Ki67DAB)) in manually selected regions containing tumor. The percent positive ACIS III score was then calculated by taking the total brown staining area and dividing it by the combined total blue and brown staining areas.

2.8. Outcome Data and Statistical Analysis. The demographic and updated outcome data for all of the patients that participated in NRG Oncology RTOG 9514 were already contained within the RTOG clinical trial database. Corresponding data for the patients in the MGH pilot trial were obtained from the MGH database, reformatted, and merged with the NRG Oncology RTOG 9514 data. Patient demographic information included age, gender, STS histology, tumor size, anatomic location, the pathologic response to neoadjuvant therapy as per the resection specimen, local recurrence, distant recurrence, and vital status at the time of the last follow-up.

For the purpose of statistical analysis, there were 3 cohorts of TMA specimens. The "pretreatment" (PRE) group consisted of specimens obtained at the time of STS diagnosis/prior to starting preoperative chemoradiation. The "posttreatment" (POST) group was specimens from the definitive surgical resection (following neoadjuvant chemoradiation). Based upon the presence of both pretreatment biopsy and surgical resection specimens for an individual patient, there was also a cohort of "matched pairs" (MPs). The patients with a pathologic complete response (PCR) were excluded from the POST and MP group analyses as there was no viable tumor for the POST TMA construction. Markers were analyzed as log-transformed continuous variables.

Assessed outcome measures included disease-free survival (DFS), distant disease-free survival (DDFS), and overall survival (OS). Failure for DFS was defined as local, regional, or distant relapse, or death due to any cause. Failure for DDFS was defined as distant relapse or death due to any cause. Failure for OS was defined as death due to any cause. DFS, DDFS, and OS were measured from the date of surgery to the date of failure or last follow-up for censored patients. The patients that progressed or died prior to surgery were excluded from analysis. Rates for DFS, DDFS, and OS were estimated by the Kaplan-Meier method. Hazard ratios were estimated by Cox models. Change of marker levels from pre- to posttreatment was compared using the nonparametric Wilcoxon signed-rank test.

3. Results

3.1. Patient Demographics and Outcome. Specimens for TMA construction were obtained for 61 patients from the combined MGH pilot trial/NRG Oncology RTOG 9514 participants. Following pathologic review, specimens from 60 patients were deemed adequate for TMA construction (37 from NRG Oncology RTOG 9514 and 23 from the MGH). Fifty-three patients had at least one marker value available. Two patients were excluded from analysis (1 not meeting inclusion/exclusion criteria; 1 disease progression prior to surgery), leaving 51 analyzable patients. In terms of the cohorts for analysis, there were 23 PRE patients, 40 POST patients, and 12 MPs.

The clinical and pathologic data for all patients are summarized in Supplementary 3. The median age for the patients represented on the TMA was 48 years (range 21–77), and 56.9% were male. Median tumor size was 14 cm (range 8.2–35), and 76.5% were located on the lower extremity/buttock. The most common STS subtypes were 45.1% undifferentiated pleomorphic sarcoma (malignant fibrous histiocytoma), 13.7% non-well-differentiated liposarcoma, 11.7% leiomyosarcoma, 5.9% malignant peripheral nerve sheath tumor, and 3.9% synovial sarcoma. Negative margin wide resection was achieved in 90.2%. Eighty-two percent of patients received all 3 cycles of preoperative MAID chemotherapy and 65% received 3 postoperative cycles. The complete follow-up and outcome data are shown in Supplementary 4. The median follow-up for

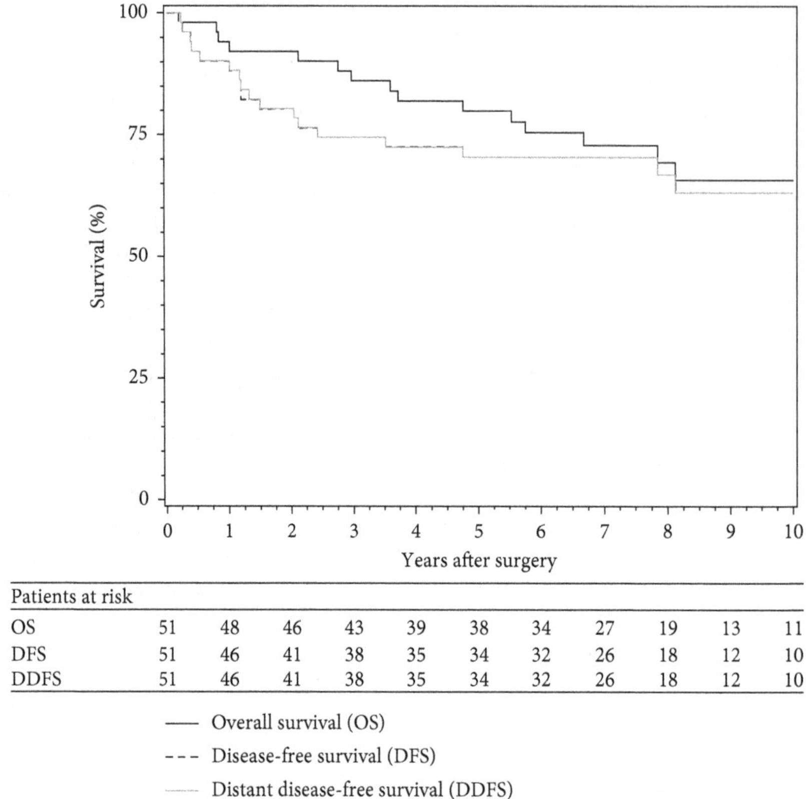

FIGURE 1: Kaplan-Meier estimates for disease-free survival, distant disease-free survival, and overall survival for deep, high-grade soft tissue sarcoma patients (with at least one biomarker value) treated with neoadjuvant chemoradiation.

surviving patients was 7.8 years (range 1.8–17.6). The 5-year estimates for DFS, DDFS, and OS were 70.4% (95% CI 57.9–83.0), 70.4% (57.9–83.0), and 79.9% (68.8–91.1), respectively (Figure 1).

3.2. Changes in Biomarker Expression following Neoadjuvant Chemoradiation. The changes in tumor biomarker expression following neoadjuvant chemoradiation in the 12 MP patients are listed in Table 1. There were statistically significant decreases in the expression of nuclear, cytoplasmic, and tumor mask CAIX ($p = 0.023, 0.039$, and 0.016, resp.), tumor mask GLUT1 ($p = 0.047$), and nuclear PARP1 ($p = 0.031$). p53 nuclear/cytoplasmic ratio also significantly increased ($p = 0.047$) following preoperative therapy. There were no significant changes in Ki67, ATM, ERCC1, XPF, or HIF-1α.

3.3. Biomarker Expression and Survival. The PRE group biomarker expression data are listed in Supplementary 5. There was no predictive association between PRE group biomarker expression and DFS, DDFS, or OS (data not shown). The POST group biomarker expression data are listed in Supplementary 6. For POST group biomarker expression, increased p53 nuclear/cytoplasmic (N/C) ratio was associated with a significantly decreased DFS (HR 4.13 (95% CI: 1.29–13.17), $p = 0.017$). Increased ERCC1 tumor mask and XPF nuclear expression were associated with an improved DFS (HR 0.30 (95% CI: 0.09–0.97), $p = 0.044$; HR 0.01 (95% CI: 0.00–0.92), $p = 0.046$, resp.). The entire POST group DFS analysis is shown in Table 2. No other POST group biomarkers were associated with DFS. Similar to DFS, increased p53 nuclear/cytoplasmic (N/C) ratio (HR 4.16 (95% CI: 1.31–13.23), $p = 0.016$) and a low expression of ERCC1 (HR 0.30 (95% CI: 0.09–0.98), $p = 0.046$) and XPF (HR 0.01 (95% CI: 0.00–0.93), $p = 0.046$) were associated with a decreased DDFS (Table 3). There was no relationship between POST biomarker expression and OS (data not shown).

4. Discussion

In light of the associated toxicity of cytotoxic chemotherapy, better predictors of poor survival in high-risk STS patients could potentially justify systemic treatment-related morbidity in a subset of this group. The tumor specimens from the MGH pilot trial and NRG Oncology RTOG 9514 provided a unique opportunity to create TMAs from a uniform cohort of high-risk STS patients with complete prospective follow-up data. The patients were also treated with almost identical neoadjuvant chemoradiation regimens. Unfortunately, there were no pretreatment expression patterns in our chosen biomarkers that correlated with DFS, DDFS, or OS. However, there were a few posttreatment biomarkers associated with the risk for distant recurrence: p53 N/C ratio, ERCC1, and XPF. If these biomarkers were associated with the risk for

TABLE 1: Changes in tumor biomarker expression following neoadjuvant chemoradiation in 12 "matched pair" large, deep, high-risk soft tissue sarcoma patients.

Marker	Pretreatment value		Posttreatment value		p value
	Mean	SD	Mean	SD	
ACIS Ki67					
Percentage	15.91	19.78	7.65	7.30	0.0674
p53					
Nuclear/cytoplasmic ratio	1.44	0.22	1.90	0.74	0.0469
ATM					
Nuclear	8349.36	1920.35	7870.75	2114.36	0.4961
Cytoplasm	3811.69	2121.29	3116.21	1035.73	0.4258
Tumor mask	5289.39	2400.71	4412.80	1205.37	0.3594
PARP1					
Nuclear	7042.80	1361.76	5533.59	1198.18	0.0313
Cytoplasm	3281.97	798.55	2293.63	471.64	0.0938
Tumor mask	4354.82	1092.11	3263.65	674.80	0.0625
ERCC1					
Nuclear	9433.46	2247.20	8586.98	1658.74	0.3594
Cytoplasm	3046.29	1563.80	2197.19	917.54	0.0977
Tumor mask	5150.35	1600.28	4206.67	1335.08	0.0977
XPF					
Nuclear	8772.27	1076.08	8880.11	2407.45	0.8457
Cytoplasm	4694.75	1556.58	4240.83	1254.75	0.3750
Tumor mask	6004.00	1598.71	5511.37	1619.80	0.4316
CAIX					
Nuclear	3939.81	1273.12	2406.95	977.10	0.0234
Cytoplasm	3931.01	1699.38	2037.18	944.15	0.0391
Tumor mask	3972.93	1569.58	2124.05	926.91	0.0156
GLUT1					
Nuclear	5389.90	2886.98	2937.34	1198.24	0.0781
Cytoplasm	4932.26	3106.79	2496.81	1116.73	0.1094
Tumor mask	5054.19	2998.35	2658.88	1128.22	0.0469
HIF-1α					
Nuclear	6267.08	1603.95	5787.91	2241.58	0.4609
Cytoplasm	3857.75	1221.78	2978.52	1433.30	0.1484
Tumor mask	4582.47	1435.49	4009.57	2108.14	0.3828

SD: standard deviation; p values are from the Wilcoxon signed-rank test on log-transformed values.

distant recurrence after neoadjuvant radiation therapy alone, then they could be tested to stratify patients for postoperative chemotherapy. There were also some intrapatient changes in tumor biomarker expression following neoadjuvant therapy that may better elucidate the biologic mechanisms underlying STS responses to chemoradiation.

In resected high-grade STSs without neoadjuvant therapy, Maseide et al. observed that the expression of CAIX correlated with decreased disease-specific survival and OS [22]. In our study, neither PRE nor POST CAIX expression was associated with outcome. Interestingly, we did observe that preoperative chemoradiation led to a significant decrease in both CAIX and GLUT1 tumor expression in the MP analysis. These findings would fit with a chemoradiation-related tumor reoxygenation phenomenon [34]. Portions of tumors (especially STS) can be hypoxic, making them less responsive to radiation. As tumor cells die in response to therapy, other hypoxic cells within the tumor will obtain more oxygen. Expression of CAIX and GLUT1 can be induced by HIF-1α [35, 36]. A decrease in HIF-1α secondary to tumor reoxygenation resulting from neoadjuvant therapy could produce the observed decreases in CAIX and GLUT1. However, we did not observe a decrease in HIF-1α in our MP group. Therefore, it is possible that the decreased expression of CAIX and GLUT1 after neoadjuvant therapy reflects altered HIF-1α signaling in response to chemoradiation, such as doxorubicin, rather than expression changes only attributable to hypoxia [37, 38].

Given the roles of PARP1, ERCC1, and XPF in the repair of DNA damage, one might expect that increased expression would enhance tumor survival. In our study, increased primary tumor POST expression of both ERCC1 and XPF was associated with an increased DFS and DDFS. This finding is somewhat similar to ERCC1 results by Rodrigo et al. in 78 high-grade "locally advanced" soft tissue sarcoma patients who received 4 cycles of neoadjuvant doxorubicin-cisplatin-ifosfamide chemotherapy [39]. Although there was no significant correlation of ERCC1 negative versus positive tumors with DFS in that study (median DFS 3.2 versus 7 years, $p \leq 0.19$), median OS for ERCC1-positive tumor was not reached as compared to 6.6 years for negative tumors ($p \leq 0.058$). We observed a decrease in PARP1 expression after neoadjuvant therapy in the MP group, but there was no correlation between PRE or POST PARP1 expression and outcome. Increased

Table 2: Correlation of posttreatment biopsy specimen tissue microarray biomarker expression with disease-free survival in 40 large, deep, high-risk soft tissue sarcoma patients treated with neoadjuvant chemoradiation.

Marker	HR (95% CI)	p value
ACIS Ki67		
Percentage	1.01 (0.60–1.68)	0.9813
p53		
Nuclear/cytoplasmic ratio	4.13 (1.29–13.17)	0.0167
ATM		
Nuclear	2.28 (0.34–15.32)	0.3971
Cytoplasm	1.86 (0.32–10.79)	0.4889
Tumor mask	1.33 (0.22–8.11)	0.7594
PARP1		
Nuclear	1.38 (0.18–10.62)	0.7596
Cytoplasm	0.53 (0.12–2.33)	0.3982
Tumor mask	0.55 (0.13–2.42)	0.4317
ERCC1		
Nuclear	0.77 (0.06–9.53)	0.8380
Cytoplasm	0.37 (0.11–1.21)	0.0991
Tumor mask	0.30 (0.09–0.97)	0.0443
XPF		
Nuclear	0.01 (0.00–0.92)	0.0457
Cytoplasm	0.25 (0.03–2.35)	0.2271
Tumor mask	0.16 (0.02–1.62)	0.1207
CAIX		
Nuclear	1.23 (0.48–3.13)	0.6713
Cytoplasm	1.33 (0.60–2.95)	0.4881
Tumor mask	1.32 (0.58–3.03)	0.5084
GLUT1		
Nuclear	1.44 (0.50–4.18)	0.4989
Cytoplasm	1.24 (0.52–2.96)	0.6322
Tumor mask	1.26 (0.50–3.20)	0.6212
HIF-1α		
Nuclear	0.59 (0.18–1.89)	0.3712
Cytoplasm	0.37 (0.12–1.16)	0.0885
Tumor mask	0.40 (0.14–1.17)	0.0945

HR: hazard ratio; CI: confidence interval.

Table 3: Correlation of posttreatment biopsy specimen tissue microarray biomarker expression with distant disease-free survival in 40 large, deep, high-risk soft tissue sarcoma patients treated with neoadjuvant chemoradiation.

Marker	HR (95% CI)	p value
ACIS Ki67		
Percentage	1.01 (0.60–1.69)	0.9691
p53		
Nuclear/cytoplasmic ratio	4.16 (1.31–13.23)	0.0159
ATM		
Nuclear	2.32 (0.35–15.59)	0.3859
Cytoplasm	1.93 (0.34–11.05)	0.4583
Tumor mask	1.37 (0.23–8.33)	0.7294
PARP1		
Nuclear	1.37 (0.18–10.68)	0.7611
Cytoplasm	0.52 (0.12–2.34)	0.3971
Tumor mask	0.55 (0.13–2.43)	0.4313
ERCC1		
Nuclear	0.78 (0.06–9.75)	0.8479
Cytoplasm	10.37 (0.11–1.22)	0.1038
Tumor mask	0.30 (0.09–0.98)	0.0455
XPF		
Nuclear	0.01 (0.00–0.93)	0.0462
Cytoplasm	0.27 (0.03–2.43)	0.2415
Tumor mask	0.17 (0.02–1.69)	0.1304
CAIX		
Nuclear	1.21 (0.47–3.12)	0.6885
Cytoplasm	1.32 (0.59–2.94)	0.5005
Tumor mask	1.31 (0.57–3.02)	0.5214
GLUT1		
Nuclear	1.44 (0.50–4.18)	0.4984
Cytoplasm	1.24 (0.52–2.97)	0.6250
Tumor mask	1.27 (0.50–3.20)	0.6168
HIF-1α		
Nuclear	0.59 (0.18–1.90)	0.3717
Cytoplasm	0.37 (0.12–1.17)	0.0913
Tumor mask	0.40 (0.14–1.17)	0.0951

HR: hazard ratio; CI: confidence interval.

PARP1 expression has been associated with decreased DFS and DDFS in other cancers, such as serous ovarian carcinoma and breast cancer [40, 41]. As previously noted, doxorubicin therapy has been associated with decreases in PARP1, which may explain our PARP1 findings [17].

Another interesting finding was the increase in p53 N/C ratio following neoadjuvant therapy in the MP group combined with an increased POST p53 N/C ratio correlating with a decreased DFS and DDFS. These results raise the possibility that chemoradiation may have increased the expression of preexisting mutant p53. Mutant p53, with loss of function, can have a positive feedback loop with respect to p53 expression, resulting in increased nuclear accumulation [42]. It also has a higher N/C ratio as there is less cytoplasmic background due to saturation of the camera from the strong nuclear expression. Use of the N/C ratio helps to normalize differences on a case-by-case basis, and it also relates to changes in localization of the protein. The fact that the p53 N/C ratio findings for DFS and DDFS were statistically significant supports a hypothesis that sarcomas with mutant p53 may be at increased risk of metastasis. Alternatively, it is conceivable that the increased accumulation of p53 following neoadjuvant therapy reflects activation of wild-type p53 that accumulates in the nucleus following DNA damage. In this scenario, the presence of wild-type p53 would correlate with worse outcome after treatment, which has been reported for preclinical mouse models of breast cancer treated with doxorubicin [43]. Future studies that include p53 gene sequencing and evaluation of the p53 N/C ratio after neoadjuvant therapy will be needed to differentiate between these two possibilities.

There are several limitations to our study. The first is that, although this is a very homogeneous, uniformly treated subset of "high-risk" STSs, the total number of patients is very small. This would potentially diminish the ability to identify any statistically significant associations between biomarker expression and outcome. As with many pathologic specimen-based analyses, we were only able to acquire adequate specimens to construct the TMA from 59 out of 112 potential patients from the combined MGH/NRG Oncology RTOG 9514 trials. Many institutions were unwilling to release the archival diagnostic pathologic material. The original pretreatment biopsy specimens were frequently very limited in size, often just a core needle biopsy, and some were performed at institutions not participating in either trial (prior to the referral of the patient for trial enrollment). When limited samples from a large tumor are used to construct a TMA, it is also possible that tumor heterogeneity will not be adequately represented. This is especially true for the rather diminutive pretreatment core needle biopsy specimens. Alternatively, one could contend that using a single small core needle biopsy specimen from a newly diagnosed sarcoma would be more representative of what would happen in a "real-world" clinical practice where only a very small, somewhat random biopsy sample from the tumor would be available to perform biomarker testing for pretreatment prognostication. If there was a complete pathologic response to neoadjuvant therapy (which was 27% in NRG Oncology RTOG 9514), it also meant that there was no POST tumor specimen to analyze [5]. Although we "lumped together" the different STS subtypes due to the small number of available cases, there are likely inherent differences in biomarker expression amongst the various histologies. The small number of matched pair specimens also limited the ability to identify intrapatient changes in tumor biomarker expression following neoadjuvant therapy. Finally, although there was a fairly long median follow-up, the overall small sample size combined with very good patient survival means that there were relatively few adverse outcome events, which limited the statistical power of our study.

In conclusion, the PRE expression of none of our candidate pretreatment biomarkers was not associated with survival in this cohort of STS patients treated with neoadjuvant chemoradiation. Therefore, we remain unable to identify a subset of truly high-risk STS patients at the time of diagnosis who would be optimal candidates for neoadjuvant chemoradiation prior to surgical resection. Some tumor biomarker expression pattern changes after neoadjuvant chemoradiation do support the concepts of tumor reoxygenation or altered HIF-1α signaling. In addition, we observed nuclear accumulation of p53 after neoadjuvant therapy, which may reflect a response of p53 to DNA damage. Hopefully, our clinically well-annotated, high-risk STS TMAs will be an extremely useful collaborative resource for future candidate biomarker analyses, either for prognostication or to assess the suitability for novel targeted therapies.

Disclosure

Alex Klimowicz is currently at Boehringer Ingelheim Pharmaceuticals, Inc, Ridgefield, CT, USA. The Pennsylvania Department of Health specifically declaims responsibility for any analyses, interpretations, or conclusions.

Acknowledgments

The authors would like to acknowledge the following at the Tom Baker Cancer Centre, Calgary, AB, Canada: Brant Pohorelic for RTOG 9514 specimen CAIX, ERCC1, GLUT1, HIF-1α, p53, PARP1, and XPF staining and image analysis; Elizabeth Kornaga for Ki67 staining and analysis on the ACISIII; and both Elizabeth Kornaga and Michelle Dean for methodology manuscript development. This project was supported by Grant nos. U10CA21661, U10CA180868, U10CA180822, U10CA37422, and U24CA180803 from the National Cancer Institute (NCI). This project was also funded, in part, under a grant with the Pennsylvania Department of Health.

References

[1] Sarcoma Meta-Analysis Collaboration, "Adjuvant chemotherapy for localised resectable soft-tissue sarcoma of adults: meta-analysis of individual data. Sarcoma meta-analysis collaboration," *The Lancet*, vol. 350, no. 9092, pp. 1647–1654, 1997.

[2] S. Frustaci, F. Gherlinzoni, A. De Paoli et al., "Adjuvant chemotherapy for adult soft tissue sarcomas of the extremities and girdles: results of the Italian randomized cooperative trial," *Journal of Clinical Oncology*, vol. 19, no. 5, pp. 1238–1247, 2001.

[3] N. Pervaiz, N. Colterjohn, F. Farrokhyar, R. Tozer, A. Figueredo, and M. Ghert, "A systematic meta-analysis of randomized controlled trials of adjuvant chemotherapy for localized resectable soft-tissue sarcoma," *Cancer*, vol. 113, no. 3, pp. 573–581, 2008.

[4] T. F. DeLaney, I. J. Spiro, H. D. Suit et al., "Neoadjuvant chemotherapy and radiotherapy for large extremity soft-tissue sarcomas," *International Journal of Radiation Oncology, Biology, Physics*, vol. 56, no. 4, pp. 1117–1127, 2003.

[5] W. G. Kraybill, J. Harris, I. J. Spiro et al., "Phase II study of neoadjuvant chemotherapy and radiation therapy in the management of high-risk, high-grade, soft tissue sarcomas of the extremities and body wall: Radiation Therapy Oncology Group Trial 9514," *Journal of Clinical Oncology*, vol. 24, no. 4, pp. 619–625, 2006.

[6] N. J. Look Hong, F. J. Hornicek, D. C. Harmon et al., "Neoadjuvant chemoradiotherapy for patients with high-risk extremity and truncal sarcomas: a 10-year single institution retrospective study," *European Journal of Cancer*, vol. 49, no. 4, pp. 875–883, 2013.

[7] W. G. Kraybill, J. Harris, I. J. Spiro et al., "Long-term results of a phase 2 study of neoadjuvant chemotherapy and radiotherapy in the management of high-risk, high-grade, soft tissue sarcomas of the extremities and body wall: Radiation Therapy Oncology Group Trial 9514," *Cancer*, vol. 116, no. 19, pp. 4613–4621, 2010.

[8] J. Gerdes, L. Li, C. Schlueter et al., "Immunobiochemical and molecular biologic characterization of the cell proliferation-associated nuclear antigen that is defined by monoclonal antibody Ki-67," *American Journal of Pathology*, vol. 138, no. 4, pp. 867–873, 1991.

[9] P. F. Choong, M. Akerman, H. Willen et al., "Prognostic value of Ki-67 expression in 182 soft tissue sarcomas. Proliferation–a marker of metastasis?," *APMIS*, vol. 102, no. 12, pp. 915–924, 1994.

[10] R. L. Huuhtanen, C. P. Blomqvist, T. A. Wiklund et al., "Comparison of the Ki-67 score and S-phase fraction as prognostic variables in soft-tissue sarcoma," *British Journal of Cancer*, vol. 79, no. 5-6, pp. 945–951, 1999.

[11] H. Taubert, A. Meye, and P. Wurl, "Soft tissue sarcomas and p53 mutations," *Molecular Medicine*, vol. 4, no. 6, pp. 365–372, 1998.

[12] H. Taubert, P. Wurl, M. Bache et al., "The p53 gene in soft tissue sarcomas: prognostic value of DNA sequencing versus

immunohistochemistry," *Anticancer Research*, vol. 18, no. 1, pp. 183–187, 1998.

[13] P. Wurl, H. Taubert, A. Meye et al., "Prognostic value of immunohistochemistry for p53 in primary soft-tissue sarcomas: a multivariate analysis of five antibodies," *Journal of Cancer Research and Clinical Oncology*, vol. 123, no. 9, pp. 502–508, 1997.

[14] J. H. Lee and T. T. Paull, "Activation and regulation of ATM kinase activity in response to DNA double-strand breaks," *Oncogene*, vol. 26, no. 56, pp. 7741–7748, 2007.

[15] M. B. Kastan, Q. Zhan, W. S. El-Deiry et al., "A mammalian cell cycle checkpoint pathway utilizing p53 and GADD45 is defective in ataxia-telangiectasia," *Cell*, vol. 71, no. 4, pp. 587–597, 1992.

[16] M. J. Schiewer, J. F. Goodwin, S. Han et al., "Dual roles of PARP-1 promote cancer growth and progression," *Cancer Discovery*, vol. 2, no. 12, pp. 1134–1149, 2012.

[17] T. Zaremba, H. Thomas, M. Cole, E. R. Plummer, and N. J. Curtin, "Doxorubicin-induced suppression of poly (ADP-ribose) polymerase-1 (PARP-1) activity and expression and its implication for PARP inhibitors in clinical trials," *Cancer Chemotherapy and Pharmacology*, vol. 66, no. 4, pp. 807–812, 2010.

[18] K. Kirschner and D. W. Melton, "Multiple roles of the ERCC1-XPF endonuclease in DNA repair and resistance to anticancer drugs," *Anticancer Research*, vol. 30, no. 9, pp. 3223–3232, 2010.

[19] A. Italiano, A. Laurand, A. Laroche et al., "ERCC5/XPG, ERCC1, and BRCA1 gene status and clinical benefit of trabectedin in patients with soft tissue sarcoma," *Cancer*, vol. 117, no. 15, pp. 3445–3456, 2011.

[20] W. S. Sly and P. Y. Hu, "Human carbonic anhydrases and carbonic anhydrase deficiencies," *Annual Review of Biochemistry*, vol. 64, no. 1, pp. 375–401, 1995.

[21] C. C. Wykoff, N. J. Beasley, P. H. Watson et al., "Hypoxia-inducible expression of tumor-associated carbonic anhydrases," *Cancer Research*, vol. 60, no. 24, pp. 7075–7083, 2000.

[22] K. Maseide, R. A. Kandel, R. S. Bell et al., "Carbonic anhydrase IX as a marker for poor prognosis in soft tissue sarcoma," *Clinical Cancer Research*, vol. 10, no. 13, pp. 4464–4471, 2004.

[23] P. Vaupel, "The role of hypoxia-induced factors in tumor progression," *Oncologist*, vol. 9, no. 5, pp. 10–17, 2004.

[24] M. Endo, U. Tateishi, K. Seki et al., "Prognostic implications of glucose transporter protein-1 (glut-1) overexpression in bone and soft-tissue sarcomas," *Japanese Journal of Clinical Oncology*, vol. 37, no. 12, pp. 955–960, 2007.

[25] G. L. Semenza, "HIF-1: mediator of physiological and pathophysiological responses to hypoxia," *Journal of Applied Physiology*, vol. 88, no. 4, pp. 1474–1480, 2000.

[26] R. Sullivan and C. H. Graham, "Hypoxia-driven selection of the metastatic phenotype," *Cancer and Metastasis Reviews*, vol. 26, no. 2, pp. 319–331, 2007.

[27] T. S. Eisinger-Mathason, M. Zhang, Q. Qiu et al., "Hypoxia-dependent modification of collagen networks promotes sarcoma metastasis," *Cancer Discovery*, vol. 3, no. 10, pp. 1190–1205, 2013.

[28] K. Shintani, A. Matsumine, K. Kusuzaki et al., "Expression of hypoxia-inducible factor (HIF)-1 alpha as a biomarker of outcome in soft-tissue sarcomas," *Virchows Archiv*, vol. 449, no. 6, pp. 673–681, 2006.

[29] M. Zhang, Q. Qiu, Z. Li et al., "HIF-1 alpha regulates the response of primary sarcomas to radiation therapy through a cell autonomous mechanism," *Radiation Research*, vol. 183, no. 6, pp. 594–609, 2015.

[30] J. Kononen, L. Bubendorf, A. Kallioniemi et al., "Tissue microarrays for high-throughput molecular profiling of tumor specimens," *Nature Medicine*, vol. 4, no. 7, pp. 844–847, 1998.

[31] M. A. Rubin, R. Dunn, M. Strawderman, and K. J. Pienta, "Tissue microarray sampling strategy for prostate cancer biomarker analysis," *American Journal of Surgical Pathology*, vol. 26, no. 3, pp. 312–319, 2002.

[32] S. Otsuka, A. C. Klimowicz, K. Kopciuk et al., "CXCR4 overexpression is associated with poor outcome in females diagnosed with stage IV non-small cell lung cancer," *Journal of Thoracic Oncology*, vol. 6, no. 7, pp. 1169–1178, 2011.

[33] R. L. Camp, G. G. Chung, and D. L. Rimm, "Automated subcellular localization and quantification of protein expression in tissue microarrays," *Nature Medicine*, vol. 8, no. 11, pp. 1323–1327, 2002.

[34] R. F. Kallman and M. J. Dorie, "Tumor oxygenation and reoxygenation during radiation therapy: their importance in predicting tumor response," *International Journal of Radiation Oncology, Biology, Physics*, vol. 12, no. 4, pp. 681–685, 1986.

[35] N. V. Iyer, L. E. Kotch, F. Agani et al., "Cellular and developmental control of O_2 homeostasis by hypoxia-inducible factor 1 alpha," *Genes & Development*, vol. 12, no. 2, pp. 149–162, 1998.

[36] S. Kaluz, M. Kaluzova, S. Y. Liao, M. Lerman, and E. J. Stanbridge, "Transcriptional control of the tumor- and hypoxia-marker carbonic anhydrase 9: a one transcription factor (HIF-1) show?," *Biochimica et Biophysica Acta*, vol. 1795, no. 2, pp. 162–172, 2009.

[37] Y. Cao, J. M. Eble, E. Moon et al., "Tumor cells upregulate normoxic HIF-1 alpha in response to doxorubicin," *Cancer Research*, vol. 73, no. 20, pp. 6230–6242, 2013.

[38] B. J. Moeller, Y. Cao, C. Y. Li, and M. W. Dewhirst, "Radiation activates HIF-1 to regulate vascular radiosensitivity in tumors: role of reoxygenation, free radicals, and stress granules," *Cancer Cell*, vol. 5, no. 5, pp. 429–441, 2004.

[39] R. S. Rodrigo, A. Nathalie, T. Elodie et al., "Topoisomerase II-alpha protein expression and histological response following doxorubicin-based induction chemotherapy predict survival of locally advanced soft tissues sarcomas," *European Journal of Cancer*, vol. 47, no. 9, pp. 1319–1327, 2011.

[40] H. Brustmann, "Poly(adenosine diphosphate-ribose) polymerase expression in serous ovarian carcinoma: correlation with p53, MIB-1, and outcome," *International Journal of Gynecological Pathology*, vol. 26, no. 2, pp. 147–153, 2007.

24

A Longitudinal Study of Functional Outcomes in Patients with Limb Salvage Surgery for Soft Tissue Sarcoma

Eunsun Oh,[1,2] Sung Wook Seo,[3] and Kwang Joon Han[3]

[1]*Department of Radiology, Soonchunhyang University Seoul Hospital, 59 Daesagwan-ro, Youngsan-gu, Seoul 04401, Republic of Korea*
[2]*Department of Radiology, Samsung Medical Center, Sungkyunkwan University School of Medicine, 81 Ilwon-Ro, Gangnam-gu, Seoul 06351, Republic of Korea*
[3]*Department of Orthopedic Surgery, Samsung Medical Center, Sungkyunkwan University School of Medicine, 81 Ilwon-Ro, Gangnam-gu, Seoul 06351, Republic of Korea*

Correspondence should be addressed to Sung Wook Seo; sungwseo@skku.edu

Academic Editor: Peter C. Ferguson

Background. Many studies have reported on the surgical outcomes of soft tissue sarcoma. However, there was no longitudinal cohort study. Because time is the most valuable factor for functional recovery, adjusting time value was the key for finding the causal relationship between other risk factors and postoperative function. Therefore, existing cross-sectional studies can neither fully explain the causal relationship between the risk factors and the functional score nor predict functional recovery. The aim of this study was to determine important predictive factors that affect postoperative functional outcomes and longitudinal changes in functional outcomes in patients who had undergone limb-sparing surgery (LSS) for soft tissue sarcoma (STS). *Methods.* Between January 2008 and December 2014, we retrospectively enrolled 150 patients who had undergone LSS for STS and had been assessed for postoperative functional outcomes with questionnaires. To evaluate functional outcomes, we used the Musculoskeletal Tumor Society (MSTS) score and Toronto Extremity Salvage Score (TESS). Multivariate generalized estimating equation (GEE) analysis was used to identify the predictive factors, including size, stage, and anatomic location of tumor, bone resection, flap reconstruction, age, and time after surgery. Each continuous variable such as age and time after surgery was explored for statistically significant cutoff points using the Wilcoxon rank sum test. *Results.* Functional scores significantly improved until the second year after surgery and plateaued for the rest of the 5-year period. Age ($p < 0.0001$), bone resection ($p = 0.0004$), and time after surgery ($p < 0.0001$) were identified as significant predictive factors. The functional score was significantly higher in patients younger than 47 years old. *Conclusions.* Functional outcomes can improve until the second year after surgery. Patients who were older than 47 and underwent bone resection may have poor final functional outcomes.

1. Introduction

Soft tissue sarcomas (STSs) are rare malignant tumors, representing approximately 1% of all adult cancers [1]. Limb salvage surgery (LSS) is the preferred treatment for patients with STS rather than amputation [2, 3]. Multidisciplinary treatment that combines surgery with or without adjuvant radiation therapy has been widely applied with local control, but without any measurable decrease in disease-free survival and overall survival [4, 5]. However, surgical success can be assessed not only by oncological outcomes but also functional outcomes. Thus, functional outcomes after LSS are important to both surgeons and patients.

Many studies have reported predictors of functional outcomes for patients who have undergone LSS for STS. They evaluated functional outcomes at specific points, such as 6 months [6, 7] or 1 year [8] after surgery, or at an uncertain postoperative time point such as final follow-up [9]. These studies have limitations in not using longitudinal data with more than 2 time points and by not examining various predictors of postoperative functional outcomes for periods exceeding 5 years. With such reports, surgeons are not able to inform patients about the functional recovery period and final outcome after surgery.

Therefore, the purpose of our study was to determine important predictive factors that affect postoperative functional outcomes and longitudinal changes in functional outcomes in patients who had undergone LSS.

2. Materials and Methods

2.1. Study Design and Patients. The institutional review board approved this retrospective Health Insurance Portability and Accountability Act (HIPAA) compliant study (2015-10-176-001). Informed patient consent was waived. A retrospective cohort study of 212 patients who had undergone LSS for STS at our medical center between January 2008 and December 2014 was performed. All patients were assessed for postoperative functional outcomes with questionnaires. The functional outcomes were measured every 3 ± 1 months for 1 year postoperatively and every 6 ± 2 months from 2 to 5 years after surgery during their outpatient clinic visits. We included patients who had filled out questionnaires at least 2 times during a minimum follow-up period of 2 years. We excluded patients who already had functional disability at the operative site ($n = 24$) or contralateral side ($n = 33$) before surgery or accidental trauma irrelevant to the disease ($n = 5$). Therefore, a total of 150 patients were included in this study.

2.2. Measurements. To evaluate functional outcomes, we used the Musculoskeletal Tumor Society (MSTS) score and Toronto Extremity Salvage Score (TESS). The MSTS score evaluates functional impairment after treatment and consists of 6 categories: pain, function, and emotional acceptance in the upper and lower extremities; supports, walking, and gait in the lower extremity; and hand positioning, dexterity, and lifting ability in the upper extremity [10]. It is measured by clinical physician through a standardized physical examination. Each category is rated on a scale of 0 to 5. The total score is calculated from the sum of each category and converted to a percentage value. The TESS evaluates performance of activities of daily living [11]. The upper and lower extremity versions of the TESS have 29-item and 30-item questionnaires, respectively. Each item is rated on a scale of 0 to 5. The point score is obtained, and the percentage is calculated. We used the translation and cross-cultural adaptation of the Korean version of TESS [12]. Kim et al. [12] demonstrated that two bilingual translators translated the original version of the TESS questionnaire into Korean then translated back into English. The Korean version of TESS was reviewed by a committee to develop the consensus. The Korean version of TESS was administered to 126 patients to examine its comprehensibility, reliability, and validity.

Several known predictors of functional outcome include patient age, size and grade of tumor, irradiation, and presence of bone and motor nerve resection [6]. Based on these, we defined several potential predictive factors that could have an influence on functional outcomes: size, stage and anatomic location of tumor, bone resection (no/yes), flap reconstruction (no/yes), postoperative radiation (no/yes), patient age, and time after surgery. The size of tumor was based on maximum diameter in centimeters. To assign a stage to a patient with STS, we adopted the 7th edition of the *American Joint Committee on Cancer (AJCC) Cancer Staging Manual* [13], which is widely accepted as an important surgical consideration. We divided tumor stage into 3 groups: group 1, stages I and IIA; group 2, stages IIB and III; and group 3, stage IV. The anatomic location of tumor was classified into upper extremity, lower extremity, and trunk.

2.3. Statistical Analysis. All statistical analyses were performed using statistical software (SAS version 9.4, SAS Institute, Cary, NC, USA; R version 3.1.0, R Development Core Team, Vienna, Austria). A box plot was applied to explore the statistical distribution of functional scores in the MSTS and TESS. Multivariate generalized estimating equation (GEE) analysis was used to identify the predictive factors that could affect the functional outcomes. Longitudinal data were repeated, and measures were obtained from the same subjects. High correlation within the same patient pool indicated that longitudinal relationships could not be analyzed by common regression methods, which presumed the independence of data [14, 15]. Therefore, the GEE analysis was the appropriate statistical methodology. For the significant predictors of functional outcome by multivariate GEE analysis, the optimal cutoff was chosen as the point with the most significant Wilcoxon rank sum test p value for all possible cutoff points. For all statistical analysis, differences were considered to be significant if the p value was less than 0.05.

3. Results

The characteristics of all 150 patients, comprising 81 men (54%) and 69 women (46%), are listed in Table 1. The mean age at the time of surgery was 47 years (range 10–90). The distribution graphics of functional scores in the MSTS and TESS are shown in Figures 1 and 2. The functional scores in the MSTS and TESS significantly improved until the second year after surgery and then remained stable for the rest of the 5-year period. The optimal cutoff was chosen as 24 months, based on the most significant Wilcoxon rank sum test p value for all possible cutoff points.

Table 2 shows the results of multivariate GEE analysis of the effective predictive factors of functional outcomes. Among all factors, time after surgery was significantly related to both MSTS ($p = 0.001$) and TESS ($p = 0.0004$). There were significant differences in functional scores by age in the MSTS and TESS ($p < 0.0001$). Older patients scored lower than younger patients in functional outcomes. The optimal cutoff was chosen as 47 years old, based on the most significant Wilcoxon rank sum test p value for all possible cutoff points.

There were also significant differences in functional scores according to bone resection in the MSTS and TESS ($p < 0.0001$). Patients who had undergone bone resection surgery scored lower in both MSTS (6.1%) and TESS (19.3%) than those who had not undergone bone resection. Thus,

TABLE 1: Clinical and demographic characteristics of patients ($n = 150$).

Characteristic	Number	Percentage (%)
Patient attributes		
Age[a] (years)	47.04 ± 17.19	
Gender		
Male	81	54
Female	69	46
Tumor attributes		
Size[a]	6.81 ± 5.79	
Stage group		
Group 1	78	52
Group 2	67	44.67
Group 3	5	3.33
Anatomic location		
Upper extremity	38	25.33
Lower extremity	102	68
Trunk	10	6.67
Surgery attributes		
Bone resection		
No	117	78
Yes	33	22
Flap reconstruction		
No	102	68
Yes	48	32
Postoperative radiation		
No	102	68
Yes	48	32

[a]Mean ± standard deviation.

even when postoperative time is considered, patients with bone resection had a 20% lower functional recovery.

4. Discussion

This study is the first to determine predictive factors associated with postoperative functional outcomes through a longitudinal study using the GEE approach to explain trends over time. In our study, we found that age, bone resection, and time after surgery were significant predictive factors of functional outcomes. Moreover, functional outcomes in the MSTS and TESS over a 5-year follow-up tended to improve until the second year.

Our study demonstrated that functional outcomes in the MSTS and TESS improved until the second year after surgery, and plateaued for the rest of the 5-year period. Previous studies used a minimum follow-up period of 6 months [6, 7] or 1 year [8, 16] for evaluation of functional outcomes, at which point functional scores are known to plateau. However, in our study, 24 months was the significant cutoff point for functional outcomes; functional scores before 24 months were not appropriate to evaluate the final functional outcome after surgery. Time after surgery was an independent predictive factor of functional outcome in our study. Therefore, time after surgery could be a confounding factor when comparing functional scores that were measured at different time points.

This study indicated that age was another independent predictive factor of functional outcomes. Older patients showed less improvement than younger patients. This may be because older patients tended to have more comorbidity. Additionally, there was a significant difference at a cutoff point of age 47.

Bone resection was another independent predictive factor of functional outcomes. Davis et al. [6] showed that bone resection was significantly related to increased disability on the MSTS using univariate and multivariate analysis and the TESS using only univariate analysis. In our study, patients who had undergone bone resection showed poorer functional outcomes on the MSTS and TESS than those without resection, regardless of time after surgery. This suggested that wide bone resection including muscle resulted in significant functional disability. Based on these data, surgeons can expect a poor functional outcome when performing bone resection, and further study is needed to solve this problem.

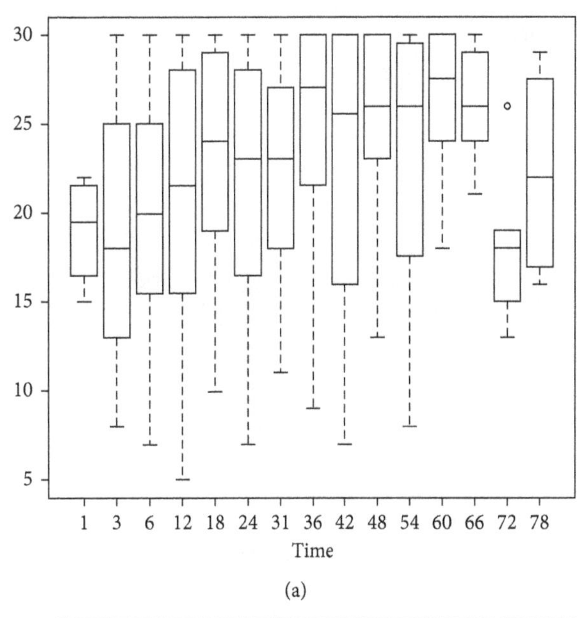

(a)

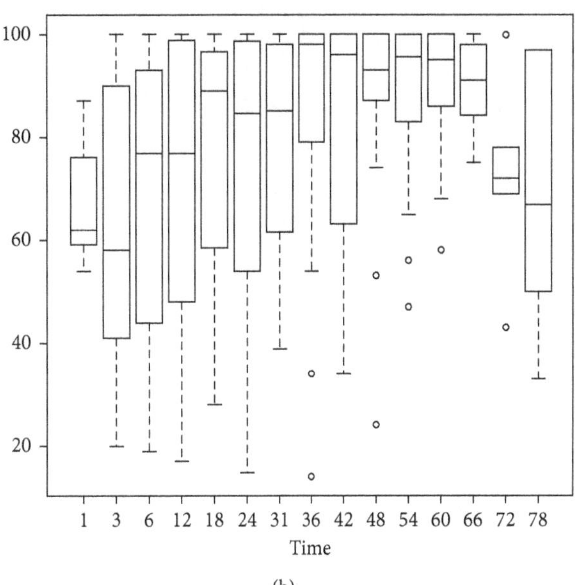

(b)

FIGURE 1: Box plot of overall (a) MSTS and (b) TESS during the entire follow-up period.

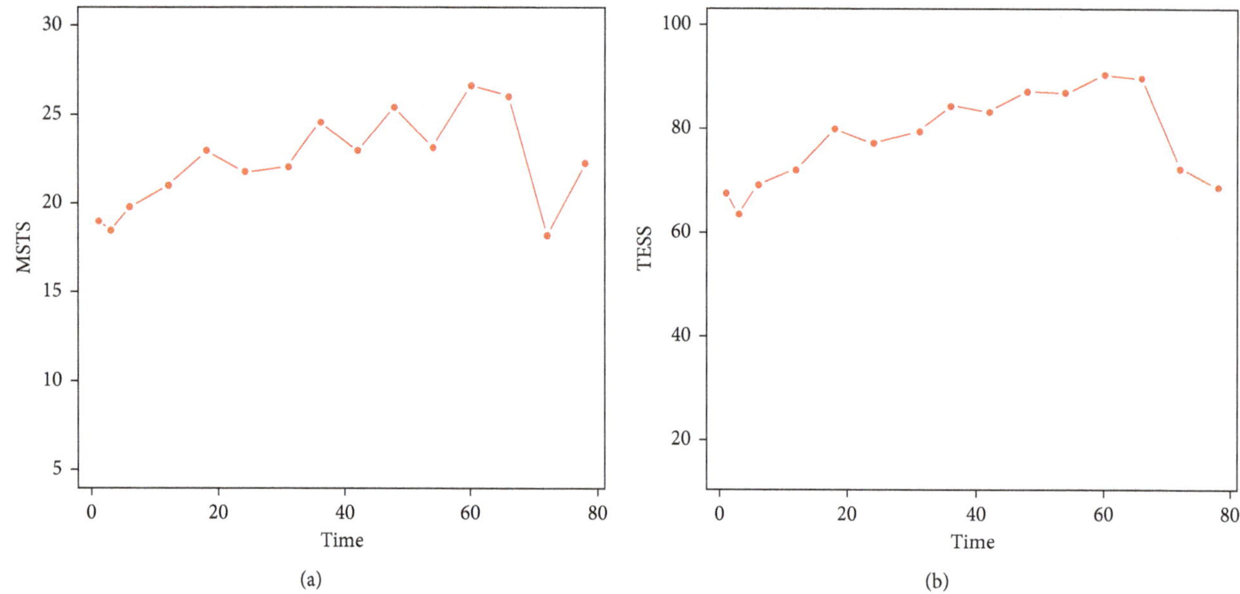

FIGURE 2: Mean plot of overall (a) MSTS and (b) TESS during the entire follow-up period.

TABLE 2: Multivariate generalized estimating equation (GEE) analysis of predictors of functional outcome in MSTS and TESS.

Variables[a]		MSTS			TESS		
		Estimate	Standard error	p value (95% CI)	Estimate	Standard error	p value (95% CI)
Intercept		29.39	1.84	<0.0001 (25.78, 33.00)	101.81	7.20	<0.0001 (87.68, 115.94)
Time		0.05	0.01	0.001 (0.02, 0.08)	0.21	0.06	0.0004 (0.09, 0.33)
Age		−0.15	0.02	<0.0001 (−0.21, −0.10)	−0.54	0.10	<0.0001 (−0.75, −0.33)
Size		−0.01	0.08	0.86 (−0.18, 0.15)	−0.13	0.29	0.64 (−0.72, 0.45)
Stage group							
Group 3	3	−2.86	1.83	0.11 (−6.46, 0.73)	−10.90	6.53	0.09 (−23.72, 1.90)
Group 2	2	−0.76	0.93	0.41 (−2.60, 1.06)	−4.50	3.40	0.18 (−11.18, 2.17)
Group 1	1	0	0		0	0	
Anatomic location							
Trunk	3	3.14	1.85	0.08 (−0.48, 6.77)	16.90	8.11	0.03 (1.00, 32.79)
Lower extremity	2	0.59	1.07	0.57 (−1.51, 2.71)	0.89	4.34	0.83 (−7.62, 9.41)
Upper extremity	1	0	0		0	0	
Bone resection		−6.13	1.24	<0.0001 (−8.57, −3.68)	−19.28	4.38	<0.0001 (−27.89, −10.68)
Flap reconstruction		−0.11	1.00	0.91 (−2.08, 1.86)	2.34	3.94	0.55 (−5.38, 10.07)
Postoperative radiation		−1.14	1.26	0.36 (−3.62, 1.32)	−6.07	4.65	0.19 (−15.18, 3.04)

[a]Bone resection: 0 = no, 1 = yes; flap reconstruction: 0 = yes, 1 = no; CI: confidence interval.

The size and stage of tumor indicated the degree of impairment in adjacent structures as well as the extent of tumor removal, and could have an effect on functional outcomes after surgery. In contrast with our expectation, the size and stage of tumor did not have a significant effect on the MSTS and TESS. The reason is that patients with advanced stage and large tumor size died during the follow-up and the patients were not available for assessment, we suggested. Therefore, further prospective study and randomized controlled trials should be performed to clarify the significance of size and stage of tumor.

Our study has several limitations. First, the number of patients followed for more than 5 years declined rapidly, and it was difficult to calculate an accurate value based on more than 5-year follow-up results. Second, we did not evaluate the preoperative functional score, local tumor recurrence, metastasis, surgical complications, indication and extent of bone resection, and type and methods of flap reconstruction, which can affect subsequent treatment and potential functional outcomes. It was a fundamental limitation of our study, and we will need more research in the future. Third, in the case of upper extremity tumors, we did not divide their locations into dominant arm and non-dominant arm. This may have had an impact on the potential functional outcomes. Fourth, the number of low grade tumors was much higher than that of high grade tumors, resulting in a relatively high level of functional outcome. Finally, MSTS and TESS were designed primarily as a simple way to measure the function of a single extremity. These systems had potential limitations in understanding the overall quality of life. Therefore, more research is needed to measure a broader understanding of the patients' overall recovery.

In conclusion, functional outcomes in patients who undergo LSS for STS can improve until the second year after surgery. The clinician can reassure patients that functional outcome improves gradually, and that final functional outcome will be better than early postoperative outcome. In addition, there is a significant difference in functional outcome between patients younger and older than 47 years of age. Patients who underwent bone resection may have a poor final outcome.

Disclosure

Kwang Joon Han is the co-first author.

Authors' Contributions

Sung Wook Seo was the guarantor of integrity of the entire study; all authors framed the study concepts/study design and participated in data acquisition or data analysis/interpretation; Eunsun Oh and Kwang Joon Han drafted and revised the manuscript for important intellectual content; all authors approved the final version of manuscript; Eunsun Oh was involved in literature research; all authors were involved in statistical analysis; and Eunsun Oh and Sung Wook Seo edited the manuscript.

Acknowledgments

This study was supported by Samsung Medical Center Grant SMX1170501 and by the Soonchunhyang University Research Fund.

References

[1] R. Siegel, D. Naishadham, and A. Jemal, "Cancer statistics, 2013," *CA: A Cancer Journal for Clinicians*, vol. 63, no. 1, pp. 11–30, 2013.

[2] V. O. Lewis, "What's new in musculoskeletal oncology," *Journal of Bone and Joint Surgery American volume*, vol. 91, no. 6, pp. 1546–1556, 2009.

[3] R. Veth, R. van Hoesel, M. Pruszczynski, J. Hoogenhout, B. Schreuder, and T. Wobbes, "Limb salvage in musculoskeletal oncology," *Lancet Oncology*, vol. 4, no. 6, pp. 343–350, 2003.

[4] S. A. Rosenberg, J. Tepper, E. Glatstein et al., "The treatment of soft-tissue sarcomas of the extremities: prospective randomized evaluations of (1) limb-sparing surgery plus radiation therapy compared with amputation and (2) the role of adjuvant chemotherapy," *Annals of Surgery*, vol. 196, no. 3, pp. 305–315, 1982.

[5] J. C. Yang, A. E. Chang, A. R. Baker et al., "Randomized prospective study of the benefit of adjuvant radiation therapy in the treatment of soft tissue sarcomas of the extremity," *Journal of Clinical Oncology*, vol. 16, no. 1, pp. 197–203, 1998.

[6] A. M. Davis, S. Sennik, A. M. Griffin et al., "Predictors of functional outcomes following limb salvage surgery for lower-extremity soft tissue sarcoma," *Journal of Surgical Oncology*, vol. 73, no. 4, pp. 206–211, 2000.

[7] S. Kolk, K. Cox, V. Weerdesteyn et al., "Can orthopedic oncologists predict functional outcome in patients with sarcoma after limb salvage surgery in the lower limb? A nationwide study," *SARCOMA*, vol. 2014, Article ID 436598, 11 pages, 2014.

[8] C. H. Gerrand, J. S. Wunder, R. A. Kandel et al., "The influence of anatomic location on functional outcome in lower-extremity soft-tissue sarcoma," *Annals of Surgical Oncology*, vol. 11, no. 5, pp. 476–482, 2004.

[9] J. Y. Kim, A. Youssef, V. Subramanian et al., "Upper extremity reconstruction following resection of soft tissue sarcomas: a functional outcomes analysis," *Annals of Surgical Oncology*, vol. 11, no. 10, pp. 921–927, 2004.

[10] W. F. Enneking, W. Dunham, M. C. Gebhardt, M. Malawar, and D. J. Pritchard, "A system for the functional evaluation of reconstructive procedures after surgical treatment of tumors of the musculoskeletal system," *Clinical Orthopaedics and Related Research*, no. 286, pp. 241–246, 1993.

[11] A. M. Davis, J. G. Wright, J. I. Williams, C. Bombardier, A. Griffin, and R. S. Bell, "Development of a measure of physical function for patients with bone and soft tissue sarcoma," *Quality of Life Research*, vol. 5, no. 5, pp. 508–516, 1996.

[12] H. S. Kim, J. Yun, S. Kang, and I. Han, "Cross-cultural adaptation and validation of the Korean Toronto Extremity Salvage Score for extremity sarcoma," *Journal of Surgical Oncology*, vol. 112, no. 1, pp. 93–97, 2015.

[13] S. B. Edge, D. R. Byrd, C. C. Compton, A. G. Fritz, F. L. Greene, and A. Trotti, *AJCC Cancer Staging Manual*, Springer, New York, NY, USA, 7th edition, 2010.

[14] H. Y. Shi, M. Khan, R. Culbertson, J. K. Chang, J. W. Wang, and H. C. Chiu, "Health-related quality of life after total hip replacement: a Taiwan study," *International Orthopaedics*, vol. 33, no. 5, pp. 1217–1222, 2009.

[15] J. W. Hardin and J. M. Hilbe, *Generalized Estimating Equations*, Chapman & Hall/CRC, Boca Raton, FL, USA, 2nd edition, 2003.

[16] R. S. Bell, B. O'Sullivan, A. Davis, F. Langer, B. Cummings, and V. L. Fornasier, "Functional outcome in patients treated with surgery and irradiation for soft tissue tumours," *Journal of Surgical Oncology*, vol. 48, no. 4, pp. 224–231, 1991.

25

Outcome for Advanced or Metastatic Soft Tissue Sarcoma of Nonextremities Treated with Doxorubicin-Based Chemotherapy

Shoko Marshall,[1] Kenji Nakano,[1] Yoshiya Sugiura,[2] Shinichiro Taira,[1] Makiko Ono,[1] Junichi Tomomatsu,[1] and Shunji Takahashi[1]

[1]*Department of Medical Oncology, Cancer Institute Hospital, Japanese Foundation for Cancer Research, Tokyo, Japan*
[2]*Department of Pathology, Cancer Institute Hospital, Japanese Foundation for Cancer Research, Tokyo, Japan*

Correspondence should be addressed to Shunji Takahashi; s.takahashi-chemotherapy@jfcr.or.jp

Academic Editor: Quincy Chu

Background. Doxorubicin is the key drug for treatment of advanced soft tissue sarcoma (STS). The appropriate dosage of doxorubicin, regarding monotherapy or the role of combination therapy, is unclear. *Methods.* We retrospectively reviewed patients with advanced or metastatic STS of nonextremities who were treated with doxorubicin-based chemotherapies in our institution. Time to treatment failure (TTF), overall survival (OS), overall response, and prognostic factors for OS were evaluated. *Results.* Seventy-five patients were enrolled. The median TTF was 4.7 months, and the median OS was 20.1 months. The overall response rate was 20%. Doses of doxorubicin monotherapy did not show significant difference either in TTF or in OS. There were no significant differences in OS between combination therapy and monotherapy, but the TTF with combination therapy was better than monotherapy. The overall response for combination therapy indicated a better response rate. Less number of involved organs, no bulky mass, and a normal CRP level were independent favorable prognostic factors for OS. *Conclusions.* Combination therapy showed better response and TTF than monotherapy but did not show better OS. Possible prognostic factors for OS were indicated. This retrospective study was approved by the institutional review board. This trial is registered with UMIN000028787.

1. Introduction

Soft tissue sarcomas (STSs) are a rare form of cancer which originate in various sites of the body [1]. STSs originating in the nonextremities can involve various sites of the body, and complete surgical resection can be difficult in some cases. Therefore, STSs of nonextremities origin are reported to have a worse prognosis when compared to STSs originating in the extremities [2, 3]. Systemic chemotherapy is often administered, and doxorubicin is currently a key drug used for treatment of advanced STS. Doxorubicin monotherapy and combination chemotherapy containing doxorubicin are options for treating advanced or metastatic STSs. The optimal dose of doxorubicin in regard to doxorubicin monotherapy remains unclear, and the role of combination therapy is controversial. The purpose of this study is to reveal the optimal dose of doxorubicin and the role that combination therapy plays in STSs originating in the nonextremities. The other purpose of this study is to reveal the clinical factors which predict prognosis in doxorubicin therapy for advanced or metastatic STS of nonextremities.

2. Materials and Methods

We retrospectively reviewed patients with advanced or metastatic STS of nonextremities who received doxorubicin-based chemotherapies at the Department of Medical Oncology in our institution from October 2005 to April 2016. A histopathological diagnosis was done by a biopsy or surgery which was reviewed by a well-trained pathologist in our institution. The regimens included a single agent of doxorubicin, a combination mostly with cyclophosphamide/vincristine/dacarbazine (CYVADIC), or ifosfamide (AI). The dose of doxorubicin monotherapy varied from 60 mg/m^2 to 75 mg/m^2, and CYVADIC consisted of 50 mg/m^2 doxorubicin, 1.5 mg/m^2 vincristine (max 2.0 mg/body, Day 1), 250 mg/m^2 dacarbazine (Day 1–5), and 500 mg/m^2 cyclophosphamide (Day 2), and AI consisted of 30 mg/m^2 doxorubicin (Day 1–2) and 2 g/m^2 ifosfamide (Day 1–5). The treatment regimen and the doxorubicin dose were chosen by a physician's choice. The doxorubicin monotherapy was chosen for the purpose of extending the patient's life, whereas the combination therapy was chosen with the purpose of shrinking the tumor. The patient's age, PS, organ functions, and risks such as the risk of myelosuppression were taken into consideration when determining the treatment regimen and the dose of chemotherapy. Clinical evidence in regard to the benefit of OS is based on some randomized clinical trials, such as EORTC62012. These trials in turn possibly affected the preference of physicians' choices regarding the use of doxorubicin monotherapy. The doxorubicin-based chemotherapy was discontinued until progressive disease (PD), unacceptable adverse events, or the cumulative dose was reached up to 450 mg/m^2. Imaging studies were performed every 2 to 3 months, or whenever the patients' presented with exacerbated symptoms. Objective responses, according to Response Evaluation Criteria in Solid Tumors (RECIST) version 1.1, were assessed by computed tomography (CT) or magnetic resonance imaging (MRI). Time to treatment failure (TTF) and overall survival (OS) were assessed by the Kaplan–Meier method. A univariate log-rank analysis was used to assess potential prognostic factors for OS, and the independent significant factors were investigated by multivariate Cox regression analyses for which the p value was less than 0.05.

3. Results

Between October 2005 and April 2016, a total of 75 patients were enrolled for analysis. The baseline characteristics of the patients treated with the doxorubicin-based chemotherapy are shown in Table 1. The patients consisted of 53% males, and the median age was 55 years (range: 21–75). Most of the patients had good performance status, and only 3 patients had ECOG performance status of 2. The locations of the primary tumor were the head and neck (19%), the thorax (9%), the abdomen (31%), the retroperitoneum (25%), the genital organs (5%), and others (5%). Others included breast, subcutaneous, groin, and the back. Regarding the number of involved organs, 29% of patients had only 1 involved organ and 36% of patients had more than 3 involved organs. The sites of the involved organs when doxorubicin therapy was administered included the head and neck (15%), intra-abdomen (40%), retroperitoneum (20%), lungs (47%), liver (29%), bone (24%), and lymph nodes (21%). Other sites of involved organs include the adrenal glands, subcutaneous, muscles, the pancreas, the renal, the spleen, the heart, the intestine, the ovaries, the

Table 1: The baseline characteristics of the patients treated with the doxorubicin-based chemotherapy.

	No. (%)
Sex	
Male	40 (53)
Female	35 (46)
Age	
Median age, years	55 (21–75)
ECOG performance status	
0	57 (76)
1	15 (20)
2	3 (4)
Location of the primary tumor	
Head and neck	14 (19)
Thorax	7 (9)
Abdomen	23 (31)
Retroperitoneum	19 (25)
Genital organs	4 (5)
Others	4 (5)
Unknown	4 (5)
Number of involved organs	
1	22 (29)
2	26 (35)
3	13 (17)
4	10 (13)
≧5	4 (5)
Site of involved organs, no. (%)	
Head and neck	11 (15)
Intra-abdomen	30 (40)
Retroperitoneum	15 (20)
Lung	35 (47)
Liver	22 (29)
Bone	18 (24)
Lymph node	16 (21)
Others	29 (39)
Maximum length	
Median (cm)	5.3 (0–21.7)
>5 cm	40 (53)
Pretreatment	
Operation	49 (65)
Radiation	21 (28)
Chemotherapy	8 (11)
None	18 (24)
Histopathology type	
Leiomyosarcoma	17 (23)
Liposarcoma	15 (20)
Spindle cell sarcoma, NOS	14 (19)
Pleomorphic sarcoma	6 (8)
Synovial sarcoma	5 (7)
Others*	18 (24)

*Others include angiosarcoma, undifferentiated pleomorphic sarcoma, solitary fibrous tumor, low-grade fibromyxoid sarcoma, malignant peripheral nerve sheath tumor, breast phyllodes tumor, round cell sarcoma with CIC rearrangement, neuroblastoma, malignant extrarenal rhabdoid tumor, and myxofibrosarcoma.

uterus, the prostate, and the bladder. The median maximum length of the tumor when doxorubicin-based chemotherapy was initiated was 5.3 cm (range: 0–21.7), and 53% had a mass which was measured to be more than 5 cm in diameter. The majority of patients received pretreatment consisting of mostly surgery (65%), radiation therapy (28%), and systemic therapy such as imatinib, sunitinib, gemcitabine, a combination of gemcitabine and docetaxel, ifosfamide, paclitaxel, and AI (11%). However, 24% of the patients had no treatment for advanced diseases before the doxorubicin-based chemotherapy. Histopathologically, 23% of the patients were diagnosed with leiomyosarcoma and 20% were diagnosed with liposarcoma, respectively, followed by spindle cell sarcoma (19%), pleomorphic sarcoma (8%), and synovial sarcoma (7%). The others were diagnosed as angiosarcoma, undifferentiated pleomorphic sarcoma, solitary fibrous tumor, low-grade fibromyxoid sarcoma, malignant peripheral nerve sheath tumor, breast phyllodes tumor, round cell sarcoma with CIC rearrangement, neuroblastoma, malignant extrarenal rhabdoid tumor, and myxofibrosarcoma. Doxorubicin monotherapy was performed on 51% of the patients, including 55% of the patients with 60 mg/m^2 and 42% with 75 mg/m^2. One patient received 50 mg/m^2 doxorubicin as a single agent due to having a previous medical history of a brain hemorrhage. Forty-nine percent of the patients had combination therapy, mostly with CYVADIC (81%), and AI was administered to 14%. The baseline characteristics of patients according to combination therapy or dose of doxorubicin were similar, except for the median age; the patients who had combination therapy were younger (median age 50 years, range: 21–74) compared to those with doxorubicin monotherapy (63 years, range: 24–72). The median total dose of doxorubicin was 300 mg/m^2.

The median follow-up time was 14.3 months. Of the enrolled patients, 48 were alive and 15% were maintaining the treatment effect or under the treatment at the data cutoff of April 2016. Nine percent were keeping more than stable disease (SD) after the doxorubicin-based chemotherapy, including one partial response (PR) and one complete response (CR), respectively. One patient showed PR after the treatment but moved on to the second-line therapy, without break by the physician's decision. The median TTF was 4.7 months (Figure 1), and the median OS was 20.1 months (Figure 2). The overall response rate was 20%, including CR with 4%, and they all were treated with CYVADIC therapy. Forty-one percent had SD, and 36% had PD (Table 2). Out of 64 patients who discontinued the chemotherapy with doxorubicin, 66% received post-anticancer therapy. An operation was performed on 7%, 29% had radiation therapy, and 76% received systemic therapy. One patient with retroperitoneum liposarcoma underwent a resection of peritoneal dissemination twice, 4 and 6 months after doxorubicin chemotherapy. Another patient with a malignant rhabdoid tumor with liver and bilateral ovaries metastasis underwent resection of pubic tumor twice, 4 and 9 months after administering 5 courses of CYVADIC. The other patient with synovial sarcoma with multiple lung metastases had 4 courses of CYVADIC and underwent a partial resection of both the right and left lung and resection of the left upper lobe. The patient also had a resection of liver metastasis 6 months later. These patients had a relapse a few months after their last surgery. Postsystemic

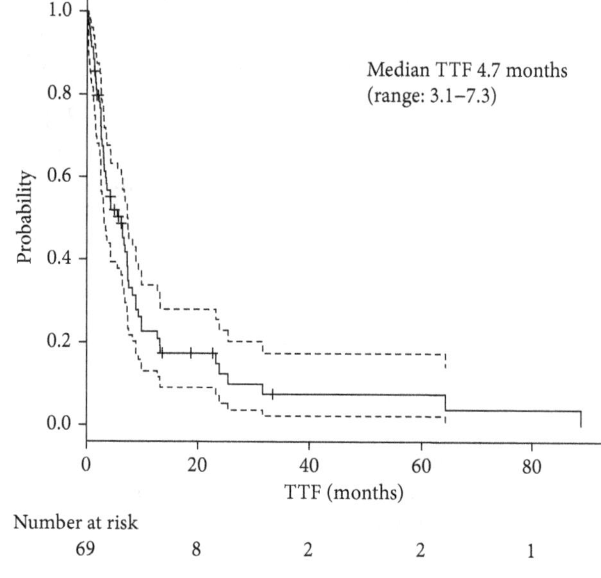

FIGURE 1: Median TTF.

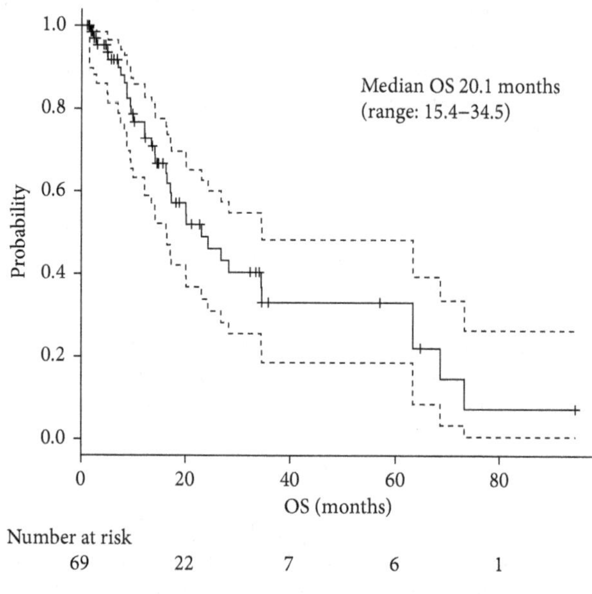

FIGURE 2: Median OS.

TABLE 2: Overall response rate.

Best overall response	No. (%)
Complete response	3 (4)
Partial response	12 (16)
Overall response	15 (20)
Stable disease	31 (41)
Progressive disease	27 (36)
Not evaluable or not assessed	2 (3)

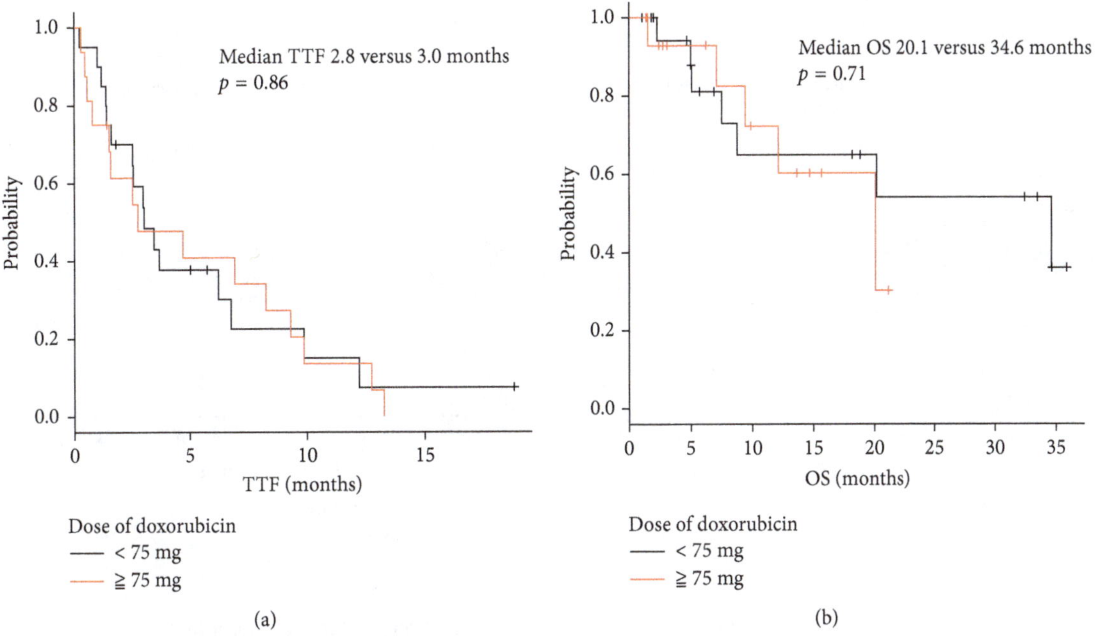

FIGURE 3: Difference of (a) TTF and (b) OS in doses of doxorubicin monotherapy.

TABLE 3: Tumor response for different doses of doxorubicin monotherapy.

Best overall response	Doxorubicin ≧ 75 mg/m^2 (n = 16), no. (%)	Doxorubicin < 75 mg/m^2 (n = 22), no. (%)
Complete response	0 (0)	0 (0)
Partial response	2 (13)	2 (6)
Overall response	2 (13)	2 (6)
Stable disease	5 (31)	14 (44)
Progressive disease	8 (50)	6 (19)
Not evaluable or not assessed	1 (6)	0 (0)

therapy included pazopanib (40%), ifosfamide (17%), irinotecan (17%), gemcitabine (7%), and other agents. Reasons for doxorubicin-based chemotherapy discontinuation were mostly due to progressive disease (94%); only 2 patients (3%) stopped the treatment because of adverse events (decreased cardiac function and anorexia), and 2 patients (3%) stopped the treatment due to the patient's request.

Doses of doxorubicin monotherapy administering 75 mg/m^2 or less than 75 mg/m^2 did not show significant difference either in TTF or in OS (Figure 3). The tumor response for different doses of doxorubicin monotherapy was also similar between 75 mg/m^2 and less than 75 mg/m^2 (Table 3). There were no significant differences in OS between doxorubicin-based combination therapy and doxorubicin monotherapy, but TTF of patients treated with combination therapy was better than doxorubicin monotherapy (Figure 4). The overall response for combination therapy was 30% compared to 11% doxorubicin monotherapy showing a better response rate (Table 4). Sex, age, PS, number of involved organs (≧3 organs), sites of involved organs, bulky mass (≧5 cm), presence of previous treatment, neutrophil to lymphocyte ratio (NLR), Hb (<11.6 g/dl), LDH (≧222 mg/dl), ALP (≧322 IU/l), and CRP (≧0.14 mg/dl) were investigated as prognostic factors for OS by univariate analysis (Table 5). Good PS (PS 0), less number of involved organs (<3), no bulky mass, and normal CRP level were favorable prognostic factors for OS. On multivariate analysis, less number of involved organs, no bulky mass, and normal CRP level were independent favorable prognostic factors, with a hazard ratio of 0.31 (95% CI: 0.15–0.65, p = 0.0019), 0.27 (95% CI: 0.12–0.60, p = 0.0013), and 0.43 (95% CI: 0.20–0.93, p = 0.032), respectively (Table 5).

4. Discussion

Locally advanced or metastatic STS of nonextremities is generally considered to be incurable and has poor prognosis. Salvage therapies such as systemic therapy and operation and radiation therapies are usually performed to such patients, and doxorubicin remains the most active single agent in STS for systemic chemotherapy. However, the optimal dose of doxorubicin in regard to doxorubicin monotherapy is unclear, neither is the role of combination therapy, especially when it is restricted to nonextremities STS. A number of trials comparing doxorubicin as a single agent

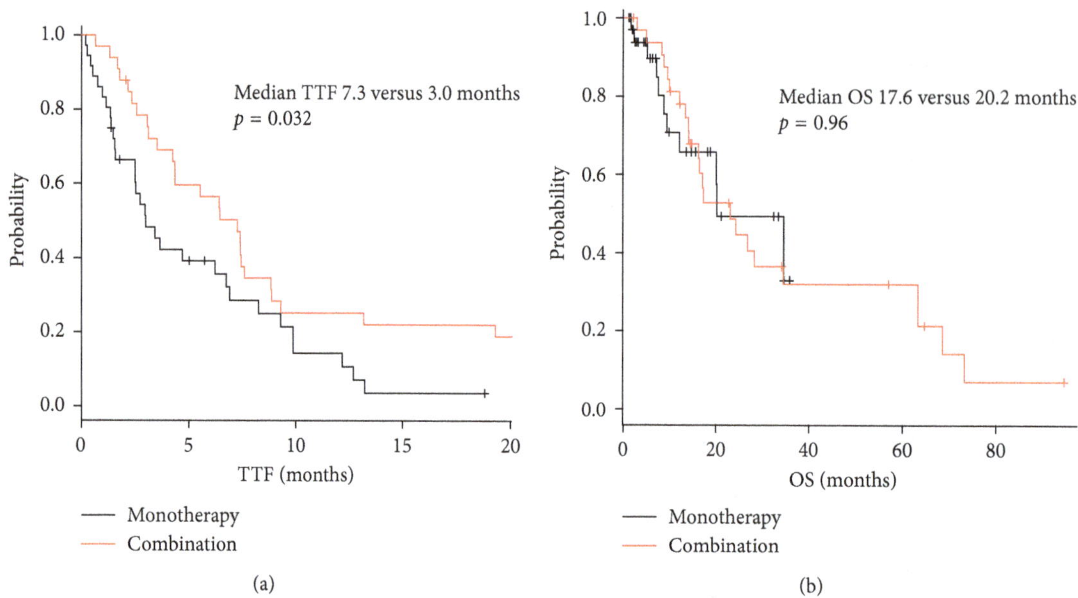

Figure 4: Difference of (a) TTF and (b) OS in combination therapy and monotherapy.

Table 4: Overall response rate for doxorubicin monotherapy and combination therapy.

Best overall response	A single agent ($n = 38$), no. (%)	Combination therapy ($n = 37$), no. (%)
Complete response	0 (0)	3 (8)
Partial response	4 (11)	8 (22)
Overall response	4 (11)	11 (30)
Stable disease	19 (50)	12 (32)
Progressive disease	14 (37)	13 (35)
Not evaluable or not assessed	1 (3)	1 (3)

with combination chemotherapy were performed, and a few studies showed a better overall response rate. However, according to those trials, combination chemotherapy has not indicated survival advantage compared to a single-agent chemotherapy [4–7]. In our analysis, median TTF was 4.7 months, and median OS was 20.1 months, with an overall response of 20%. Sixty-six percent of patients had post-treatment and among those patients, 36% had surgery or radiotherapy, which was comparatively high. Some of the cases were metastatic, but it is possible that oligometastatic cases in which salvage surgeries could be the option were included. This inclusion of oligometastatic cases could have contributed to our OS. Combination therapy showed a better overall response and longer TTF, but neither combination therapy nor difference in doses of doxorubicin monotherapy showed any significant difference in OS, which was in agreement with previous trials. Most of the patients discontinued doxorubicin-based chemotherapy because of PD, and there were only two cases which stopped the chemotherapy because of adverse effects. We also compared doses of a single agent of doxorubicin (75 mg/m^2 or less than 60 mg/m^2), but there was no significant difference in TTF nor in OS. We tried to reveal prognostic factors for OS. There have been previously reported favorable and unfavorable prognostic factors. For example, Van Glabbeke et al. reported good PS, absence of liver metastases, long time lapse since initial diagnosis, and young age as favorable prognostic factors of survival time for advanced patients treated with anthracycline-containing regimens [8]. There is also a report that found young age, liposarcoma, and synovial histology as favorable prognostic factors and bone involvement as an unfavorable prognostic factor for those with advanced soft tissue sarcoma treated on palliative therapy [9]. Lymphopenia is also reported as an unfavorable prognostic factor for sarcomas and other advanced carcinomas [10]. We included sex, age, PS, number of involved organs, sites of involved organs, bulky mass, pretreatment, and NLR, Hb, LDH, ALP, and CRP levels to investigate for prognostic factors, and on multivariate analysis, less number of involved organs, no bulky mass, and normal CRP level were found to be favorable prognostic factors in regard to OS. In our non-extremities advanced or metastatic cases, most of the patients had good PS; therefore, PS did not show as a prognostic factor, and sites of organs were not found to be positive, but the number of involved organs and bulky mass were relevant as prognostic factors. The three favorable prognostic factors, identified in this study, are considered of value in point of restricting to advanced or metastatic STS of nonextremities.

We acknowledge that there are several limitations in this study since this was a retrospective study. Some of the

Table 5: Prognostic factors by univariate analysis and multivariate analysis.

Prognostic factors	Univariate analysis	Multivariate analysis	
	p	Relative risk (95% CI)	p
Male	0.55	—	—
Age (<40)	0.15	—	—
PS (0)	0.012	—	0.54
Number of involved organs (<3)	0.013	0.31 (0.15–0.65)	0.0019
Head and neck	0.28	—	—
Intra-abdomen	0.25	—	—
Retroperitoneum	0.17	—	—
Lung	0.34	—	—
Liver	0.30	—	—
Bone	0.60	—	—
Lymph node	0.84	—	—
No bulky mass (<5 cm)	0.009	0.27 (0.12–0.60)	0.0013
Pretreatment	0.73	—	—
Normal, N/l	0.44	—	—
Normal Hb level (≧11.6 g/dl)	0.18	—	—
Normal LDH level (<222 mg/dl)	0.61	—	—
Normal ALP level (<322 IU/l)	0.12	—	—
Normal CRP level (<0.14 mg/dl)	0.020	0.43 (0.20–0.93)	0.032

decisions were made by individual physicians. For example, when imaging studies were performed, they may influence TTF. Furthermore, chemotherapy regimens and the dose of chemotherapy were chosen by a physician's choice. As a result, the dose of doxorubicin, in our study, was lower than the standard dose, in a high proportion of the patients. A further investigation which includes a prospective randomized study is needed.

5. Conclusion

In conclusion, doses of doxorubicin and doxorubicin monotherapy or combination therapy did not show significant differences in OS, but combination therapy showed a better overall response rate and longer TTF compared to monotherapy. Furthermore, less number of involved organs, no bulky mass, and normal CRP level were found to be independent favorable prognostic factors.

References

[1] M. J. Kransdorf, "Malignant soft-tissue tumors in a large referral population: distribution of diagnoses by age, sex, and location," *American Journal of Roentgenology*, vol. 164, no. 1, pp. 129–134, 1995.

[2] A. Ferrari, G. Bisogno, R. Alaggio et al., "Synovial sarcoma of children and adolescents: the prognostic role of axial sites," *European Journal of Cancer*, vol. 44, no. 9, pp. 1202–1209, 2008.

[3] N. Iqbal, N. K. Shukla, S. U. Deo et al., "Prognostic factors affecting survival in metastatic soft tissue sarcoma: an analysis of 110 patients," *Clinical and Translational Oncology*, vol. 18, no. 3, pp. 310–316, 2016.

[4] A. Santoro, T. Tursz, H. Mouridsen et al., "Doxorubicin versus CYVADIC versus doxorubicin plus ifosfamide in first-line treatment of advanced soft tissue sarcomas: a randomized study of the European Organization for Research and Treatment of Cancer Soft Tissue and Bone Sarcoma Group," *Journal of Clinical Oncology*, vol. 13, no. 7, pp. 1537–1545, 1995.

[5] P. Lorigan, J. Verweji, Z. Papai et al., "Phase III trial of two investigational schedules of ifosfamide compared with standard-dose doxorubicin in advanced or metastatic soft tissue sarcoma: A European organization for research and treatment of cancer soft tissue and bone sarcoma group study," *Journal of Clinical Oncology*, vol. 25, pp. 3144–3150, 2007.

[6] ESMO/European Sarcoma Network Working Group, "Soft tissue and visceral sarcomas: ESMO Clinical Practice Guidelines for diagnosis, treatment and follow-up," *Annals of Oncology*, vol. 25, no. 3, pp. iii102–iii112, 2014.

[7] I. Judson, J. Verweij, H. Gelderblom et al., "Doxorubicin alone versus intensified doxorubicin plus ifosfamide for first-line treatment of advanced or metastatic soft-tissue sarcoma: a randomized controlled phase 3 trial," *The Lancet Oncology*, vol. 15, no. 4, pp. 415–423, 2014.

[8] M. Van Glabbeke, A. T. Van Oosterom, J. W. Oosterhuis et al., "Prognostic factors for the outcome of chemotherapy in advanced soft tissue sarcoma: an analysis of 2,185 patients treated with anthracycline-containing first-line regimens—a European Organization for Research and Treatment of Cancer Soft Tissue and Bone Sarcoma Group Study," *Journal of Clinical Oncology*, vol. 17, no. 1, pp. 150–157, 1999.

Permissions

All chapters in this book were first published in SARCOMA, by Hindawi Publishing Corporation; hereby published with permission under the Creative Commons Attribution License or equivalent. Every chapter published in this book has been scrutinized by our experts. Their significance has been extensively debated. The topics covered herein carry significant findings which will fuel the growth of the discipline. They may even be implemented as practical applications or may be referred to as a beginning point for another development.

The contributors of this book come from diverse backgrounds, making this book a truly international effort. This book will bring forth new frontiers with its revolutionizing research information and detailed analysis of the nascent developments around the world.

We would like to thank all the contributing authors for lending their expertise to make the book truly unique. They have played a crucial role in the development of this book. Without their invaluable contributions this book wouldn't have been possible. They have made vital efforts to compile up to date information on the varied aspects of this subject to make this book a valuable addition to the collection of many professionals and students.

This book was conceptualized with the vision of imparting up-to-date information and advanced data in this field. To ensure the same, a matchless editorial board was set up. Every individual on the board went through rigorous rounds of assessment to prove their worth. After which they invested a large part of their time researching and compiling the most relevant data for our readers.

The editorial board has been involved in producing this book since its inception. They have spent rigorous hours researching and exploring the diverse topics which have resulted in the successful publishing of this book. They have passed on their knowledge of decades through this book. To expedite this challenging task, the publisher supported the team at every step. A small team of assistant editors was also appointed to further simplify the editing procedure and attain best results for the readers.

Apart from the editorial board, the designing team has also invested a significant amount of their time in understanding the subject and creating the most relevant covers. They scrutinized every image to scout for the most suitable representation of the subject and create an appropriate cover for the book.

The publishing team has been an ardent support to the editorial, designing and production team. Their endless efforts to recruit the best for this project, has resulted in the accomplishment of this book. They are a veteran in the field of academics and their pool of knowledge is as vast as their experience in printing. Their expertise and guidance has proved useful at every step. Their uncompromising quality standards have made this book an exceptional effort. Their encouragement from time to time has been an inspiration for everyone.

The publisher and the editorial board hope that this book will prove to be a valuable piece of knowledge for researchers, students, practitioners and scholars across the globe.

List of Contributors

Clara Chen, Wan-Yu Tseng, Shanmugapriya Saravanan and Rahul Dhanda
Department of Information Technology, Health Economics and Outcomes Research, McKesson Specialty Health, The Woodlands, TX, USA

Rohit Borker and Michelle D. Hackshaw
GlaxoSmithKline, Philadelphia, PA 19112, USA

James Ewing
Department of Information Technology, Health Economics and Outcomes Research, McKesson Specialty Health, The Woodlands, TX, USA
Texas Oncology, Dallas, TX, USA
Baylor Charles A. Sammons Cancer Center, Dallas, TX, USA
Baylor University Medical Center at Dallas, Dallas, TX, USA

Eric Nadler
Department of Information Technology, Health Economics and Outcomes Research, McKesson Specialty Health, The Woodlands, TX, USA
Texas Oncology, Dallas, TX, USA
Baylor Charles A. Sammons Cancer Center, Dallas, TX, USA
Baylor University Medical Center at Dallas, Dallas, TX, USA
Texas Oncology, Baylor Sammons Cancer Center, 3410Worth Street, Dallas, TX 75246, USA

Sheila Thampi, Katherine K. Matthay, Robert Goldsby and Steven G. DuBois
Department of Pediatrics, UCSF School of Medicine and UCSF Benioff Children's Hospital, 505 Parnassus Avenue M649, San Francisco, CA 94143, USA

W. John Boscardin
Department of Medicine and Epidemiology and Biostatistics, UCSF School of Medicine 505 Parnassus Avenue, San Francisco, CA 94143, USA

S. J. Neuhaus, D. Thomas and J. Desai
Australasian Sarcoma Study Group, Melbourne, VIC 3002, Australia

C. Vuletich, J. von Dincklage and I. Olver
Cancer Council Australia, Sydney, NSW 2000, Australia

Frédéric Amant
Department of Obstetrics and Gynecology, UZ Gasthuisberg, Katholieke Universiteit Leuven, Herestraat 49, 3000 Leuven, Belgium

Domenica Lorusso
Gynecologic Oncology Unit, Fondazione IRCCS National Cancer Institute, Via Venezian 1, 20133 Milan, Italy

Alexander Mustea
Department of Gynecology and Obstetrics, University Hospital Greifswald, Ferdinand-Sauerbruch-Strasse, 17475 Greifswald, Germany

Florence Duffaud
Department of Medical Oncology, La Timone University Hospital, 264 rue Saint Pierre, 13385 Marseille, France

Patricia Pautier
Département de Medecine, Institut Gustave-Roussy, 114 rue Edouard Vaillant, 94805 Villejuif Cedex, France

Melissa H. Tang, David J. Castle and Peter F. M. Choong
St. Vincent's Hospital Melbourne, 35 Victoria Parade, Fitzroy, VIC 3065, Australia

Kenneth R. Gundle, Amy M. Cizik, Stephanie E. W. Punt, Ernest U. Conrad III and Darin J. Davidson
Department of Orthopaedics and Sports Medicine, University of Washington Medical Center, 1959 Pacific Street NE, Seattle, WA 98195, USA

Neyssa Marina
Department of Pediatrics, Stanford University and Lucile Packard Children's Hospital, 1000Welch Road, Suite 300, Palo Alto, CA 94304-1812, USA

Linda Granowetter
Department of Pediatrics, New York University, Langone Medical Center, New York, NY 10016, USA

Holcombe E. Grier
Pediatric Hematology-Oncology, Dana Farber and Boston Children's Hospital, 44 Binney Street, Boston, MA 02115, USA

Richard B. Womer
Division of Oncology, Children's Hospital of Philadelphia, Philadelphia, PA 19104, USA

R. Lor Randall
Sarcoma Services, Huntsman Cancer Institute and Primary Children's Medical Center Department of Orthopaedics, University of Utah, Salt Lake City, UT 84112, USA

Karen J. Marcus
Department of Radiation Oncology, Boston Children's Hospital/Dana Farber Cancer Institute Brigham and Women's Hospital, Harvard Medical School, Boston, MA 02115, USA

Elizabeth McIlvaine and Mark Krailo
Department of Preventive Medicine, University of Southern California, Los Angeles, CA 90027, USA
Children's Oncology Group Statistics, Monrovia, CA 91016, USA

Monica Panca and Erikas Sladkevicius
Catalyst Health Economics Consultants, 34b High Street, Northwood, Middlesex HA6 1BN, UK

Julian F. Guest
Catalyst Health Economics Consultants, 34b High Street, Northwood, Middlesex HA6 1BN, UK
School of Biomedical Sciences, King's College, London SE1 1UL, UK

Nicholas Gough
Palliative Care Department, Royal Marsden Hospital, London SW3 6JJ, UK

Mark Linch
Sarcoma Unit, Royal Marsden Hospital, London SW3 6JJ, UK

Christina Kåbjörn Gustafsson and Pierre Åman
Sahlgrenska Cancer Center, Department of Pathology, Institute of Biomedicine, University of Gothenburg, 40530 Gothenburg, Sweden

Katarina Engström
Department of Oncology, Institute of Medical Sciences, University of Gothenburg, Gothenburg, Sweden

Satoshi Nagano, Masahiro Yokouchi, Hiromi Sasaki, Hirofumi Shimada, Ichiro Kawamura, Junichi Kamizono, Takuya Yamamoto and Setsuro Komiya
Department of Orthopaedic Surgery, Graduate School of Medical and Dental Sciences, Kagoshima University, 8-35-1 Sakuragaoka, Kagoshima City, Kagoshima 890-8520, Japan

Takao Setoguchi
The Near-Future Locomotor Organ Medicine Creation Course (Kusunoki Kai), Graduate School of Medical and Dental Sciences, Kagoshima University, 8-35-1 Sakuragaoka, Kagoshima City, Kagoshima 890-8520, Japan

Yasuhiro Ishidou
Department of Medical Joint Materials, Graduate School of Medical and Dental Sciences, Kagoshima University, 8-35-1 Sakuragaoka, Kagoshima City, Kagoshima 890-8520, Japan

Hideki Kawamura
Infection Control Team, Kagoshima University Hospital, 8-35-1 Sakuragaoka, Kagoshima City, Kagoshima 890-8520, Japan

Daniel M. Sullivan
Chemical Biology and Molecular Medicine, H. Lee Moffitt Cancer Center and Research Institute, 12902 Magnolia Drive, Tampa, FL 33612, USA

Christopher L. Cubitt
Chemical Biology and Molecular Medicine, H. Lee Moffitt Cancer Center and Research Institute, 12902 Magnolia Drive, Tampa, FL 33612, USA
Translational Research Lab, H. Lee Moffitt Cancer Center and Research Institute, 12902 Magnolia Drive, Tampa, FL 33612, USA

Jiliana Menth and Jana Dawson
Translational Research Lab, H. Lee Moffitt Cancer Center and Research Institute, 12902 Magnolia Drive, Tampa, FL 33612, USA

Gary V. Martinez, Parastou Foroutan and David L. Morse
Small Animal Imaging Lab, H. Lee Moffitt Cancer Center and Research Institute, 12902 Magnolia Drive, Tampa, FL 33612, USA

G. Douglas Letson
Sarcoma Program, H. Lee Moffitt Cancer Center and Research Institute, 12902 Magnolia Drive, Tampa, FL 33612, USA

Damon R. Reed
Chemical Biology and Molecular Medicine, H. Lee Moffitt Cancer Center and Research Institute, 12902 Magnolia Drive, Tampa, FL 33612, USA
Sarcoma Program, H. Lee Moffitt Cancer Center and Research Institute, 12902 Magnolia Drive, Tampa, FL 33612, USA

Marilyn M. Bui
Sarcoma Program, H. Lee Moffitt Cancer Center and Research Institute, 12902 Magnolia Drive, Tampa, FL 33612, USA
Anatomic Pathology Department, H. Lee Moffitt Cancer Center and Research Institute, 12902 Magnolia Drive, Tampa, FL 33612, USA

Stein J. Janssen, Eva A. J. van Rein, Nuno Rui Paulino Pereira, Kevin A. Raskin, Francis J. Hornicek, Santiago A. Lozano-Calderon and Joseph H. Schwab
Department of Orthopaedic Surgery, Orthopaedic Oncology Service, Massachusetts General Hospital, Harvard Medical School, Boston, MA, USA

Marco L. Ferrone
Department of Orthopaedic Surgery, Orthopaedic Oncology Service, Brigham and Women's Hospital, Harvard Medical School, Boston, MA, USA

Laura Bellanova, Thomas Schubert, Olivier Cartiaux, Xavier Banse and Pierre-Louis Docquier
Computer Assisted and Robotic Surgery (CARS), Institut de Recherche Expérimentale et Clinique (IREC), Université catholique de Louvain Tour Pasteur +4, Avenue Mounier, 53, 1200 Brussels, Belgium

Frédéric Lecouvet
Département D'imagerie Médicale, Cliniques Universitaires Saint-Luc 10, Avenue Hippocrate, 1200 Brussels, Belgium

Christine Galant
Département de Pathologie, Cliniques Universitaires Saint-Luc 10, Avenue Hippocrate, 1200 Brussels, Belgium

Lena Fauske
Department of Oncology, Oslo University Hospital, Norwegian Radium Hospital, Nydalen, 0424 Oslo, Norway

Oyvind S. Bruland
Department of Oncology, Oslo University Hospital, Norwegian Radium Hospital, Nydalen, 0424 Oslo, Norway
Institute of Clinical Medicine, University of Oslo, Blindern, 0316 Oslo, Norway

Ellen Karine Grov
Faculty of Health Sciences, Department of Nursing, Oslo and Akershus University College of Applied Sciences, St. Olavs plass, 0130 Oslo, Norway

Hilde Bondevik
Institute of Health and Society, Department of Health Sciences, University of Oslo, Blindern, 0317 Oslo, Norway

Khin Thway and Cyril Fisher
Sarcoma Unit, Royal Marsden Hospital, London SW3 6JJ, UK

Jayson Wang
Department of Histopathology, Royal Marsden Hospital, London SW3 6JJ, UK

John Swansbury and Toon Min
Clinical Cytogenetics, Royal Marsden Hospital, Sutton, Surrey SM2 5NG, UK

William W. Tseng
Department of Surgery, Section of Surgical Oncology, University of Southern California, Los Angeles, CA 90033, USA
Hoag Memorial Hospital Presbyterian, Newport Beach, CA 92663, USA

Shruti Malu, Minying Zhang, Jieqing Chen, Geok Choo Sim and Gregory Lizée
Department of Melanoma Medical Oncology, The University of Texas MD Anderson Cancer Center, Houston, TX 77030, USA

Wei Wei
Department of Biostatistics, The University of Texas MD Anderson Cancer Center, Houston, TX 77030, USA

Davis Ingram and Dina C. Lev
Department of Cancer Biology, The University of Texas MD Anderson Cancer Center, Houston, TX 77030, USA

Neeta Somaiah
Department of Sarcoma Medical Oncology, The University of Texas MD Anderson Cancer Center, Houston, TX 77030, USA

Raphael E. Pollock
Division of Surgical Oncology, The James Comprehensive Cancer Center, Ohio State University Medical Center, Columbus, OH 43210, USA

Laszlo Radvanyi
Lion Biotechnologies, Woodland Hills, CA 91637, USA
Department of Immunology, H. Lee Moffitt Cancer Center, Tampa, FL 33612, USA

Patrick Hwu
Department of Melanoma Medical Oncology, The University of Texas MD Anderson Cancer Center, Houston, TX 77030, USA
Department of Sarcoma Medical Oncology, The University of Texas MD Anderson Cancer Center, Houston, TX 77030, USA

Stacie Hudgens
Clinical Outcomes Solutions, Tucson, AZ, USA

Anna Forsythe and David D'Adamo
Purple Squirrel Economics, New York, NY, USA

Ilias Kontoudis
Eisai Ltd., Hertfordshire, UK

Ashley Bird
UT Southwestern Medical Center, Dallas, TX, USA

Hans Gelderblom
Department of Medical Oncology, Leiden University Medical Center, Leiden, Netherlands

Ae Rang Kim
Center for Cancer and Blood Disorders, Children's National Health System, 111 Michigan Ave NW, Washington, DC 20010, USA

Douglas R. Stewart
Clinical Genetics Branch, Division of Cancer Epidemiology and Genetics, National Cancer Institute, 9609 Medical Center Drive, Room 6E450, Bethesda, MD 20892, USA

Karlyne M. Reilly
Rare Tumors Initiative, OD, CCR, National Cancer Institute, 37 Convent Drive, Bethesda, MD 20814, USA

David Viskochil
University of Utah, 295 Chipeta Way, Salt Lake City, UT 84108, USA

Markku M. Miettinen
Center for Cancer Research, National Cancer Institute, 10 Center Drive, Room 2S235C, Building 10, Bethesda, MD 20892, USA

Brigitte C. Widemann
National Cancer Institute, Pediatric Oncology Branch, 10 Center Drive, Room 1-3742, Building 10, Bethesda, MD 20892, USA

David Thorn and Christoph Mamot
Division of Medical Oncology, Cantonal Hospital Aarau, 5001 Aarau, Switzerland

Fatime Krasniqi
Division of Medical Oncology, University Hospital Basel, 4031 Basel, Switzerland

Frank Metternich and Sven Prestin
Division of Ear, Nose and Throat, Head and Neck Surgery, Cantonal Hospital Aarau, 5001 Aarau, Switzerland

Hussein Sweiti, Fabian Bormann and Matthias Schwarzbach
Department of Surgery, Clinical Center Frankfurt H¨ochst, Frankfurt, Germany

Noor Tamimi
Department of Trauma and Orthopedic Surgery, BG Trauma Center, Frankfurt, Germany

Markus Divo
Institute for Pathology, Clinical Center Frankfurt H¨ochst, Frankfurt, Germany

Daniela Schulz-Ertner
Radiological Institute, Agaplesion Markus Hospital, Frankfurt, Germany

Marit Ahrens
Department of Hematology and Oncology, University Hospital Frankfurt, Frankfurt, Germany

Ulrich Ronellenfitsch
Department of Vascular and Endovascular Surgery, Heidelberg University Hospital, Heidelberg, Germany

Gaetano Apice, Antonio Pizzolorusso, Massimo Di Maio, Annarosaria De Chiara, Flavio Fazioli, Giampaolo De Palma, Nicola Mozzillo and Francesco Perrone
Istituto Nazionale Tumori IRCCS "Fondazione G. Pascale", Via Mariano Semmola, 80131 Napoli, Italy

Giovanni Grignani and Danilo Galizia
Institute for Cancer Research and Treatment, Strada Provinciale, km 3.95, Candiolo, 10060 Turin, Italy

Vittorio Gebbia and Carlo Arcara
Medical Oncology Unit, La Maddalena Hospital, Via San Lorenzo Colli 312/d, 90146 Palermo, Italy

Angela Buonadonna
Departments of Radiation Oncology and Medical Oncology, CRO, National Cancer Institute, Via Franco Gallini 2, 33081 Aviano, Italy

Xiaodong Mu and Johnny Huard
Department of Orthopaedic Surgery, University of Texas Health Science Center at Houston, Houston, TX 77030, USA
Center for Regenerative Sports Medicine, Steadman Philippon Research Institute, Vail, CO 81657, USA

Rashmi Agarwal, Daniel March, Adam Rothenberg, Jessica Tebbets and Kurt Weiss
Cancer Stem Cell Laboratory, Department of Orthopaedic Surgery, University of Pittsburgh, Pittsburgh, PA 15213, USA

Clifford Voigt
Department of Orthopaedic Surgery, Lenox Hill Hospital, New York, NY 10075, USA

John M. Kane III
Roswell Park Cancer Institute, Buffalo, NY, USA

Anthony Magliocco
H. Lee Moffitt Cancer Center, Tampa, FL, USA

Qiang Zhang and Jonathan Harris
NRG Oncology Statistics and Data Management Center, Philadelphia, PA, USA

Dian Wang
Rush University Medical Center, Chicago, IL, USA

Alex Klimowicz
Tom Baker Cancer Centre, Calgary, AB, Canada

Jeff Simko
University of California, San Francisco, CA, USA

Thomas De Laney
Massachusetts General Hospital, Boston, MA, USA

William Kraybill
The Ohio State University, Columbus, OH, USA

David G. Kirsch
Duke University Medical Center, Durham, NC, USA

Eunsun Oh
Department of Radiology, Soonchunhyang University Seoul Hospital, 59 Daesagwan-ro, Youngsan-gu, Seoul 04401, Republic of Korea
Department of Radiology, Samsung Medical Center, Sungkyunkwan University School of Medicine, 81 Ilwon-Ro, Gangnam-gu, Seoul 06351, Republic of Korea

Sung Wook Seo and Kwang Joon Han
Department of Orthopedic Surgery, Samsung Medical Center, Sungkyunkwan University School of Medicine, 81 Ilwon-Ro, Gangnam-gu, Seoul 06351, Republic of Korea

Shoko Marshall, Kenji Nakano, Shinichiro Taira, Makiko Ono, Junichi Tomomatsu and Shunji Takahashi
Department of Medical Oncology, Cancer Institute Hospital, Japanese Foundation for Cancer Research, Tokyo, Japan

Yoshiya Sugiura
Department of Pathology, Cancer Institute Hospital, Japanese Foundation for Cancer Research, Tokyo, Japan

Index

www.ingramcontent.com/pod-product-compliance
Lightning Source LLC
Chambersburg PA
CBHW080521200326
41458CB00012B/4284

* 9 7 8 1 6 3 2 4 2 9 1 3 1 *